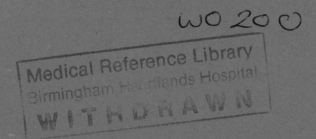

Rob & Smith's
Operative Surgery

Pediatric Surgery

Fifth edition

Rob & Smith's
Operative Surgery

General Editors

David C. Carter MD, FRCS(Ed), FRCS(Glas)
Regius Professor of Clinical Surgery, Royal Infirmary,
Edinburgh, UK

R. C. G. Russell MS, FRCS
Consultant Surgeon, Middlesex Hospital and Royal National
Throat, Nose and Ear Hospital, London, UK

Henry A. Pitt MD
Professor and Vice Chairman, Department of Surgery,
Johns Hopkins Hospital, Baltimore, Maryland, USA

Consulting Editor

Hugh Dudley CBE, ChM, FRCS(Ed), FRACS, FRCS
Emeritus Professor, St Mary's Hospital, London, UK

Art Editor

Gillian Lee FMAA, HonFIMI, AMI, RMIP
15 Little Plucketts Way, Buckhurst Hill, Essex, UK

Other volumes available in the series

Cardiac Surgery 4th Edition
Stuart W. Jamieson and Norman E. Shumway

The Ear 4th Edition
John C. Ballantyne and Andrew Morrison

**General Principles, Breast and Extracranial
Endocrines** 4th Edition
Hugh Dudley and Walter J. Pories

Genitourinary Surgery 5th Edition
Hugh N. Whitfield

Gynaecology and Obstetrics 4th Edition
J. M. Monaghan

The Hand 4th Edition
Rolfe Birch and Donal Brooks

Head and Neck 4th Edition
Ian A. McGregor and David J. Howard

Neurosurgery 4th Edition
Lindsay Symon, David G. T. Thomas and Kemp Clark

Nose and Throat 4th Edition
John C. Ballantyne and D. F. N. Harrison

Ophthalmic Surgery 4th Edition
Thomas A. Rice, Ronald G. Michels and Walter W. J. Stark

Orthopaedics 4th Edition
George Bentley and Robert B. Greer III

Plastic Surgery 4th Edition
T. L. Barclay and Desmond A. Kernahan

Surgery of the Colon, Rectum and Anus 5th Edition
L. P. Fielding and S. M. Goldberg

Surgery of the Upper Gastrointestinal Tract 5th Edition
G. G. Jamieson and H. T. Debas

Thoracic Surgery 4th Edition
The late J. W. Jackson and D. K. C. Cooper

Trauma Surgery 4th Edition
Howard R. Champion, John V. Robbs and Donald D. Trunkey

Vascular Surgery 5th Edition
C. W. Jamieson and J. S. T. Yao

Rob & Smith's
Operative Surgery

Pediatric Surgery

Fifth edition

Edited by

Lewis Spitz PhD, FRCS, FRCS(Ed), FAAP(Hon)
Nuffield Professor of Paediatric Surgery, Institute of Child Health, University of London, and Consultant
Paediatric Surgeon, Great Ormond Street Hospital for Children, London, UK

Arnold G. Coran MD
Professor of Surgery and Head of the Section of Pediatric Surgery, University of Michigan Medical School,
and Surgeon-in-Chief, C.S. Mott Children's Hospital, Ann Arbor, Michigan, USA

CHAPMAN & HALL MEDICAL
London · Glasgow · Weinheim · New York · Tokyo · Melbourne · Madras

Published by Chapman & Hall, 2–6 Boundary Row, London SE1 8HN, UK

Chapman & Hall, 2–6 Boundary Row, London SE1 8HN, UK

Blackie Academic & Professional, Wester Cleddens Road,
Bishopbriggs, Glasgow G64 2NZ, UK

Chapman & Hall GmbH, Pappelallee 3,
69469 Weinheim, Germany

Chapman & Hall USA, One Penn Plaza, 41st Floor,
New York, NY 10119, USA

Chapman & Hall Japan, ITP-Japan, Kyowa Building, 3F, 2-2-1 Hirakawacho,
Chiyoda-ku, Tokyo 102, Japan

Chapman & Hall Australia, Thomas Nelson Australia,
102 Dodds Street, South Melbourne, Victoria 3205, Australia

Chapman & Hall India, R. Seshadri, 32 Second Main Road, CIT East,
Madras 600 035, India

© 1995 Chapman & Hall

Typeset in 10/11 Garamond ITC by Genesis Typesetting, Laser Quay, Rochester, Kent

Printed in Great Britain by Hartnolls, Bodmin, Cornwall

ISBN 0 412 59110 3

A catalogue record for this book is available from the British Library

Library of Congress Catalog Card Number: 94-68719

∞ Printed on acid-free text paper, manufactured in accordance with
ANSI/NISO Z39. 48-1992

Contributors

I. A. Aaronson MA, FRCS
Professor of Urology and Pediatrics, Medical University of South Carolina, 171 Ashley Avenue, Charleston, South Carolina 29423-2280, USA

F. E. Abyholm MD, DDS, PhD
Head, Department of Plastic Surgery, Rikshospitalet University Hospital, Pilestredet 32, 0027 Oslo, Norway

C. T. Albanese MD
Assistant Professor of Surgery, Division of Pediatric Surgery, University of Pittsburgh School of Medicine, and Children's Hospital of Pittsburgh, Pittsburgh, Pennsylvania 15213-2583, USA

R. P. Altman MD
Surgeon-in-Chief, Babies' Hospital, Columbia-Presbyterian Medical Center, 3959 Broadway, New York, New York 10032, USA

R. J. Andrassy MD, FACS, FAAP
A. G. McNeese Professor of Surgery and Pediatrics and Chief of Pediatric Surgery, M. D. Anderson Cancer Center, Houston, Texas 77030, USA

K. W. Ashcraft MD
Chief of Urology, The Children's Mercy Hospital, 2401 Gillham Road, Kansas City, Missouri 64108, USA

S. W. Beasley MS, FRACS
Consultant Surgeon, Royal Children's Hospital, Flemington Road, Parkville, Victoria, Australia 3052

A. Bianchi MD, FRCS, FRCS(Ed)
Consultant Neonatal and Paediatric Surgeon, Royal Manchester Children's Hospital, Pendlebury, Manchester M27 1HA, UK

D. A. Bloom MD
Chief of Pediatric Urology, Professor of Surgery (Urology), University of Michigan, Ann Arbor, Michigan 48109-0330, USA

S. A. M. Boddy MS, FRCS
Consultant Paediatric Surgeon, St George's Hospital, London SW17 0QT, UK

J. Boix-Ochoa
Professor of Pediatric Surgery, Autonomous University of Barcelona, and Chairman, Department of Paediatric Surgery, Children's Hospital, Vall d'Hebron, Barcelona 08035, Spain

R. J. Brereton FRCS
Consultant Paediatric Surgeon, Chelsea and Westminster Hospital, London SW10 9NH, UK

F. D. Burstein MD
Co-Director, Center for Craniofacial Disorders, Scottish Rite Children's Hospital, Atlanta, Georgia 30342, USA

J. M. Casasa
Head of Gastrointestinal Surgery, Department of Paediatric Surgery, Autonomous University of Barcelona, and Children's Hospital, Vall d'Hebron, Barcelona 08035, Spain

R. E. Cilley MD
Assistant Professor of Surgery and Pediatrics, Division of Pediatric Surgery, Department of Surgery, Pennsylvania State University College of Medicine, The Milton S. Hershey Medical Center, Hershey, Pennsylvania 17033, USA

S. R. Cohen MD
Co-Director, Center for Craniofacial Disorders, Scottish Rite Children's Hospital, Atlanta, Georgia 30342, USA

R. C. M. Cook MA, BM, FRCS
Consultant Paediatric Surgeon, Royal Liverpool Children's NHS Trust, Alder Hey, Liverpool L12 2AP, UK

D. R. Cooney MD
H. William Clatworthy Jr. Professor of Pediatric Surgery, The Ohio State University, and Surgeon-in-Chief, Columbus Children's Hospital, 700 Children's Drive, Columbus, Ohio 43205, USA

A. G. Coran MD
Professor of Surgery and Head of the Section of Pediatric Surgery, University of Michigan Medical School, and Surgeon-in-Chief, C.S. Mott Children's Hospital, Ann Arbor, Michigan 48109-0245, USA

D. C. G. Crabbe MD, FRCS
Senior Registrar, Department of Paediatric Surgery, Great Ormond Street Hospital for Children, London WC1N 3JH, UK

S. Cywes MMed, FACS, FRCS, FRCS(Ed), FRCPS(Glas), FAAP
Professor of Paediatric Surgery, University of Cape Town and Chief Surgeon, Institute of Child Health, Red Cross Children's Hospital, 7700 Rondebosch, South Africa

R. C. Dauser MD
Assistant Professor of Neurosurgery, Texas Children's Hospital, Houston, Texas 77030, USA

M. Davenport FRCS
Senior Surgical Registrar, Department of Paediatric Surgery, Institute of Child Health, University of London, London WC1N 1EH, UK

P. W. Dillon MD
Associate Professor of Surgery and Pediatrics, Division of Pediatric Surgery, Department of Surgery, Pennsylvania State University College of Medicine, The Milton S. Hershey Medical Center, Hershey, Pennsylvania 17033, USA

P. K. Donahoe MD
Marshall K. Bartlett Professor of Surgery, Pediatric Surgical Services, Massachusetts General Hospital, Boston, Massachusetts 02114, USA

D. P. Doody MD
Associate Visiting Surgeon, Division of Pediatric Surgery, Massachusetts General Hospital, Boston, Massachusetts 02114, USA

J. W. Duckett MD
Professor of Urology, School of Medicine, University of Pennsylvania, Children's Hospital of Philadelphia, Philadelphia, Pennsylvania 19104, USA

P. G. Duffy FRCSI
Consultant Paediatric Urologist, Great Ormond Street Hospital for Children, London WC1N 3JH, UK

S. H. Ein MDCM, FRCS(C), FACS, FAAP
250 Lawrence Avenue West, Suite 315, Toronto, Ontario, Canada M5M 1B2

D. M. Evans FRCS
Consultant Hand Surgeon, Royal National Orthopaedic Hospital, Stanmore, Middlesex, UK

J. N. G. Evans DLO, FRCS
Consultant Ear, Nose and Throat Surgeon, Great Ormond Street Hospital for Children, London WC1N 3JH, UK

R. M. Filler MD, FRCS(C)
Surgeon-in-Chief, The Hospital for Sick Children, 555 University Avenue, Toronto, Ontario, Canada M5G 1X8

J. A. Fixsen MChir, FRCS
Consultant Orthopaedic Surgeon, Great Ormond Street Hospital for Children, London WC1N 3JH, UK

J. D. Frank FRCS
Consultant Paediatric Surgeon and Urologist, Directorate of Children's Services, Bristol Royal Hospital for Sick Children, Bristol BS2 8BJ, UK

M. W. L. Gauderer MD
Professor of Pediatric Surgery and Pediatrics and Chief, Division of Pediatric Surgery, Case Western Reserve University, Cleveland, Ohio 44106, USA

J. J. Grosfeld MD
Surgeon-in-Chief, James Whitcomb Riley Hospital for Children, 702 Barnhill Drive, Indianapolis, Indiana 46202-5200, USA

M. L. Gustafson MD
Surgical Research Fellow, Pediatric Research Laboratories, Massachusetts General Hospital, Boston, Massachusetts 02114, USA

B. H. Harris MD
Chief of Pediatric Surgery, New England Medical Centre, 750 Washington Street, Boston, Massachusetts 02111-1526, USA

D. M. Heimbach MD
Professor of Surgery, University of Washington Burn Center, Harborview Medical Centre, 325 9th Avenue, Seattle, Washington 98104, USA

W. H. Hendren MD, FACS, FRCSI(Hon)
Chief of Surgery, Children's Hospital, 300 Longwood Avenue, Boston, Massachusetts 02115, USA

R. J. Hernandez MD
Professor of Pediatric Radiology, University of Michigan Medical Center, Ann Arbor, Michigan 48109-0030, USA

B. A. Hicks MD
Assistant Professor of Surgery, Division of Pediatric Surgery, The University of Texas Southwestern Medical Center, Dallas, Texas, USA

R. B. Hirschl MD
Assistant Professor of Surgery, Section of Pediatric Surgery, University of Michigan Medical School, and Pediatric Surgeon, C.S. Mott Children's Hospital, Ann Arbor, Michigan 48109-0245, USA

E. R. Howard MS, FRCS
Consultant Paediatric Hepatobiliary Surgeon, Kings' College Hospital, London SE5 9RS, UK

J. M. Hutson MD, FRACS
Professor of Surgery, University of Melbourne and Director, Department of General Surgery, Royal Children's Hospital, Parkville, Victoria 3052, Australia

T. R. Karl MD
Consultant Cardiac Surgeon, Royal Children's Hospital, Melbourne, Victoria, Australia

F. M. Karrer MD
Associate Professor of Surgery, The Children's Hospital, 1950 Ogden Street B323, Denver, Colorado 80218, USA

E. M. Kiely FRCSI, FRCS
Consultant Paediatric Surgeon, Great Ormond Street Hospital for Children, London WC1N 3JH, UK

S. H. Kim MD
Visiting Surgeon, Division of Pediatric Surgery, Massachusetts General Hospital, Boston, Massachusetts 02114, USA

C. F. Koopmann Jr MD, FACS
Professor and Associate Chair, Department of Otolaryngology, Head and Neck Surgery, and Chief, Pediatric Otolaryngology, University of Michigan Medical Center, Ann Arbor, Michigan 48109, USA

T. M. Krummel MD
John W. Oswald Professor of Surgery, Pennsylvania State University, Children's Hospital, Hershey Medical Center, Hershey, Pennsylvania 17033, USA

J. R. Lilly MD
Professor of Surgery, The Children's Hospital, 1950 Ogden Street B323, Denver, Colorado 80218, USA

D. A. Lloyd MChir, FRCS, FACS, FCS(SA)
Professor of Paediatric Surgery, University of Liverpool, and Consultant Paediatric Surgeon, Alder Hey Children's Hospital, Liverpool L12 2AP, UK

T. E. Lobe MD
Chairman, Section of Pediatric Surgery, University of Tennessee and Le Bonheur Children's Medical Center, Memphis, Tennessee 38105, USA

R. I. MacPherson MD, FRCP(C)
Medical University of South Carolina, 171 Ashley Avenue, Charleston, South Carolina 29425, USA

N. P. Madden MA, FRCS
Consultant Paediatric Surgeon, Chelsea and Westminster Hospital and St Mary's Hospital, London, UK

P. S. J. Malone BSc, MCH, FRCSI
Consultant Paediatric Urologist, Wessex Regional Centre for Paediatric Surgery, Southampton General Hospital, Tremona Road, Southampton SO9 4XY, UK

M. V. Marx MD
Assistant Professor of Radiology, University of Michigan Medical Center, Ann Arbor, Michigan 48109-0030, USA

R. M. Merion MD, FACS
Associate Professor of Surgery and Chief, Division of Transplantation, University of Michigan Medical School, Ann Arbor, Michigan 48109-0331, USA

P. J. Milla MSc, FRCP
Reader of Paediatric Gastroenterology, Gastroenterology Unit, Institute of Child Health, London WC1N 1EH, UK

C. R. Moir MD, BSc, FRCS(C), FACS
Consultant in Pediatric Surgery, Mayo Foundation, Rochester, Minnesota 55905, USA

P. Mollard
Chirurgie Urinaire et Genitale de l'Enfant, Hôpital Debrousse, 29 rue Soeur Bouvier, 69322 Lyon cedex 05, France

P. D. E. Mouriquand MD
Consultant in Paediatric Surgery, Addenbrooke's Hospital, Cambridge CB2 2QQ, UK

K. M. Muraszko MD
Assistant Professor of Pediatric Neurosurgery, C.S. Mott Children's Hospital, University of Michigan, Ann Arbor, Michigan 48109-0338, USA

J. A. O'Neill MD
Surgeon-in-Chief, The Children's Hospital of Philadelphia, Philadelphia, Pennsylvania 19104, USA

H. B. Othersen MD
Professor of Surgery and Pediatrics, and Chief, Pediatric Surgery, Children's Hospital, Medical University of South Carolina, Charleston, South Carolina 29425-2270, USA

A. Peña MD
Chief, Division of Pediatric Surgery, Schneider Children's Hospital, New Hyde Park, New York 11042, USA

W. J. Pokorny MD
Professor of Surgery and Pediatrics, Baylor College of Medicine, Houston, Texas 77030, USA

T. Pranikoff MD
Lecturer in Surgery, Fellow in Extracorporeal Life Support, University of Michigan Medical School, Ann Arbor, Michigan 48109-0245, USA

P. Puri MS, FACS
Consultant Paediatric Surgeon and Director, Children's Research Centre, Our Lady's Hospital for Sick Children, Crumlin, Dublin 12, Ireland

P. G. Ransley FRCS
Consultant Urological Surgeon, Great Ormond Street Hospital for Children, London WC1N 1EH, UK

F. J. Rescorla MD
Associate Professor, Section of Pediatric Surgery, James Whitcomb Riley Hospital for Children, 702 Barnhill Drive, Indianapolis, Indiana 46202-5200, USA

A. M. K. Rickwood MA, FRCS
Paediatric Urological Surgeon, Royal Liverpool Children's NHS Trust, Alder Hey, Liverpool L12 2AP, UK

M. L. Ritchey MD, FACS, FAAP
Associate Professor and Chief of Pediatric Urology, Department of Surgery, Division of Pediatric Surgery, University of Texas Health, Science Center, Houston, Texas 77030, USA

H. Rode MMed(Surg), FCS(SA), FRCS(Ed)
Associate Professor, Department of Paediatric Surgery, Institute of Child Health, Red Cross Children's Hospital, 7700 Rondebosch, South Africa

M. I. Rowe MD
Professor of Surgery, Division of Pediatric Surgery, University of Pittsburgh School of Medicine, and Children's Hospital of Pittsburgh, Pittsburgh, Pennsylvania 15213-2583, USA

K. H. Sartorelli MD
Instructor in Surgery, The Children's Hospital, 1950 Ogden Street B323, Denver, Colorado 80218, USA

A. F. Scharli MD
Professor of Surgery, Department of Pediatric Surgery, Children's Hospital, 6000 Lucerne 16, Switzerland

C. C. Schulman MD, PhD
Professor of Urology, University Clinics of Brussels, Erasmus Hospital, 8088 route de Lennik, B-1070 Brussels, Belgium

M. Z. Schwartz MD
Chairman, Department of Surgery, Surgeon-in-Chief, Children's National Medical Centre, Department of Surgery, 111 Michigan Avenue NW, Washington, DC 20010, USA

R. C. Shamberger MD
Associate in Surgery, Children's Hospital, 300 Longwood Avenue, Boston, Massachusetts 02115, USA

N. J. Sherman MD, FACS, FAAP
Associate Clinical Professor of Surgery (Pediatric), Univerity of Southern California, California 91790, USA

C. D. Smith MD
Associate Professor of Pediatric Surgery, Children's Hospital, Medical University of South Carolina, Charleston, South Carolina 29425-2270, USA

L. Spitz PhD, FRCS, FRCS(Ed), FAAP(Hon)
Nuffield Professor of Paediatric Surgery, Institute of Child Health, University of London, and Consultant Paediatric Surgeon, Great Ormond Street Hospital for Children, London WC1N 1EH, UK

J. Stark MD, FRCS
Cardiothoracic Unit, Great Ormond Street Hospital for Children, London WC1N 3JH, UK

C. J. H. Stolar MD
Attending Surgeon, Babies' Hospital, Columbia-Presbyterian Medical Center, 3959 Broadway, New York, New York 10032, USA

M. D. Stringer BSc, MRCP, MS, FRCS
Department of Paediatric Surgery, Clarendon Wing, The General Infirmary at Leeds, Belmont Grove, Leeds LS2 9NS, UK

S. Stylianos MD
Attending Pediatric Surgeon, Babies' Hospital, Columbia-Presbyterian Medical Center, 3959 Broadway, New York, New York 10032, USA

E. Sumner MA, FRCA
Consultant Paediatric Anaesthetist, Great Ormond Street Hospital for Children, London WC1N 3JH, UK

E. P. Tagge MD
Assistant Professor of Paediatric Surgery, Children's Hospital, Medical University of South Carolina, Charleston, South Carolina 29425-2270, USA

K.-C. Tan FRCS(Ed)
Consultant Surgeon, Liver Transplant Surgical Service, King's College Hospital, London SE5 9RS, UK

D. H. Teitelbaum MD
Assistant Professor of Pediatric Surgery, University of Michigan Medical School, C.S. Mott Children's Hospital, Ann Arbor, Michigan 48109-0245, USA

J. Wan MD
Attending Pediatric Urologist, Children's Hospital of Buffalo, 2109 Bryani Street, Buffalo, New York 14222, USA

T. R. Weber MD
Department of Pediatric Surgery, Cardinal Glennon Children's Hospital, St Louis, Missouri 63104, USA

J. R. Wesley MD
Clinical Professor of Surgery Chair, Division of Pediatric Surgery, University of California, Davis Medical Center, Sacramento, California 95817, USA

E. S. Wiener MD, FACS, FAAP
Department of Surgery, The Children's Hospital of Pittsburgh, 3705 Fifth Avenue, Pittsburgh, Pennsylvania 15213-2583, USA

C. B. Williams FRCP
London Clinic Endoscopy, The Clinic, 20 Devonshire Place, London W1N 2DH, UK

V. M. Wright FRCS, FRACS
Consultant Paediatric Surgeon, Queen Elizabeth Hospital for Children, London E2 8PS, UK

Contributing Medical Artists

Diane Bruyninckx MMAA, AIMI
20 Van Halmaelelei,
B-2930 Brasschaat, Belgium

Joanna Cameron BA(Hons), MMAA
11 Pine Trees, Portsmouth Road,
Esher, Surrey KT10 9JF, UK

Angela Christie MMAA
14 West End Avenue, Pinner,
Middlesex HA5 1BJ, UK

Peter Cox RDD, MMAA, AIMI
Canon Frome Court,
Canon Frome, Ledbury,
Herefordshire HR8 2TD, UK

Marc Donon
2 rue Leriche, 75015 Paris, France

Patrick Elliott BA(Hons), ATC, MMAA, AIMI
46 Stone Delf,
Sheffield S10 3QX, UK

Mark Iley BA(Hons)
12 High Street, Great Missenden,
Buckinghamshire HP16 9AB, UK

Diane Kinton BA(Hons)
Gillian Lee Illustrations,
15 Little Plucketts Way, Buckhurst Hill,
Essex IG9 5QU, UK

Gillian Lee FMAA, HonFIMI, AMI
Gillian Lee Illustrations,
15 Little Plucketts Way, Buckhurst Hill,
Essex IG9 5QU, UK

Marks Creative Consultants
4 Harrison's Rise, Croydon,
Surrey CR0 4LA, UK

Gillian Oliver MMAA, AIMI
15 Bramble Road, Hatfield,
Hertfordshire AL10 9RZ, UK

Paul Richardson BA(Hons)
54 Wellington Road,
Orpington, Kent BR5 4AQ, UK

Philip Wilson FMAA, AIMI
Flat 2, 136 High Street,
Purley, Surrey CR8 2AD, UK

Contents

Preface

The new edition of *Pediatric Surgery* has been extensively revised and greatly expanded to take account of recent developments in the specialty and is still the only comprehensive operative text in the field.

We have been fortunate in attracting contributions from a wide range of recognized authorities in specific topics. There has been a 30% increase in individual authors. This expansion has particularly involved pediatric surgeons from the United States.

The number of chapters has now reached 100. Among the new chapters we have included are those on vascular access, reflecting the increased workload of pediatric surgeons in this field, surgical access to the thorax and abdomen, cervical esophagostomy, extra-corporeal membrane oxygenation, patent ductus arteriosus, the expanding field of laparoscopy, the management of burns and the principles of fetal surgery, organ transplantations and interventional radiology. We have greatly expanded the amount of space devoted to indications for surgery, postoperative complications and preoperative and postoperative management.

All our authors have responded remarkably well to the very tight schedule imposed on them and, as a result, all the chapters reflect contemporary technical innovations and provide current data on results and up-to-date references for further reading.

Most of the artwork has been redrawn to a consistently high standard by a team of medical artists under the direction of Gillian Lee.

We hope that both trainees in pediatric surgery and established pediatric surgeons will find this textbook useful as a guide when performing a wide range of procedures.

Lewis Spitz
Arnold Coran
October 1994

Transfer of the surgical neonate

A. F. Scharli MD
Professor of Pediatric Surgery, Department of Pediatric Surgery, Children's Hospital, Lucerne, Switzerland

Lewis Spitz PhD, FRCS, FRCS (Ed), FAAP (Hon)
Nuffield Professor of Paediatric Surgery, Institute of Child Health, University of London, and Consultant Paediatric Surgeon, Great Ormond Street Hospital for Children, London, UK

Centralization of perinatal care to regional centers could significantly reduce the mortality and morbidity associated with life-threatening congenital anomalies. The availability of fully equipped intensive care facilities, medical and nursing personnel experienced in the management of critically ill infants, the easy access to allied specialties such as cardiology, renal and respiratory units, and the on-site provision of radiology and pathology services specifically devoted to pediatric care in these centers improve the treatment of the neonate undergoing surgery. In these centers future pediatric surgeons may be trained in the complex field of neonatal surgery[1].

The range of congenital anomalies that may be diagnosed before birth is increasing. Patients who are diagnosed with such an anomaly are transported to the unit in one of two ways: while still *in utero*; or as a neonate.

Transfer *in utero*

Advantages

The advantage of transfer *in utero* is that both mother and infant are in a highly specialized center where even the most complex problems may be handled. Delivery can be planned and surgery can proceed without delay, which may be a particular advantage in gastroschisis or ruptured exomphalos. The immediate access to intensive care and extracorporeal membrane oxygenation may benefit infants with diaphragmatic hernia.

Disadvantages

The unit may be a considerable distance away from the mother's home and family and she may have to remain in hospital for some time before the delivery[2], which could cause distress and feelings of isolation.

Transfer of neonates

It is generally accepted that the risks to the neonate of properly organized transport are minimal: certainly they are lower than those of treating the patient in a small local hospital which may lack the experienced personnel or facilities for dealing with complex neonatal surgery[3].

Many regional centers have a retrieval service for collecting critically ill neonates. A fully equipped team, comprising a doctor capable of effecting neonatal and pediatric resuscitation and an experienced intensive care nurse, travel to the local hospital where the infant is resuscitated and stabilized before transfer. Transport can then be effected in a controlled, unhurried manner avoiding high-speed travel[4].

Stabilization before transfer

The condition of the neonate must be stabilized before transfer is considered. The procedures needed for optimal stabilization are discussed below.

Oxygenation

Adequate oxygenation, including the use of endotracheal intubation and mechanical ventilatory support when required (e.g. in diaphragmatic hernia, respiratory distress syndrome or necrotizing enterocolitis) is essential[5]. It is possible to initiate extracorporeal membrane oxygenation locally and to effect transfer in a specially designed ambulance. A tension pneumothorax will require decompression; drainage of a tension pneumoperitoneum may be life-saving and will permit satisfactory ventilatory support.

Vascular access

Durable vascular access, including central venous and arterial access if necessary, should be secured.

Stabilizing circulatory dynamics

Blood, plasma or electrolyte infusion and vasoactive drugs are used to stabilize the circulation and blood pressure.

Thermoregulation

Monitoring thermal stability is particularly important in the extremely preterm infant. A skin–core temperature differential greater than 3–5°C indicates poor peripheral perfusion. The neonate with exposed viscera from a gastroschisis or major omphalocele (exomphalos) is particularly at risk of developing hypothermia; heat loss can be reduced by wrapping the exposed surface in plastic wrap.

Correction of fluid and electrolyte imbalances

Imbalances in fluid and electrolytes, especially acidosis, must be corrected.

Nasogastric decompression

Infants with intestinal obstruction require nasogastric decompression to avoid the risk of aspiration during transportation. Fine-bore nasogastric tubes have a tendency to kink or curl up and are inefficient in decompressing the stomach: an 8-Fr tube (term infants) or a 6-Fr tube (preterm infants) is more appropriate. The nasogastric tube should be aspirated regularly and left open on free drainage at all times.

Use of antibiotics

Broad-spectrum antibiotics should be administered therapeutically for infants with necrotizing enterocolitis and prophylactically for those with gastroschisis, exomphalos or myelomeningocele.

Choice of transport

The method of transport is largely dependent on the distance between hospitals, geographical circumstances and weather conditions. Safe transfer can be effected equally well by ambulance, helicopter or fixed-wing aircraft.

Transfer equipment

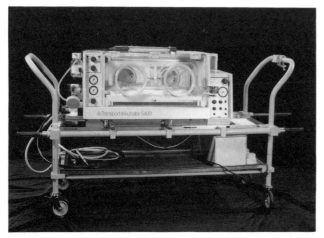

1 A portable incubator fitted with built-in air/oxygen cylinders and a ventilator is essential for maintaining a neutral thermal environment and providing respiratory support throughout the journey. As an additional precaution the neonate may be wrapped in an aluminium foil swaddler. Facilities for continuous monitoring of heart rate, respiratory rate and pressures and pulse oximetry are desirable to minimize handling. Maintenance fluids and essential drugs may be delivered by battery-operated syringe pumps.

Table 1 Equipment and drugs essential in transport of the neonate

Drugs	Equipment
Epinephrine (adrenaline) 1:1000	Endotracheal tubes (variety)
Atropine 500 µg/ml	Airways and masks (variety)
Calcium chloride	Laryngoscope and forceps
Lidocaine (lignocaine) 100 mg/ 10 ml	Nasogastric tubes (variety)
Sodium bicarbonate 8.4%	Syringes 1, 2 and 5 ml
Dextrose 50%	Needles
Isoprenaline 2 mg/2 ml	Intravenous infusion set
Pancuronium 4 mg/2 ml	Intravenous cannulas (variety)
Diazepam/midazolam 10 mg/ 2 ml	Blood glucose testing strips
Suxamethonium 100 mg/2 ml	Adhesive dressings
Dopamine 200 mg/5 ml	Chest drains and Heimlich valves
Dobutamine 250 mg/20 ml	Self-inflating bag (Ambubag)
	Suction catheters
	Swabs
	Scalpels
	Artery forceps
	Gloves

Equipment and emergency drugs that should be carried are shown in *Table 1*.

The decision as to whether ventilatory support will be necessary during transfer should be made before beginning the journey as endotracheal intubation is extremely difficult to perform in a moving vehicle. Carers should err on the side of caution and intubate whenever support may be required. Nasotracheal intubation requires special expertise but the tube can be fixed securely and is therefore unlikely to become dislodged during the journey. Ventilation by facemask is an ineffective means of assisted respiration and introduces gas into the gastrointestinal tract, resulting in abdominal distension which may further aggravate respiratory embarrassment.

Check list

The following items should be transported to the special regional unit with the patient: a copy of neonatal records and list of drugs administered, including vitamin K; a specimen of maternal blood (10 ml), which will be tested for the presence of passively acquired maternal antibodies by hematologists at the regional center in preparing blood for transfusion; copies of all radiographs and results of other investigations (hematology, biochemistry, microbiology, pathology); a legally valid consent form, signed by one or both parents, authorizing surgery.

Transport audit

To determine the efficiency of the transfer system, a critical audit is necessary. This should include documentation of the characteristics of the patient (birth weight, physical condition, reason for referral), stabilization measures taken (vascular access, oxygenation, ventilatory support, cardiovascular support), transport-related complications and the outcome of treatment. Shenai *et al.*[6] have reported an increase in pretransport stabilization measures from 12% to 58%, an increase in assisted ventilation from 10% to 33% and a decrease in neonatal mortality from 17% to 7%.

Surgical conditions requiring special care during transport

Esophageal atresia and tracheoesophageal fistula

These conditions always carry a high risk of aspiration and cyanosis, which may be prevented by frequent aspiration of saliva and placing the neonate in a lateral position. For long journeys or in preterm infants, endotracheal intubation is advisable. The patient should be given 1 mg vitamin K intramuscularly.

Gastroschisis and ruptured omphalocele

Extreme and rapid heat and fluid loss from the exposed viscera are avoidable if the intestines are placed in a moist plastic bag. The bowel should be supported to avoid traction and intestinal ischemia. Wrapping the entire abdomen prevents further heat loss. Intravenous fluids with plasma and glucose should be supplied in sufficient amounts to counteract hypovolemia and hypoglycemia. Temperature and blood glucose levels should be checked frequently.

Myelomeningocele

The exposed neural tissue should be covered with a moist saline dressing.

Necrotizing enterocolitis

The mostly preterm infants suffering from necrotizing enterocolitis are usually in a critical condition with symptoms of shock and septicemia. Assisted ventilation provides sufficient tissue oxygenation. Administration of fluid and antibiotics is indicated. Drainage of a tension pneumoperitoneum will facilitate ventilatory support and should be initiated before transfer but may be required during the journey.

Sacrococcygeal teratoma

This tumor is increasingly being diagnosed before birth. Most fetal teratomas present with an enlarged uterus due to the tumor and associated polyhydramnios by 20–32 weeks' gestation. Rapidly growing tumors tend to produce placentamegaly and hydrops of the fetus and may lead to death *in utero*.

References

1. Connolly HV, Fetcho S, Hageman JR. Education of personnel involved in the transport program. *Crit Care Clin* 1992; 8: 481–90.

2. Kollee LA, Brand R, Schreuder AM, Ens-Dokkum MH, Veen S. Five-year outcome of preterm and very low birth weight infants: a comparison between maternal and neonatal transport. *Obstet Gynecol* 1992; 80: 635–8.

3. Kronick JB, Kissoon N, Frewen TC. Guidelines for stabilizing the condition of the critically ill child before transfer to a tertiary care facility. *Can Med Assoc J* 1988; 139: 213–20.

4. Spitz L, Wallis M, Graves HF. Transport of the surgical neonate. *Arch Dis Child* 1984; 59: 284–8.

5. Kanter RK, Tompkins JM. Adverse events during interhospital transport: physiologic deterioration associated with pretransport severity of illness. *Pediatrics* 1989; 84: 43–8.

6. Shenai JP. Neonatal transport. Outreach educational program. *Pediatr Clin North Am* 1993; 40: 275–85.

Preoperative and postoperative management of the neonate

Craig T. Albanese MD
Assistant Professor of Surgery, Division of Pediatric Surgery, University of Pittsburgh School of Medicine, and Children's Hospital of Pittsburgh, Pittsburgh, Pennsylvania, USA

Marc I. Rowe MD
Professor of Surgery, Division of Pediatric Surgery, University of Pittsburgh School of Medicine, and Children's Hospital of Pittsburgh, Pittsburgh, Pennsylvania, USA

The neonate, infant, child and adolescent differ significantly from each other and from the adult. The most distinctive and rapidly changing physiologic characteristics occur during the neonatal period due to the newborn infant's adaptation to the extrauterine environment, differences in the physiologic maturity of individual neonates, the small size of these patients, and the demands of growth and development. Recent advances in neonatal care have resulted in the survival of increasing numbers of extremely low birthweight infants. Extreme prematurity predisposes these tiny, fragile infants to physiologic derangements in temperature regulation, fluid and electrolyte homeostasis, bilirubin metabolism, intracranial hemorrhage and hyaline membrane disease. For these reasons this chapter will emphasize the management of the neonate undergoing surgery. Neonates can be classified according to their level of maturation (gestational age) and development (weight) as:

1. Term infants. The normal full-term infant has a gestational age of 38 weeks or more and a body weight over 2500 g.
2. Low birthweight (LBW) infants.
   (a) Preterm infants. The preterm infant has a gestational age of less than 38 weeks with a birth weight appropriate for that age.
   (b) Small for gestational age (SGA) infants. The SGA infant has a gestational age of more than 38 weeks, but a body weight under 2500 g.
3. Very low birthweight (VLBW) infants (also called extremely preterm infants or 'micropremie'). These infants are generally born at less than 32 weeks gestation with a body weight less than 1500 g.

4. Large for gestational age (LGA) infants. The birth weight of these infants is greater than 4000 g if term, or greater than the 90th percentile for gestational age.
5. Post-term infants. These infants have a gestational age of 42 weeks or longer.

The physiologic differences between preterm, SGA and VLBW infants are detailed below.

Preterm infant

Preterm infants are born before 38 weeks of gestation and have a body weight appropriate for that age; if the gestational age is not accurately known, prematurity can be confirmed by physical examination. The principal features of preterm infants are a head circumference below the 50th percentile, a thin, semi-transparent skin, absence of plantar creases, soft malleable ears (little cartilage), absence of breast tissue, undescended testes (testicular descent begins around the 32nd week of gestation) with a flat scrotum in boys and relatively enlarged labia minora and small labia majora in girls.

Several physiologic abnormalities exist in preterm infants. Episodes of apnea and bradycardia are common and may occur spontaneously or as non-specific signs of problems such as sepsis and hypothermia. Prolonged apnea with significant hypoxemia leads to bradycardia and ultimately to cardiac arrest. All preterm infants should therefore undergo electrocardiographic pulse monitoring, with the alarm set at a minimum pulse rate

5

of 90 beats per minute, and apnea monitoring. In the neonate with respiratory difficulties chest radiography will help to detect hyaline membrane disease and cardiac failure. The lungs and retinas of preterm infants are very susceptible to high oxygen levels, and even relatively brief exposures may result in various degrees of hyaline membrane disease and retinopathy of prematurity. Infants receiving oxygen therefore require continuous pulse oximetry monitoring, with the alarm set between 85% and 92%. Shunting across a patent ductus arteriosus or foramen ovale is not uncommon. The direction of the shunt is determined by body weight and the underlying physiologic or organic disorder. Most shunts are left-to-right, with resultant cardiac failure. Right-to-left shunts are present in neonates with congenital diaphragmatic hernia, meconium aspiration and sepsis. Right-to-left shunting (persistent fetal circulation) does not occur in infants weighing less than 1200 g because they lack the vascular musculature necessary to produce pulmonary hypertension.

The preterm infant may be unable to tolerate oral feeding because they have a weak suck reflex, and intragastric tube feeds or total parenteral nutrition may be required. Bilirubin metabolism may be impaired, and so the serum bilirubin should be monitored for rising levels of unconjugated bilirubin. Preterm infants have higher requirements for glucose, calcium and sodium than term infants, as well as a propensity for hypothermia, intraventricular hemorrhage and metabolic acidosis (renal tubular).

Very low birthweight (VLBW) infant

Owing to the advances in neonatal intensive care increasing numbers of VLBW infants are surviving. Long-term venous access or surgical therapy for necrotizing enterocolitis are the most common reasons for pediatric surgeons being involved with these patients.

Physiologically VLBW infants are similar to the 'ordinary' preterm infant. However, most (if not all) of the problems mentioned above are accentuated (electrolyte abnormalities, hypothermia, hyperbilirubinemia) or are found with greater frequency (retinopathy of prematurity, intraventricular hemorrhage, patent ductus arteriosus, oxygen requirement with resultant hyaline membrane disease). Extreme prematurity of the gastrointestinal tract and its tendency to develop necrotizing enterocolitis if presented with enteral formulas too early mean that most of these infants require total parenteral nutrition for several weeks.

Small for gestational age (SGA) infant

Although the body weight is low, the body length and head circumference of the SGA infant are appropriate for the gestational age. Such an infant is the product of a pregnancy complicated by any one of several placental, maternal, or fetal abnormalities which result in intrauterine growth retardation. The SGA infant is older and developmentally more mature than a preterm infant of equivalent weight, and faces different physiologic problems. Because of the longer gestational period and resultant well developed organ systems, the metabolic rate of the SGA infant is much higher in proportion to the body weight than a preterm infant of similar weight. Fluid and caloric requirements are therefore increased. Intrauterine malnutrition results in a relative lack of body fat and decreased glycogen stores and, coupled with their relatively large surface area and high metabolic rate, greatly predispose these neonates to hypothermia and hypoglycemia. Close monitoring of the blood sugar level is therefore essential. Polycythemia is common and the hematocrit level should be monitored. Persistently high central hematocrits (> 65%) may necessitate plasma exchange transfusions to avoid the potential risks of hyperviscosity. These infants also have an increased risk of meconium aspiration syndrome. Because of the adequate length of gestation retinopathy of prematurity, intraventricular hemorrhage and hyaline membrane disease are relatively uncommon.

Metabolic considerations in the care of the neonate

Thermoregulation

Neonates are susceptible to heat loss because of their large surface area, low body fat relative to body weight, small mass to act as a heat sink and high thermoneutral temperature zone. Heat loss may occur by evaporation, conduction, convection and radiation (the most difficult to control). The amount of evaporative heat loss increases as the gestational age decreases. Neonates generate heat by metabolizing their brown fat reserves (non-shivering thermogenesis) rather than by shivering. This has practical consequences because brown fat may be rendered inactive by pressors or anesthetic and neuromuscular blocking agents, and may be depleted by poor nutritional intake. When an infant is exposed to cold, metabolic work increases above basal levels and calories are consumed to maintain the body temperature. If prolonged, this depletes the limited energy reserves and predisposes to hypothermia and increased mortality.

The optimal thermal environment (thermoneutrality) is defined as the range of ambient temperatures in which an infant, at a minimal metabolic rate, can maintain a constant normal body temperature by vasomotor control. The environmental temperature must be maintained near the appropriate thermoneutral zone for each individual. Thermoneutrality is determined by weight and postnatal age using standard nomograms: 34–35°C for LBW infants up to 12 days of age, 31–32°C at 6 weeks of age. Neonates weighing 2000–3000 g have a thermoneutral zone of 31–34°C at birth and 29–31°C at 12 days.

The environmental temperature of the neonate is best controlled in an incubator by monitoring the ambient temperature and maintaining it at thermoneutrality. A servo system regulates the incubator temperature according to the patient's skin temperature, monitored by a skin probe. Radiant warmers can not prevent heat loss by convection and lead to higher insensible water loss. The normal skin temperature for a full-term infant is 36.2°C and for an LBW 36.5°C. Increased metabolic activity can be detected by comparing skin and rectal temperatures, which normally differ by 1.5°C. A decreasing skin temperature with a constant rectal temperature suggests that the metabolic rate has increased to maintain the core temperature.

In a cold environment (such as the operating room or radiography department) heat loss may be reduced by wrapping the head, extremities, and as much of the trunk as possible in wadding, plastic sheets or aluminum foil. A plastic sheet placed beneath the infant increases the humidity of the microenvironment between it and the sheet. After draping, the infant is covered by a large adhesive plastic sheet which retains evaporative heat and water and prevents the patient from becoming wet during the operation. Any exposed intestine (e.g. gastroschisis) should be wrapped in plastic. An overhead infrared heating lamp is focused on the infant during induction of anesthesia and preparation for operation, and again at the termination of the operation. Solutions used for skin cleansing should be warmed.

Glucose homeostasis

The fetus receives glucose from its mother by facilitated transplacental diffusion; very little is derived from fetal gluconeogenesis. The limited liver glycogen stores are rapidly depleted within 2–3 h after birth, and the blood glucose level then depends on the neonate's capacity for gluconeogenesis, the adequacy of substrate stores, and energy requirements. The risk of developing hypoglycemia is high in LBW (especially SGA) infants, those born to toxemic or diabetic mothers, and those requiring surgery who are unable to take oral nutrition and who have the additional metabolic stresses of their disease and the surgical procedure.

The clinical features of hypoglycemia are non-specific and include a weak or high-pitched cry, cyanosis, apnea, jitteriness or trembling, apathy and seizures. The differential diagnosis includes other metabolic disturbances or sepsis. Over 50% of infants with symptomatic hypoglycemia suffer significant neurologic damage. Neonatal hypoglycemia is defined as a serum glucose level less than 1.66 mmol/l in the full-term infant and less than 1.11 mmol/l in the LBW infant. However, neurologic abnormalities have been reported with higher blood glucose levels. Older children, particularly those with depleted stores and severe metabolic demands, are also at risk of hypoglycemia.

All pediatric surgical patients, particularly neonates, are therefore monitored for hypoglycemia. To avoid delay, blood glucose levels can be rapidly determined in the neonatal unit using blood glucose reagent strips. This may be correlated at intervals with serum glucose determinations, the frequency depending on the stability of the patient. Any intravenous fluids administered should contain at least 10% dextrose and, if non-dextrose containing solutions such as blood or plasma are being administered, close monitoring of the blood glucose level is essential. Hypoglycemia should be treated urgently with intravenous 50% dextrose, 1–2 ml/kg, and maintenance intravenous dextrose, 10–15%, 80–100 ml/kg for each 24 h.

Hyperglycemia is commonly a problem of VLBW infants on parenteral nutritional support since they have a lower insulin response to glucose. Hyperglycemia may lead to intraventricular hemorrhage and renal water and electrolyte loss from glycosuria. Prevention of hyperglycemia is by small and gradual incremental changes in the glucose concentration and infusion rate.

Calcium and magnesium homeostasis

The fetus receives calcium by active transport across the placenta, 75% of the total requirement being transferred after the 18th week of gestation. Hypocalcemia, defined as a serum level of ionized calcium below 1.0 mg/100ml, is most likely to occur 24–48 h after birth. Causes include decreased calcium stores, decreased renal phosphate excretion and relative hypoparathyroidism secondary to suppression by high fetal calcium levels. LBW infants are at great risk (particularly if they are preterm), as are those born of a complicated pregnancy or delivery (e.g. diabetic mother) or those receiving bicarbonate infusions. Exchange transfusions or the rapid administration of citrated blood may also lead to hypocalcemia. The symptoms of hypocalcemia are non-specific (as with hypoglycemia) and include jitteriness, high-pitched crying, cyanosis, vomiting, twitching and seizures. Diagnosis is confirmed by determining the serum calcium level: the ionized fraction of the serum calcium may be low, however, resulting in clinical hypocalcemia without a great reduction in total serum calcium.

Hypocalcemia is prevented by adding calcium gluconate to daily maintenance therapy, 1–2 g per 24 h intravenously or 2 g per 24 h by mouth. Symptomatic hypocalcemia is treated by intravenous administration of 10% calcium gluconate in a dose of 1–2 ml/kg over 10 min; the rate should not exceed 1 ml/min.

Infants at risk for hypocalcemia are also at risk for hypomagnesemia; the two conditions may coexist. If there is no response to attempted correction of a documented calcium deficiency, hypomagnesemia should be suspected and serum magnesium levels measured. Hypomagnesemia is corrected by administering 50% magnesium sulfate, 0.2 mEq/kg every 6 h intravenously, followed by oral magnesium sulfate 30 mEq/day.

Although most seizures that occur in the neonatal period have a cerebral cause and are not secondary to hypoglycemia or hypocalcemia, hypocalcemia should be suspected in high-risk infants, particularly after surgery. Immediate blood glucose determination and serum glucose and calcium measurements should therefore be performed in a 'jittery' neonate. Treatment should be prompt, with intravenous glucose when hypoglycemia is suspected, followed by intravenous calcium if symptoms persist.

Blood volume

Total blood, plasma, and red cell volumes are higher during the first few hours of life than at any other time in an individual's life. The levels may be further increased if a significant placental transfusion takes place at delivery (delayed cord clamping). Several hours after birth plasma shifts out of the circulation and total blood and plasma volumes decrease. The high red blood cell volume persists, decreasing slowly to reach adult levels by the seventh postnatal week. Age-related estimations of blood volume are summarized in *Table 1*.

Table 1   Estimation of blood volume

Age	Blood volume (ml/kg)
Preterm infants	85–100
Term infants	85
1–3 months	75
3 months to adult	70

Adapted from Rowe[1].

In the neonate, polycythemia is defined as a central venous hematocrit greater than 65%. This may be associated with high blood viscosity which is further increased by a fall in body temperature. Partial exchange transfusion may be indicated since hyperviscosity may be an etiologic factor of several disorders (for example, central nervous system dysfunction or necrotizing enterocolitis).

Jaundice

Heme pigments, notably hemoglobin, are catabolized in the spleen and liver to produce bilirubin. The bilirubin is conjugated with glucuronic acid in the liver, forming a water-soluble substance which is excreted via the biliary system into the intestine. In the fetus the lipid-soluble, unconjugated (indirect) bilirubin is cleared across the placenta. In the fetal intestine beta-glucuronidase hydrolases conjugated bilirubin, which is then reabsorbed for transplacental clearance. Circulating unconjugated bilirubin is bound to albumin.

The neonate's capacity for conjugating bilirubin is not fully developed and may be exceeded by the bilirubin load, resulting in transient physiologic jaundice which reaches a maximum at the age of 4 days but returns to normal levels by the sixth day. Usually the maximum bilirubin level does not exceed 170 μmol/l. Physiologic jaundice is particularly likely to occur in SGA and preterm infants in whom higher and more prolonged hyperbilirubinemia may be encountered.

High serum levels of unconjugated bilirubin may cross the immature blood–brain barrier in the neonate and can act as a neural poison leading to kernicterus. This condition, in its most severe form, is characterized by athetoid cerebral palsy and sensorineural hearing loss. Predisposing factors are hypoalbuminemia, acidosis, cold stress, hypoglycemia, caloric deprivation, hypoxemia and competition for bilirubin binding sites by drugs (e.g. furosemide, digoxin or gentamicin) or free acids.

Clinical jaundice is apparent at serum bilirubin levels of 120–135 μmol/l. A rapid rise early in the neonatal period suggests hemolysis, secondary to inherited enzyme defects or to maternal–neonatal blood group incompatibilities. Prolonged hyperbilirubinemia is often associated with an increase in conjugated bilirubin due to biliary obstruction or hepatocellular dysfunction. Breast milk jaundice commonly appears between 1 and 8 weeks of age. Mild indirect hyperbilirubinemia occurs with pyloric stenosis and quickly disappears after pyloromyotomy. Intestinal obstruction can intensify jaundice by increasing the enterohepatic circulation of bilirubin. Finally, jaundice is an early and important sign of septicemia.

If hemolysis is suspected, serial hematocrit estimations, reticulocyte counts, peripheral blood smears and a Coomb's test are appropriate. Evaluation of neonatal sepsis includes hematocrit, white blood cell count and differential platelet count, chest radiography and cultures of blood, urine and cerebrospinal fluid.

Phototherapy is widely used prophylactically in high-risk neonates to decrease the serum bilirubin levels by photodegradation of bilirubin in the skin to water-soluble products. It is continued until the total serum bilirubin level is less than 170 μmol/l and falling. The timing of phototherapy is based on the level of indirect bilirubin and the weight of the patient. Exchange transfusion is indicated if the indirect bilirubin level exceeds 340 µmol/l. The precise indications vary according to the individual patient, and in VLBW infants exchange transfusion is indicated at much lower serum bilirubin levels. Factors increasing the risk of kernicterus also influence the indications for exchange transfusion.

Vitamin K

The routine administration of vitamin K to all neonates to prevent hypoprothrombinemia and hemorrhagic disease is established practice. This may be overlooked during the activities attendant on major congenital anomalies or conditions requiring urgent surgical evaluation. When in doubt, 1.0 mg of vitamin K should be administered by intramuscular or intravenous injection.

Energy requirements

The pediatric patient requires a relatively large energy intake because of the high basal metabolic rate, requirements for growth and development, energy needs to maintain body heat, and the limited energy reserve these patients possess. These requirements vary according to age and environmental factors, and are significantly increased by cold stress, surgical procedures, infections and injuries (particularly burns). Energy requirements are increased 10–25% by surgery, more than 50% by infection, and 150% by burns. Energy reserves are limited in the neonate, whose liver glycogen stores are consumed in the first 3 h of life, and to an even greater extent in the preterm and SGA infant.

Table 2 Energy requirements of various age groups

	Energy required per 24 h (J)
Basal metabolism: full-term infant	
Birth	134
2 weeks	202
1 year	168
Teen	97
Growth calories	
Birth	139
3 months	76
6 months	50
1 year	50
Teen	76
Total calories (maintenance and growth)	
Neonatal term (0–4 days)	462–504
Low birthweight infant	504–546
3–4 months	420–445
5–12 months	420
1–7 years	378–315
7–12 years	315–252
12–18 years	252–126

The energy needs are calculated according to the requirements for basal metabolism plus growth (*Table 2*). Consideration must also be given to the adequacy of energy reserves and the presence of stress factors such as cold, infection and trauma, including surgery.

Fluid and electrolyte management

Effective fluid and electrolyte management involves: (1) calculating the fluid and electrolyte requirements for maintaining metabolic functions; (2) replacing losses (evaporative, third space, external); and (3) considering pre-existing fluid deficits or excesses. Taking these factors into consideration a tentative program is devised for fluid and electrolytes administered for a finite period of time, usually 8 h, but shorter intervals are necessary for critically ill patients. The response of the patient is monitored and the program adjusted accordingly.

Calculating maintenance needs

The neonate's basic maintenance requirement for water is the volume required for growth, renal excretion (renal water) and replacing losses from the skin, lungs and stools. Stool water loss has been estimated at 5–10 ml per 420 J expended, the lower figure applying to those patients not being fed. In the surgical patient with postoperative ileus, stool water loss is usually insignificant. Growth is inhibited during periods of severe stress and is also not a major factor under these conditions. The basal fluid maintenance requirement is therefore renal water plus insensible loss. Requirements during the first day of life are unique because of the greatly expanded extracellular fluid volume in the neonate, which decreases after 24 h, and because neonates with intestinal obstruction are not hypovolemic as a result of intrauterine adjustments across the placenta. During the first 24 h basic maintenance fluid should not exceed 90 ml/kg in preterm infants weighing less than 1000 g or less than 32 weeks gestational age, or 75 ml/kg in larger infants.

The basic electrolyte and energy requirements are provided by NaCl (2–3 mEq/kg/day: up to 5 mEq/kg/day for preterm infants) in 5% or 10% dextrose, with the addition of potassium (2–3 mEq/kg/day) once urine production has been established. Calcium gluconate (1–2 g/l fluid) may be added, especially in preterm infants.

Renal water

The volume of water required for excretion by the kidney depends on the renal solute load and the renal concentrating ability of the individual. The solute load that the kidneys must excrete is derived from the endogenous tissue catabolism and exogenous protein and electrolyte intake. The osmolar load is thus reduced by growth and increased by tissue necrosis, high osmolar feeds and infusions. The volume of fluid administered should be sufficient to allow excretion of the solute load at an isotonic urine osmolality of 280 mOsmol/dl. It is important to understand that there is no 'normal' urine output for neonates: the authors found that during the first three postoperative days the osmolar load in neonates ranged between 8.8 and 33.4 mOsmol/kg per 24 h (mean 16.47). The calculated ideal urine output, representing the renal water required to excrete this load, averaged between 2 and 3 ml/kg/h.

Insensible loss

Invisible continuing loss of water occurs from the lungs (respiratory water loss) and through the skin (trans-epithelial water loss), and constitutes the insensible water loss (IWL). Respiratory water loss (RWL) accounts for approximately one-third of IWL in infants older than 32 weeks of gestational age and is approximately 5 ml/kg body weight per 24 h at a relative humidity of 50%. Transepithelial water loss (TEWL) for a full-term infant in a thermoneutral environment is approximately 7 ml/kg body weight. The insensible water loss for a full-term infant in the thermoneutral environment at 50% relative humidity is therefore 12 ml/kg per 24 h.

The main factors that affect IWL are the gestational age of the infant and the relative humidity of the environment. For infants of 25–27 weeks' gestation TEWL has been estimated at 128 ml/kg per 24 h at 50% relative humidity. The relative humidity has a marked inverse effect on TEWL, which decreases to almost zero as the relative humidity approaches 100%. Plastic sheets may be used to increase the relative humidity around the infant and reduce TEWL by 50–70%. Conversely, radiant warmers and phototherapy lights increase IWL by 50% in infants weighing less than 1500 g and by 80% in those weighing more than 1500 g.

Management program

The most commonly used method of calculating fluid requirements is based on body weight. However, because of the many factors affecting maintenance requirements, there is no close or constant relationship between body weight and fluid and electrolyte needs. Thus, the authors have developed a dynamic approach to fluid management in the neonate undergoing surgery. This requires two components: an initial volume that is safe for the patient's status (termed the 'bogey' volume) and a monitoring system to assess the effects of the initial bogey volume and make appropriate adjustments.

The initial bogey volume is essentially a 'best guess' volume and, from the surgical experience at the Children's Hospital of Pittsburgh, has ranged from 80 to 160 ml/kg/day depending on age and the particular surgical disorder (e.g. 80 ml/kg/day for a neonate undergoing colostomy on day 1 of life; 160 ml/kg/day for one being treated for a gastroschisis). In the older child (over 10 kg in weight), fluid calculations are based on body weight according to the guidelines outlined in *Table 3*.

Table 3   Calculation of maintenance fluid requirements

Body weight (kg)	Fluid volume per 24 h
1–10	100 ml/kg
11–20	1000 ml + 50 ml for each kg over 10 kg
> 20	1500 ml + 20 ml for each kg over 20 kg

Calculation of additional losses

External losses from the intestinal drainage, fistulas and drainage tubes are directly measured and replaced volume for volume with an appropriate electrolyte solution. In neonates it is wise to measure the electrolytes in the fluid to more accurately guide replacement. Protein-rich losses (e.g. from chest tubes) are replaced with an albumin solution or fresh frozen plasma. Internal losses into body cavities or tissues (third space losses) cannot be measured, and adequate replacement of these losses depends on careful monitoring of the patient's response.

Monitoring the fluid and electrolyte program

Clinical features

Severe isotonic and hypovolemic dehydration results in poor capillary filling and collapse of peripheral veins. The skin is cool and mottled, with reduced turgor; the mucous membranes are dry and the anterior fontanelle is sunken. These findings occur with 10% body fluid losses in an infant of more than 28 days of age and 15% in a neonate. Hypertonic dehydration is more difficult to detect clinically because the decrease in circulating blood volume is considerably less than the total loss of body fluids. Signs of shock occur late and central nervous system signs, including lethargy, stupor and seizures, predominate.

Body weight

Serial measurements of body weight are a useful guide to total body water in the neonate. Fluctuations over a 24-h period are primarily related to loss or gain of fluid; 1 g body weight being approximately equal to 1 ml water. Errors will occur if changes in clothing, dressings, tubes and standard IV boards are not accounted for, and if weighing scales are not regularly calibrated.

Urine volume and composition

If the volume of fluid administered is inadequate, urine volume falls and its concentration increases: if excess fluid is administered the opposite occurs. The authors aim to achieve a urine output which will maintain a urine osmolality of approximately 280 mOsmol/dl (specific gravity 1.009–1.012); in neonates this usually results in a urine output of 2 ml/kg/h. For infants and older children, hydration is adequate if the urine output is 1–2 ml/kg/h with an osmolality of 280–300 mOsmol/kg. Serial hematocrit determinations, in the absence of hemolysis or bleeding, also suggest a loss or gain of plasma water.

When the osmolar load is large, for example with extensive tissue destruction or with infusion of high osmolar solutions (e.g. gastrointestinal or intravenous contrast fluids), urine flow may have to be increased to provide adequate renal clearance. Accurate measurements of urine flow and concentration are fundamental to the management of critically ill infants and children, and in this situation insertion of an indwelling urinary catheter is recommended.

The specific gravity of the urine is a reliable indicator of hypertonicity (> 1.012) and hypotonicity (< 1.008) but is unreliable if urine is in the isotonic range (1.009–1.011). When fluid monitoring is critical, urine osmolality estimations provide more precise information than specific gravity. An increase in osmolality suggests that too little water or too much electrolyte (usually sodium) has been given. A fall is osmolality suggests that sodium replacement is inadequate or that too much water is being administered. An unexpected change in osmolality, particularly an increase, requires immediate determination of serum levels of electrolytes, blood urea nitrogen and glucose values and a calculation of the osmolality. Serum osmolality can be measured directly or calculated by the formula:

$$\text{Osmolality} = \text{serum sodium} \times 1.86 + \frac{\text{blood urea nitrogen}}{2.8} + \frac{\text{glucose}}{18} + 5$$

From this it is possible to determine whether the rise in osmolality is due to an increase in serum sodium, the development of hyperglycemia or a high blood urea nitrogen. Occasionally the measured serum osmolality is higher than the calculated osmolality. This suggests that the increase in serum osmolality is due to some unidentified osmolar active substance such as a metabolic byproduct resulting from sepsis, shock or radio-opaque contrast material.

A rising blood urea nitrogen level and falling urine output may be due to acute renal failure or prerenal oliguria with azotemia resulting from hypovolemia. The distinction between these two states is important for appropriate treatment. Initially, the response to a fluid challenge of 20 ml/kg 5% dextrose and sodium chloride solution over 1 h is monitored. If oliguria persists the sodium, creatinine and osmolality levels in both the blood and urine are determined, and the fractional excretion of sodium (Fe_{Na}) is calculated using the formula:

$$Fe_{Na} = \frac{\text{Urine sodium/serum sodium}}{\text{Urine creatinine/serum creatinine}} \times 100$$

A normal Fe_{Na} is 2–3%. A value below 2% implies prerenal azotemia, one above 3% implies renal failure.

Perioperative management

In the neonate undergoing surgery fluid, serum electrolyte and acid–base abnormalities are corrected before operation, except in the case of immediate emergency surgery. Intraoperative fluid requirements consist of the estimated maintenance requirement plus replacement of pre-existing deficits (if uncorrected) and replacement of estimated intraoperative electrolyte and blood losses. The need for intraoperative blood transfusion is determined by the clinical condition, pulse, blood pressure, haematocrit and urine output of the patient in relation to measured losses in sponges and suction bottles.

General considerations

Gastrointestinal decompression

The importance of gastric decompression in the neonate undergoing surgery cannot be overemphasized. The distended stomach carries the risk of aspiration and pneumonia, and may impair diaphragmatic excursions, resulting in respiratory distress. With congenital diaphragmatic hernia, ventilation is progressively impaired as the herniated intestine becomes distended with air and fluid. With gastroschisis, omphalocele and diaphragmatic hernia the ability to reduce the prolapsed intestine into the abdominal cavity is impaired by intestinal distension. This may be alleviated by adequate orogastric or nasogastric tube decompression. A double-lumen sump tube, such as the Replogle tube, is preferred, utilizing low continuous suction. If a single-lumen tube is used intermittent aspiration is required. The correct position of the tube in the stomach is confirmed by carefully measuring the tube before insertion, by noting the nature of the aspirate and by radiography. The tube should be carefully taped to avoid displacement. The use of gastrostomy tubes for postoperative gastric decompression is decreasing in popularity, but should be considered when prolonged postoperative gastric or intestinal stasis is anticipated.

Antimicrobial therapy

Deficiencies in the neonate's immune system render it vulnerable to major bacterial insults. Prophylactic antimicrobial therapy is advised for infants undergoing major surgery, particularly of the gastrointestinal tract or genitourinary system. Adequate coverage is provided by combining a penicillin (e.g. ampicillin) or first-generation cephalosporin (e.g. cefazolin) with an aminoglycoside (usually gentamicin or tobramycin). Clindamycin is added when anaerobic coverage is deemed necessary. Alternatively, single-drug therapy using a broad-spectrum cephalosporin (e.g. cefoxitin) may be appropriate. Antibiotics are commenced before operation and may be discontinued after surgery at the surgeon's discretion.

Diagnostic studies

Most tests pose an additional burden to the already stressed neonate, and diagnostic studies should be restricted to those essential for diagnosis and proper management. The volume of blood drawn for laboratory tests should be documented as these small volumes cumulatively represent significant loss in a small infant. The authors believe that a complete blood count with a differential and platelet count, and a blood specimen for type and cross-match (in the case of major neonatal surgery) are all that are indicated before surgery. In the first 12 h of life electrolyte levels simply reflect the mother's electrolytes. Coagulation studies are rarely necessary.

When the patient is transferred to other departments for investigational procedures, monitoring and resuscitation equipment should be available with a surgeon in attendance. All studies should be done with minimal disturbance, taking steps to prevent heat loss. Before using hyperosmolar radio-opaque contrast materials intravenous fluids must be administered and fluid deficits corrected, regardless of the route of administration. To counteract the osmotic effect of the contrast medium an intravenous infusion of sodium chloride 34 mEq/l at twice the maintenance rate should be given during the radiographic study and for 2–4 h afterwards. During this period the patient should be carefully monitored as described above.

Transport

Whenever possible, a trained team including a nurse and a physician with the necessary expertise for intubation and respiratory support should transport neonates, using a portable incubator. Exposed viscera must be protected as described above. Vital functions should be constantly monitored. When intestinal obstruction is present intravenous fluids and continuous gastric decompression must be provided. Unless fluid losses have been high, intravenous fluids may not be required for neonates during short journeys, but an intravenous infusion may be needed to provide glucose requirements.

Reference

1. Rowe PC, ed. *The Harriet Lane Handbook*, 11th edn. Chicago: Year Book Medical Publishers, 1987; 25.

Further reading

Albanese CT, Nour BM, Rowe MI. Anesthesia block nonshivering thermogenesis in the neonatal rabbit. *J Pediatr Surg* 1994 (in press).

Bell EF, Oh W. Fluid and electrolyte balance in very low birth weight infants. *Clin Perinatol* 1979; 6: 139–50.

Krummel TM, Lloyd DA, Rowe MI. The postoperative response of the term and preterm newborn infant to sodium administration. *J Pediatr Surg* 1985; 20: 803–9.

Oh W, ed. Symposium on the newborn. *Pediatr Clin North Am* 1982; 29: 1055–298.

Rowe MI. Fluid and electrolyte management. In: Welch KJ, Randolph JG, Ravitch MM, O'Neill JA, Rowe MI, eds. *Pediatric Surgery*, 4th edn. Chicago: Year Book Medical Publishers, 1986: 22–30.

Rowe MI, Pettit BJ. Management of the critically ill patient. In: Welch KJ, Randolph JG, Ravitch MM, O'Neill JA, Rowe MI, eds. *Pediatric Surgery*, 4th edn. Chicago: Year Book Medical Publishers, 1986: 31–50.

Scanlon JW. The very-low-birth-weight infant. In: Avery GB, Fletcher MA, MacDonald MG, eds. *Neonatology: Pathophysiology and Management of the Newborn*, 4th edn. Philadelphia: JB Lippincott Company, 1994; 399–416.

Smith CA, Nelson MN. *The Physiology of the Newborn Infant*, 4th edn. Springfield: Charles C. Thomas.

Pediatric anesthesia

Edward Sumner MA, FRCA
Consultant Paediatric Anaesthetist, Great Ormond Street Hospital for Children, London, UK

Pediatric anesthesia is recognized as an independent specialized subject. It is generally accepted that the term applies to infants and children up to the age of 3 years.

The biochemical, physiologic and psychologic needs peculiar to young children are best met in a children's environment. The recommended policy is to concentrate pediatric surgery and intensive care in children's departments and children's hospitals, so that each centre for neonatal surgery serves a population of about two million. This is feasible because transport of sick infants, even over very long distances, by surface or air, is now routine and safe even for intubated and ventilated patients.

The differences between adult and pediatric anesthesia are related to differences in anatomy and physiology – differences which are most marked in the very young. Neonates with a gestational age as low as 26 weeks with weights of 600 g are now surviving so that the implications of the traditional neonatal period of 28 days of life in terms of development have become meaningless: the neonatal period is now defined as up to 44 weeks after conception (*Figure 1*).

The weight of the infant and an assessment of the function of its various bodily systems are more important guides than the age from birth. For a given gestation age, the morbidity and mortality are greater the lower the birth weight.

Thus all children should be accurately weighed on admission to hospital. Much of the surgery in children aged up to 3 years is for congenital defects and it is important to remember that such defects are often multiple. For example, a cleft palate or tracheoesophageal fistula is very often associated with a cardiac defect.

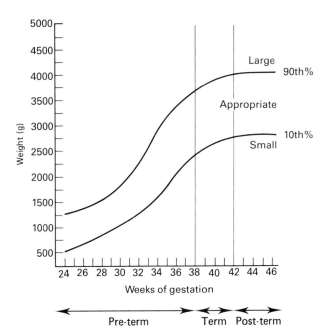

Figure 1 Percentile chart showing appropriate weight for gestational age

Physiologic differences between neonates and older children

Infants have poor respiratory reserve and respiratory failure is a common sequel to pathology in any system[1]. Total pulmonary resistance at 25 cmH$_2$O/l/s is five times that of the adult.

Lung compliance is very low (6 ml/cmH$_2$O compared with 160 ml/cmH$_2$O in the adult) but the infant chest wall is a very compliant structure so that small infants have great difficulty in maintaining a normal functional residual capacity (FRC) in states where pulmonary compliance is further reduced. The chest wall provides no counter-resistance to the collapsing forces of the lungs as it will do later in life. Hence, the response to constant distending pressure in the form of positive end expiratory pressure (PEEP) or continuous positive airway pressure (CPAP) is strikingly beneficial in this age group.

After birth an eight-fold increase in the number of alveoli occurs and the adult number is reached by the age of 6 years. The resistance of the airways (and thus the work of breathing) remains high, until finally the airways begin to enlarge from about the same time as the full complement of alveoli are present.

Closing volume occurs within tidal breathing until 6 years of life so that there is an increase in physiologic right-to-left shunt during this period and an even greater effect on oxygenation should the FRC fall, as it does with pulmonary disease or during anesthesia.

The resistance of the nasal passages in neonates is relatively great (45% of the total). They are obligatory nose breathers, so respiratory obstruction may occur if the nares are blocked, for example by choanal atresia or by too large a nasogastric tube. This facility of nose breathing can be used with great effect to apply distending pressure in the form of CPAP using one nasal prong.

Alveolar ventilation and oxygen consumption per unit body weight are twice that of the adult, as manifest by the alarming rate at which cyanosis appears if ventilatory problems arise.

Respiration during the early months of life is purely diaphragmatic (the bucket-handle effect of ribs becomes operational towards the end of the first year of life) so that respiratory failure may ensue if diaphragm movement is restricted, for example by abdominal distension or with phrenic palsy. Attempts to increase alveolar ventilation can be made only by increasing the respiratory rate, which explains why a rising respiratory rate is such a good sign of increased respiratory distress in infants. Phrenic palsy may occur as part of a birth injury, but is more commonly associated with damage to the phrenic nerve during thoracic or cardiac surgery.

The circulation of the neonate is labile and may revert to the fetal pattern with blood flowing from right to left through a patent ductus arteriosus (DA) and/or through the foramen ovale (FO) if subject to conditions which

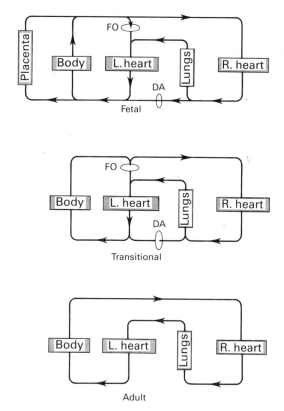

Figure 2   Transitional circulation: FO, foramen ovale; DA, ductus arteriosus

promote pulmonary vasoconstriction: a state known as transitional circulation. This state, previously known as persistent fetal circulation, is a transitional state between the fetal circulation including the placenta and that of the adult when the right and left sides are quite separate (see Figure 2).

The duct may reopen with exposure to hypoxia or fluid overload, until it is firmly closed by fibrosis after 3–4 weeks. Attempts can be made to close the duct pharmacologically, using small doses of a prostaglandin synthetase inhibitor such as salicylate or, more commonly, indomethacin, with a fair chance of success. Conversely, prostaglandin E$_2$ may be infused to maintain ductal patency where this is essential, for example in severely cyanosed infants with pulmonary artery atresia, until a systemic–pulmonary shunt of the Blalock type may be created surgically.

The lability of the pulmonary vasculature is caused by abundant arteriolar smooth muscle, extending more peripherally than in later life (due to a failure of normal regression of the muscle in the first few hours of life). These arterioles constrict in response to hypoxia, hypercapnia or acidosis via an adrenergic mechanism (this response is abolished after sympathectomy).

Some infants develop this state of persistent pulmonary hypertension of the neonate following a rise in pulmonary vascular resistance and a right-to-left shunt through the ductus arteriosus or patent foramen ovale.

Such a condition, with a shunt of 80% and critical hypoxemia, occurs commonly in hyaline membrane disease, congenital diaphragmatic hernia, meconium aspiration, β-hemolytic streptococcal infections and post-maturity.

If left untreated these infants will die in a vicious cycle of cyanosis, acidosis and falling cardiac output. Steps must be taken to reverse the high pulmonary vascular resistance: a high inspiratory oxygen concentration (FIO_2), hyperventilation if possible and pH > 7.4. In the past, vasodilating drugs such as tolazoline, prostacyclin or glyceryl trinitrate have been used, but nowadays inhaled nitric oxide is the treatment of choice[2]. Some centers use extracorporeal membrane oxygenation (ECMO) for this condition.

Neonates do attempt to maintain core temperature at 37°C but may not succeed because of an initial low basic metabolic rate, a large surface-to-weight ratio, immature sweat function and an inability to adapt to adverse conditions. Superficial thermoreceptors exist in the trigeminal area of the face; hence a cold stimulus causes an increase in metabolic heat production from hydrolysis of triglycerides in brown fat, causing a great increase in oxygen consumption which may make existing hypoxia worse. Brown fat is distributed over the back and provides thermal lagging for the major intrathoracic vessels. The metabolic response to cold is inhibited by general anesthesia, hypoxia, hypoglycemia and prematurity. Neonates are nursed in the neutral thermal environment at which their oxygen demands are minimal, as low as 31°C for a 3 kg term baby and up to 36°C for those with low birthweight (*see Figure 3*). If preterm infants are allowed to cool there is increased mortality and morbidity. They are more likely to

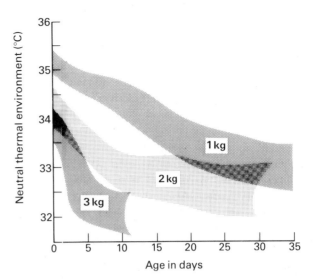

Figure 3   Neutral thermal environment for three groups of infants of differing birth weight

develop hyaline membrane disease, acidosis, hypoxia, coagulopathy, intraventricular hemorrhage and a subsequent slower rate of brain growth.

Some heat loss is inevitable in the operating theater, but this can be minimized by using warm wrappings, aluminum swaddlers, aluminum foil to the head and limbs to reflect radiant heat, a heated mattress, an overhead heater during induction of anesthesia and by maintaining an ambient temperature of 24°C without draughts and using heated, humidified, anesthetic gases[3].

1 A thermostatically controlled hot-air mattress is particularly effective in maintaining the temperature of small patients and is routinely used for patients under 1 year of age.

The mean cord hemoglobin concentration is approximately 18 g/dl at birth and rises by 1–2 g/dl in the first days of life because of low fluid intake and a decrease in extracellular fluid volume. After that, the level declines (*see Figure 4*) and causes the physiologic anemia of infancy. Premature babies have a greater fall because of lower red cell production and survival. At birth 70% of the hemoglobin is HbF, which has a greater affinity for oxygen, possibly because of a relative insensitivity to 2,3-diphosphoglycerate which itself lowers the oxygen affinity of the hemoglobin molecule. HbF is replaced by HbA by 3 months of age, at which time sickle tests are needed in susceptible children. A hemoglobin concentration < 10 g/dl is always abnormal and should be investigated. Non-emergency surgery is usually delayed pending investigation of severe anemias.

The blood volume of an infant with a normal hemoglobin is estimated to be 80–85 ml/kg. In premature infants it is greater, perhaps as much as 100 ml/kg. The blood volume of the neonate is more variable than that of the older infant and depends on the magnitude of the placental transfusion. Difficulties may arise if blood replacement is based on a percentage of the estimated blood volume.

Carbohydrate reserves of the normal neonate are relatively low and, as most glycogen is synthesized after 36 weeks gestation, those of preterm infants may be very low. Blood sugar levels should average 2.7–3.3 mmol/l (50–60 mg/dl) and hypoglycemia of less than 1.6 mmol/l (30 mg/dl) is treated by infusion of 10% dextrose, or a

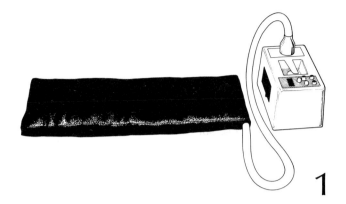

1

bolus of 1 ml/kg 25% dextrose if urgent correction of hypoglycemia is indicated. Four-hourly testing with blood glucose testing strips is mandatory, as only very severe hypoglycemia is symptomatic. There is no agreement as to the hypoglycemia effect of preoperative starvation but 4 h between the last drink and induction of anesthesia is the very maximum, and small children should be woken for a drink of 5% dextrose solution if they are first on a morning list. Children below 15 kg weight are at the greatest risk from hypoglycemia.

Maturity of liver enzyme systems is complete by 2 months of age. Synthesis of vitamin K dependent clotting factors II, VII, IX and X is suboptimal until then. Minimal levels of clotting factors occur on the second or third day of life and this is partially prevented by routine intramuscular administration of vitamin K_1 to all neonates.

Hepatic immaturity also means that drugs detoxicated in the liver, such as barbiturates and opiates, should be used with extreme caution. The conjugation of bilirubin is very inefficient and uncoupling of a least one of the two molecules occurs at times of stress such as hypoxia or acidosis. After liver maturity is reached most drugs are well tolerated becuase of the high metabolic rate of the young child.

The neonate has no diuretic response to a water load for the first 48 h of life. By the end of the first week dilute urine can be produced, but the output falls before the full load has been excreted.

Fluid maintenance requirements for full-term infants start at 20–40 ml/kg per 24 h on day 1, increasing by 20 ml/kg each day until the levels shown in *Table 1* are reached by the end of the first week of life[4].

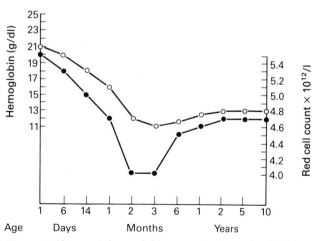

Figure 4 Changes in hemoglobin concentration and red cell count in the first 10 years of life: ○, hemoglobin; ●, red cell count

Table 1   Basic fluid requirements of neonates 7 days after birth

Birth weight (g)	Volume/24 h (ml/kg)
< 1000	180
1000–2500	150
> 2500	120

Fluid retention associated with surgery is usually severe and restriction to the requirements suggested for the neonatal period is necessary during and after operation. All intravenous fluids for maintenance in infancy should contain dextrose 4% or 10% depending on blood sugar, usually in combination with 0.2 N (0.18%) saline solution, although hyperglycemia becomes a risk for low birthweight neonates undergoing surgery if dextrose solutions are continued during the operation.

Assessment of the patient

Fitness for general anesthesia and surgery must be assessed in the light of the urgency of surgery. It frequently involves weighing up the risks related to an associated medical problem against the benefits of surgery. This requires cooperation between the anesthetist and the surgeon. Many centers run preoperative clinics in which medical problems can be identified, appropriate investigations performed, and treatment instituted. The parents and patients can be given the necessary instructions for admission to hospital, which is especially important for day-case patients.

No cold surgery should be undertaken on any patient with an acute intercurrent illness. Operation should be deferred until 1 month after the last symptoms of respiratory tract infection, croup or the acute exanthems have subsided. After bronchiolitis, pulmonary abnormalities of increased resistance and reduced compliance may persist for as long as 1 year. In patients with chronic respiratory disease lung function is assessed by measuring airway resistance, compliance and lung volumes, and by ventilation/perfusion scans. Baseline blood gas estimations may show metabolic alkalosis compensating for respiratory acidosis, or a raised $Pa\text{CO}_2$ if there is incipient respiratory failure.

Patients with values 50% of the predicted normal may be expected to develop respiratory problems after the operation and those with only 30% of predicted values with a resting $Pa\text{CO}_2$ above 40 mmHg (5.3 kPa) will undoubtedly need postoperative respiratory support.

Preoperative antibiotic prophylaxis against subacute bacterial endocarditis is usually necessary in patients with corrected or uncorrected congenital heart disease, particularly if they are to be intubated. Penicillin G, 1 mega unit intravenously with induction of anesthesia, or amoxycillin, 1–3 g orally 1 h before operation may be given. For Gram-negative organisms associated with intestinal and genitourinary surgery, gentamicin sulphate, 2 mg/kg, combined with metronidazole, 7.5 mg/kg, intravenously is more appropriate.

The history, including exercise tolerance, and physical examination should reveal any problems such as respiratory obstruction or failure, and alert the anesthetist to the possibility of technical problems such as difficult intubation, for example in patients with Pierre–Robin syndrome or Still's disease.

Many pediatric centers perform minor surgery of all specialities (up to 15% of cases) on a day-case basis. This arrangement is more cost effective, more convenient for the parents and has obvious psychologic advantages for the child. Anesthetic techniques of premedication, intubation, inhalational or intravenous anesthesia, local blocks and postoperative analgesia are the same as for hospitalized patients. Facilities must be available, however, to admit the child overnight if the anesthesia or surgery has not been straightforward or if the parents feel they cannot manage the child at home.

Neonates of less than 46 weeks since conception should not be treated on a day-stay basis, even for minor surgery, if they have a history of previous apneic attacks. There is a risk of apnea recurring up to 24 h after the operation.

Infants and small children are vulnerable to the psychologic stress of being in hospital and undergoing surgery. They are totally dependent on their parents, and prolonged separation in the early months of life may cause problems with maternal bonding. Children between 2 and 4 years of age are especially vulnerable as they may have unreasonable fears about hospitals and surgery but may not yet have developed the intellectual mechanisms to deal with these fears. Full preparation with a kindly and sympathetic approach is therefore required. In most children over 6 kg in weight this is often supplemented by preoperative sedation.

Premedication

There is no ideal agent for premedication. The aim is to achieve mild sedation for most children since a dose required to produce sleep in most will cause oversedation in a few. In recent years preoperative medication has become less important with parents always being present at induction and the universal use of topical lidocaine (lignocaine) plus prilocaine (EMLA cream) to allow painless intravenous induction of anesthesia. Opioid premedication is rarely used since intramuscular injections are so disliked and intraoperative and postoperative analgesia are usually managed by specific measures involving regional analgesia or intravenous opioid infusions.

Premedication drugs include: atropine sulphate, 0.02 mg/kg orally or intramuscularly; trimeprazine, 2–3 mg/kg orally; temazepam, 0.5–1 mg/kg orally; and chloral hydrate, 30–50 mg/kg orally.

Special equipment

Specialized apparatus with low resistance to breathing (less than $30\,cmH_2O/l/s$ during quiet breathing) and minimal dead space is necessary as infants already have a high airway resistance and a rather higher ratio of dead space to tidal volume than adults[4].

2 Ayre's T-piece with Jackson Rees' modification has almost universal approval for small infant anesthesia. The T-piece has been extensively studied and no rebreathing with spontaneous or controlled ventilation occurs unless the fresh gas flow is reduced below 220 ml/kg/min. No circuit should be used at the limit of its function, so in practice at least 4 liters fresh gas flow is used.

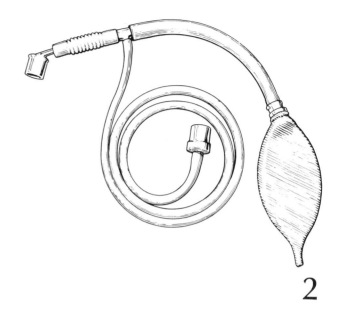

2

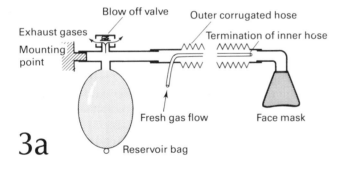

3a

Blow off valve
Exhaust gases
Mounting point
Outer corrugated hose
Termination of inner hose
Fresh gas flow
Reservoir bag
Face mask

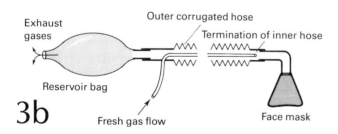

3b

Exhaust gases
Outer corrugated hose
Termination of inner hose
Reservoir bag
Fresh gas flow
Face mask

3a, b Scavenging of polluting expired gases is most safely achieved by an indirect, active system, with nothing directly connected to the expiratory limb of the T-piece. The Bain coaxial circuit (*Illustration 3a*), modified for pediatric use (*Illustration 3b*), is also very useful for many pediatric procedures, particularly those involving the head and neck.

Circle systems for use in children such as the Bloomquist and Ohio are popular in North America. The author prefers the clear plastic cuffed face masks to the Rendell–Baker type because they are a better fit to the face, and in practice the dead space is less because of streaming of the fresh gas flow within the mask. A firm fit also enables distending pressure to be applied to spontaneously breathing patients, which prevents stridor, promotes gas exchange, and prevents reduction in functional residual capacity.

4 Non-cuffed tracheal tubes with, for example, a Cardiff or a standard 15 mm connector are used down to 2.5 mm inside diameter.

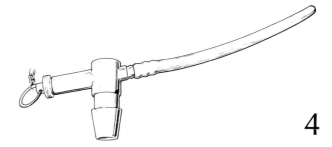

4

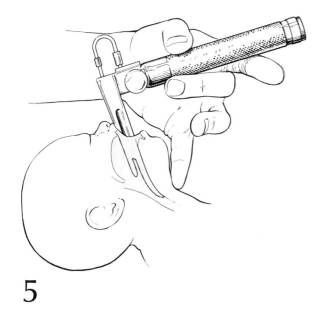

5

5 The infant larynx lies higher in the neck (opposite the fourth cervical vertebra) and more anterior than in the adult and, as the epiglottis is relatively large, laryngoscopy is best performed with a small straight-bladed laryngoscope, the tip of which picks up the epiglottis.

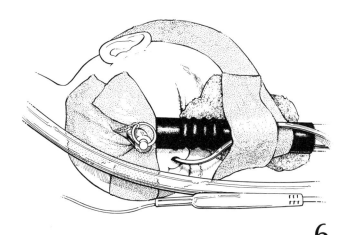

6

6 A small airway is put in the mouth alongside the tube to splint it and to prevent lateral movement. Perfect sizing, positioning and fixation of the tracheal tube is central to pediatric anesthesia and intensive care. The oral tube is fixed to the face by two pieces of strapping, with, if possible, a secondary fixation to the forehead.

Nasal fixation is similar with primary strapping to the face and secondary fixation to the forehead, thus preventing accidental dislodgement of the tube by pulling or twisting. The metal Tunstall correction is popular in the UK.

The correct size of tube is that which allows a small air leak between it and the mucosa of the cricoid at a peak inspiratory pressure of 25 cmH$_2$O. The cricoid ring is the narrowest part of the upper airway in a child and is easily damaged by too large a tracheal tube, resulting in postoperative stridor or even subglottic stenosis (1 mm of mucosal edema in the infant cricoid will reduce the airway by 60%).

Cuffed tracheal tubes are used for children aged 8 years and older.

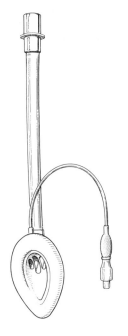

7

7 The Brain laryngeal mask airway is used as an alternative to intubation in many cases[5].

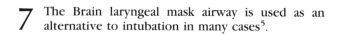

General principles

The general principles of pediatric anesthesia have not changed significantly in recent years. Even though neonates may be intubated awake this is now achieved after general anesthesia. All infants weighing < 5 kg are usually intubated for anesthesia however minor the surgery, to allow controlled ventilation. Awake intubation is associated with a greater incidence of hypoxemia and may be a factor allowing intraventricular cerebral hemorrhage in vulnerable neonates.

The metabolic studies of Anand *et al.*[6] clearly show that even neonates mount harmful stress responses to surgery that are obtunded by opioid analgesias or regional anesthesia. Such responses may contribute to morbidity and mortality.

Induction agents

Induction of anesthesia is usually achieved either by inhalation or intravenous administration. Halothane continues to be a popular agent as it is readily accepted by children. Isoflurane is more irritant to the airway than halothane, but the newer agent sevoflurane may prove to be a useful induction agent. Thiopental (thiopentone sodium) in doses of 4–5 mg/kg is the preferred agent for intravenous use and has become the standard by which all others are judged. Ketamine (1–2 mg/kg intravenously) is a good agent for cardiac surgery patients as it may enhance cardiac output. Propofol (3 mg/kg), the non-barbiturate induction agent, is very short acting and may therefore be of some advantage for day-case patients.

Muscle relaxants

Sensitivity of the neuromuscular junction to non-depolarizing muscle relaxants exists during the first 2–3 weeks of life. This, together with wide individual variation, makes careful titration of dose with effect mandatory.

The progress of action of the relaxants is monitored with a peripheral nerve stimulator using the 'train of four' response, although the post-tetanic count is the more sensitive. Atracurium besylate is the relaxant of choice for neonates as its metabolism is independent of hepatic and renal function and it may be given by bolus (0.5 mg/kg) or continuous infusion[7] (9 μg/kg/min). The short acting non-depolarizing relaxant mivacurium inactivated by plasma cholinesterase is also given by infusion.

The reported resistance to succinylcholine (suxamethonium) in the neonate is caused by the dilution of a given dose in the larger extracellular fluid volume of the neonate.

Prevention of aspiration

Cricoid pressure to prevent aspiration of regurgitated gastric contents is as effective in infants as it is in adults if correctly applied and is used when indicated, for example in patients with pyloric stenosis or bowel obstruction.

Ventilation

Many machines exist for intraoperative mechanical ventilation of chidren. T-piece occluding machines such as the Penlon 200 series with the Newton valve are satisfactory for many cases.

All mechanical ventilators must have a reliable alarm system. Hand ventilation is essential during thoracic surgery in infants or in other situations of changing pulmonary compliance or if there is tracheal compression. Controlled ventilation with distending pressure should be used for all neonates because the respiratory depressant effect of inhalational anesthesia is so great at this stage, but older infants may be allowed to breathe spontaneously via a tracheal tube, laryngeal mask or face mask for periods of 30–45 min. Halothane or isoflurane is used. The metabolites of halothane may cause sensitization and severe liver failure in postpubertal patients but only very rarely in children. Halothane may preserve blood flow to the liver better than other agents and is thus not contraindicated in children with liver disease.

Analgesic supplements

Agents such as fentanyl (2–10 μg/kg) or morphine (0.1–0.2 mg/kg) are given during surgery if a regional technique is not used. Great care must be taken when these agents are given to neonates unless postoperative mechanical ventilation is planned. Older infants and children tolerate up to 10 μg/kg fentanyl and this provides excellent analgesia.

Regional anesthesia

Central or peripheral nerve blocks usually, but not necessarily, associated with light general anesthesia are routine in pediatric anesthesia. They obviate the need for opioid analgesia in high risk groups such as ex-premature infants and, where analgesia is provided on a preemptive basis, subsequent analgesic requirements are reduced. All techniques such as spinal or extradural blocks with catheters are used even in neonates[8] and have the advantage of lasting into the postoperative period. Sacral, lumbar and thoracic roots up to T10 may be blocked by caudal analgesia using 0.25% plain bupivacaine. A dose of 0.5 ml/kg is sufficient to block sacral roots, but 1.25 ml/kg will be needed to block up to T10.

Fluid maintenance

Neonates often do not require clear fluids as maintenance during surgery and fluids to flush drugs may be enough. Otherwise, inappropriate secretion of antidiuretic hormone, shifts from circulating blood volume to the third space, and poor renal function will result in severe fluid overload.

Blood losses approaching 10% of the estimated blood volume are replaced by colloid in the form of plasma if the hemoglobin is $> 15\,g/dl$, otherwise by whole blood. Older patients may be given intraoperative fluids at $6-10\,ml/kg/h$ as, for example, 4% dextrose and 0.18% saline.

Monitoring

All techniques of monitoring adult anesthesia are entirely appropriate even for the neonate, but the precordial or esophageal stethoscope is unsurpassed as a means of drawing the anesthetist closer to the patient and of providing valuable respiratory and cardiovascular information. A monaural earpiece also enables the anesthetist to keep in touch with the conversation going on around him. This, together with pulse oximetry, electrocardiography and automatic blood pressure monitoring (e.g. Dinamap) are minimal monitoring standards for all patients.

Direct measurements of arterial and central venous pressures may be required for major cases. Care must be taken with flushing devices and those of the Intraflo type are unsuitable for use in small infants, in whom a syringe pump at $0.5-1\,ml/h$ should be used. Temperature is measured by a nasopharyngeal probe. The normal difference between core and peripheral temperature is $2°C$ and peripheral cooling in infants is a very sensitive guide to cardiac output and the adequacy of cardiac filling. Transcutaneous Po_2 and Pco_2 electrodes are not frequently used in the operating theater because at least 20 min is necessary before stability occurs and they may be affected in a non-linear way by anesthetic gases.

Modern pulse oximetry has revolutionized the monitoring of oxygenation by non-invasive means and is used routinely for all patients. Oxygen saturation may also be useful to limit oxygenation in neonates at risk from retinopathy of prematurity before the retina is fully vascularized.

Capnometry, measuring endtidal Pco_2, is essential as it provides a continuous guide to the adequacy of ventilation and in neurosurgery as an early warning of air embolism. The Hewlett-Packard type which does not sample is more appropriate for very small infants, and the pediatric curette can be further modified so that any increase in dead space is kept to an absolute minimum.

Postoperative care

Pain management

Since it was discovered that postoperative pain in children was being seriously undertreated, a great deal of interest has been given to the subject of acute pain relief in pediatrics. Many centers have established Acute Pain Services with physicians and nurses to treat, audit and research this problem. Neonates present a unique problem of assessment and of treatment since they are so sensitive to the respiratory depressant effects of opioid analgesia. Regional techniques should be used where possible, including simple wound infiltration with $0.25\,ml/kg$ of 0.25% bupivacaine. Paracetamol is safe and effective for neonates in doses of $10-15\,mg/kg$ orally or rectally or codeine phosphate, $1\,mg/kg$ intramuscularly, is surprisingly effective. For robust infants and older children postoperative analgesia is based on morphine infusions. These obviate the need for intramuscular injections, the peaks and troughs of bolus opioid administration ($1\,mg/kg$ in 50 ml 5% dextrose provides $20\,\mu g/kg/ml$) and for neonates $5-10\,\mu g/kg/h$ and older children $20-30\,\mu g/kg/h$ are suitable doses. Children of school age manage patient controlled analgesia (PCA) and self administer boluses of morphine from a special PCA pump. Younger children benefit from nurse controlled analgesia (NCA) using the same pump which delivers a low dose background infusion which can be supplemented by boluses as judged necessary by the nurse. For safety, NCA requires a longer lock-out period[9]. Continuous epidural infusions of bupivacaine, with or without an opioid, are increasingly used in pediatric practice.

Respiratory support

After surgery, infants are extubated when fully awake once spontaneous respiration is judged to be adequate. Because of the low respiratory reserve at this age, however, respiratory failure may ensue. Acute respiratory failure is a clinical diagnosis based on a rising respiratory rate ($> 60/min$), pulse rate, cardiac output and oxygen dependence and on an assessment of the work of breathing as shown by intercostal recession, tracheal tug, nasal flaring, restlessness and grunting. The inability to clear secretions or apnoeic attacks are further pointers. Blood gas levels may confirm the clinical impression and are measured to determine baseline values.

Distending pressure in the form of CPAP is indicated when an infant cannot maintain a Pao_2 of $50\,mmHg$ ($6.7\,kPa$) in 60% oxygen.

Mechanical ventilation is necessary if, after an

adequate trial of CPAP, the Pa_{O_2} remains > 60 mmHg (7.8 kPa) but the pH is < 7.25 or if the Pa_{O_2} is < 50 mmHg (6.7 kPa) on 100% oxygen. CPAP may be administered via a tight fitting facemask or nasal prong in an attempt to avoid tracheal intubation.

Prolonged intubation requires nasal plain PVC (polyvinyl chloride) tubes of the Portex type. All the complications of blockage, dislodgement and subglottic stenosis can be avoided by meticulous care. The tube must be of a size to allow ventilation, but also some leakage of air around it, or damage to the mucosa of the cricoid will result. Intubation may be continued if necessary for many weeks without resorting to tracheostomy.

The art of ventilating babies with modern infant ventilators such as the Bear Cub BP 2000 consists of using the facilities of the machines to minimize the factors such as high inspired oxygen concentrations and barotrauma known to be associated with bronchopulmonary dysplasia[10].

Infant lungs are particularly liable to be damaged by intubation and mechanical ventilation, with factors such as high inspired oxygen concentrations and high peak airway pressures being incriminated in the production of bronchopulmonary dysplasia. The lung architecture is progressively deranged with fibrosis and formation of cysts, which in turn demands higher oxygen and ventilator pressures to maintain adequate gas exchange. Unless the factors known to produce bronchopulmonary dysplasia are minimized, the condition will progress until ventilation becomes impossible. Machines must have the facility to allow high respiratory rates, square wave formation, variable inspiration:expiration ratio, control of peak pressures and full humidification. They should also have an alarm system for disconnection and power failure, a facility for constant distending pressure and the ability to wean the patient from the ventilator by using intermittent mandatory ventilation.

Many infant ventilators also have the facility for patient triggered ventilation which may be useful in weaning difficult children.

Constant distending pressure, whether used with intermittent positive pressure ventilation (PEEP) or spontaneous breathing (CPAP), will improve the relation between FRC and closing volume in the lungs, and reduce right-to-left intrapulmonary shunting. By keeping the small airways distended it will also cause a fall in pulmonary resistance and in the work of breathing.

PEEP of up to 10 cmH₂O is used routinely after cardiopulmonary bypass and in other patients with increased pulmonary water. The distending pressure may save surfactant but, as PEEP is increased, pulmonary vascular resistance rises and there is an increased incidence of pneumothorax.

Formulae are of little help in setting up patients on ventilation because of the internal compliance of the machine and its tubing: 10 ml/kg tidal volume or 20–25 cmH₂O pressure are reasonable initial settings. Inspired oxygen concentration should be set at the level the child needed before mechanical ventilation was instituted.

All children ventilated in an intensive care unit require analgesia such as a morphine infusion at least at the start, but later they may be ventilated with simple sedation such as diazepam, 0.2 mg/kg intravenously, or chloral hydrate, 30 mg/kg by nasogastric tube. It is increasingly necessary, however, to paralyse patients with severe pulmonary disease who need limitation of peak airway pressure and changes in the inspiration:expiration ratio, for example, with infusion of atracurium or vecuronium. There is evidence that gas exchange may be improved in such paralysed patients so that they may need mechanical ventilation for a shorter period than those not paralysed.

Weaning takes place when cardiovascular stability has been achieved with a peak pressure of < 30 cmH₂O, giving a Pa_{CO_2} of < 45 mmHg (5.8 kPa) and a Pa_{O_2} > 100 mmHg (13 kPa) with an Fi_{O_2} < 0.6. Distending pressure is used with intermittent mandatory ventilation (IMV), which is the most convenient way of weaning from full ventilator support. IMV with the Bear Cub BP 2000 ventilator is ideal, with continuous fresh gas flow and favourable inspiration:expiration ratios during the reduction in mandatory breaths. The patient must be able to manage on 15–20 mandatory breaths before being ready to be weaned. The number of mandatory breaths is gradually reduced (the rate depending on the clinical progress of the infant) until the ventilator is delivering no breaths and the patient is on CPAP.

Patients are extubated when coping on 3 cmH₂O CPAP. Those with stiff lungs who are CPAP-dependent may continue on CPAP after extubation, using a nasal prong[5]. No patient is left to breathe through a tracheal tube without distending pressure since, without the physiologic levels of CPAP, the FRC will fall with increased resistance to gas flow, increased work of breathing and increased right-to-left intrapulmonary shunting.

Invasive and non-invasive blood gas analysis is essential for setting up and maintaining patients on mechanical ventilation, but plays very little part in monitoring them during the weaning process when clinical observation of respiratory rate and effort is more important.

High frequency jet ventilation or oscillation, negative pressure ventilation and ECMO are used in various centers for difficult patients or cases of extreme respiratory failure.

References

1. Hatch D, Fletcher M. Anaesthesia and the ventilatory system in infants and young children *Br J Anaesth* 1992; 68: 398–410.

2. Frostell C, Fratacci M-D, Wain JC, Jones R, Zapol WM. Inhaled nitric oxide: a selective pulmonary vasodilator reversing hypoxic pulmonary vasoconstriction. *Circulation* 1991; 83: 2038–47.

3. Spear RM. Anesthesia for premature and term infants: perioperative implications. *J Pediatr* 1992; 120: 165–76.

4. Hatch DJ, Sumner E, Hellman J. *The Surgical Neonate: Anaesthesia and Intensive Care*, 3rd edn. London: Edward Arnold, 1994.

5. Mizushima A, Wardall GJ, Simpson DL. The laryngeal mask airway in infants. *Anaesthesia* 1992; 47: 849–51.

6. Anand KJ, Hansen DD, Hickey PR. Hormonal–metabolic stress responses in neonates undergoing cardiac surgery. *Anesthesiology* 1990; 73: 661–70.

7. Guodsuozian NG, Shorter G. Myoneural blocking agents in infants: a review. *Paediatr Anaesth* 1992; 2: 3–16.

8. Dalens B, Chrysotstome Y. Intervertebral epidural anaesthesia in paediatric surgery: success rate and adverse effects in 650 consecutive procedures. *Paediatr Anaesth* 1991; 1: 107–17.

9. Lloyd-Thomas AR. A pain service for children. *Paediatr Anaesth* 1994; 4: (in press).

10. Goldsmith JP, Karotkin EH. *Assisted Ventilation of the Neonate*, 2nd edn. Philadelphia: Saunders, 1988.

Illustrations by Peter Cox

Vascular access

Mark D. Stringer BSc, MRCP, MS, FRCS
Consultant Paediatric Surgeon, United Leeds Teaching Hospitals Trust and St James's University Hospital Trust, Leeds, UK

History

During the last 30 years vascular access in children, and particularly chronic venous access, has evolved to become one of the most common operations in pediatric surgery. It is now critically important in the management of many patients (both in hospital and at home) requiring parenteral nutrition, chemotherapy, repeated blood sampling or regular blood product replacement therapy. There currently exists a vast array of access devices composed of various materials; external and totally implantable devices with single or multiple lumen catheters may be inserted into veins or arteries located peripherally or centrally. These variables must be tailored to the child's size, circumstances, therapeutic requirements, and anticipated duration of treatment. Despite the advances in vascular access technology, these procedures are potentially dangerous and should not be undertaken if safer, more simple alternatives are possible.

Principles and justification

Peripheral venous access in infants and children is usually obtained by inserting a short 14–26-gauge cannula into a superficial vein in an upper or lower limb. In addition to easily visible veins, useful sites include the long saphenous vein anterior to the medial malleolus at the ankle, the cephalic vein at the wrist, the interdigital vein between the fourth and fifth metacarpals on the dorsum of the hand, the external jugular vein (rarely practical in the mobile patient), the superficial temporal vein of the scalp in small infants, and occasionally superficial veins on the trunk.

Essential techniques for the pediatric surgeon include: operative insertion of a central venous catheter for long-term use; percutaneous insertion of a central venous catheter for short and long-term use; percutaneous insertion of a central venous catheter in the infant via a peripheral vein; emergency intraosseous venous access; and arterial puncture and cannulation.

Other aspects of venous access such as hemodialysis and hemofiltration, diagnostic vascular access, and extracorporeal membrane oxygenation are beyond the scope of this chapter.

Preoperative

Before elective central venous access the risks and complications of the procedure should be discussed with the child's parents. Blood should be grouped and held and cross-matched blood must be available if a coagulopathy is present; the platelet count and clotting parameters should be optimized before surgery but the benefits and risks in an individual patient need to be balanced. Adequate assistance, lighting and instruments (including a range of catheter sizes and suction apparatus in open procedures) must be available. Magnifying loupes are useful in small infants. With the variety of vascular access devices currently available, the surgeon should be familiar with specific directions supplied with commercial kits.

Operating theater traffic should be kept to a minimum. The patient is positioned supine on a radiolucent operating table with facilities for fluoroscopy and radiation protection. A diathermy plate is positioned well away from the operative field and, after thorough antiseptic skin preparation using a chlorhexidine or povidone-iodine based solution, the patient is draped. During the procedure, handling of the catheter should be kept to a minimum.

Anesthesia

Many patients requiring chronic vascular access are relatively unfit with oncologic or metabolic problems. Although percutaneous techniques are possible under sedation in infants and older children, central vascular access usually requires a general anesthetic. Monitoring of oxygen saturation, temperature, blood pressure and cardiac rhythm are standard. The airway must be closely watched when extending and rotating the head. After the operation most patients require only simple analgesics but larger incisions for implantable ports demand stronger analgesia and/or local anesthesia.

Operations

OPERATIVE INSERTION OF A CENTRAL VENOUS CATHETER FOR LONG-TERM USE

1   The catheters used are commonly known as Broviac and Hickman catheters; these Silastic (silicone elastomer) catheters are available with single or multiple lumens and a size range of 2.7–12 Fr. A Dacron cuff around the extravascular subcutaneous portion of the line allows tissue ingrowth and subsequent catheter fixation.

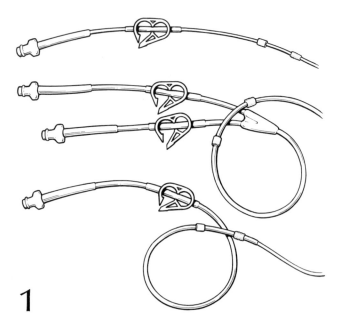

1

Internal jugular vein

2 The patient is positioned supine with a soft radiolucent roll under the scapulae and the head extended and turned to the contralateral side. After thorough skin preparation of the operative field, which includes the planned catheter exit site, the ipsilateral nipple and the neck, the drapes are secured with adhesive plastic or sutures.

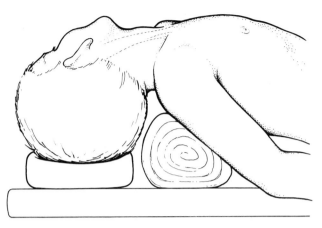

2

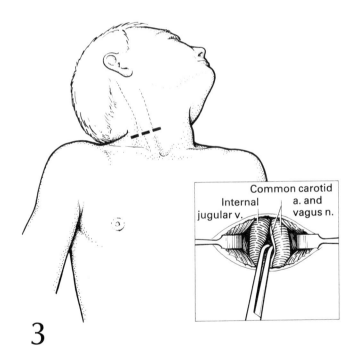

3

3 A short skin crease incision is made about 2–3 cm above the clavicle over the diverging clavicular and sternal heads of sternomastoid. The incision is deepened through platysma and the cervical fascia with needle diathermy and the two heads of the sternomastoid are then separated by blunt dissection. Small retractors are inserted and the internal jugular vein exposed. Picking up and incising the fascia investing the vein makes its subsequent dissection easier. Using a Mixter blunt right-angled forceps a plane is developed on either side of the vein and then the instrument is passed around the vein, but never as a blind maneuver. A thin Silastic vessel loop is used to sling the vein and, using this gently as a retractor, a second vessel loop can be passed and a 1–2 cm length of vessel exposed between the slings. It is rarely necessary to ligate any venous branches at this level. The retractors can be removed and the slings relaxed whilst the catheter tunnel is made.

4 Various exit sites over the chest wall are possible but, in girls, the developing breast and strap lines should be avoided. A 0.5 cm skin incision is made and a track of sufficient size to accommodate the catheter cuff is developed using a hemostat. Either a blunt tunneling rod to which the catheter is attached or a hollow tunneler is used to pass the catheter subcutaneously to the cervical wound. Soaking the Dacron catheter cuff with aqueous antiseptic may be useful and positioning it near the middle of the tunnel enables subsequent fine adjustments of catheter position. The distal catheter is placed on antiseptic-soaked gauze swabs surrounding the cervical incision and then flushed with normal saline and clamped. The catheter is cut to length and the tip bevelled. On the right, the distance to the mid right atrium is estimated by a point just above the nipple line and, on the left, just below.

The prepared section of vein is elevated between the two slings and, using fine non-toothed forceps and microvascular scissors, a short transverse venotomy, equal to the catheter diameter, is made. The catheter is introduced into the vein with the bevel facing posteriorly and the assistant gently relaxes the lower sling to allow distal passage of the catheter and then tightens it to prevent back bleeding. The catheter should pass freely and, once inserted, free bidirectional flow should be confirmed. The venotomy is closed around the catheter with one or two 6/0 polypropylene (Prolene) vascular sutures, care being taken to avoid narrowing the vein, and hemostasis is checked with the slings relaxed. A purse-string suture around the catheter should be avoided because this may cause catheter shearing.

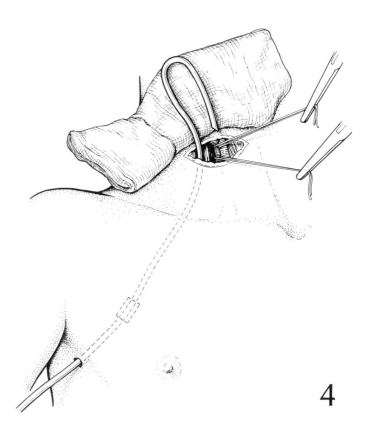

4

5 The catheter tip position in the mid right atrium is checked with fluoroscopy. The sternomastoid muscle is loosely tacked together with an absorbable suture and the cervical wound is closed in two layers using an absorbable fine subcuticular suture for the skin. The catheter exit site incision is approximated around the catheter with a 4/0 monfilament suture and firmly tied (without compression) to the catheter to aid fixation. The catheter is flushed with heparinized saline (10 units/ml heparin). The exit site is dressed with gauze and a semipermeable, transparent adhesive plastic dressing. Adhesive tape is also used to secure the external part of the catheter and, in infants, an elasticated string vest is sometimes useful.

Unless soiled, the dressing is changed after 1 week and the exit suture is removed after 10 days. It is advisable to avoid using both internal jugular veins within 3 weeks of each other.

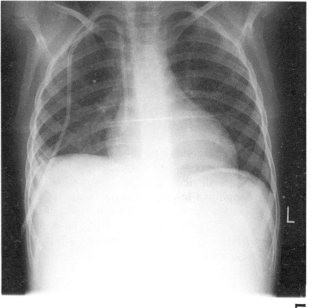

5

Alternative sites of operative insertion

The external jugular vein is easily visible and requires minimal dissection, but its use is limited by the caliber of the vein and the occasional difficulty of negotiating the junction with the subclavian vein.

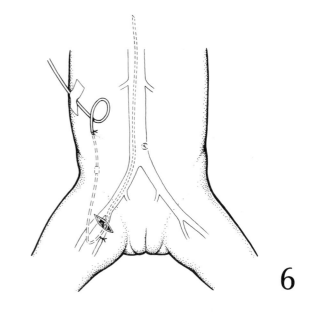

6

6 The long saphenous vein is approached by a short transverse incision 1 cm below the groin skin crease and medial to the femoral artery. The vein is isolated with a proximal ligature and tied distally. The catheter tip is positioned in the right atrium and exits over the lateral abdomen.

The femoral vein is especially useful for short-term access but may be used as a route for long-term catheters.

The axillary vein is easily approached by an axillary incision and dissection but size can be restricting.

The common facial vein is a large anterior tributary of the internal jugular vein in infants that may be entered midway between the angle of the mandible and the clavicular head.

The cephalic vein is accessed in the deltopectoral groove but tends to be small in young children.

In some children who have required repeated, chronic venous access complicated by central vein thrombosis, other routes have included the azygos (via a limited right extrapleural thoracotomy), intercostal, lumbar, epigastric, iliac, and hepatic veins, the inferior vena cava and the right atrium. In these difficult cases, venography may be helpful.

Ports

7 Totally implantable vascular access devices or 'ports' have a catheter connected to a small reservoir which is implanted subcutaneously. A thick silicone membrane forming the roof of the port can be repeatedly injected percutaneously using a 22-gauge side-fenestrated, non-coring (Huber) needle. The ports are manufactured from stainless steel, titanium or hard plastic and are available in different shapes and sizes. One variety is designed to be implanted in the arm with central venous access through a peripherally inserted catheter. These devices are ideally suited to children requiring long-term intermittent venous access such as those with malignant tumors, cystic fibrosis, or hematologic diseases. The absence of an external component and the ability to swim are important advantages to some children.

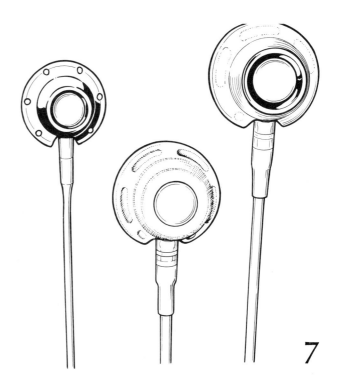

7

8 At the predetermined reservoir site, which must be
   easily accessible and rest on a firm surface such as
the anterolateral chest wall, the skin incision is
deepened with diathermy. Hemostasis must be meticulous. A subcutaneous pocket is developed beneath the
superficial fascia in such a way as to avoid placing the
port directly under the skin incision. Devices with a
preconnected catheter are easier to insert. The catheter
must be tunneled from the reservoir pocket to the site
of venous access, such as the internal jugular vein in the
neck. Before implanting the port it is helpful to place
non-absorbable sutures through the muscular fascia and
the circumference of the port; when tied, these will
provide three-point fixation of the device. The port is
flushed with saline, ensuring there are no kinks in the
catheter. The distal catheter is cut to length (see above)
and inserted by a cutdown or percutaneous technique.
After confirming the catheter tip position by fluoroscopy, the port is flushed with heparinized saline and the
skin incision is closed in two layers with an absorbable
subcuticular skin suture.

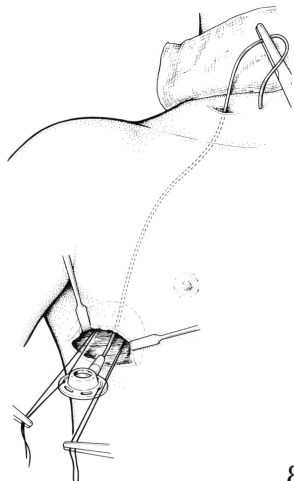

   Each injection must access the port vertically through
the centre of the silicone diaphragm, such that the
needle touches the baseplate. As the needle is
withdrawn, the port should be held in place and positive
injection pressure applied to prevent reflux of blood
into the catheter. A careful aseptic injection technique
must always be used and the system flushed periodically.

8

Removal

Most external catheters and all ports require a short
general anesthetic for removal. With the former, the
Dacron cuff can usually be dissected free with a
hemostat and fine scissors via the exit site incision
which is then closed with Steristrips.

PERCUTANEOUS INSERTION OF A CENTRAL VENOUS CATHETER FOR SHORT-TERM AND LONG-TERM USE

To many pediatric surgeons, the percutaneous infra-clavicular subclavian vein approach using the Seldinger technique is the preferred method of obtaining long-term central venous access, not least because it is relatively quick, reliable, repeatable and comfortable for the patient[1]. Insertion usually requires a general anesthetic, however, and to the long list of vascular access-related problems are added the potential complications of a blind procedure.

9a, b The patient is positioned supine in the Trendelenburg position with a small roll between the scapulae. The skin is prepared and draped, and the needle, attached to a 5 ml syringe, is inserted 0.5 cm below the clavicle, just lateral to its midpoint. The needle is advanced towards a spot 1 cm above the suprasternal notch, skirting the undersurface of the clavicle. In older children the needle should be directed more towards the sternal notch. The needle is slowly advanced whilst continuously aspirating the syringe and if the vein is not encountered, the needle is slowly withdrawn and reinserted in a slightly different direction. Temporarily stopping positive pressure mechanical ventilation may reduce the risk of pneumothorax. A flashback of venous blood signals entry into the vein and the needle should be advanced 2 mm more to ensure complete entry. Once blood can be freely aspirated, the syringe is removed and the flexible J-tipped guidewire inserted. Ideally, the guidewire is advanced to the mid right atrium under fluoroscopic control (if this induces ectopic beats it should be withdrawn slightly).

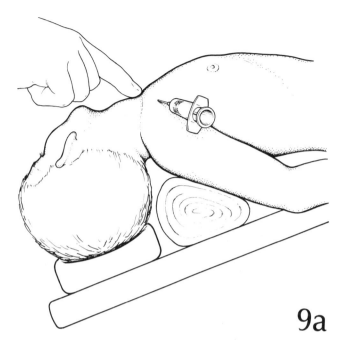

9a

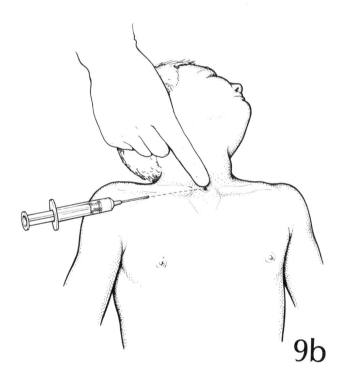

9b

10 A small (0.5 cm) incision is made in the tension lines of the skin alongside the wire insertion site and a second small incision is made over the anterolateral chest wall. The catheter is passed subcutaneously on a tunneling trocar from the second incision and brought out through the upper incision, postioning the catheter cuff at the midpoint of the tunnel. If the length of guidewire remaining outside the patient is subtracted from its total length, the appropriate catheter length can now be determined. The vein dilator and peel-away sheath are threaded over the wire and advanced *only* as far as the superior vena cava. The wire and vein dilator are then removed and the catheter inserted as the outer sheath is peeled away. Catheter position is checked by radiography (and a pneumothorax excluded) and free bidirectional flow confirmed. The catheter is secured with a monofilament suture at the exit site and the upper incision is closed with a single absorbable suture.

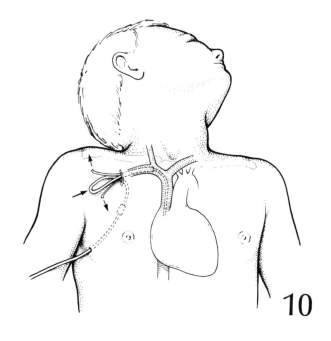

11 Because of the central venous anatomy in the infant, successful catheter placement is slightly more likely from the left subclavian vein than from the right[2].

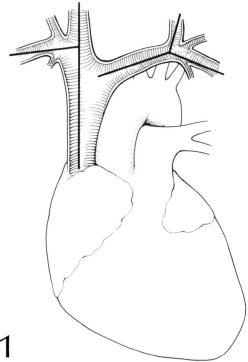

Percutaneous internal jugular vein puncture provides a useful route for short-term central venous access, especially in older infants and children, and it has fewer complications than subclavian vein puncture. It is particularly valuable during major surgery for monitoring central venous pressure, administering irritant drugs and enabling rapid transfusion. The high approach using a Seldinger technique is described.

12 The anesthetized patient is positioned supine with 20° of Trendelenburg tilt, with a rolled towel under the shoulders to extend the neck, and with the head turned away from the side of catheterization. After preparing and draping the skin, a pilot venepuncture is performed with a 23-gauge needle at a site immediately lateral to the carotid artery and medial to sternomastoid at the level of the cricoid cartilage. The needle is angled towards the ipsilateral nipple at about 15° to the skin. After locating the internal jugular vein, it is re-entered with a 22-gauge cannula through which a J-tipped guidewire is passed. The cannula is removed and a catheter is advanced over the guidewire into the vein. The guidewire is removed and the catheter tip is advanced into a central position and sutured in place. The catheter position can be checked radiologically. If arterial puncture inadvertently occurs, the needle is withdrawn and the area is compressed for up to 5 min.

The femoral and axillary veins can be similarly punctured percutaneously for short-term venous access.

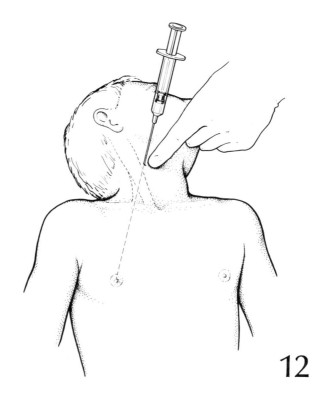

12

PERCUTANEOUS INSERTION OF A CENTRAL VENOUS CATHETER IN THE INFANT VIA A PERIPHERAL VEIN

13 Percutaneous insertion of these fine Silastic central venous catheters can be easily performed in the nursery under sterile conditions without sedation. Cannulation is without serious mechanical complications and the catheters are easily removed. However, blood sampling is difficult or impossible and occlusion is not uncommon. These single-lumen, small-diameter catheters are particularly useful in neonates requiring venous access for periods of up to 1–2 months[3]. The 30-cm line with an outer diameter of 0.6 mm has a maximum crystalloid flow rate of about 6 ml/min.

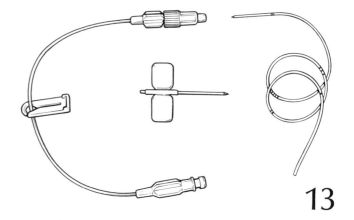

13

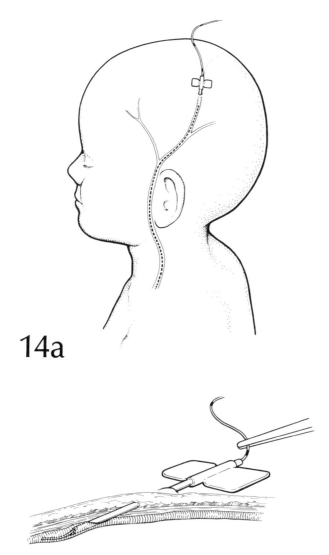

14a

14b

14a, b Popular insertion sites include the median cubital vein at the elbow, the long saphenous vein anterior to the medial malleolus and the superficial temporal vein. The distance from the chosen vein to the right nipple is measured as a guide to the length of catheter that should be inserted. Good nursing assistance is essential. After antiseptic preparation of the skin, venepuncture is performed with a 19-gauge butterfly needle and the fine Silastic feeding line is inserted into the needle and threaded up the vein using fine non-toothed forceps. The progress of the catheter may be interrupted at venous junctions but manipulating the limb will usually allow it to be advanced further. Once inserted to the desired distance, the butterfly needle is withdrawn and the line is connected to the infusion system via an inner blunt metal cannula and flushed with heparinized saline. Gentle suction on a 2 ml syringe should allow blood to be aspirated if the catheter tip lies in a large vein. The external catheter is firmly secured with a small piece of gauze covered by a transparent adhesive (non-circumferential) dressing. The position of the catheter tip should be checked radiologically by injecting 0.5 ml intravenous contrast material; it should ideally lie within the mid right atrium.

EMERGENCY INTRAOSSEOUS VENOUS ACCESS

15 This route provides immediate vascular access during life-threatening emergencies in young children when rapid venous access cannot be achieved (cardiac arrest, shock, burns and trauma). Contraindications include fracture or infection near the insertion site. After antiseptic preparation the skin is punctured with a scalpel blade. The intraosseous needle is inserted into the medullary cavity of the proximal tibia through the middle of its flat anteromedial surface, 1–3 cm below the tibial tuberosity (depending on the size of the child). The infusion needles (14–18 Fr) have an inner occluding stylet designed to facilitate bone penetration and should be inserted almost perpendicularly to the bone but angled slightly away from the growth plate. Upon entering the marrow cavity, the resistance suddenly decreases. The needle should then stand firmly in the bone, it should be possible to aspirate bone marrow or flush the needle easily without extravasation, or both. The needle flange is adjusted to skin level and taped in position. The patient's leg should be restrained with a support behind the knee. Crystalloids, blood products and drugs may be administered[4], but blood sampling may occlude the needle.

The infusion needle should be removed once secure conventional access has been obtained if potential complications (extravasation, compartment syndrome, fractures, osteomyelitis, fat embolism) are to be avoided. The distal femur and distal tibia are alternative sites in children.

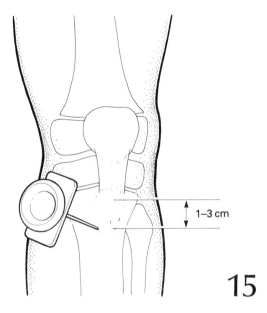

1–3 cm

15

ARTERIAL PUNCTURE AND CANNULATION

Intra-arterial access is used to provide continuous monitoring of systemic arterial blood pressure and to enable repeated arterial sampling for blood gas measurements.

16a, b The radial artery is the preferred site for both percutaneous and cutdown cannulation. The presence of adequate collateral flow must first be checked by the Allen test: both arteries are occluded at the wrist and, after releasing the ulnar artery alone, the hand should flush pink (most hands have an ulnar dominant palmar arch). A small gauze roll is placed under the supinated, extended wrist and the palm is taped to a padded surface, keeping the fingers exposed in order to assess the distal circulation. The skin is cleaned with antiseptic and a small quantity of local anesthetic is injected subcutaneously over the radial artery just proximal to the transverse crease at the wrist. The skin is punctured with a no. 11 scalpel blade and a 22 or 24-gauge Teflon cannula with a needle stylet is selected, according to the size of the child. The artery position is verified by palpation. Two techniques are used. In the first, the needle and Teflon cannula are advanced at about 30° to the skin until a flashback of blood is seen in the needle hub and the cannula is then advanced into the artery. In the transfixion method the artery is transfixed by the needle and cannula. The needle is then removed and the cannula is gently withdrawn until arterial blood appears when it is advanced up the artery lumen.

In the cutdown technique a small transverse incision over the artery allows the vessel to be punctured and cannulated under direct vision, with the option of proximodistal vessel control. The catheter hub is sutured in place and the skin is sutured around the cannula.

Arterial cannulas require continuous perfusion with 0.5–1.0 ml/h heparinized saline. Because of the risk of serious complications (ischemia, embolism, hemorrhage, sepsis), arterial access requires an even higher level of vigilance and should be used for the shortest possible time. The cannula should be removed if signs of digital ischemia develop. Alternative sites for arterial access include pedal, umbilical, femoral, brachial and axillary arteries but complications are more frequent than with radial artery cannulas[5].

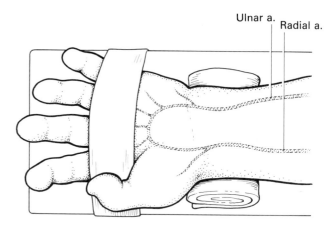

16a

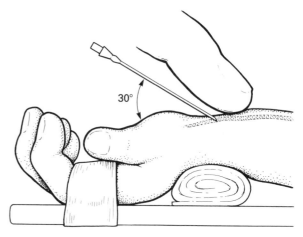

16b

Postoperative care

Care of the catheter and exit site is crucial to successful line maintenance. The line must be securely attached to the patient at all times. Several approaches reduce the risk of sepsis: the number of lumens and the duration of catheter use should be kept to a minimum; a meticulous aseptic technique (which many parents can be taught to perform well) is necessary when accessing the catheter; infusates should be prepared according to strict sterile protocols; and trained nursing staff should be assigned to catheter care in hospital. Although prophylactic antibiotics may be indicated in specific individuals, their routine use has not been shown to reduce catheter-related sepsis[6]. Totally implantable devices are reported to be associated with fewer septic complications.

Clinical suspicion of catheter-related sepsis, which occurs in up to 30% of patients, should be investigated by blood cultures taken via the catheter and from a separate peripheral venepuncture, together with swabs from the catheter exit site. Catheter-related sepsis often responds to antibiotic therapy but exit site infections only occasionally and tunnel infections rarely. Failure to respond to appropriate antibiotic therapy or infections with organisms such as *Candida* species, necessitate removal of the line.

Catheter occlusion can be minimized by regular flushing with heparinized saline. Protocols vary according to the device in use. If infusion or aspiration become difficult, the catheter position should be checked radiologically to ensure it has not migrated. Thrombolytic agents may successfully clear an occluding thrombus and dilute hydrochloric acid is occasionally useful in removing parenteral nutrition precipitates. Completely blocked non-infected lines can be replaced by a cutdown on the existing catheter track close to the previous venotomy. There is usually a fibrous capsule surrounding the catheter which can be gently exposed with hemostats and stay sutures allowing a new line to be threaded down the old track.

Catheter-related thrombosis can be confirmed by echocardiography and is usually treated by removing the catheter (unless it is used to administer thrombolytic therapy) and anticoagulating the patient.

Fractured Broviac or Hickman catheters can often be successfully repaired using commercially available kits.

Complications are reduced by correct positioning of the catheter tip, preferably in the mid or upper right atrium. A left sided superior vena cava should be suspected if a central venous catheter takes an abnormal course down the left side of the mediastinum; there is a greater risk of complications in this situation.

Complications

There are a vast number of vascular access-related complications, but they broadly fall into three groups as shown in *Table 1*.

Table 1 Complications of central venous access

Mechanical
  Insertion: pneumothorax, arterial puncture, hemorrhage, air
              embolism, malposition, cardiac arrhythmia, brachial
              plexus injury
  Dislodgment/migration
  Fracture
  Erosion/perforation: cardiac tamponade, hydrothorax, port
                        erosion
  Occlusion

Catheter-related sepsis
  Local: tunnel, exit site
  Septicemia
  Endocarditis, osteomyelitis

Catheter-related thrombosis

The commonest infecting organisms are *Staphylococcus epidermidis* and *Staphylococcus aureus*, but Gram-negative bacteria and *Candida* species are not infrequent sources.

Recent developments in vascular access have included retrograde tunneling of catheters to prevent dislodgment, new catheter materials, use of a second proximal catheter cuff impregnated with antimicrobial silver ions, sonographic guidance during catheter insertion and positioning, and safer connecting devices for catheter access. It remains to be seen which of these will merit adoption into routine use.

Acknowledgments

Illustrations 1 and *7* are reproduced by courtesy of Bard Access Systems Inc, and *Illustration 13* by courtesy of Vygon (UK) Ltd.

References

1. Gauderer MWL. Vascular access techniques and devices in the pediatric patient. *Surg Clin North Am* 1992; 72: 1267–84.

2. Cobb LM, Vincour CD, Wagner CW, Weintraub WH. The central venous anatomy in infants. *Surg Gynecol Obstet* 1987; 165: 230–4.

3. Stringer MD, Brereton RJ, Wright VM. Performance of percutaneous silastic central venous feeding catheters in surgical neonates. *Pediatr Surg Int* 1992; 7: 79–81.

4. Guy J, Haley K, Zuspan SJ. Use of intraosseous infusion in the pediatric trauma patient. *J Pediatr Surg* 1993; 28: 158–61.

5. Cilley RE. Arterial access in infants and children. *Semin Pediatr Surg* 1992; 1: 174–80.

6. Mughal MM. Complications of intravenous feeding catheters. *Br J Surg* 1989; 76: 15–21.

Cleft lip and palate

Frank E. Åbyholm MD, DDS
Head, Department of Plastic Surgery, Rikshospitalet National Hospital, Oslo, Norway

Cleft lip and palate is one of the most common facial deformities, the incidence among white people being around two per 1000 live births. There are racial variations with the incidence and in the occurrence of the different cleft types.

The defects range from the most minor notch of the lip or the uvula to complete unilateral or bilateral clefts of lip, alveolus and palate. The clefts are usually classified on an embryologic basis, with clefts located anterior to the incisive foramen being known as clefts of the primary palate, while clefts posterior to the incisive foramen are known as clefts of the secondary palate. The fusion of the primary palate, lip and alveolus begins early in the third week of fetal life, and the fusion of the secondary palate, hard and soft palate, takes place during weeks 7–11.

Classification

1a–c The clefts vary in severity, laterality and symmetry and may occur in a number of different combinations: (1) clefts of the primary palate may be incomplete or complete, unilateral or bilateral, symmetric or asymmetric (*Illustration 1a*); (2) clefts of the secondary palate may be incomplete or complete (*Illustration 1b*); and (3) combined clefts may be incomplete or complete, unilateral or bilateral, symmetric or asymmetric (*Illustration 1c*).

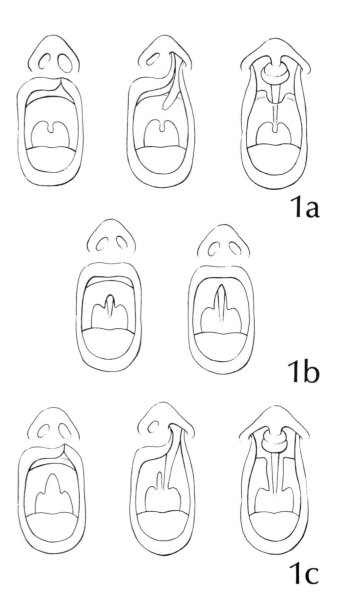

1a

1b

1c

General principles

In order to achieve an optimal end result in patients with cleft lip and palate a number of factors are of fundamental importance.

Team work

A complete cleft lip and palate is a severe malformation which greatly influences appearance, speech, mastication, hearing, facial growth, feeding, breathing and the psychologic state of child and parents. A large team is therefore necessary for the overall management of a child with a cleft, and the cleft team must have at least the following members: plastic surgeon, orthodontist, prosthodontist, otorhinolaryngologist, speech therapist, pediatrician, psychologist, geneticist and social worker.

Long-term treatment plan

The treatment of cleft lip and palate should be viewed as a whole. The treatment commences shortly after birth and continues to the age of 18 years in children with severe clefts. The cleft team should be responsible for the follow-up of the patient throughout this period.

The outcome of the surgical repair of the cleft lip and palate is directly related to surgical techniques, the skill of individual surgeons, the complete program of surgery and the timing of the various operations. Poorly performed primary surgery carries a high risk of iatrogenic disturbances of subsequent orofacial growth and development, increasing the risk of secondary facial and dental deformities and speech impairment.

A complete cleft treatment program will reflect the compromise that has to be made between the claims of the different members of the team. For example, the orthodontist would prefer to have the hard palate closed relatively late to avoid the risk of interfering with maxillary growth. The speech therapist, however, would like the palate closed early in order to secure normal development of speech. The otorhinolaryngologist would likewise advocate an early closure of the palate to improve tubar function.

There are a large number of surgical techniques available for closure of the lip and palate, and the timing of the different procedures shows great variation. There are scarcely two centers in the world that have the same surgical program for patients with cleft lip and palate.

Centralization

Work on cleft lip and palate should not be a matter of secondary importance, but the main task for those involved. A cleft center should therefore treat sufficient patients a year to ensure that all members of the team gain enough experience with all the problems related to the severe cleft types. Centralization is a key word where the care of patients with cleft lip and palate is concerned.

Preoperative

Anesthesia is delivered through an endotracheal tube passed through the mouth and fixed in the midline. Distortion of the upper lip must be avoided. The lower pharynx is packed with a moistened gauze pack to prevent aspiration of blood (the tube has no inflatable cuff). The eyelids are closed with tape. During the operation the blood loss is continuously monitored and is replaced when it exceeds 10% of the estimated blood volume.

Operation

Position of patient

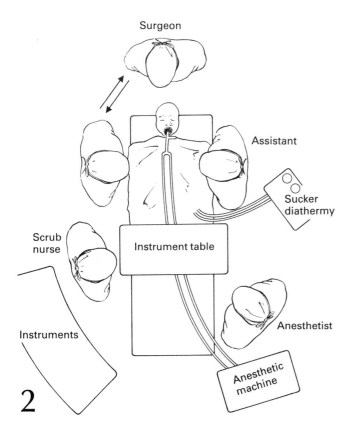

2 The child is positioned supine on the operating table with the head at the upper end and the neck slightly hyperextended toward the lap of the surgeon who is seated at the head of the table.

PRIMARY SURGERY

Lip repair

3a–i The lip repair is performed at the age of 3 months. For closure of the lip a Millard procedure is used (*Illustrations 3a–e*). In complete clefts of lip and palate the anterior hard palate is closed simultaneously with a single layer vomer flap plasty.

The incisions are marked with Bonney's blue. Local anesthetic (0.5% lidocaine (lignocaine) with epinephrine (adrenaline) 1:500 000) is infiltrated into all layers of both lip segments and under the planned vomer flap. This reduces the bleeding to a minimum, and blood transfusions are very seldom required. The labial muscle is isolated on each side of the cleft and dissected free for about 5 mm. The vomer flap is elevated, mobilized and turned as a book page across the cleft and sutured beneath the mucoperiosteal palatal flap, raw side against raw side. The nasal floor is thus reconstructed from the posterior part of the hard palate to the nostril sill.

The labial muscle is sutured across the cleft using 4/0 polyglycolic acid (Dexon) sutures. The skin is closed with 6/0 polypropylene (Prolene) and the mucosa with 5/0 polyglycolic acid sutures.

Millard's repair has the advantage of being a flexible technique which can be modified during the course of the operation. The Cupid's bow is preserved and the scars lie in a good position following the line of the philtrum which greatly facilitates secondary corrections.

Other well known techniques for primary lip closure that are widely used include the Le Mesurier repair (*Illustrations 3f and 3g*) and the Tennison repair (*Illustrations 3h and 3i*).

Some centers prefer to leave the hard palate open during childhood in order to avoid interfering with maxillary growth and therefore limit the primary operations to lip closure and soft palate closure.

Bilateral cleft lip repair

If a bilateral lip repair is combined with a vomer flap of the hard palate the operation must be performed in two stages, closing one side at a time with an interval of 5 weeks between the operations. This is because the blood supply to the premaxilla is received through the posterior septal arteries, running along the sides of the nasal septum. A bilateral vomer flap could interfere with the blood supply to such a degree as to cause atrophy of the premaxilla. If the vomer flap is omitted, however, bilateral lip closure may be performed. As these patients always need secondary corrections of their lips, the primary repair should be as gentle as possible avoiding unnecessary scarring that will complicate secondary surgery.

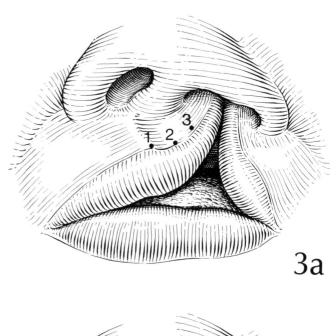

3a

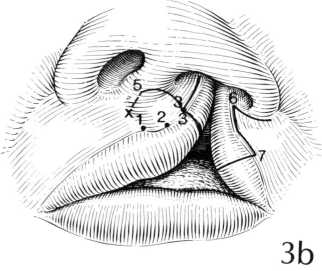

3b

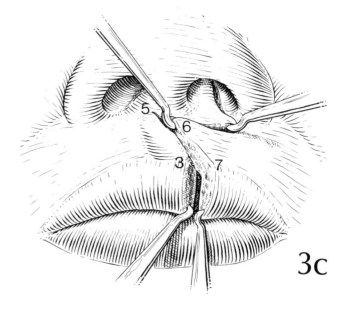

3c

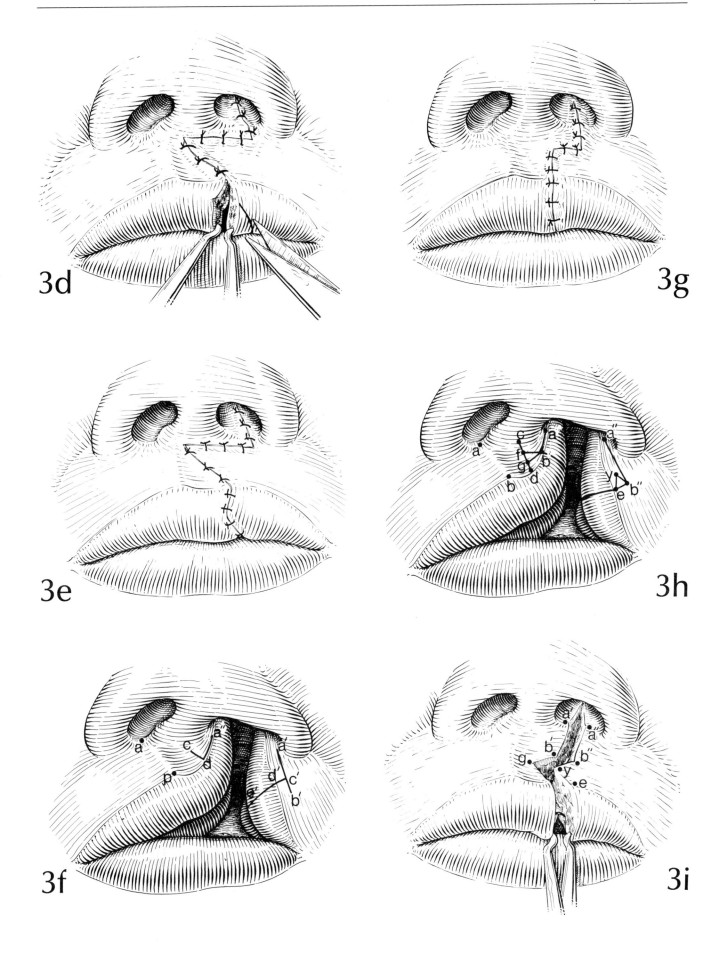

3d

3e

3f

3g

3h

3i

Palatal repair

The timing for palatal repair must take into consideration speech, maxillary growth and hearing.

4a–c The palatal cleft is closed at the age of 12 months using a modified von Langenbeck technique.

A self-retaining mouth gag is used. The operating field is infiltrated with local anesthetic containing epinephrine to reduce bleeding.

The incisions are made along the cleft at the junction between the oral and nasal mucosa. Mucoperiosteal flaps are bluntly dissected free from the bony palatal shelves. In all clefts of the palate the palatal muscles have to be reconstructed. By elevating the mucoperiosteal flaps the pathologic insertion of the musculus levator veli palatini to the posterior edge of the hard palate can be visualized. This muscle has to be freed and reconstructed as a sling across the cleft in order to obtain a functional soft palate. In order to mobilize the palatal mucoperiosteal flaps, relaxing incisions have to be made along the alveolar ridge on the border between the oral mucoperiosteum and gingiva on both sides. The neurovascular palatine bundles are identified and kept intact.

The suturing starts with the nasal layer. The levator muscle is sutured separately, and the mucoperiosteal flaps are closed using everting mattress sutures. Only absorbable suture material is used.

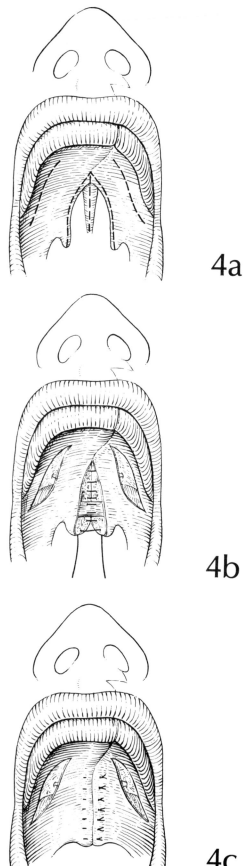

4a

4b

4c

5a–d There are many techniques available for closure of the palate. One of the most commonly used techniques is the pushback procedure. This procedure achieves lengthening of the palate which is reputed to improve speech. The technique gives excellent access to the palatal muscles but has the disadvantage of causing excessive scarring and more fistula problems.

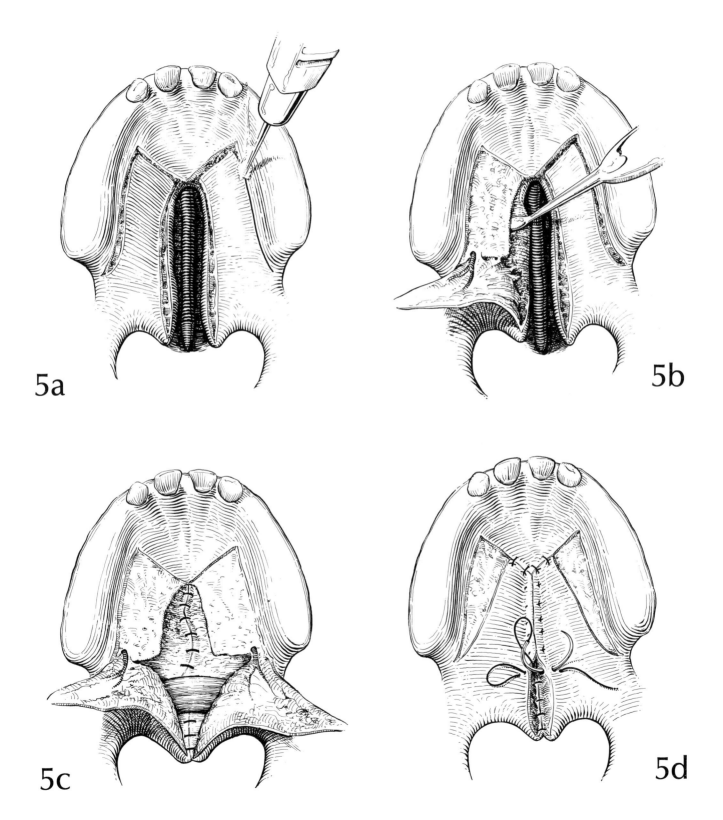

5a

5b

5c

5d

SECONDARY SURGERY

Columella lengthening in bilateral complete clefts

6a–c Patients with bilateral complete clefts will, at the age of 3–4 years, have a short columella and a broad nose with flaring nostrils. This deformity has to be corrected at the age of 4–5 years. A Millard forked flap procedure is used. The prolabium, which at birth was very small, has at this stage grown considerably and there is plenty of tissue available for columella lengthening.

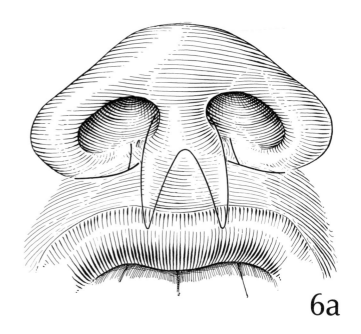

6a

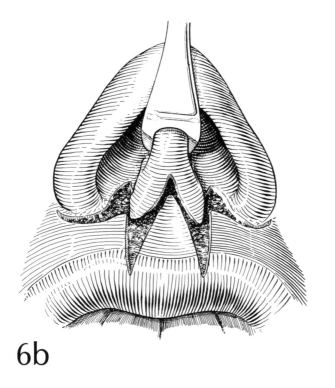

6b

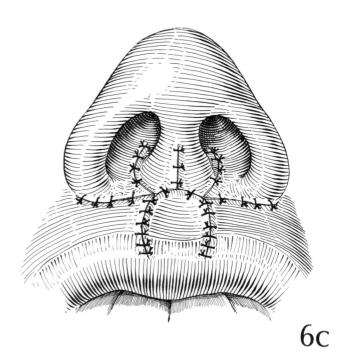

6c

Secondary bone grafting

7a–d Full dental rehabilitation in cleft patients is possible by means of bone grafting to the alveolar cleft at the age of 8–11 years with subsequent orthodontic treatment. Only autologous cancellous bone chips are used. A suitable donor site is the anterior iliac crest. When designing the flaps for covering the bone graft it is important to ensure that only attached gingiva covers the marginal part of the graft. Only then can a normal periodontium be expected around the erupting tooth. By this method full dental rehabilitation is possible in over 90% of the cleft alveolar cases making dental bridges or prostheses unnecessary. Bone grafting to the alveolar cleft at the age of 8–11 years does not have any negative effect on maxillary growth.

Primary bone grafting to the alveolar cleft, simultaneously with the lip closure, has been performed in several cleft centers and is still used today to some extent. The major side effect reported in the literature is a significant long-term inhibition of maxillary growth. Primary bone grafting has therefore been abandoned in most centers.

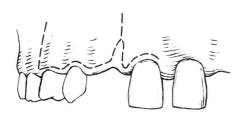

7a

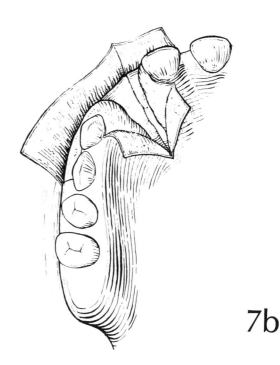

7b

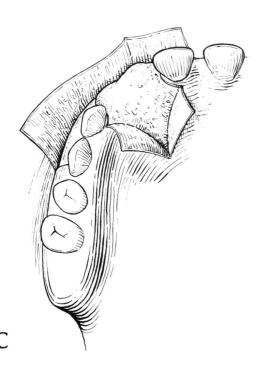

7c

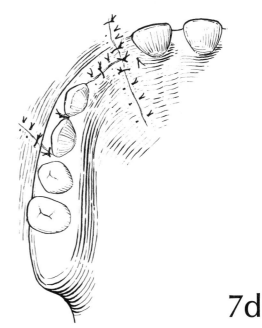

7d

Secondary nose correction

The typical secondary nose deformity seen in patients with complete cleft lip and palate has the following characteristics: septum deviation, alar cartilage asymmetry, deficient alar base support and broad nostril sill on the cleft side and deviation of the columella. This deformity represents a major challenge to the surgeon.

8a–d A rim incision on both sides combined with a transcolumellar incision gives excellent access to the deformed alar cartilage and the deviated septum. The shape and size of the alar cartilages are corrected and the septum is straightened. If extra cartilage is needed for the reconstruction, choncal grafts are preferred.

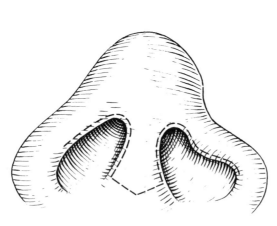

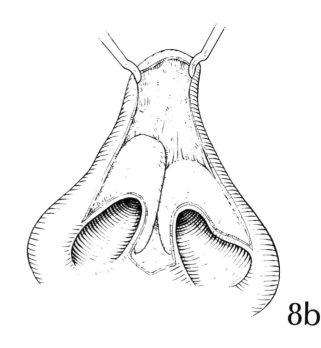

8a

8b

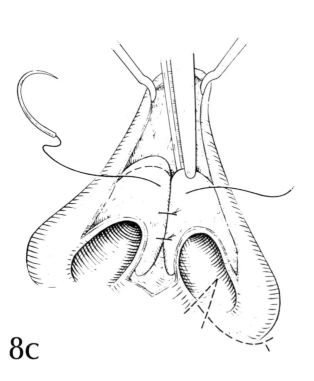

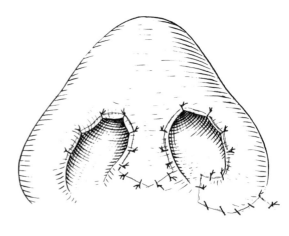

8c

8d

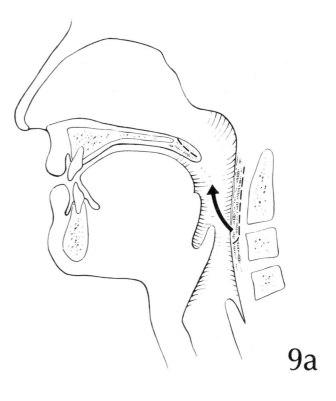

9a

Pharyngeal flap/pharyngoplasty

After primary cleft palate repair 15–20% of the patients will have nasal speech due to velopharyngeal incompetence to such a degree as to require a secondary operation to narrow the pharyngeal space.

9a, b A commonly used technique is creation of a superiorly based pharyngeal flap. A flap is dissected out from the posterior pharyngeal wall, elevated and sutured into the soft palate, creating a soft tissue bridge between the soft palate and the posterior pharyngeal wall. An opening to the epipharynx is left on both sides.

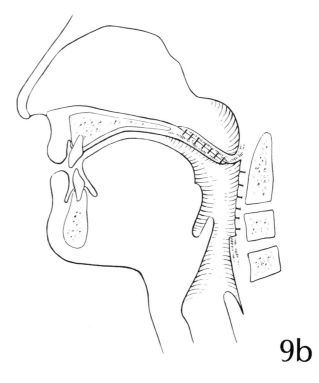

9b

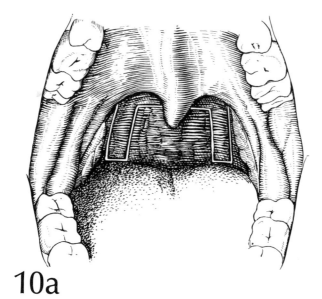

10a

10a–e Another widely used technique is pharyngoplasty. Two lateral pharyngeal flaps are dissected out from the posterior pillars of the fauces. They are superiorly based and contain palatopharyngeus muscle. A horizontal incision is made on the posterior pharyngeal wall, and the flaps are rotated and sutured to the edges of this incision and joined end-to-end in the midline.

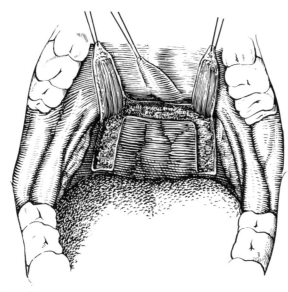

10b

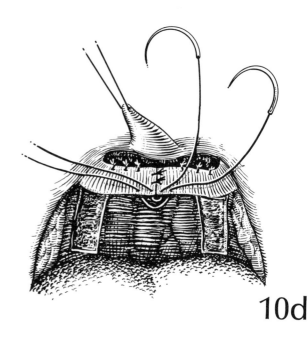

10d

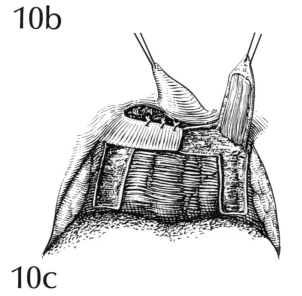

10c

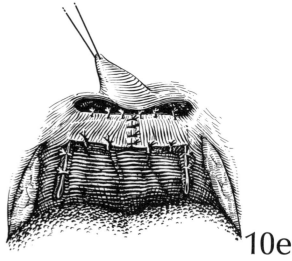

10e

Outcome

Patients with cleft lip and palate need a long-term treatment plan which covers all aspects related to the cleft including appearance, feeding, mastication, speech, hearing, facial growth, breathing and psychologic problems for children and parents.

In the treatment of cleft lip and palate it is important that a chosen program is carried out consistently over years. Introduction of new techniques or timing of procedures should only be done after careful consideration. Accurate documentation and long-term follow-up are essential.

Every surgical procedure used in primary cleft repair has advantages and some negative aspects. When planning and performing primary cleft surgery it is important to be aware of the secondary problems that will arise as a result of the treatment, and to have a long-term treatment plan for solving these problems.

The treatment of a child with cleft lip and palate is not a 'one man show'. Close cooperation between the various members of the cleft team is mandatory if a satisfactory end result is to be achieved.

Further reading

Åbyholm FE, Borchgrevink HC, Eskeland G. Cleft lip and palate in Norway. III Surgical treatment of CLP patients in Oslo 1954–75. *Scand J Plast Reconstr Surg* 1981; 15: 15–28.

Bergland O, Semb G, Åbyholm FE. Elimination of the residual alveolar cleft by secondary bone grafting and subsequent orthodontic treatment. *Cleft Palate J* 1986; 23: 175–205.

David DJ, Bagnall AD. Velopharyngeal incompetence. In: McCarthy JG, ed. *Plastic Surgery*. Vol 4. Philadelphia: Saunders, 1990: 2903–21.

Hotz M, Gnoinski W, Perko M, Nussbaumer H, Hof E, Haubensak, eds. *Early Treatment of Cleft Lip and Palate*. Toronto: Huber, 1986.

Millard DR. *Cleft Craft: The Evolution of its Surgery*. Vol I. *The Unilateral Deformity*. Boston: Little, Brown, 1976: 449–86.

Randall P, LaRossa D. Cleft palate. In: McCarthy JG, ed. *Plastic Surgery*. Vol 4. Philadelphia: Saunders, 1990: 2723–52.

Ranula

Charles F. Koopmann Jr MD, FACS
Professor and Associate Chair, Department of Otolaryngology-Head and Neck Surgery, and Chief, Pediatric Otolaryngology, University of Michigan Medical Center, Ann Arbor, Michigan, USA

History

Ranulas are histologically benign lesions which present in the floor of the mouth. They arise from the sublingual salivary glands and have also been called by such terms as mucoceles, mucous extravasation cysts and simple mucous retention cysts[1,2]. Ranulas may be 'simple' or 'plunging', the latter being much more difficult to manage. Until the 1960s little was written in the medical literature about this entity. Early statements suggested that ranulas were found mainly in African tribes or dogs[3]. The lack of knowledge of the pathophysiology led to varied recommendations for treatment (radiation, grommet insertion, marsupialization and total excision) which resulted in a high incidence of recurrence (an average of three operations in 1979[4]) and high morbidity. Since the sublingual gland has been recognized as the site of origin, treatment has been much more successful.

Principles and justification

The sublingual gland has been identified as the site of origin of ranulas because of its high protein fluid content and the observation that excision of the sublingual glands markedly reduces recurrence.

1 The simple ranula (a simple cyst) probably represents obstruction of the duct and has an epithelial lining. However, the more common variety (the plunging ranula) probably represents mucous extravasation and is thus a pseudocyst without an epithelial lining but with a lining of connective tissue or granulation tissue. The plunging ranula therefore dissects deeply into the soft tissue and fascial planes of the neck.

Trauma to the sublingual gland may be an important etiologic factor in ranulas that develop later in life. Crysdale *et al.*[5] reported that persistent ranulas occurred in 5% of patients undergoing submandibular duct relocation surgery. Ligation of the sublingual gland duct in some laboratory animals has also led to lesions which are identical to naturally occurring ranulas[6].

The modalities for treatment have varied because of the initial misunderstanding about the cause of ranulas. Some of the methods of therapy have included: simple incision, marsupialization or fistulization with or without packing of the intraoral wound, destruction of the 'lining', grommet insertion, radiation therapy, excision of the sublingual gland with or without drainage or excision of the pseudocyst, and total surgical excision (via an intraoral or cervical approach). In the rare cases of well encapsulated simple cysts of less than 1 cm diameter with an epithelial lining and no history of trauma, intraoral excision of the cyst will often be successful.

If the lesion is a pseudocyst without an epithelial lining, if the ranula is recurrent, if the cyst is greater than 1 cm in diameter, if there is a history of antecedent trauma, and especially if the ranula is 'plunging', then excision (usually intraoral) with removal of the ipsilateral sublingual gland is preferred. In extensive plunging ranulas a cervical neck incision may be used to give good access to both the sublingual and the submandibular glands. However, whether an intraoral or cervical approach is used, extensive dissection of the cyst in an attempt to remove all of the cyst lining is unnecessary when the sublingual gland is removed.

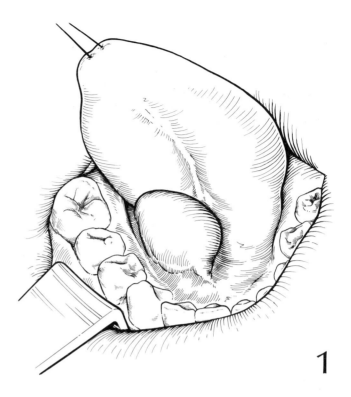

1

Differential diagnosis

The differential diagnosis of ranula (especially 'plunging' types) must include cystic hygroma, thyroglossal duct cyst, second branchial cleft cyst, enteric cyst, dermoid or epidermoid cyst, or inflammatory lesions. Malignant neoplasms such as squamous cell carcinoma are very unlikely in children.

2   Cystic hygromas arise from aberrant development of fetal lymphatic tissue in the neck and may extend into the floor of the mouth, tongue, or submandibular space. These lesions are usually easily compressible, transilluminate well, and are multilocular. They grow progressively, especially during upper respiratory infections, and may present with dangerous airway compromise. The differentiation between a cystic hygroma and ranula is difficult when the lesion is located in the superior anterior neck with extension into the sublingual or submandibular spaces.

Thyroglossal duct cyst tracts usually have well defined borders, may elevate when the tongue is protruded, are close to the midline (20% are lateral), may enlarge during upper respiratory infections, are usually at the level of the hyoid bone, and are associated with the strap muscles.

Second branchial cleft cysts are usually located along the anterior border of the sternocleidomastoid muscle at the level of the angle of the mandible and may enlarge with upper respiratory infections.

An epidermoid inclusion cyst is usually superficial, adherent to the skin, may be in the sublingual space, and may be difficult to differentiate from a ranula radiographically. Lipomas grow slowly, are not fluctuant, and do not grow in response to inflammation. Dermoid cysts may be similar to epidermoid cysts but have different signals radiographically on magnetic resonance imaging. Benign cervical lymph nodes are rarely found in the floor of the mouth. Inflammatory lesions secondary to sialadenitis or oral inflammatory processes will usually involve several spaces in the neck. Computed tomographic (CT) findings are usually somewhat different from those of a ranula.

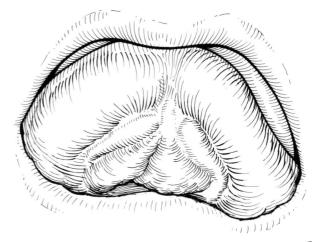

2

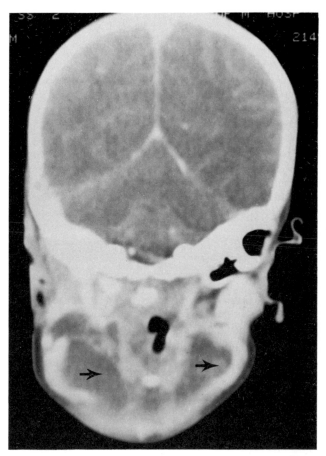

3a

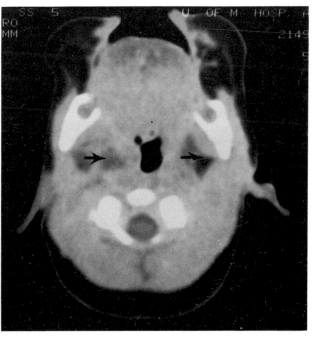

3b

3a, b Computed tomographic scans are extremely useful in differentiating ranulas from the above lesions. A 'plunging ranula' has a water content on CT scan while dermoid and epidermoid cysts have high protein and fat contents, lipomas have a low attenuation, and the thyroglossal and branchial cleft cysts have different locations in the neck. An anterior cervical cystic hygroma will generally contain septae while a plunging ranula is usually a single cavity. The demonstration of a unilocular, cystic mass in the sublingual space will usually be either a ranula or an epidermoid cyst. Since all 'plunging' ranulas arise from the sublingual glands, the lesions must involve or adjoin the sublingual space in every case. If no sublingual space extension or abutment occurs, the diagnosis of 'plunging' ranula is very unlikely[7,8].

Magnetic resonance imaging may be useful in verifying the cystic nature of the lesion, in providing information about the thickness and vascularization of the cyst wall, and for determining the relationship between the cyst and the surrounding tissues so that surgical planning may be more precise[9].

Preoperative

Anesthesia

These patients must have a general anesthesia with either oral or nasal endotracheal intubation. The author prefers nasotracheal intubation which gives complete access to the oral cavity and the floor of the mouth. The patient should not be given a long-acting muscle relaxant (again the author prefers that *no* relaxants be administered) as it is desirable to be able to monitor tongue 'twitches' as an indication of the close proximity of the motor nerves to the tongue. The hypopharynx should be packed with a gauze pack.

Operation

4a–d After suitable general endotracheal anesthesia is performed a mouth gag (usually a Jennings type) is utilized to hold the mouth open. An alternative in cases where the mouth does not accommodate the gag is to place a small dental bite block posteriorly or an assistant can retract the mouth with a Weider retractor or a small Army-Navy retractor. The tongue can be retracted with a heavy silk suture through the tongue tip.

Both Wharton's (submandibular) duct orifices are identified and the ipsilateral orifice is usually cannulated with a lacrimal probe to lessen the chance of injury. Three or four stay sutures (3/0 silk) can be placed around the planned mucosal incision. The mucosa is incised with coagulation unipolar or bipolar cautery. Avoidance of injury to the lingual and hypoglossal nerves is also paramount. Here the surgeon can use one of two approaches. The first is to make an incision in the floor of the mouth directly over the gland with the duct cannulated with a rigid lacrimal probe. The second is to make an incision in the lingual gingival sulcus at the first molar on the ipsilateral side, extending across the midline as far as is necessary for adequate exposure. A full-thickness flap of mucoperiosteum is elevated from the lingual surface of the mandible to the floor of the mouth. This will allow the sublingual gland to bulge against the periosteum which is incised, causing the gland to herniate through the incision and make its excision much easier[10].

If the lesion is well encapsulated and appears to have a distinct wall, the intraoral excision without removal of the ipsilateral sublingual gland is warranted. If the lesion is not well encapsulated but has several loculations which are ruptured, the ipsilateral sublingual gland should be removed also via the intraoral approach. After removal of the cyst and sublingual gland the intraoral incision is closed with interrupted 3/0 or 4/0 polyglactin (Vicryl) sutures.

If the ranula is 'plunging' and very large a cervical incision may be considered. This approach allows the surgeon to have a wider access to the cyst and sublingual gland because the excision of the submandibular gland makes exposure of these structures easier and also makes identification of the lingual nerve more obvious. Again, even in the external approach, extensive dissection of the cervical cyst is usually not necessary[11]. The neck incision is drained with a suction drain, such as a Jackson-Pratt drain system. The subcutaneous tissue is closed with a 3/0 polyglactin or chromic suture and the skin is closed with a running 4/0 subcuticular suture.

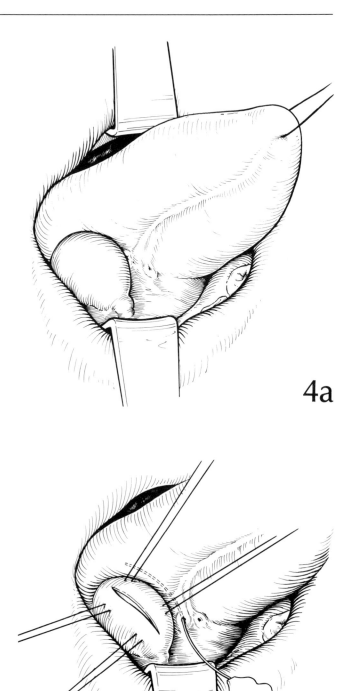

4a

4b

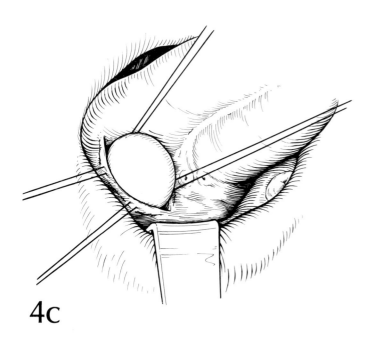

4c

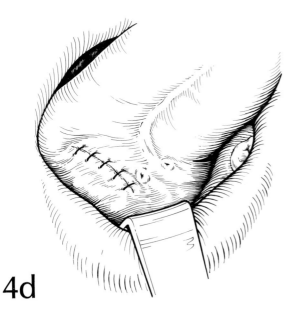

4d

Postoperative care

The patient should refrain from having a nipple or pacifier as it may traumatize the incision site. Oral feedings are usually initiated 8–12 h after surgery using a red rubber catheter for gavage feedings for 24–48 h. If an external approach is employed the Jackson-Pratt drain is hooked to wall suction for 24 h and then placed to bulb (or grenade) suction for 24 h before being removed.

Outcome

The use of the above approaches has been very successful both in this author's hands and in others in the literature.

References

1. Batsakis JG, McClatchey KD. Cervical ranulas. *Ann Otol Rhinol Laryngol* 1988; 97: 561–2.

2. Roediger WEW, Kay S. Pathogenesis and treatment of plunging ranulas. *Surg Gynecol Obstet* 1977; 144: 862–4.

3. Mair IWS. Schewitsch I, Svendsen E, Haugeto OK. Cervical ranula. *J Laryngol Otol* 1977; 93: 623–8.

4. Van den Akker HP, Bays RA, Becker AE. Plunging or cervical ranula. Review of the literature and report of 4 cases. *J Maxillofac Surg* 1978; 6: 286–93.

5. Crysdale WS, Mendelsohn JD, Conley S. Ranulas – mucoceles of the oral cavity: experience in 26 children. *Laryngoscope* 1988; 98: 296–8.

6. Harrison JD, Garrett JR. Experimental salivary mucoceles in cat: a histochemical study. *J Oral Pathol* 1975; 4: 297–306.

7. Charnoff SK, Carter BL. Plunging ranula: CT diagnosis. *Radiology* 1986; 158: 467–8.

8. Coit WE, Harnsberger HR, Osborn AG, Smoker WRK, Stevens MH, Lufkin RB. Ranulas and their mimics: CT evaluation. *Radiology* 1987; 163: 211–16.

9. Vogl TJ, Steger W, Ihrler S, Ferrera P, Grevers G. Cystic masses in the floor of the mouth: value of MR imaging in planning surgery. *Am J Roentgenol* 1993; 161: 183–6.

10. Galloway RH, Gross PD, Thompson SH, Patterson AL. Pathogenesis and treatment of ranula: report of three cases. *J Oral Maxillofac Surg* 1989; 47: 299–302.

11. Parekh D, Stewart M, Joseph C, Lawson HH. Plunging ranula: a report of three cases and review of the literature. *Br J Surg* 1987; 74: 307–9.

Thyroglossal cyst and fistula

R. J. Brereton FRCS
Consultant Paediatric Surgeon, Chelsea and Westminster Hospital, London, UK

Principles and justification

Development of thyroid gland and thyroglossal tract

The thyroid gland develops as a median thickening of the floor of the pharynx, between the first and second branchial arches, and descends to its final position in the neck, leaving the thyroglossal duct extending caudally from the foramen cecum of the tongue to the pyramidal lobe of the gland, passing anterior, through or posterior to the body of the hyoid bone. The lateral lobes of the gland receive contributions from the fourth branchial clefts, which form the medullary C cells. Thereafter the duct normally disappears. Thyroid remnants may be found along the course of the thyroglossal duct[1,2].

Thyroglossal cysts

Thyroglossal cysts, the most common anterior cervical swelling in children, most frequently arise just inferior to the level of the hyoid bone. Occasionally the duct deviates anterosuperiorly once it has passed the hyoid bone, giving rise to a thyroglossal cyst in the submental triangle, where it may be mistaken for a dermoid cyst. Although dermoid cysts may occur below the hyoid bone, they are more common in the submental triangle and can be distinguished from thyroglossal cysts by their softer 'putty-like' consistency. Very occasionally, aberrant thyroid glandular tissue is found along the course of the thyroglossal duct.

Thyroglossal fistulas

A thyroglossal fistula usually results from rupture or incision of an inflamed thyroglossal cyst, but the orifice often appears quite low down on the neck. Recurrent discharge and inflammation are common symptoms.

Preoperative

Assessment and preparation

In thyroid hypoplasia, a small central area of aberrant ectopic thyroid tissue may be mistaken for a thyroglossal cyst and it is recommended that the precise location of the thyroid gland is determined, using isotope scanning or ultrasound examination, before undertaking surgery, as removal of the aberrant tissue may be followed by hypothyroidism[3]. The incidence of such aberrant tissue is, however, low (about 1% of all thyroglossal abnormalities[4]) and it is easily recognizable when the lesion is exposed.

Occult staphylococcal infection is common in these cysts, and perioperative antibiotic cover using a penicillinase-resistant agent such as flucloxacillin or fusidic acid is usually indicated.

Anesthesia

General anesthesia using an orotracheal or nasotracheal tube is recommended.

Operations

EXCISION OF THYROGLOSSAL CYST

The aim of surgery is to remove the entire duct, including the central part of the body of the hyoid bone, to the level of the foramen cecum[1,2]. Because side branches may arise from the duct within the muscles of the tongue, the intraglossal part of the duct should be removed with a surrounding cuff of muscle approximately 0.5 cm in diameter. Complete excision is essential to prevent recurrence and eliminate the risk of malignant degeneration[5]. All thyroglossal cysts, however small, should be excised as soon as possible because delay invariably leads to infection, which makes subsequent surgery more difficult, morbidity and recurrence rates higher and cosmetic results less satisfactory. The operation may be performed on a day-case basis on certain patients who are free of infection, but hemostasis must be meticulous.

Position of patient

The patient is placed supine with the head extended and the shoulders elevated on a small sandbag.

Incision

1 A short (usually less than 3 cm) transverse incision is made in a skin crease over the main prominence of the cyst. Some authors recommend infiltration of the skin with epinephrine (adrenaline) to prevent hemorrhage.

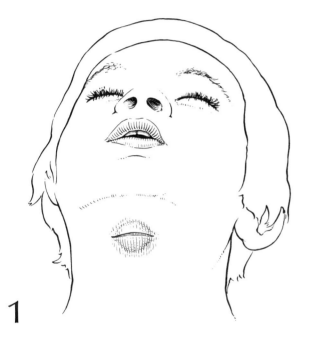

1

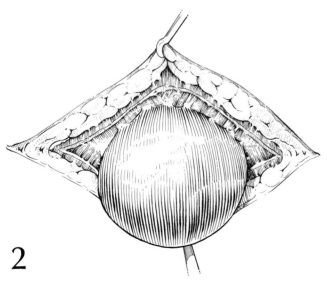

2 The subcutaneous fat, platysma and deep cervical fascia are cut in the line of the incision with a diathermy needle and the cyst freed from its superficial attachments by a combination of sharp and blunt dissection. Meticulous hemostasis is essential so that the operative field is not obscured.

2

Dissection

3 The thyroglossal tract is identified at its deep attachment to the cyst and followed between the sternohyoid muscles to the hyoid bone. The centrum of the hyoid bone is freed from the sternohyoid muscles below and the mylohyoid and geniohyoid muscles above with a diathermy needle. The thyrohyoid membrane is separated from the posterior aspect of the centrum using artery forceps, a closed pair of scissors or a McDonald dissector. Small bone-cutting forceps or strong Mayo scissors are then used to divide the body of the hyoid 5 mm to either side of the midline. This maneuver is facilitated by grasping and steadying the bone with Kocher artery forceps.

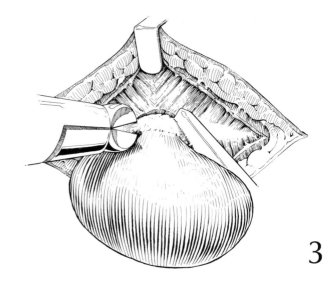

3

4 A cylinder of geniohyoid and genioglossus muscles 0.5–1.0 cm wide (depending on the size of the patient), including the duct, is excised to the foramen cecum: this is best performed using needle diathermy. It has been suggested that the dissection is made easier if the anesthetist uses his or her finger to depress the foramen cecum into the wound, but this is seldom of practical value and is a potential danger to the anesthetist. Meticulous hemostasis using diathermy will prevent postoperative respiratory obstruction due to hematoma formation.

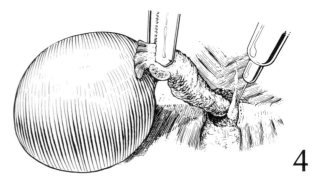

4

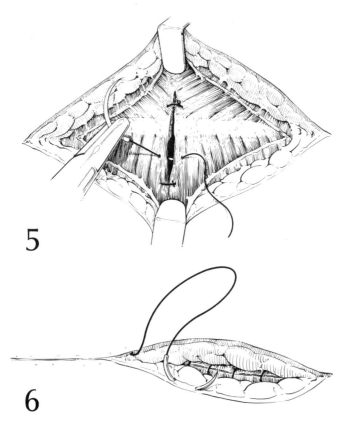

5

6

Wound closure

5 The muscles are approximated in the midline using sutures of 3/0 polyglycolic acid or chromic catgut to aid hemostasis. It is not necessary to reconstitute the hyoid bone because its cut ends tend to be approximated by the muscle sutures.

6 The fascia and platysma are closed with a continuous suture of 3/0 or 4/0 polyglycolic acid or chromic catgut and the same suture is used in the subcutaneous layer to appose the skin edges. Alternatively, the skin edges may be approximated with self-adhesive wound tapes. The use of non-absorbable skin sutures or clips is not recommended as their removal causes anxiety and discomfort. If adequate hemostasis has been secured, no drains or dressings are required.

EXCISION OF THYROGLOSSAL FISTULA

Treatment is similar to that for an uncomplicated thyroglossal cyst. All traces of the fistula must be excised to the foramen cecum.

Position of patient

The patient should be positioned as for excision of a thyroglossal cyst (page 57).

Incision

7 A small elliptical incision is made around the orifice of the fistula (sinus) in the neck.

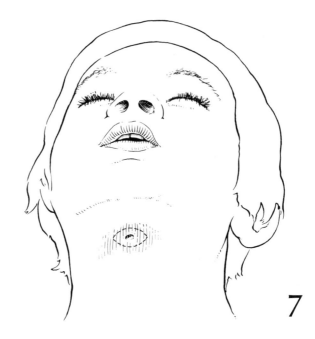

7

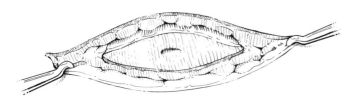

8

8 The ellipse of skin (including the sinus or fistulous tract) is traced through the subcutaneous tissues towards the hyoid bone.

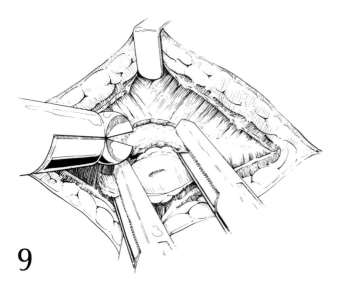

9

Resection

9 The centrum of the hyoid bone is resected with the fistulous tract.

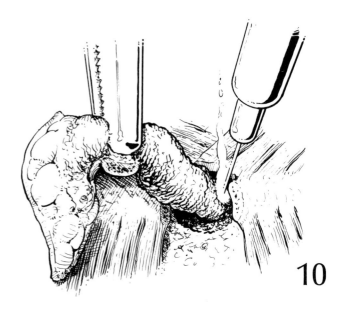

10 A core of geniohyoid and genioglossus muscles, including the tract, is excised up to the level of the foramen cecum.

Wound closure

The wound is closed as for a thyroglossal cyst. It may be necessary to insert a drain if perfect hemostasis cannot be guaranteed or if there is florid inflammatory edema.

Postoperative care

It is important to ensure that the airway does not become obstructed by reactionary hemorrhage. Infection is common and spreading cellulitis may cause airway compression, so oral antibiotics should be continued for 2–3 days after the procedure. The child is allowed home on the day after surgery.

Outcome

If the thyroglossal duct is excised with the cyst, recurrence is unlikely[1,2,6]. Cysts may recur, however, sometimes as much as 10 years later, in more than 20% of patients treated by local excision only. This rate is reduced to 5% by removing the central part of the hyoid bone with the cyst. The recurrence rate of a thyroglossal fistula is higher than that for the uncomplicated cyst.

References

1. Sistrunk WE. The surgical treatment of cysts of the thyroglossal tract. *Ann Surg* 1920; 71: 121–3.

2. Sistrunk WE. Techniques of removal of cysts and sinuses of the thyroglossal duct. *Surg Gynecol Obstet* 1928; 46: 109–12.

3. Pulito AR, Shaw A. Median ectopic thyroid gland. *J Pediatr Surg* 1973; 8: 73–4.

4. Gross RE. Thyroglossal cysts and sinuses. In: Gross RE, ed. *The Surgery of Infancy and Childhood*. Philadelphia: WB Saunders, 1953: 936–59.

5. Lui AHF, Littler ER. Thyroid carcinoma originating in a thyroglossal cyst: report of a case. *Am Surg* 1970; 36: 546–8.

6. Brereton RJ, Symonds E. Thyroglossal cysts in children. *Br J Surg* 1978; 65: 507–8.

Branchial cysts, sinuses and fistulas

John R. Wesley MD
Clinical Professor of Surgery, Chair, Division of Pediatric Surgery, University of California, Davis Medical Center, Sacramento, California, USA

Principles and justification

Cysts, sinuses and fistulas of the neck derived from branchial cleft remnants are common in the pediatric age group. Sinuses and fistulas are encountered more commonly in infants and children, while branchial cysts occur more often in older children and young adults. Remnants of the first and second branchial apparatus are most common, with abnormalities of the second cleft outnumbering those of the first by 6:1[1]. Abnormalities of the third and fourth branchial apparatus are rare, but recent case reports and reviews indicate that they may be more common than previously supposed[2].

1 A simple knowledge of head and neck embryology is helpful in understanding these abnormalities. The branchial arches appear by the 15th day of fetal life and present as bar-like ridges separated by grooves or clefts. Five paired ectodermal clefts and five endodermal pouches separate the six branchial arches. A closing membrane lies at the interface of the pouches and clefts. The four clinically significant arches and clefts are shown.

The pathogenesis of branchial cleft anomalies is controversial, and may occur as any combination of sinus, fistula and cyst. Incomplete obliteration of the branchial apparatus, primarily the cleft, is accepted as the most likely etiology. Most branchial anomalies arise from the second branchial apparatus as the second branchial arch overgrows the second, third and fourth branchial clefts, and finally fuses with the lateral branchial wall. As the arches coalesce during the growth

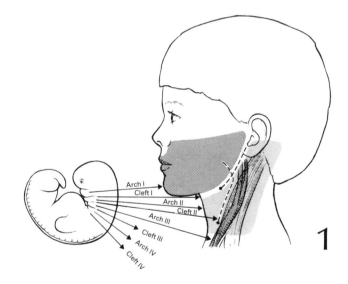

of the embryo, part of the first branchial cleft remains open as the eustachian tube and auditory canal. The second branchial cleft normally closes completely; however, either branchial cleft may form a sinus tract or cyst as it coalesces.

2 Remnants of the first branchial cleft occur along an imaginary line extending from the auditory canal behind and below the angle of the mandible to its mid point. Second branchial cleft remnants are found anywhere along an imaginary line extending from the tonsillar fossa down to a point on the lower one-third of the anterior border of the sternocleidomastoid muscle.

Although branchial apparatus anomalies may present at any age, most branchial sinuses present clinically soon after birth or before the age of 10 years.

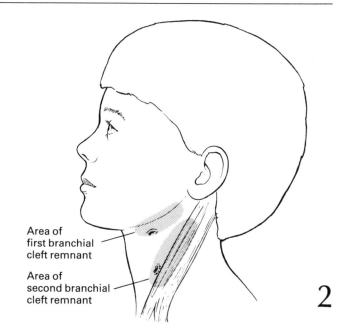

Area of
first branchial
cleft remnant

Area of
second branchial
cleft remnant

2

3 The more common second branchial cleft sinus presents as a pinpoint opening on the anterior border of the sternocleidomastoid muscle, one-quarter to one-third of its length cephalad from the sternal end. The defect is usually characterized by the appearance of small drops of clear fluid at the opening or by the occurrence of infection in the tract itself. The anomaly may be either unilateral or bilateral, and may be familial. Tracts that have an exterior opening occasionally become infected, though infection is a more common problem in sinuses and cysts in the older age group. Cysts of the first branchial cleft usually present as enlarging masses near the lower pole of the parotid gland and are more commonly seen in older children and young adults. Cysts of the second branchial cleft usually present in children and young adults as a mass at the mandibular angle along the anterior border of the sternocleidomastoid muscle, often associated with upper respiratory infection.

Case reports and recent reviews suggest that cysts or acute infections arising from a third or fourth branchial pouch sinus are rare but well-defined entities that offer diagnostic and therapeutic challenges not encountered with the anomalies of the first and second branchial remnants. These lesions present as an air-containing inflammatory lateral neck mass in the neonate or as acute suppurative thyroiditis in the infant or child. The etiology for both presentations is a fistulous track from the pyriform sinus, most commonly on the left side, occurring as a result of a persistent remnant from the third or fourth branchial pouch. This condition should always be suspected in a neonate presenting with an

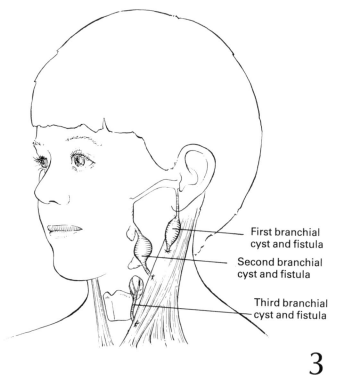

First branchial
cyst and fistula

Second branchial
cyst and fistula

Third branchial
cyst and fistula

3

inflammatory lesion containing air in the left side of the neck. Similarly, acute suppurative thyroiditis is rare and its presence should prompt consideration of a pyriform sinus fistula as the etiology. Treatment of the acute infection should be followed by surgical extirpation in all cases.

Preoperative

Assessment and preparation

Cysts and sinuses of the first and second branchial clefts are diagnosed by their clinical appearance on careful physical examination. No special diagnostic imaging is indicated. The operation may be performed at any age, usually at the time of diagnosis, the main consideration in neonates being the availability of sophisticated pediatric anesthesia. The use of sclerosing solutions is contraindicated and may be dangerous. If infection is present, a course of antibiotics should be administered first. With respect to cysts or sinuses suspected to be of third or fourth branchial pouch origin, barium studies may demonstrate the presence of a pyriform sinus fistula, particularly after a course of antibiotics and resolution of the surrounding inflammation. Computed axial tomography has also proved useful in diagnosing lesions of a third or fourth branchial pouch origin[3,4]. If imaging techniques are not successful after resolution of the inflammation, then the next time the inflammation recurs, compression of the pus-filled cyst during endoscopy may reveal the origin of the fistula as pus exudes from the pyriform sinus.

Anesthesia

Endotracheal inhalation general anesthesia, preferably by a pediatric anesthetist, is preferred.

Operations

Position of patient and preparation

The patient is placed in the supine position with a sandbag beneath the shoulders and a soft ring headrest beneath the cranium so that the neck is extended. The head of the table is raised slightly to diminish venous blood pressure in the head and neck. The chin is turned away from the side of the lesion, and the skin is prepared with 10% povidone-iodine solution. The field is draped with four towels held to the contours of the neck with plastic barrier drapes with one adhesive edge (Steri-drape 1010). An electrocautery grounding plate is applied to the thigh.

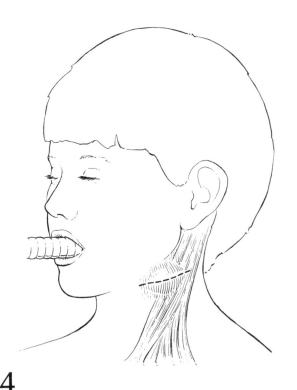

4

Exposure of cyst

4 The most common branchial cyst is derived from the second branchial cleft. The skin incision is made over the cyst along Langer's lines or in a natural skin crease in order to obtain the best cosmetic result. The length of the incision will vary with the size of the cyst.

Infiltration of the overlying skin and adjacent tissues with dilute norepinephrine (noradrenaline) (1:1000 in isotonic saline) is optional, but generally unnecessary. A scalpel is used to incise the skin only, and subsequent dissection is accomplished by lifting the tissues off the underlying structures with Adson's tissue forceps and dissecting with a fine hemostat and electrocautery. The incision is carried through the subcutaneous tissues and platysma to the level of the cyst. The cyst is exposed by retracting the skin and muscle flaps, best accomplished with a self-retaining or ring retractor.

5 The deep cervical fascia is divided next to the anterior border of the sternocleidomastoid muscle, allowing the belly of the muscle to be retracted away from the cyst. Exposure is extended anteriorly and medially by retraction of the sternohyoid muscle. The fascia and soft tissue overlying the cyst are lifted and incised carefully to expose the superficial aspect of the cyst.

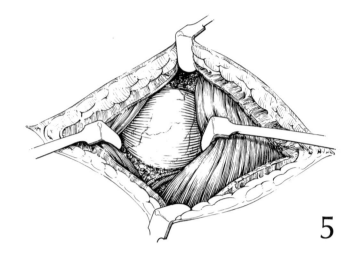

5

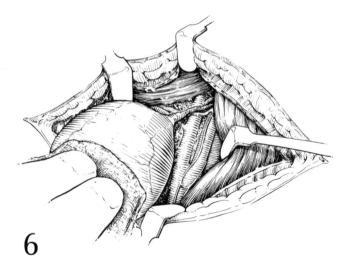

6

DISSECTION AND REMOVAL OF A SECOND BRANCHIAL CLEFT CYST

6 Great care is taken to avoid rupture of the cyst, as a tense cyst wall is easier to define and dissect than a collapsed cyst. Adjacent structures are separated from the cyst by blunt and electrocautery dissection along the cyst wall, special care being taken along the deep aspect of the cyst where the jugular vein and carotid arteries are in intimate relation. The pedicle of the cyst generally lies posterior to the jugular vein, most often coursing between the carotid artery bifurcation. It is then dissected cephalad towards the tonsillar pillar, where it is clamped and suture ligated with fine non-absorbable suture. Meticulous hemostasis is obtained and the wound irrigated with 1% povidone-iodine solution before closure.

DISSECTION AND REMOVAL OF A FIRST BRANCHIAL CLEFT CYST

7 During dissection of the less common first branchial cleft cyst, care must be taken to avoid damage to the adjacent facial nerve in cases where there is a tract leading up to or into the external auditory meatus. Not uncommonly, the deep or superficial lobes of the parotid gland must be mobilized. A neurosurgical nerve stimulator is often helpful during the dissection.

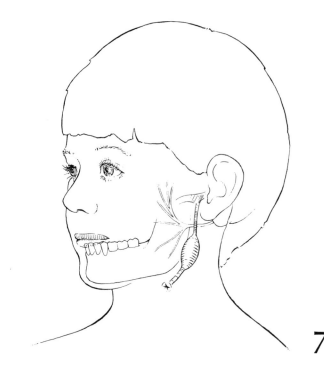

7

DISSECTION AND REMOVAL OF A THIRD OR FOURTH BRANCHIAL POUCH CYST AND SINUS

In instances where the cyst presents as acute thyroiditis or an air-containing inflammatory lateral neck mass suggesting a third or fourth branchial pouch origin, preoperative resolution with antibiotics should be followed by barium studies to allow visualization of the pyriform sinus tract common to each of these anomalies. Exploration of the neck with excision of the entire tract to the level of the pyriform sinus is necessary to prevent recurrence. Operative endoscopy at the start of the operation may enable cannulation of the tract from above, which greatly facilitates localization of the tract during resection[5].

8 The thyroid gland is exposed through a standard collar incision, and the left lobe is mobilized. The recurrent and superior laryngeal nerves and parathyroid glands should be identified and protected. If no discrete cyst or tract is found, the fistula may be located at the laryngeal level near the cricothyroid membrane[6]. The fibers of the inferior constrictor muscle are bluntly spread to expose the pyriform recess. Extreme caution should be exercised in this region to preserve the external branch of the superior laryngeal nerve. The tract usually passes inferiorly, external to the recurrent laryngeal nerve along the trachea to the superior pole of the thyroid. It may end blindly near the gland or actually penetrate the capsule to terminate in the parenchyma of the left thyroid lobe. Thyroid lobectomy or resection of the superior pole is carried out as indicated by the extent of the cyst.

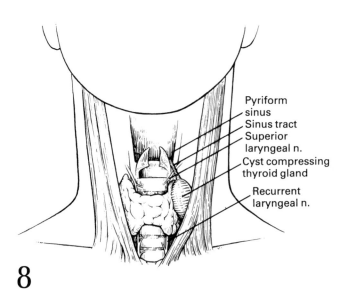

Pyriform sinus
Sinus tract
Superior laryngeal n.
Cyst compressing thyroid gland
Recurrent laryngeal n.

8

EXCISION OF A SECOND BRANCHIAL CLEFT SINUS

9a, b The operation to excise a second branchial cleft sinus begins with an elliptical transverse incision at the sinus opening, and cephalad dissection of the tract to its furthest extent, generally at the level of the tonsillar pillar. The dissection is kept directly on the tract to avoid injury to contiguous structures, e.g. the internal jugular vein, the bifurcation of the carotid artery and the hypoglossal nerve. The operation can almost always be carried out through a single elliptical incision if the tract is kept under gentle traction, and the anesthetist places a gloved finger in the tonsillar fossa and exerts downward pressure towards the field of dissection. In addition, the anesthetist's finger helps to localize the tonsillar fossa at the end point of dissection, where the sinus tract is suture ligated and divided. Dissection of the sinus tract may be facilitated by passing a fine silver probe or piece of heavy nylon suture the length of the tract and clamping this in position as the dissection progresses.

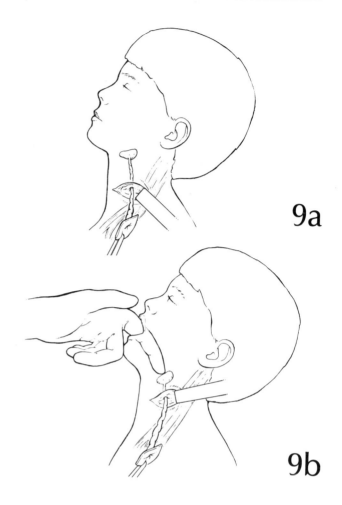

9a

9b

MINOR BRANCHIAL REMNANTS

A branchial arch remnant may also occur along the lower anterior border of the sternocleidomastoid muscle near the sternoclavicular joint, and typically consists of a small cartilaginous mass presenting in the subcutaneous tissue. The lesion is usually visible and palpable, and bilateral occurrences are common. An accompanying sinus or cyst is seldom present, and infection is uncommon. Excision may be carried out for cosmetic reasons or may be delayed indefinitely.

Preauricular sinuses or pits are common and have been attributed to vestiges of the first branchial cleft. These lesions probably relate to the infolding and fusion associated with formation of the ear. Asymptomatic lesions require no treatment; draining sinuses and infected cysts require antibiotic treatment, incision and drainage if they fail to resolve, and later excision to prevent recurrence.

Wound closure

10 The cervical fascia and platysma are closed with interrupted sutures of 4/0 polyglycolic acid. When the dissection is carefully performed and the cyst or sinus is not infected, the incision may be closed without using a drain. The skin is closed with a running 5/0 subcuticular absorbable suture or pull-out nylon suture. Steristrips and a clear plastic dressing (Opsite) are applied as a wound dressing.

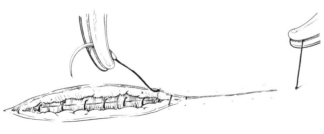

10

Postoperative care

The operations described are carried out as outpatient procedures, unless unusual difficulties are encountered or unless a drain is placed. Antibiotics (penicillin or a cephalosporin) are continued for 1–5 days after operation, depending on the presence of infection or degree of contamination. An occlusive dry sterile dressing is kept in place for 48 h, after which the patient is permitted to bathe and shower normally. If a drain is placed, it is removed after 24 h or whenever drainage has ceased. The patient is seen 7 days after operation for a wound check.

Outcome

The outcome for the procedures described is usually excellent, both functionally and cosmetically. Operative damage to related anatomical structures is rare and should not occur provided that the surgeon has adequate knowledge of the anatomy, and that meticulous hemostasis is obtained during dissection to ensure a clear field. Failure to excise the cyst or sinus completely may lead to its recurrence, in which case the patient should be treated with antibiotics and a thorough diagnostic re-evaluation initiated.

References

1. Albers GD. Branchial anomalies. *JAMA* 1963; 183: 399–409.

2. Rosenfeld RM, Biller HF. Fourth branchial pouch sinus: diagnosis and treatment. *Otolaryngol Head Neck Surg* 1991; 105: 44–50.

3. Faerber EN, Swartz JD. Imaging of neck masses in infants and children. *Crit Rev Diagn Imaging* 1991; 31: 283–314.

4. Herman TE, McAlister WH, Siegel MJ. Branchial fistula: CT manifestations. *Pediatr Radiol* 1992; 22: 152–3.

5. Makino S-I, Tsuchida Y, Yoshioka H, Saito S. The endoscopic and surgical management of pyriform fistulae in infants and children. *J Pediatr Surg* 1986; 21: 398–401.

6. Miller D, Hill JL, Sun CC, O'Brien DS, Haller JA Jr. The diagnosis and management of pyriform sinus fistulae in infants and young children. *J Pediatr Surg* 1983; 18: 377–81.

Illustrations by Marks Creative Consultants

External angular dermoid cyst

R. J. Brereton FRCS
Consultant Paediatric Surgeon, Chelsea and Westminster Hospital, London, UK

Principles and justification

The external angle of the orbit is one of the more common sites for a congenital dermoid cyst. In infancy and childhood there are few conditions that cause diagnostic confusion. The cyst lies in a shallow, saucer-like depression in the bone but occasionally it is deeper, almost surrounded by bone. A tiny pit is invariably present in the base of the bony depression through which the cyst receives its blood supply. Rarely, the pit is deeper and a dumb-bell extension of the cyst erodes the orbital plate of the frontal bone and thereby lies in contact with the dura mater of the anterior cranial fossa.

The treatment is complete excision of the cyst.

Preoperative

A plain radiograph may be reassuring but it is usually difficult to be certain of the size and depth of the defect in the frontal region. If there is genuine concern about an intracranial extension, a computed tomographic scan or magnetic resonance imaging should be arranged as these lesions merit removal by planned craniotomy.

Anesthesia

General anesthesia via endotracheal tube is recommended.

Operation

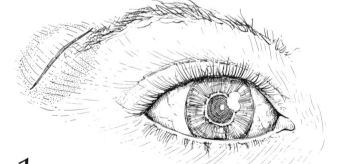

1

1 Alcoholic antiseptics should *not* be used for preoperative skin preparation. Rather than a head towel, the use of a circumcision towel is advised. In most cases the cyst can be totally excised through an incision 1.5 cm long placed just above the hairline of the eyebrow on the affected side. The eyebrow should not be removed by shaving. Hemorrhage from the surrounding vessels may be profuse, so facilities for electrocoagulation must be available. The use of needle point cutting diathermy is recommended for making the incision.

2 The cyst is exposed by blunt dissection of the fibers of the eyebrow muscle using a pair of mosquito artery forceps. Meticulous hemostasis is necessary. A small margin of periosteum of the frontal bone, beyond the edges of the cyst, is cleared.

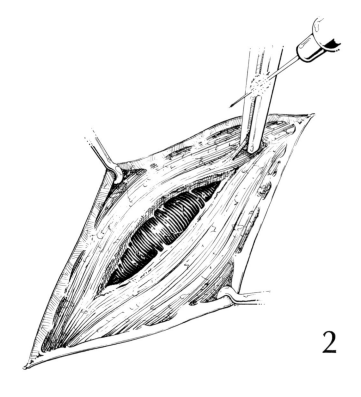

2

3a, b A fringe of periosteum 1 mm wide is incised around the entire circumference of the cyst with needle diathermy. The periosteum is stripped from the bone and used to hold the cyst. Instruments should not be applied directly to the cyst because this usually causes it to rupture, making removal more difficult. Using blunt or sharp dissection, the periosteum from the saucer-like depression in the frontal bone is elevated along with the cyst. Should the cyst rupture, simple excision of the remaining lining along with the periosteum from the frontal depression will suffice.

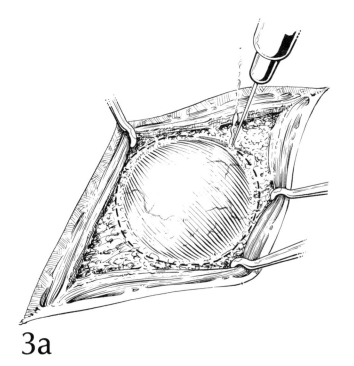

3a

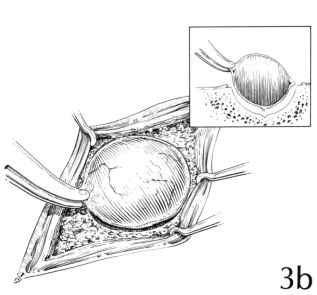

3b

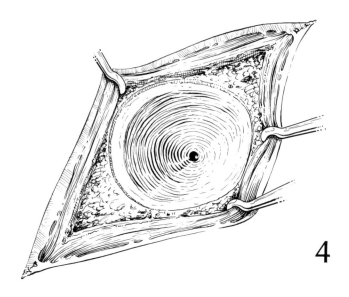

4   The feeding vessels passing through the pit of the bony depression are coagulated. Very rarely the pit has to be packed with bone wax to secure hemostasis, but bleeding from other areas of the depression in the frontal bone which has been denuded of its periosteum is not a problem.

4

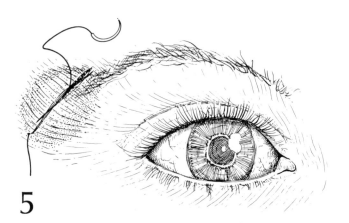

5

5   The wound is closed with a subcuticular suture to the skin.

In the rare event of an intracranial extension an osteoplastic craniotomy will be required because the intracranial portion may be the larger of the two elements. It is not safe to attempt removal by simply nibbling away the orbital plate of the frontal bone.

Postoperative care

Most patients can be treated on a daycase basis. Complications are rare. Hematomas will not occur if hemostasis was meticulous. Keloid may develop in the scars of black-skinned children.

Illustrations by Marks Creative Consultants

Sternocleidomastoid torticollis

Ronald B. Hirschl MD
Assistant Professor of Surgery, Section of Pediatric Surgery, University of Michigan Medical School, and
Pediatric Surgeon, C.S. Mott Children's Hospital, Ann Arbor, Michigan, USA

Principles and justification

Sternocleidomastoid torticollis is the term used to describe the presence of a shortened, fibrosed sternocleidomastoid muscle, which results in traction of the mastoid process toward the sternoclavicular joint[1]. The head is therefore rotated away from and tilted toward the involved sternocleidomastoid muscle.

The etiology of torticollis remains unclear. Light microscopic examination of the involved sternocleidomastoid muscle demonstrates replacement of muscle bundles by dense fibrous tissue[2]. Approximately 30% of patients presenting with sternocleidomastoid torticollis have a history of breech presentation at birth, with 60% involved in a complicated birth[3]. Recent evidence suggests that sternocleidomastoid torticollis may be the manifestation of an intrauterine positional disorder with development of sternocleidomastoid compartment syndrome. Bilateral sternocleidomastoid fibrosis is present in 2–3% of cases[4].

About 50–70% of patients present at age 1–8 weeks with a hard 1–3-cm painless, discrete mass, or pseudotumor, located within the substance of the middle or inferior portion of the sternocleidomastoid muscle[5]. This is often, but not always, accompanied by torticollis with the face turned away from and the head tilted toward the side with the pseudotumor. Approximately one-third of neonates and infants present with torticollis and diffuse fibrosis of the sternocleidomastoid muscle rather than a pseudotumor[4]. Passive neck range-of-motion exercises, which emphasize rotation towards and side-flexing away from the affected sternocleidomastoid muscle, should be performed by the parents under the guidance of a physiotherapist. The parents should place toys and other desirable objects on the ipsilateral side in order to encourage turning towards that side. With physiotherapy, resolution of the sternocleidomastoid pseudotumor and/or fibrosis is usually observed over the following 4–8 months in at least 70% of patients[4]. Operative intervention is not necessary in most (> 90%) neonates and infants[6]. Acquired plagiocephaly with flattening of both the frontal area on the ipsilateral side and the occipital region on the contralateral side may be noted in the first few months of life, but usually resolves spontaneously by 1 year of age after the infant begins to sit up[7].

Persistence of torticollis beyond 1 year of age or presentation in children older than 1–2 years of age is more often refractory to conservative management. Operation is indicated in children older than 1 year of age if physiotherapy has failed[7]. Facial hemihypoplasia, which involves flattening and underdevelopment of the malar eminence and downward displacement of the eye, ear and mouth on the affected side, may appear as early as 6 months of age, but most often appears after 3–4 years[6]. The development of facial hemihypoplasia is an indication for operative intervention, as potential resolution of skeletal abnormalities and subsequent normal growth and development of the facial skeleton will occur only after prompt operative correction of the torticollis.

Preoperative

Assessment and preparation

Preoperative evaluation includes assessment to exclude other causes of abnormal head posture. Compensatory head positions due to the presence of ocular nystagmus or strabismus and vestibular disorders are quite rare and are usually associated with a normal sternocleidomastoid muscle. Occasionally, however, sternocleidomastoid fibrosis may coexist with 'ocular torticollis'[8]. Cervical spine radiologic evaluation is necessary to exclude congenital osseous deformity of the cervical spine and Klippel–Feil syndrome or potential C1–C2 cervical spine subluxation. The diagnosis of a sternocleidomastoid pseudotumor and torticollis in a neonate or infant presenting with a sternocleidomastoid mass can almost always be made on the basis of physical examination, history and clinical progression[4]. Only occasionally should ultrasonographic evaluation be necessary to differentiate such a sternocleidomastoid pseudotumor from a mass secondary to lymphadenopathy or neoplasm.

Photographic and/or computed tomographic evaluation for hemihypoplasia should be performed in any patient in whom torticollis persists beyond 6 months of age and as a baseline before operative intervention. Radiologic evaluation of the hips and lower extremities should be performed because of the relatively high incidence (28%) of congenital dysplasia of the hip and abnormalities of the lower extremities in patients with torticollis[7].

Anesthesia

General anesthesia with endotracheal intubation is required. The endotracheal tube should be adequately secured and placed appropriately to allow sterile preparation of the entire neck and full rotation of the neck in both directions.

Operation

Position of patient

The patient is placed supine with a roll transversely under the shoulders in order to provide neck extension. The bed is flexed so that the head of the patient remains in a 30° upright position in order to decrease venous bleeding. The head is turned slightly to the side opposite the affected sternocleidomastoid muscle. A sponge doughnut is placed under the head to maintain its position. The prepared field should include the entire neck, extending up to just above the mandible, down to the areas of both shoulders, and to the infraclavicular regions bilaterally. Crumpled drapes are placed in the posterior aspect of the junction of the neck and shoulders bilaterally. Drapes are then placed along the inferior border of the mandible, at the level of the clavicle, and bilaterally along the posterolateral aspect of the neck.

Incision

1 An approximately 3-cm, transverse, curvilinear incision is made in a skin crease one or two fingerbreadths above the clavicle.

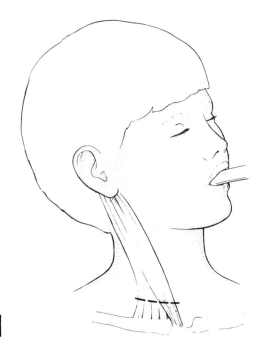

1

2 The platysma is divided. Subplatysmal flaps are developed along the sternocleidomastoid muscle for 1–2 cm superiorly and to the level of the clavicle inferiorly. Division of the external jugular vein may be necessary. The posterior aspect of the sternocleidomastoid muscle is then dissected free from the underlying carotid sheath structures at the point where the sternal and clavicular heads converge.

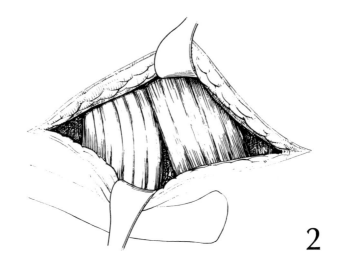

2

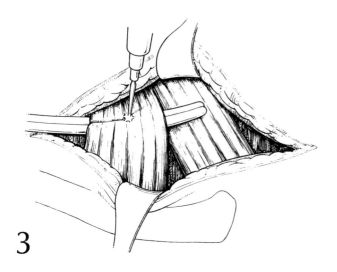

3

3 The sternal and clavicular heads, including the underlying investing cervical fascia, are divided at this level using electrocautery, with care taken to ensure hemostasis. The spinal accessory nerve is usually located superior to this region.

4 The ends of the transected sternocleidomastoid muscle are then dissected free from the underlying carotid sheath structures. Limited dissection is performed superiorly while more extensive dissection is performed inferiorly down to the level of the sternum and clavicle.

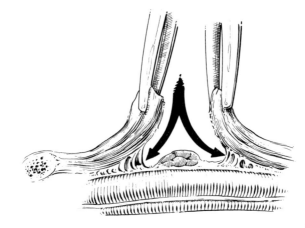

4

5 The head is turned from side to side and the depth of the wound palpated to ensure that all contracted tissue is released. If tight lateral structures, such as the deep cervical fascia lateral to the sternocleidomastoid muscle, are identified, these should be divided under direct vision. Although unusual, fascial tissue involved with the omohyoid muscle and the carotid sheath may occasionally require division.

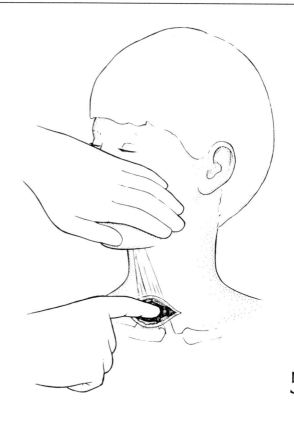

5

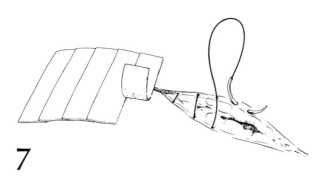

6

6 The platysma muscle is then reapproximated with interrupted 3/0 polyglactin (Vicryl) sutures.

7

7 The skin is approximated with a running 5/0 polyglactin subcuticular suture. Steristrips are placed perpendicular to the incision in overlying fashion such that a dressing is formed.

The patient is maintained in a 30° head-up position during and after recovery.

Postoperative care

For the first 48 h after operation the patient remains supine in the 30° head-up position without the use of a pillow. Careful assumption of the erect posture with initial assistance is then allowed. Physiotherapy with resumption of passive neck range-of-motion exercises is then reinstituted and continued for the following 6 months[9]. Full neck range of motion should be achieved by 7–10 days after operation. Older children must undergo retraining of the neck righting reflexes in front of a mirror over the following months. Occasionally, a patient who is too young or not willing to cooperate with postoperative physiotherapy will require placement of a Minerva cast for 6 weeks in order to maintain the head rotated toward the operatively treated side and tilted laterally toward the opposite side.

Complications

The most common complication is postoperative bleeding. Hematoma formation over the hours to days after the procedure may require evacuation. Specific attention to hemostasis during division of the muscular fascial tissues and to potential bleeding from tributaries of the internal jugular vein should prevent this complication. The risk of airway compromise secondary to postoperative bleeding is low. Injury to the spinal accessory or facial nerve is unusual.

Follow-up

In the 90% or more of patients who are managed without operative intervention, follow-up should include monitoring to ensure resolution of the sternocleidomastoid pseudotumor, residual sternocleidomastoid fibrosis and torticollis. Specifically, close follow-up should ensure the early detection of facial hemihypoplasia in those patients with persistent torticollis after 6 months of age[6].

After operation, recurrent torticollis is observed in fewer than 3% of patients[9]. Follow-up should include evaluation to ensure resolution of facial hemihypoplasia and plagiocephaly if present. In addition, because of the high incidence of residual cervical and thoracolumbar scoliosis in patients with torticollis, radiologic spine evaluation is indicated to ensure identification and appropriate follow-up of any spinal deformities[10].

References

1. Wolfort FG, Kanter MA, Miller LB. Torticollis. *Plast Reconstr Surg* 1989; 84: 682–92.

2. Middleton DS. The pathology of congenital torticollis. *Br J Surg* 1930; 18: 188–204.

3. Davids JR, Wenger DR, Mubarak SJ. Congenital muscular torticollis: sequela of intrauterine or perinatal compartment syndrome. *J Pediatr Orthop* 1993; 13: 141–7.

4. Thomsen JR, Koltai PJ. Sternomastoid tumor of infancy. *Ann Otol Rhinol Laryngol* 1989; 98: 955–9.

5. Tom LWC, Handler SD, Wetmore RF, Potsic WP. The sternocleidomastoid tumor of infancy. *Int J Pediatr Otorhinolaryngol* 1987; 13: 245–55.

6. De Chalain TMB, Katz A. Idiopathic muscular torticollis in children: the Cape Town experience. *Br J Plast Surg* 1992; 45: 297–301.

7. Morrison DL, MacEwen GD. Congenital muscular torticollis: observations regarding clinical findings, associated conditions, and results of treatment. *J Pediatr Orthop* 1982; 2: 500–5.

8. Slate RK, Posnick JC, Armstrong DC, Buncic JR. Cervical spine subluxation associated with congenital muscular torticollis and craniofacial asymmetry. *Plast Reconstr Surg* 1993; 91: 1187–97.

9. Wirth CJ, Hagena FW, Wuelker N, Siebert WE. Biterminal tenotomy for the treatment of congenital muscular torticollis. *J Bone Joint Surg [Am]* 1992; 74: 427–34.

10. Minamitani K, Inoue A, Okuno T. Results of surgical treatment of muscular torticollis for patients greater than 6 years of age. *J Pediatr Orthop* 1990; 10: 754–9.

Protruding ears

Steven R. Cohen MD
Co-Director, Center for Craniofacial Disorders, Scottish Rite Children's Hospital, Atlanta, Georgia, USA

F. D. Burstein MD
Co-Director, Center for Craniofacial Disorders, Scottish Rite Children's Hospital, Atlanta, Georgia, USA

Principles and justification

Anatomy of the external ear

1a, b The auricle is approximately 6 cm long in the adult. It lies between horizontal lines at the upper rim of the orbit and nasal spine and protrudes at about 30° from the skull[1]. The gap between the upper part of the helix and the skull is usually less than 2 cm. The cartilage has depressions and ridges that are easily seen in the overlying skin. The auricularis posterior is the thickest of three extrinsic muscles to the ear. It originates on the base of the mastoid and inserts onto the ponticulus, which is opposite the concha.

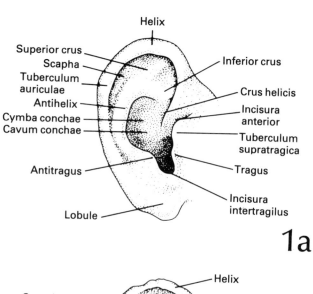

1a

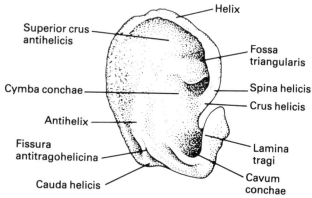

1b

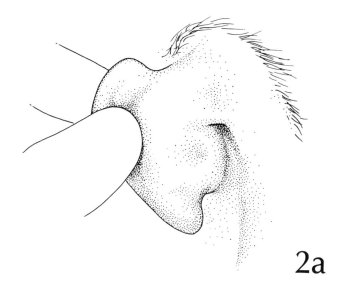

2a

2a, b Clinically, the auricularis posterior is demonstrated by pulling the ear forward. It is innervated by the posterior auricular branch of the facial nerve. The posterior auricular veins travel just deep to the great auricular nerve and are commonly encountered during deep dissection to expose the concha. To avoid bleeding the auricularis posterior muscle is best divided with electrocautery.

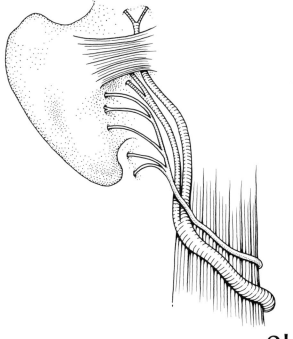

2b

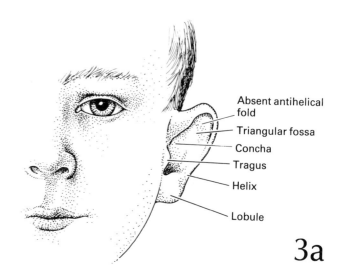

3a

Pathology of the protruding ear

3a, b During the third month of gestation the protrusion of the auricle increases; by the end of the sixth month the helical margin curls. The antihelix forms its fold and the antihelical crura appear. Anything that interferes with this process may result in prominent ears. The most common deformity arises from failure of the antihelix to fold. This widens the conchoscaphal angle to as much as 100° or more, flattening the superior crus and, in severe forms, the antihelical body and inferior crus. In extreme cases the helical rim may be absent, producing a flat, shell-like ear. The normal ear has a conchoscaphal angle of 90° or less, while the prominent ear has more obtuse angulation. Abnormalities are often bilateral and frequently present with variable degrees of symmetry.

Timing of operation

The optimum age for operation is between 5 and 7 years old. At this age the ear is nearly of adult size and the cartilage is of adequate thickness to tolerate scoring and hold sutures. Significant teasing generally has not occurred and the patients are usually well motivated and cooperative.

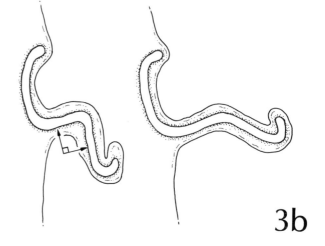

3b

Preoperative

Preoperative preparation includes photographic documentation with anterior–posterior, lateral, and posterior–anterior views. A detailed interview with the patient and the parents, with the emphasis on postoperative care, is conducted. Preoperative and postoperative photographs of children with similar deformities are often shown. Patients are asked to shampoo their hair the night before surgery. All operative procedures are done on an outpatient basis under general anesthesia. Intravenous antibiotics are routinely given before skin incision.

Operations

MUSTARDÉ'S PROCEDURE

Correction of the ear with either normal or absent antihelical fold is known as Mustardé's procedure[2].

4 The desired location of the antihelical fold and, if indicated, the amount of conchal resection, are marked using methylene blue.

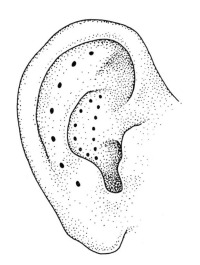

4

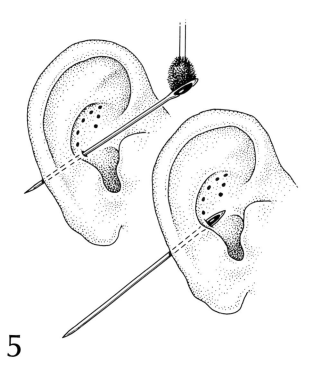

5

5 A Keith needle is used to tattoo the location of the antihelical fold as well as the posterior skin incision on the cartilage wall. Methylene blue is applied to the eyelet of the needle and the needle is pulled through the ear with the needle holder, marking anterior skin, cartilage and posterior skin.

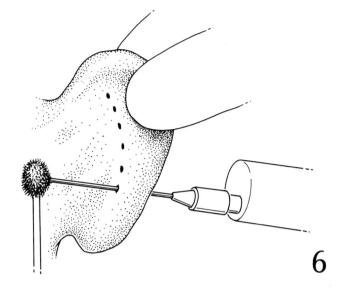

6 A 22 gauge needle may also be used.

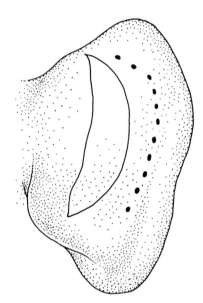

7 The proposed postauricular incision and area for conchal resection are injected with bupivacaine 0.25% and epinephrine (adrenaline) 1:400 000 concentration. An elliptical incision is made along the postauricular markings and dissection is carried out to expose the site of the proposed antihelical fold The skin excision is minimal to avoid a 'pinned back' appearance.

8 The dissection is carried out directly over the cartilage with an Iris scissor, or in the subcutaneous plane using electrocautery. The previously placed methylene blue tattoos along the line of the antihelical fold are directly visualized.

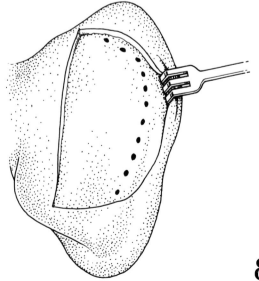

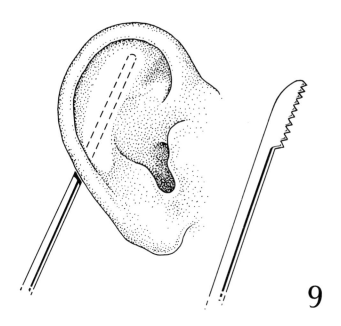

9 A small incision is made in the cartilage near the cauda helicis and a subperichondrial tunnel is made along the anterior surface of the cartilage with a Joseph elevator. An otobrader is then introduced along the same tunnel and gentle scoring of the cartilage is performed in a 5-mm wide strip until the antihelical fold can be produced with minimal fingertip pressure. Caution must be exercised to prevent lacerating the cartilage, which will result in too sharp a fold.

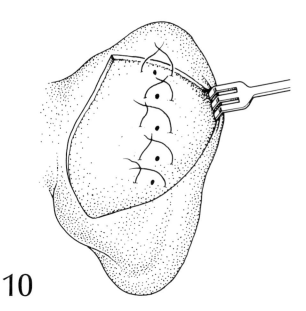

10 The tattoo marks are then used to guide the placement of permanent undyed 4/0 or 5/0 sutures (Mersilene or clear nylon are often used). These sutures are placed in a horizontal mattress fashion through the perichondrium and cartilage. The sutures are placed approximately 2 mm on either side of the tattoo marks along the antihelical fold. Generally four or five sutures are employed.

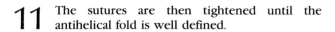

11 The sutures are then tightened until the antihelical fold is well defined.

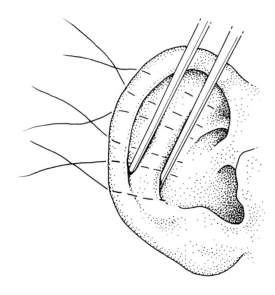

CONCHAL ALTERATION

Dieffenbach is credited with the first otoplastic attempt which consisted of excising skin from the auriculo-cephalic sulcus and suturing the conchal cartilage to the mastoid periosteum[3].

12 Conchal alteration[4] is used to supplement creation of an antihelical fold, further reducing the conchoscaphal angle when necessary. A finger is inserted into the concha, which is displaced posteriorly and superiorly toward the mastoid periosteum. A permanent 4/0 undyed Mersilene or clear nylon suture is placed in a vertical mattress fashion, first in the concha and then in the periosteum of the mastoid. Generally three sutures are utilized.

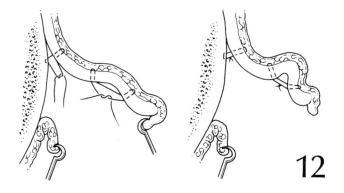

13 The conchal sutures are tied before tying the sutures used to recreate the antihelical fold.

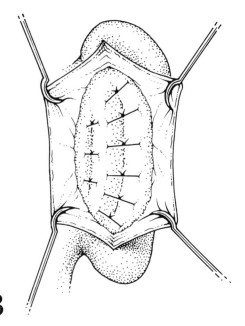

14 When conchal resection is necessary, a cartilaginous ellipse beneath the antihelical body may be excised. This is closed directly with permanent 4/0 or 5/0 undyed suture material.

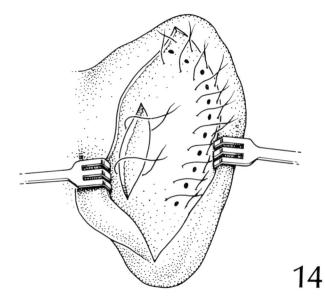

15a, b Skin closure is carried out using a continuous 5/0 plain catgut suture. When the superior or inferior poles are protruding beyond the central one-third of the ear, a dumb-bell shaped skin excision may be carried out (*Illustration 15b*).

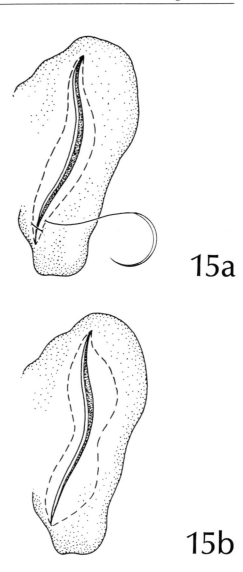

15a

15b

Dressings

16 Xeroform petrolatum dressing impregnated with an antibiotic ointment is placed within the contours of the ear and used to fill the conchal bowl. Moistened cotton is then rolled behind the ear and used to supplement the Xeroform within the conchal bowl.

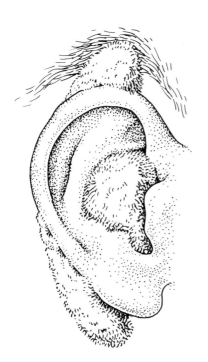

16

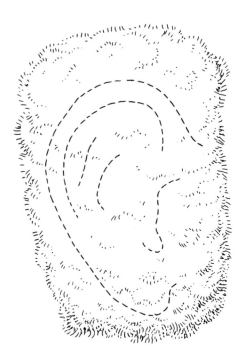

17a, b Additional cotton is packed over both ears, and the head is wrapped with soft gauze rolls and a cap of burn netting to complete the dressing. A meticulous dressing is essential to prevent subpericonchal hematoma or folding of the ear.

17a

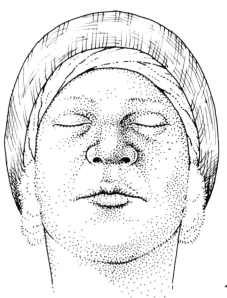

17b

Postoperative care

The dressing is removed on the third postoperative day, and the postauricular incision is cleaned with peroxide; a small amount of topical antibiotic is applied to the incision twice daily. The patient is asked to bring a terry-cloth tennis-type headband with them at the time of dressing removal and this is worn night and day for 3 days and then only at night for another 2 weeks. This prevents inadvertent trauma to the ear during sleep. The patient is allowed to wash their hair and swim after the third postoperative day. A first-generation cephalosporin is administered, beginning at the time of surgery and continuing for a total of 5 days. Contact sports are allowed after 4 weeks.

Complications

Any hematoma should be promptly drained using a 19 gauge needle to prevent organization and a 'cauliflower ear'. If this occurs a conforming dressing is reapplied for an additional 3 days.

Infection with chondritis should be suspected if there is fever, a loss of ear definition or a sudden increase in postoperative pain. Prompt drainage, culture and appropriate antibiotic therapy are essential to prevent cartilage loss.

Streptococcus and *Staphylococcus* usually account for early acute infections while *Pseudomonas* may present with chronic drainage. Rarely it may be necessary to debride devitalized cartilage and treat with intravenous antibiotics.

Late deformities are usually due to surgical error. A 'telephone ear' may result from over-zealous skin excision from the middle third of the ear with or without over-resection of the conchal cartilage. Correction involves resection of skin from the upper and lower thirds of the ear and/or adding a full-thickness skin graft to the middle third of the ear. A very sharp antihelical fold with prominent cartilage edges may result from cartilage lacerations from exaggerated pressure on the otobrader or from over-tightening of the horizontal mattress sutures used to create the fold. Some correction may be achieved by releasing one or more of these sutures. In severe cases, a thin temporalis fascia graft can be tunneled over the antihelical cartilage to soften the irregularities. Slight asymmetries may become evident after all of the postoperative edema subsides. These can usually be corrected by judicious postauricular skin excision.

Keloid formation is rare and should be treated with steroid injections and massage. Excision may require a full thickness skin graft to prevent obliteration of the postauricular sulcus with a 'plastered down appearance'.

References

1. Allison GR. Anatomy of the external ear. *Clin Plast Surg* 1978; 5: 419–22.

2. Mustardé JC. The correction of prominent ears using simple mattress sutures. *Br J Plast Surg* 1963; 16: 170–8.

3. Dieffenbach JF. *Die Operative Chirurgie*. Leipzig: Brockhaus, 1845.

4. Brent B. Reconstruction of the auricle. In: McCarthy JG, ed. *Plastic Surgery, Volume 3, The Face, Part 2*. Philadelphia: Saunders, 1990: 2094–152.

Tracheostomy

John N. G. Evans DLO, FRCS
Consultant Ear, Nose and Throat Surgeon, Great Ormond Street Hospital for Children and St Thomas' Hospital, London, UK

Principles and justification

Tracheostomy should be performed as an elective procedure. Children are usually intubated.

Indications

1. Airway obstruction
   (a) Congenital anomalies, e.g. laryngeal webs, sub-glottic stenosis;
   (b) Acute infection, e.g. epiglottitis, acute laryngo-tracheobronchitis;
   (c) Increasing laryngeal edema and evidence of mucosal damage as a consequence of naso-tracheal intubation;
   (d) Functional obstruction, e.g. recurrent laryngeal paralysis, cricoarytenoid fixation;
   (e) Tumors, e.g. hematoma, lymphangioma, papilloma;
   (f) External trauma, e.g. 'hanging' type injuries;
   (g) Extrinsic or intrinsic narrowing of the trachea.
2. Long-term respiratory support after cardiac surgery or in cases of pulmonary pathology or thoracic dystrophy.
3. Clearance of secretions.
4. As a preliminary procedure to operations on the larynx, pharynx or temporomandibular joints.

Preoperative

Anesthesia

The operation is performed under general anesthesia. In exceptional circumstances preliminary intubation of the trachea may be impossible, in which case a local anesthetic using 1% lidocaine (lignocaine) with epinephrine (adrenaline) 1:200 000 is necessary.

Operation

Position of patient

1 The neck must be hyperextended. A sandbag, or rolled towel in the case of a neonate, is placed under the shoulders. The occiput is supported by a ring. The patient is tipped into the head-up position and a diathermy pad applied.

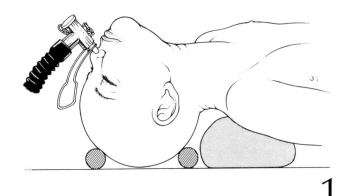

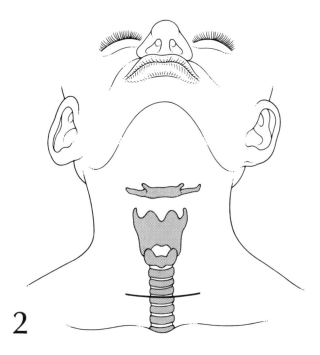

Incision

2 The neck is palpated carefully so that the hyoid bone and cricoid cartilages can be felt. The skin over the third tracheal ring is infiltrated using 1% lidocaine with 1:200 000 epinephrine. This aids hemostasis. A transverse skin incision approximately 2 cm in length is made through the infiltrated area, cutting through fat and platysma.

3 The incision is deepened in a horizontal plane until the deep cervical fascia investing the sternohyoid and sternothyroid muscles is encountered. Branches of the anterior jugular vein will be seen during this dissection; these should be coagulated with diathermy and divided.

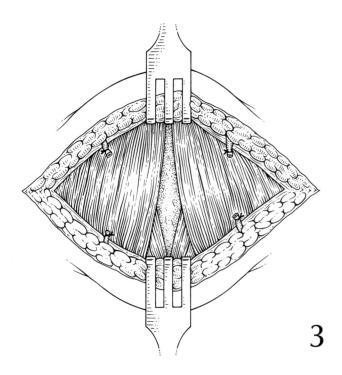

4   Having identified the strap muscles, a condensation
     of the investing layer of the deep cervical fascia will
be seen running vertically between the sternohyoid and
sternothyroid muscles. This interval is entered by blunt
scissor dissection in a vertical direction and the strap
muscles separated and retracted laterally.

Exposure of thyroid gland

Retracting of the strap muscles reveals the thyroid gland
with the thyroid isthmus joining the two lobes of the
gland. Above the isthmus the cricoid is seen, and even in
a neonate it is easy to identify by touch.

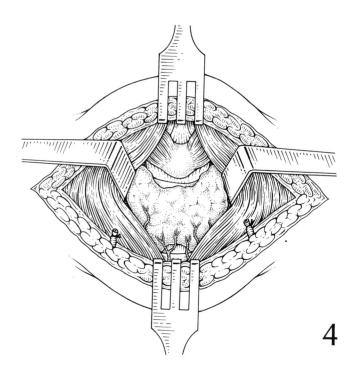

4

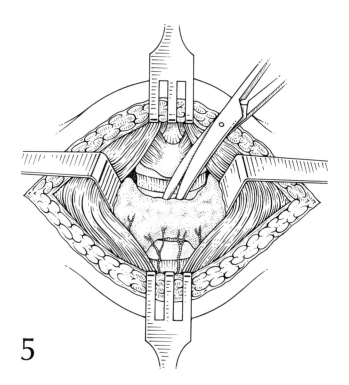

5

Dissection of thyroid isthmus

5   The size and relationship of the thyroid isthmus to
     the trachea is variable, but in almost all cases the
isthmus should be divided. A small incision is made
through the condensation of the pretracheal fascia at the
upper border of the isthmus, and the isthmus is then
separated from the underlying trachea by blunt
dissection. Branches of the inferior thyroid vein will be
encountered at the lower border of the isthmus, and
these should be coagulated with diathermy.

Division of thyroid isthmus

6 A hemostat is placed at each side of the isthmus, which is then divided, the cut ends being secured by suture ligation.

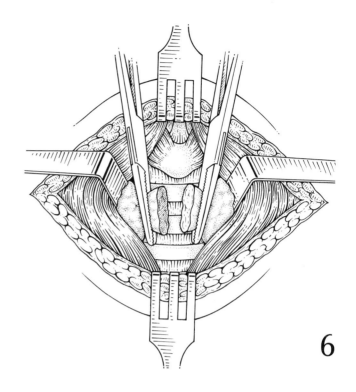

6

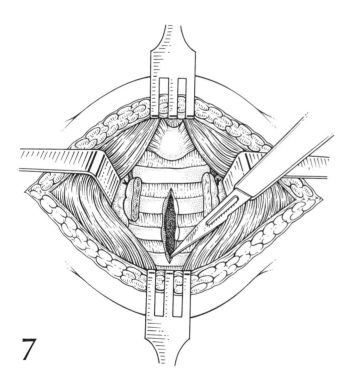

7

Opening the trachea

Careful hemostasis is achieved and the tracheal rings counted: the first tracheal ring must *not* be included in the tracheostomy.

7 For a routine tracheostomy in children a vertical incision is made in the trachea through the second, third and fourth tracheal rings. If a subsequent reconstructive operation upon the larynx is planned, the incision in the trachea is made through the third, fourth and fifth tracheal rings. Care should be taken with a low tracheostome that the end of the tracheostomy tube is clear of the carina. A small sucker should be used to prevent blood from entering the trachea.

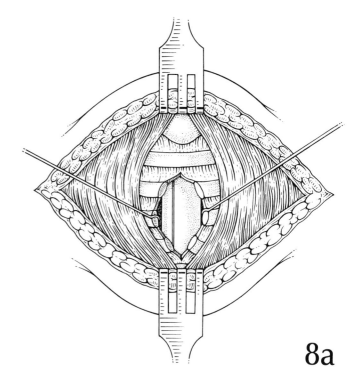

8a

8a, b Fine skin hooks are now used to distract the cut edges of the trachea. The endotracheal tube will then be clearly seen.

An alternative method of distracting the tracheal opening is to use stay sutures which are taped to the skin until the first tracheostomy tube change.

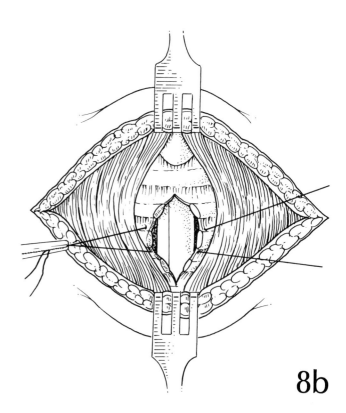

8b

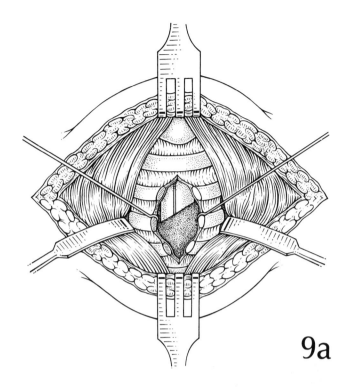

9a

Insertion of tracheostomy tube

9a, b The anesthetist is asked to withdraw the endotracheal tube gently until its proximal end is just above the tracheostome. The tracheostomy tube is then inserted into the tracheal opening.

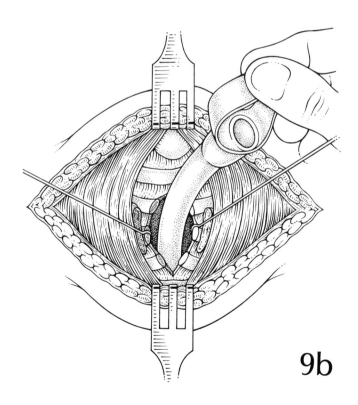

9b

Fixation of tracheostomy tube

When the tracheostomy tube is fully inserted it must be held by the assistant until it is properly secured. The skin edges are partly approximated with a suture on each side of the tube. It is essential to leave a gap around the tube to avoid postoperative surgical emphysema.

10 The sandbag is then removed from underneath the patient's shoulders and the tracheostomy tube is secured by tying the tapes with a reef knot with the *neck flexed*. It is extremely important to remember this neck flexion and to tie the tapes fairly tightly; failure to do this may result in the tube becoming dislodged. This must be avoided during the immediate postoperative period as subsequent insertion of the tracheostomy tube can be difficult in the first few postoperative days. A non-adherent dressing is applied to the wound with a keyhole to accommodate the tracheostomy tube. This dressing should be changed when necessary and kept clean.

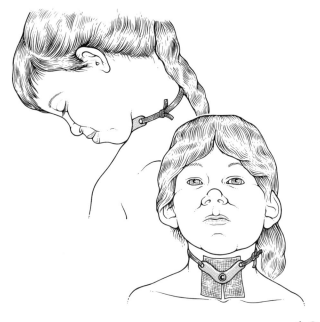

10

Postoperative care

The following must be provided at the bedside:
(a) A tracheostomy tube of the same size as that in the patient.
(b) Suction apparatus and sterile catheters with holes in the side.
(c) A tracheal dilator.
(d) A properly trained nurse.
(e) Humidification.

On return to the ward a chest radiograph should be arranged to check the length of the tracheostomy tube and its position with regard to its proximity to the carina, and to ensure that the right main bronchus has not been intubated. Suction is applied via the tracheostomy tube. This will be necessary half-hourly for the first few days after operation. Suction is facilitated by the instillation of 2 ml of sterile normal saline into the tracheostomy tube. A sterile catheter is inserted into the tracheal lumen gently but quickly, and suction is applied only as the catheter is withdrawn.

If the tracheostomy tube is properly positioned and functioning satisfactorily, respiration should be inaudible. If bubbling noises are heard, further suction is required.

Adequate humidification in a head box must be provided for neonates; this is also important for children in oxygen tents, or for older children using a thermostatically controlled humidifier connected to the tracheostomy tube. This will reduce the frequency of suction and the tenacity of secretions, and allow the tracheostomy tube to remain patent.

The tracheostomy tube is changed after the first week. If any difficulty is encountered during suction, if breathing becomes noisy despite suction, or if the child begins to phonate, then the tube must be changed immediately. This should be done with adequate help: the child's neck must be extended, good illumination is essential, and a headlight is desirable. As the tracheostomy tube is withdrawn the tracheostome should be visible and a new tube is readily inserted under direct vision. If difficulty is encountered, a tracheal dilator must be inserted into the tracheal lumen, after which subsequent intubation of the trachea should present no difficulty.

The most common cause for difficulty in suction of the trachea is displacement of the tube in front of the trachea. This is always accompanied by audible respiration and by the child being able to phonate.

Complications

Intraoperative

1. Bleeding may be encountered from an abnormally high innominate artery. Careful controlled dissection of the structures in the lower part of the neck should avoid this.
2. Damage to the cervical pleura may cause a pneumothorax; dissection lateral to the trachea should be avoided.
3. Injury to the esophagus should not occur when an elective tracheostomy is performed.

Postoperative

1. *Blocking and displacement of the tracheostomy tube*. These complications are preventable by careful nursing and attention to detail when tying tracheostomy tube tapes.
2. *Postoperative pneumonia*. This risk is small if a sterile technique of tracheal toilet is used and effective humidification maintained. Adequate physiotherapy to encourage coughing is also desirable.
3. *Surgical emphysema*. If this occurs the wound should be opened fully. It is caused by suturing the wound too tightly around the tracheostomy tube.
4. *Hemorrhage*. Erosion of the anterior wall of the trachea may well occur if a metal tracheostomy tube of the incorrect curvature is used. The overlying innominate artery may also be damaged, in which event a frequently fatal hemorrhage will result.
5. *Stenosis*. This may occur at the tracheostome if cartilage is removed during the tracheostomy, or at the tip of the tube if suction is too vigorous or incorrectly applied.
6. *Difficult decannulation*. In the absence of persisting pathology, decannulation may be facilitated by using a metal fenestrated tube which can be fitted with a blocker (Alder Hey pattern). Care must be taken to ensure that the fenestration of the tracheostomy tube is correctly positioned.
7. *Persistent tracheal fistula*. After prolonged tracheostomy, removal of the tube may result in a persistent fistula at the site of the tracheostomy. This is not serious. If it either fails to close or a persistent leak of mucus issues from it, the tract may be excised and a formal closure performed. In young children this may be done conveniently before they start school.

In an emergency, for example in the case of acute epiglottitis when sudden airway obstruction may occur and peroral endotracheal intubation may not be possible, a cricothyrotomy should be considered in preference to a crash tracheostomy which can be extremely difficult in the child whose trachea is soft and not always easy to identify.

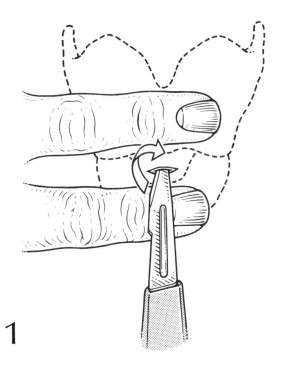

CRICOTHYROTOMY

11 The child is held with the neck extended and the left hand is placed with the first finger over the cricoid cartilage and the second over the thyroid cartilage. A transverse stab incision is made through the cricothyroid membrane. The blade of the knife is then turned vertically, establishing the airway so that a tracheal dilator or any other tube of suitable size may be inserted to preserve the airway and to enable general anesthesia to be undertaken safely. Elective tracheostomy is then performed.

11

Further reading

Duncan BW, Howell LJ, de Lorimier AA, Adzick NS, Harrison MR. Tracheostomy in children with emphasis on home care. *J Pediatr Surg* 1992; 27: 432–5.

Cystic hygroma

Craig T. Albanese MD
Assistant Professor of Surgery, Division of Pediatric Surgery, School of Medicine, University of Pittsburgh and Department of Surgery, The Children's Hospital of Pittsburgh, Pittsburgh, Pennsylvania, USA

Eugene S. Wiener MD, FACS, FAAP
Professor of Surgery, Division of Pediatric Surgery, School of Medicine, University of Pittsburgh and Department of Surgery, The Children's Hospital of Pittsburgh, Pittsburgh, Pennsylvania, USA

Cystic hygroma is a term describing a benign multilobular, multinodular cystic mass which arises from lymph ducts along the venous channels. It may occur anywhere in the body, most commonly in the neck (75%); axilla (20%); or mediastinum, retroperitoneum, pelvis and groin (5%). Neck hygromas may communicate beneath the clavicle with other axillary hygromas, mediastinal hygromas, or rarely both. The most common location in the neck is the posterior triangle.

The mass is often observed at birth and sudden enlargement may be preceded by an upper respiratory tract infection, trauma or a spontaneous hemorrhage. The majority of neck hygromas are asymptomatic initially but, depending on location, some may cause symptoms of pharyngeal or upper airway obstruction. Partial or complete regression occasionally occurs either spontaneously or after an upper respiratory tract infection, but this is too rare to warrant expectant management so excision after diagnosis is the accepted therapy. The risks of expectant management are several: infection, progressive growth and disfigurement, extension into previously uninvolved areas, dysphagia, airway compromise and erosion into vascular structures with hemorrhage. Surgical excision may be preceded by needle aspiration if acute airway compromise is present or by incision and drainage for a floridly infected cyst. The use of sclerosing agents (in lieu of surgery) has had inconsistent results. Timing of excision is usually not crucial. Asymptomatic cysts in the premature or small-for-dates child may await growth and development of the infant. For the majority of patients there is no need to defer excision.

Preoperative

Physical examination is the mainstay of the evaluation of the child with a cystic hygroma, and extension into the axilla or oral cavity must be noted. For large neck hygromas, a radiograph of the chest is required to assess mediastinal involvement (2–3%). Ultrasonography, computed tomographic scanning and magnetic resonance imaging are useful for determining the extent of disease, especially if one suspects an intraoral or mediastinal component. Magnetic resonance imaging is also useful in the diagnosis of orbital lymphangiomas. In general, however, the authors consider it unnecessary to use any of these imaging methods.

Anesthesia

General endotracheal anesthesia is always used. Blood should be available for the larger cysts or those that communicate with the pharynx, axilla or mediastinum.

Operation

The method described below is for excision of a posterior triangular, cervical cystic hygroma.

Caveats of dissection

Even if the preoperative evaluation reveals a unilocular cyst, it is not unusual to encounter multiple hygromas. These masses tend to grow along fascial planes and around neurovascular structures. Intraoperative cyst rupture increases the difficulty of dissection, since the thin-walled empty cyst is difficult to identify and the margins are obscure. Every extension of the cyst must be excised with the main mass. This is not a malignant lesion, however, so there is no need to sacrifice normal structures in the course of operation. If any tumour is to be left behind, it is imperative to leave no intact cysts. Any structures that suggest lymphatic trunks should be ligated or cauterized to minimize postoperative fluid accumulation.

Position of patient

The patient is positioned with the neck slightly hyperextended using a shoulder roll and the head is turned to the side opposite the lesion.

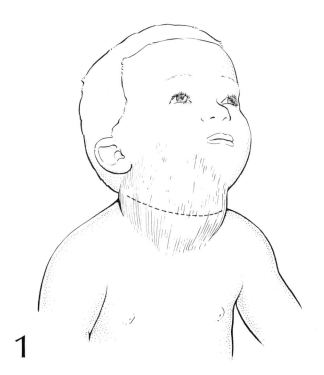

Incision

1 A transverse skin crease incision extending the length of the mass is placed over its mid portion. Antibiotics are administered within 1 h of the incision.

2 The hygroma never involves the skin, so dissection is preceded by generous subplatysmal skin flaps (arrows). The external jugular vein as well as branches of the ansa cervicalis are sacrificed.

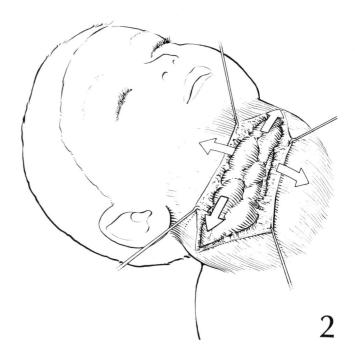

2

3a, b Dissection is usually begun at the superior margin of the mass near the ramus of the mandible. In this location, the mandibular branch of the facial nerve (arrow) is encountered. The nerve does not usually enter the lesion and can be safely dissected free.

Optical magnification is helpful. Bipolar cautery is used routinely during the entire dissection. Not only does this ensure a hemostatic dissection, but it decreases the incidence of lymph leak due to cauterization of the fine lymphatic channels.

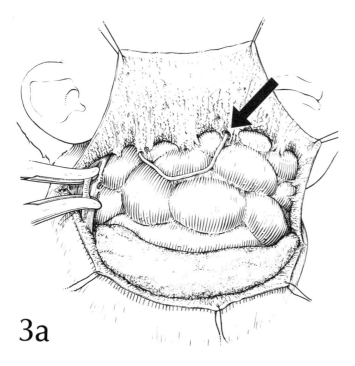

3a

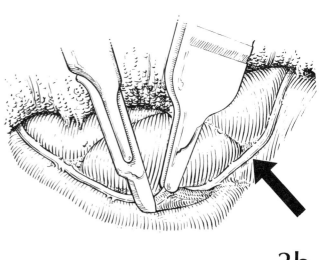

3b

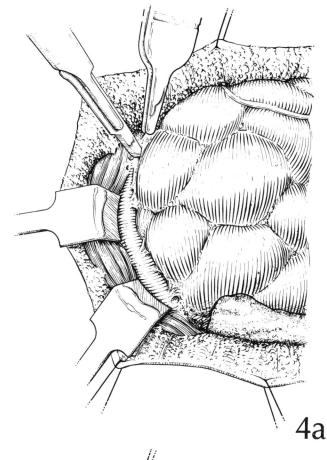

4a

4a, b The dissection proceeds medially, lifting the cyst from the surrounding alveolar tissue. It is usually necessary to divide the middle thyroid vein (arrow) as the carotid sheath is approached. The deep dissection frequently involves the contents of the carotid sheath, as well as other nearby vascular and neural structures.

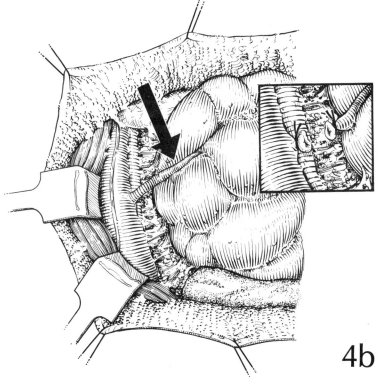

4b

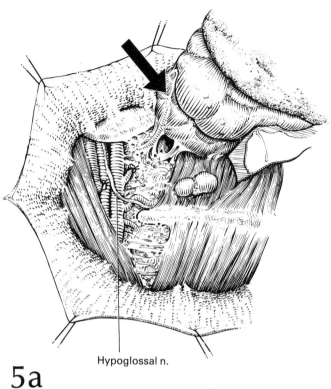

Hypoglossal n.

5a

5a, b Care is taken to preserve the hypoglossal nerve as it passes within the bifurcation of the common carotid artery. The mass must then be freed from the hyoid bone as well as the submandibular gland (arrow). It is sometimes necessary to remove the submandibular gland (sacrificing the facial artery, *Illustration 5b*) *en bloc* with the mass. The inferior border of the mass may be adherent to portions of the brachial plexus. Posteriorly the spinal accessory nerve is spared, if possible.

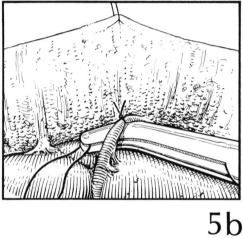

5b

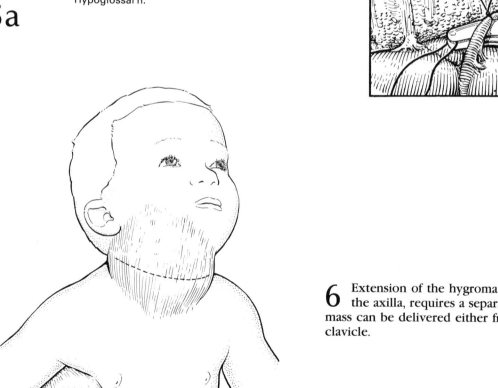

6 Extension of the hygroma under the clavicle, into the axilla, requires a separate axillary incision. The mass can be delivered either from above or below the clavicle.

6

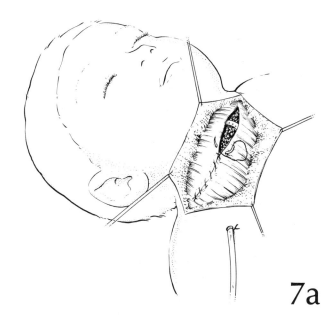

7a

7a, b The platysma is reapproximated with fine absorbable sutures and the skin with subcuticular sutures of similar material. Closed suction drainage is used in all cases.

Postoperative care

Feeding can be resumed as soon as the infant is awake and alert. Extensive intraoral dissection may temporarily impair swallowing and delay the onset of oral feeds. Removal of the drain is dictated by daily volume of drainage. Antibiotics are administered postoperatively for 5 days in neonates and for 24 h in older children.

Outcome

Recurrence is not rare, and is most likely within the first year after resection. The recurrence rate is low (10%) if all macroscopic disease is resected. When gross disease is left, recurrences occur in up to 100% of patients. Lymph leaks and nerve injuries are minimized by the use of bipolar diathermy. Lymph leaks are treated with adequate drainage and may require re-exploration.

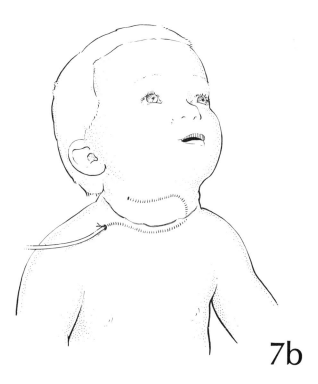

7b

Preauricular sinus

R. J. Brereton FRCS
Consultant Paediatric Surgeon, Chelsea and Westminster Hospital, London, UK

Principles and justification

The preauricular sinus is a congenital sinus situated on the anterior aspect of the helix which passes anteriorly and inferiorly through the skin to end in a racemose group of preauricular cysts. They arise from imperfect fusion of the six fetal tubercles which form the pinna. Symptoms are rare in infants. Infection commonly occurs in older children and is difficult to treat. If untreated, recurrent infection results in a preauricular ulcer. The lesion may be unilateral or bilateral and may be familial. Complete excision is necessary to effect a cure.

Preoperative

Surgery should not be undertaken if there is active acute infection. This should be treated with antistaphylococcal antibiotics, because such organisms are almost invariably the cause of the suppuration. Oblique incisions to drain pus should be avoided as they are associated with unacceptable scarring and may result in an ulcer surrounded by infected granulation tissue. In chronically infected cases, surgery should be covered by appropriate antibiotics commencing 2–3 days before the operation and continuing for several days afterwards.

The injection of a coloured dye into the duct to outline the extent of the subcutaneous gland is generally unhelpful and may be misleading as the dye seldom outlines the full extent of the lesion. Rupture of the gland with escape of the dye may result in the excision of an unnecessarily large amount of normal tissue.

Anesthesia

General anesthesia by endotracheal tube is recommended, particularly for bilateral lesions.

The preauricular region should be infiltrated with 1:1000 epinephrine (adrenaline) in saline solution or a local anesthetic agent which also serves to reduce postoperative discomfort.

Operation

Position and toweling

Any hair immediately anterior to the pinna should be shaved. For bilateral cases standard head toweling is indicated but when the lesion is unilateral a circumcision towel with a central aperture for the preauricular region suffices.

Exposure

1   A purse-string suture of 5/0 nylon or 4/0 silk is inserted around the punctum and used for holding the skin flap to be raised. An inverted L-shaped incision is made with the vertical limb running along the groove anterior to the pinna and the horizontal limb in the hairline.

The flap of skin so outlined is raised using fine-needle point diathermy which controls the hemorrhage. Damage to the preauricular nerve and vessels can be prevented by avoiding unnecessarily deep dissection immediately anterior to the pinna.

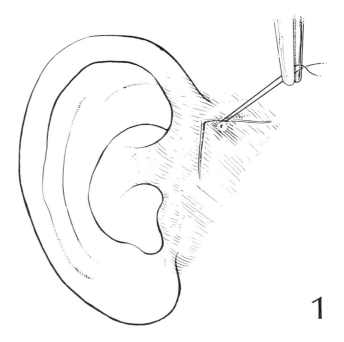

1

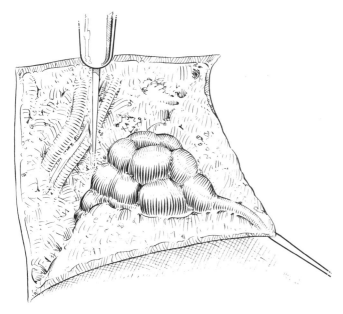

2

2   As dissection of the flap proceeds, the level of dissection is progressively deepened to avoid leaving any of the racemose gland. The gland is dissected anteriorly on the elevated flap.

Removal of the gland

3 Having dissected the gland completely from its fascial attachments it merely remains to detach the gland and its duct from the elevated skin flap. The flap is held vertically and the gland excised using a scalpel blade or needle diathermy. Care should be taken not to buttonhole the flap.

Wound closure

The flap is repositioned using two or three subcutaneous sutures of 5/0 chromic catgut and the skin edges approximated with small interrupted sutures of 6/0 polypropylene. The holding stitch is removed.

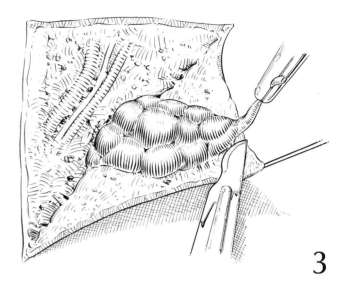

3

Postoperative care

To prevent postoperative hematoma formation the preauricular depression, crevices of the pinna and postauricular space should be lightly packed with proflavine wool and a pressure dressing of orthopedic wool and crepe bandage applied. The dressing may be kept in place by a helmet made from elastic tubular stockinette. The pressure dressing is removed after 24 h and the sutures after 5 days.

Outcome

Provided all the subcutaneous glandular tissue has been excised, a cure is assured and the cosmetic result is excellent. In patients who have suffered recurrent infections, the preauricular skin is usually very thin and scarred and the cosmetic result is less satisfactory.

Further reading

Singer R. A new technic for extirpation of preauricular cysts. *Am J Surg* 1966; 111: 291–5.

Illustrations by Marks Creative Consultants

Thoracic surgery: general principles of access

David A. Lloyd MChir, FRCS, FACS, FCS(SA)
Professor of Paediatric Surgery, University of Liverpool, and Consultant Paediatric Surgeon, Alder Hey Children's Hospital, Liverpool, UK

Principles and justification

Thoracotomy in infants and young children differs from the procedure in adults. The chest of the infant is compliant and relatively short in its longitudinal axis so a lateral transverse incision, entering the chest through the fifth intercostal space, is suitable for most operations. It is not necessary to remove or transect a rib. The posterior incision, which curves upwards around the scapula, is rarely required.

For esophageal atresia, a higher approach through the fourth or third space is needed. An approach below the fifth space is required for access to the diaphragm (bearing in mind that in the infant the liver is relatively large and elevates the right hemidiaphragm) or to the distal oesophagus on the left.

A median sternotomy is used for access to the mediastinum or to explore simultaneously both lungs.

The skin is incised with a scalpel; to minimize blood loss diathermy is used for subsequent layers.

Operations

THORACOTOMY

Position of patient and incision

1 The child lies in the full lateral position. The arm on the side of the incision lies forwards and upwards over the face or on an arm rest. A bolster placed under the chest approximately in the line of the nipples may aid the exposure. The child is firmly stabilized in position with sandbags or pads at the front and back of the chest, and adhesive strapping across the hips and perhaps the shoulders.

The skin is widely prepared with antiseptic solution. Sterile towels are placed to keep the nipple, lower scapula, spine, and costal margin visible as landmarks. A large adhesive plastic sheet membrane is applied to stabilize the towels and reduce heat loss. The lower chest wall is included in the operative field for later chest drain placement.

The lateral transverse incision starts posterior and inferior to the nipple to avoid damaging the immature breast tissue, and extends posteriorly below the inferior tip of the scapula, as far as the erector spinae muscle. The incision should be low enough not to cross the scapula even when the arm is brought down, as this may lead to an unsightly scar.

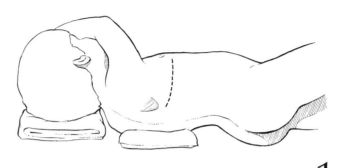

1

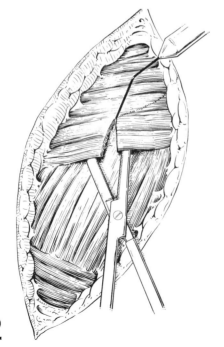

2

2 The subcutaneous tissues are divided, followed by the pectoralis major, latissimus dorsi and serratus anterior muscles. A pair of artery forceps is passed deep to the muscle to lift it while it is being cut with diathermy. Bleeding vessels are accurately picked up with toothed forceps and coagulated. The scapula is then elevated with a retractor and the ribs counted; the highest that can be palpated is usually the second rib.

Opening the chest

3 The intercostal muscles are divided with diathermy along the upper border of the rib, to avoid the neurovascular bundle. A short incision is made initially, using artery forceps to spread the muscle and, with the lungs deflated by the anesthetist, the pleural cavity is entered.

The remaining intercostal muscle is then divided with the diathermy, using a peanut swab or retractor to protect the lung.

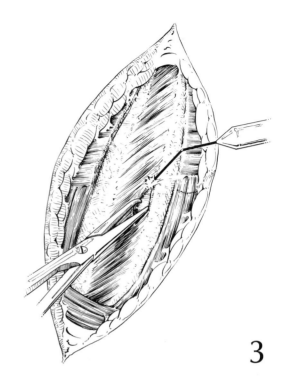

3

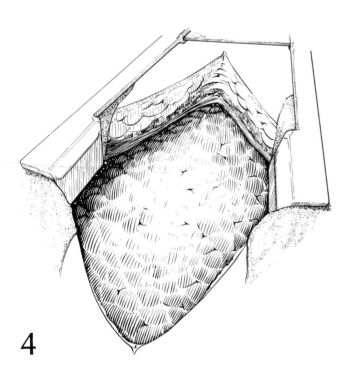

4

4 A small rib retractor (such as the Finochietto retractor) is inserted and opened slowly while dividing the intercostal muscles anteriorly and posteriorly. The chest wall muscles and subcutaneous tissues may also need to be incised further.

Extrapleural approach

5 Division of the intercostal muscles begins as shown in *Illustration 3*, using artery forceps to enter the extrapleural space in the posterior half of the incision and diathermy to incise the muscle.

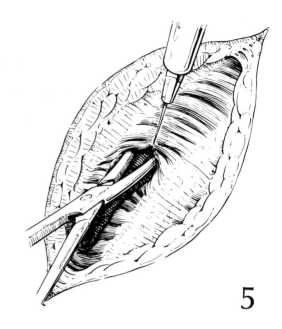

5

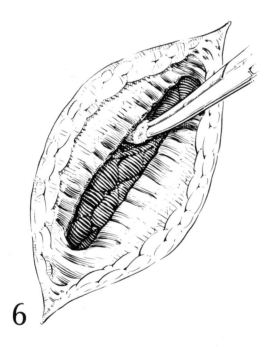

6

6 A moist peanut swab is used carefully to extend the extrapleural dissection. Anteriorly the pleura is adherent to the ribs and easily torn, and the dissection must proceed in a posterior direction.

7 A moist gauze swab is then unfolded and packed into the extrapleural space posteriorly and cranially in order to strip the pleura from the chest wall. The swab is removed, a small rib retractor is inserted, and the extrapleural dissection to the posterior mediastinum is completed under direct vision.

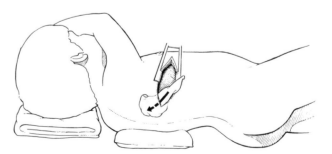

7

Wound closure

Before closing, a chest drain is inserted through a short transverse incision in the mid-axillary line, two intercostal spaces below the thoracotomy incision. The drain is passed into the chest, sutured to the skin and connected to an underwater seal.

To enhance postoperative analgesia, the intercostal nerves are infiltrated with local anesthetic posteriorly at the level of the incision and in the two spaces above and below.

8 Three or four pericostal sutures are passed around the ribs above and below the incision, taking care to avoid the intercostal vessels, and firmly tied to approximate the ribs. In the neonate an absorbable suture is used and the ribs are approximated gently. Tight apposition of these pliable ribs may result in them fusing together. If possible, the intercostal muscles and periosteum are closed, but this is not essential.

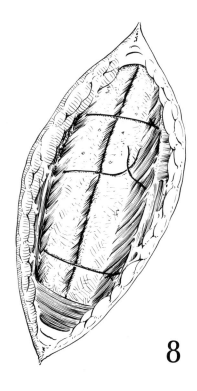

8

9 The chest wall muscles and subcutaneous layer are repaired in anatomical layers using continuous absorbable sutures; accurate closure enhances the functional and cosmetic outcome. In particular, the edges of the divided muscles must be aligned accurately. The skin is closed with an absorbable subcuticular suture or adhesive strips.

The chest drain is removed when there is no air leak and the lung has re-expanded.

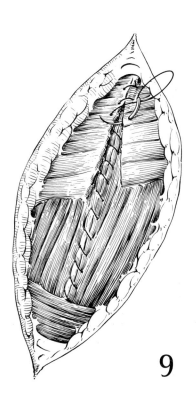

9

Subperiosteal incision

This approach, which may be used even in premature infants, preserves the intercostal muscles and provides access to the extrapleural space.

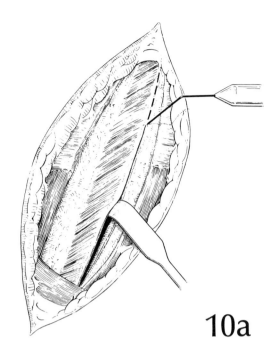

10a, b On the rib below the intercostal space to be entered, the periosteum is incised longitudinally using the diathermy. The periostium is elevated in an anterior direction off the upper border of the rib using a curved raspatory. This exposes the posterior periosteum, which is incised to enter the extrapleural space or the pleural cavity. The incision continues as above.

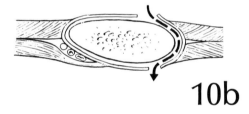

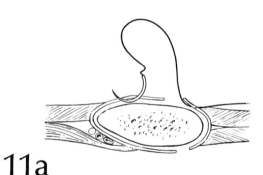

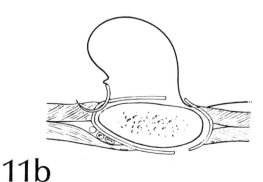

Closure of chest

11a, b To close the chest, pericostal sutures are inserted in the usual manner and are used to approximate the ribs but need not be tied. The cranial edge of the incised periosteum and intercostal muscle is sutured with an absorbable suture to the periosteum over the rib, or at the lower edge of the rib where muscle may be included. The pericostal sutures are then tied or may be removed.

MEDIAN STERNOTOMY

Position of the patient and incision

12 The child lies supine, with a bolster placed under the upper thorax to hyperextend the thoracic spine and bring the sternum forward. Slight elevation of the head of the operating table will reduce venous congestion.

The skin is incised from just below the suprasternal notch to the xiphoid cartilage.

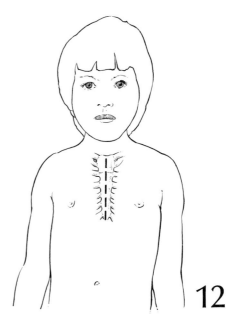

12

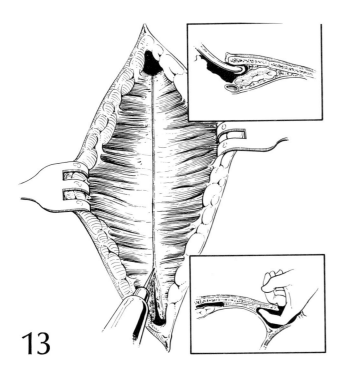

13

13 The subcutaneous tissues over the sternum are divided with diathermy. In the suprasternal notch the soft tissues are dissected off the superior and posterior aspects of the manubrium with sharp and blunt dissection. Inferiorly, the xiphoid is mobilized and divided vertically with heavy scissors or diathermy. It is possible now to enter the retrosternal plane cranially and caudally, using a peanut swab or finger to free the mediastinal structures from the back of the sternum.

Dividing the sternum

14 The sternum is divided vertically in the midline using a suitable bone saw. In the infant, shears or sturdy scissors are adequate. Ventilation should be suspended while this is done to avoid opening the pleura. Bleeding, which usually is from the periosteum or bone marrow, is controlled with diathermy and bone wax.

A self-retaining retractor is inserted and opened slowly while dissecting the soft tissues off the inner aspect of the ribs. In the infant it may be necessary to mobilize and retract the thymus gland; this is done by sharp and blunt dissection from below upwards, ligating larger vessels. Laterally, care must be taken not to damage the phrenic nerves.

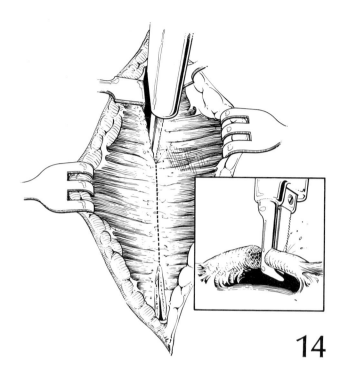

14

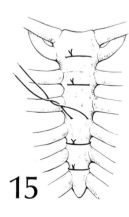

15

Wound closure

Whether or not the pleural cavity has been opened, one or two suction drainage catheters should be placed in the retrosternal space and brought out through stab incisions below and lateral to the xiphoid process, and sutured to the skin. This may not be necessary when a drain has been placed into the pleural cavity and the pleura not closed.

15 The two halves of the sternum are apposed with several strong sutures (polydioxanone in infants; nylon or wire in the older child) placed around or through the sternum and firmly tied. The subcutaneous tissues are closed with a continuous absorbable suture. The skin is approximated with a fine absorbable subcuticular suture.

Postoperative care

The drains are removed after 24 h if there is no drainage or pneumomediastinum.

Esophageal atresia with and without tracheoesophageal fistula

Lewis Spitz PhD, FRCS, FRCS(Ed), FAAP(Hon)
Nuffield Professor of Paediatric Surgery, Institute of Child Health, University of London, and Consultant
Paediatric Surgeon, Great Ormond Street Hospital for Children, London, UK

History

The first description of esophageal atresia is credited to Durston who, in 1670, described esophageal atresia in one of a conjoined twin. Thomas Gibson in 1697 accurately described the clinical features of esophageal atresia. In 1913, Richter proposed a plan of management which comprised dividing the tracheoesophageal fistula and feeding the infant by gastrostomy until the 'technical difficulties of an esophageal anastomosis' had been overcome. Ladd and Leven were independently the first to achieve long-term survival in 1939, but only by a staged approach. Haight in 1941 is credited with the first primary anastomosis.

Principles and justification

Embryology

The classic theory of esophageal development describes a tracheoesophageal septum which develops between, and finally separates, the ventral trachea from the dorsal esophagus at around the 26th day of gestation.

Kluth challenged this theory and proposed three stages of separation: an initial system of folds appears in the primitive foregut which covers the tracheoesophageal space cranially and caudally; the paired cranial folds descend while the caudal fold ascends, thereby reducing the tracheoesophageal space; approximation of the folds is followed by elongation of the trachea and esophagus.

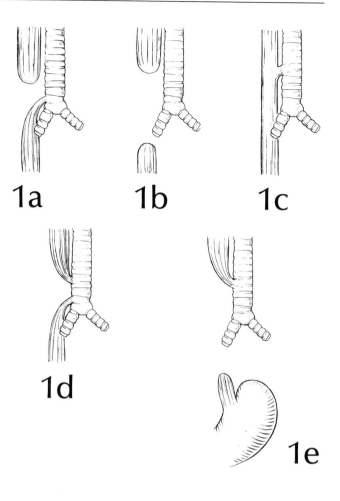

1a   1b   1c

1d

1e

Classification of esophageal atresia

1a–e The various types of esophageal atresia are: (*a*) esophageal atresia with distal fistula (85%); (*b*) esophageal atresia without fistula (7%); (*c*) H-type tracheoesophageal fistula (4%); (*d*) esophageal atresia with proximal and distal fistula (3%); and (*e*) esophageal atresia with proximal fistula (1%).

Associated anomalies

At least 50% of infants with esophageal atresia have one or more associated anomalies. Most common are cardiac malformations, particularly ventricular septal defects and tetralogy of Fallot, and these are responsible for the majority of deaths. Next most common are gastrointestinal and anorectal anomalies, followed by genitourinary tract abnormalities. The VACTERL association (V = vertebral, A = anorectal, C = cardiac, T = tracheo, E = esophageal, R = renal, L = limb) is a well known combination of defects.

A full clinical examination should be made at the outset for associated anomalies, and special investigations including echocardiography and renal ultrasonography are carried out as indicated.

Prognosis

Waterston in 1962 proposed criteria for survival which are no longer relevant. A new classification, based on experience of 372 patients treated between 1980 and 1992, is proposed (*Table 1*).

Table 1 Prognosis based on 372 patients treated for esophageal atresia 1980–1992

		Survival (%)
Group I	Birth weight > 1500 g and no major cardiac anomaly	97
Group II	Birth weight < 1500 g *or* major cardiac anomaly	59
Group III	Birth weight < 1500 g *plus* major cardiac anomaly	22

Diagnosis

Antenatal

Polyhydramnios is present in 95% of patients with isolated atresia without fistula and in 35% of cases with a distal fistula.

With expert fetal ultrasonography it is possible to visualize the blind upper esophageal pouch filling and emptying, and an inability to detect the stomach would indicate atresia without fistula.

Postnatal

A nasogastric tube (8–10 gauge) should be passed at birth in all cases where polyhydramnios was present during pregnancy. Failure to advance the tube beyond 10 cm from the nose or mouth indicates esophageal atresia.

Symptoms that develop in the neonatal period include: inability to clear secretions from the mouth; cyanotic episodes with or without attempting to feed the infant; inability to swallow; and respiratory distress.

Preoperative

Investigations

2 Plain radiography of chest and abdomen demonstrates the tube arrested in the upper mediastinum, and air in the intestine confirms the presence of a distal tracheoesophageal fistula.

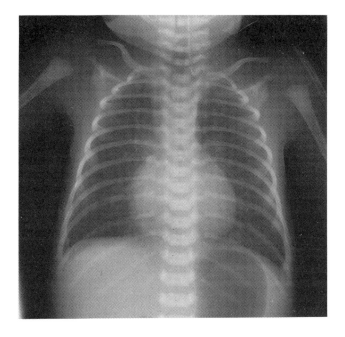

2

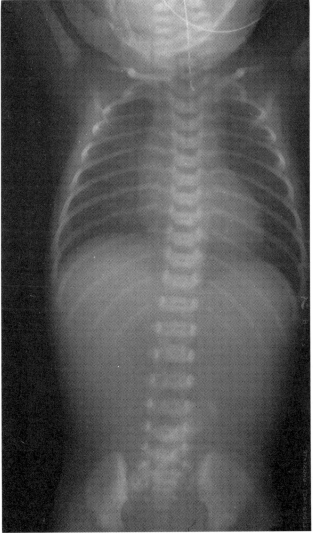

3 The absence of intestinal air suggests the diagnosis of pure esophageal atresia. Contrast studies of the upper pouch are seldom indicated. Endoscopic examination of the upper esophagus and/or bronchoscopy immediately before surgery will detect an upper pouch fistula in most cases. If contrast medium is used, the examination should be performed with extreme care by an experienced radiologist.

3

Initial management

Immediate surgery in esophageal atresia is seldom necessary; a period of 24–48 h between diagnosis and operation allows a full assessment of the neonate and, if aspiration has occurred, resolution of the pulmonary changes can be expedited with appropriate physiotherapy and antibiotics. Before operation the upper pouch is continuously aspirated using a Replogle tube attached to low-pressure suction. Intravenous 10% dextrose and 0.18% saline will maintain fluid and electrolyte balance and prevent hypoglycemia. A vitamin K analogue should be administered routinely before operation.

Neonates with respiratory distress syndrome requiring assisted ventilation and those with severe abdominal distension present special problems. To prevent perforation of the stomach and to improve respiratory support, emergency ligation of the fistula is recommended. Gastrostomy is to be avoided. If the condition of the infant permits, primary repair of the atresia can be carried out, or alternatively the repair may be postponed for 7–10 days.

Choice of operation

In most neonates with esophageal atresia and a distal tracheoesophageal fistula division of the fistula and primary anastomosis of the esophagus is possible. The anastomosis should be attempted, even if performed under extreme tension. It is important to recognize the presence of a right-sided aortic arch, best identified on an echocardiogram, as this may alter the surgical approach.

A short upper pouch on the preliminary plain radiograph may also indicate that a primary anastomosis will be difficult. The presence of a distal tracheoesophageal fistula requiring division, however, dictates the necessity for right thoracotomy, and the possibility of obtaining a satisfactory primary anastomosis should not be ruled out until the anatomy has been inspected at the time of thoracotomy.

The absence of a lower pouch fistula is usually associated with a long gap between upper and lower esophagus. This situation is usually managed by a preliminary feeding gastrostomy. If esophageal replacement is the procedure of choice, a cervical esophagostomy is necessary. The alternative is a delayed primary anastomosis after several weeks of gastrostomy feeding and upper pouch suction. The decision on when to attempt the delayed primary anastomosis is based on radiological assessment of the intervening gap. Bakes' dilators inserted into the upper and lower pouches are the best means of determining the size of the gap. In general it is not profitable to wait longer than 8–12 weeks before deciding on the need for a replacement procedure.

Preoperative

The Replogle tube or a similar large-bore tube should be in position in the upper pouch. Careful attention is paid to maintaining body temperature with a heating blanket, and to preventing heat loss by covering the infant with foil. Broad-spectrum antibiotics should be administered either preoperatively or at the time of induction.

Anesthesia

Premedication is with atropine alone. The endotracheal tube requires careful positioning to permit adequate ventilation with minimal gas flow through the fistula. The majority of pediatric anesthetists will control ventilation from an early stage following intubation. An intravenous infusion is sited in a limb other than the right upper limb.

Operation

Incision

4 The infant is positioned on the left side and stabilized with strapping or sandbags. The right arm is extended above the head and fixed. Care must be taken to ensure that the neck is flexed. A curved incision is made around the lower border of the scapula, extending from the anterior axillary line to the paravertebral region posteriorly.

Division of the subcutaneous tissues and muscles is carried out with diathermy to minimize blood loss. Following division of the muscles the scapula is elevated and the rib spaces are counted by palpation.

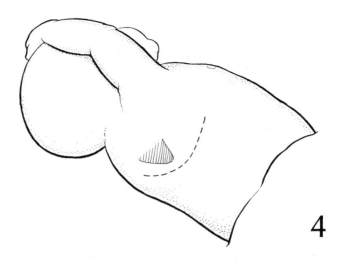

4

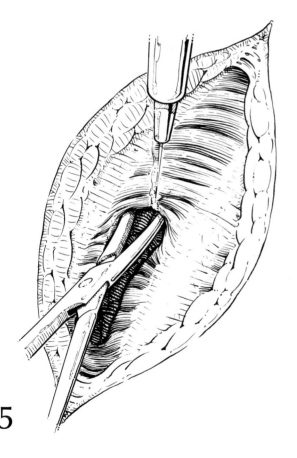

5

5 The thorax can be entered through the bed of the fifth rib, which is mobilized following incision of the overlying periosteum. An alternative and rather simpler approach is to divide the intercostal muscles of the fourth intercostal space. Whichever the approach, care is required to prevent incision of the pleura. Although the extrapleural approach is slower initially, it confers substantial benefit and should always be used in the initial thoracotomy.

6 Having exposed the pleura through the intercostal space, stripping of the pleura from the chest wall is best carried out by the gentle insertion of a gauze swab into the extrapleural space. On withdrawing the swab an extensive area of dissection will have resulted; a rib spreader can then be inserted and the ribs gently separated. Further dissection of the pleura is achieved by using moist pledgets; a pair of pledgets used simultaneously is most satisfactory.

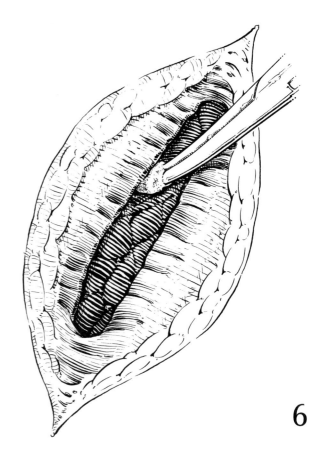

6

7 The azygos vein and the posterior mediastinum should be exposed, enabling the lower pouch, upper pouch and fistula to be seen. Anterior dissection of the pleura should be sufficient to allow the ribs to be adequately spread. Very occasionally the size or position of the fistula may make it impossible for the anesthetist to ventilate the lungs adequately. In that situation the more rapid transpleural approach to the fistula may be necessary. In order to expose the posterior mediastinum effectively lung retraction is essential, but care must be taken to ensure that the retractor does not compress the mediastinal structures.

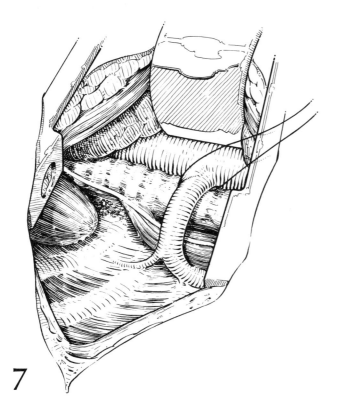

7

Mobilization of lower esophagus and division of fistula

The azygos vein is ligated and divided. The lower esophagus may be obvious, distending with each inspiration as it lies in the lower posterior mediastinum. The close proximity of the vagus to the lower esophagus helps identification.

8 Every attempt must be made during dissection to preserve the fibers of the vagus supplying the lower esophagus. The lower esophagus is dissected circumferentially just distal to the fistula and a tape is placed around it. Traction on this tape controls the fistula and enables the junction of the lower esophagus and trachea to be recognized and dissected.

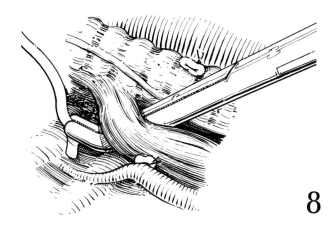

8

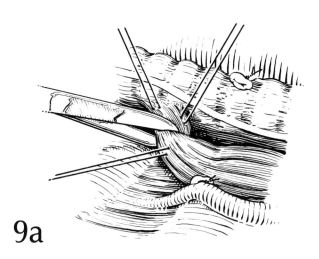

9a

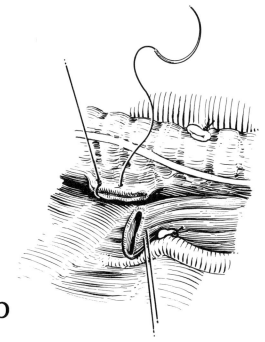

9b

9a, b After carefully defining the junction between the trachea and esophagus, two 5/0 polypropylene (Prolene) sutures are placed in the trachea at the extremities of the fistula and the fistula is divided flush with the trachea. The trachea is closed with interrupted sutures. The airtightness of the closure should be tested by filling the thoracic cavity with saline and watching for bubbles on ventilation. An alternative means of closing the fistula is to transfix it close to the trachea with a 5/0 suture.

A small tube is passed through the distal esophagus into the stomach to ensure that an adequate lumen exists and to enable air distending the stomach to be aspirated. Dissection of the lower esophagus needs care to preserve the vagal attachments and prevent damage to the adjacent thoracic duct and left pleura. A 5/0 stay suture allows traction on the lower esophagus without excessive handling with forceps. Dissection should be the minimum required to achieve an anastomosis.

Identification of upper pouch

10 If the upper pouch is not immediately visible, pressure on the Replogle tube by the anesthetist will usually advance it into the mediastinum. Dissection of the upper pouch should be sufficient to allow an opening to be made in the distal end for an anastomosis to be performed. As with the lower esophagus, branches of the vagus supplying the upper esophagus should not be disturbed. Dissection on the plane between the esophagus and trachea should be carried out with extreme care to avoid inadvertently opening the trachea. A stay suture can be placed in the muscular wall of the esophagus to facilitate its exposure and minimize the need for forceps traction. When opening the upper esophagus care should be taken to ensure that the opening is at the lowermost point; this is most reliably recognized by pushing the Replogle tube down and incising the esophagus over the tip of the tube. The size of the opening in the upper esophagus should correspond to the diameter of the lower esophagus.

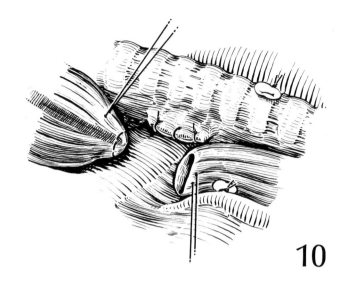

Anastomosis

11 This is achieved using interrupted 5/0 or 6/0 sutures positioned along the posterior aspect of the anastomosis, particular care being taken to ensure that both mucosa and muscle are included in each suture. It is seldom necessary to insert more than four or five sutures. Unless the two ends of the esophagus are very close together the siting of these sutures before tying is essential.

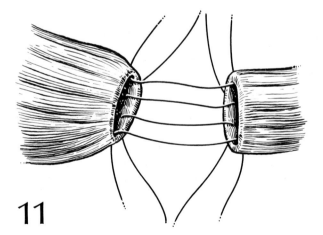

12 Following completion of the posterior layer of the anastomosis, a feeding tube should replace the Replogle tube and be advanced across the anastomosis into the stomach. The anterior layer of the anastomosis is then completed over the tube. Once the anastomosis is complete, the intraesophageal tube may be withdrawn; if it is to be left *in situ* for feeding, its mobility should be checked to ensure that a suture has not inadvertently passed through it.

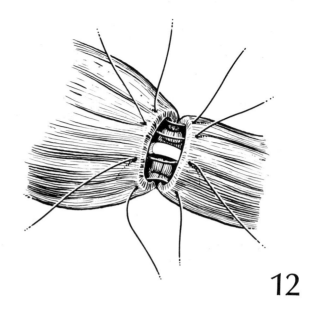

12

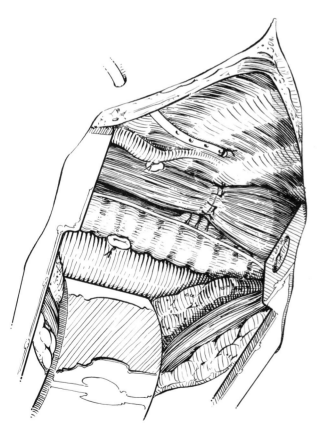

13

Wound closure

13 The lung is expanded following the placement of two pericostal 3/0 polyglactin sutures. The muscles are closed with 3/0 coated polyglycolic acid (Dexon); the subcutaneous layer with plain 4/0 polyglycolic acid, and the skin with subcuticular 5/0 polyglycolic acid.

A chest drain is only used in specific circumstances; e.g. trauma to the underlying pleura and lung, or occasionally in a very tight anastomosis. The tip of the drain should be sutured to the lateral chest wall away from the anastomotic site with 4/0 chromic catgut.

Postoperative care

The patient is nursed in the neonatal intensive care unit. Intravenous fluids are administered and antibiotic prophylaxis is continued. Feeds via the transanastomotic nasogastric tube may be commenced on the second or third day after operation. Oral feeding is gradually introduced. Regular chest physiotherapy, with nasopharyngeal suction as required, is carried out to avoid respiratory infection.

If the esophageal anastomosis has been performed under extreme tension it is recommended that the infant is electively paralyzed and mechanically ventilated for an arbitrary period of 5 days.

Complications

Mortality is directly related to the severity of associated congenital anomalies, particularly cardiac malformations.

Early anastomotic leakage within 48 h of the repair should be explored urgently with a view to secondary surgery. Late leaks can be managed conservatively in the expectation that they will seal spontaneously.

Gastroesophageal reflux should be treated conservatively, but if there is no response and the infant suffers repeated repiratory infections or apneic attacks, a surgical approach should be adopted. Tracheomalacia is a common occurrence and if severe should be treated by aortopexy, as described in the chapter on pp. 132–135.

Recurrent tracheoesophageal fistula should be suspected in the event of choking episodes associated with feeding, or recurrent bouts of pneumonia. Anastomotic strictures usually respond to repeated dilatation, but gastroesophageal reflux as an aggravating factor should be excluded.

Further reading

Beasley SW, Auldist AW, Myers NA. Current surgical management of oesophageal atresia and/or tracheo-oesophageal fistula. *Aust N Z J Surg* 1989; 59: 707–12.

Chittmittrapap S, Spitz L, Kiely EM, Brereton RJ. Oesophageal atresia and associated anomalies. *Arch Dis Child* 1989; 64: 364–8.

Kiely E, Spitz L. Is routine gastrostomy necessary in the management of oesophageal atresia? *Pediatr Surg Int* 1987; 2: 6–9.

Kluth D, Steding G, Seidl W. The embryology of foregut malformations. *J Pediatr Surg* 1987; 22: 389–93.

Louhimo I, Lindahl H. Esophageal atresia: primary results of 500 consecutively treated patients. *J Pediatr Surg* 1983; 18: 217–29.

MacKinlay GA, Burtles R. Oesophageal atresia, paralysis and ventilation in management of the wide gap. *Pediatr Surg Int* 1987; 2: 10–12.

Malone PS, Kiely EM, Brain AJ *et al*. Tracheo-oesophageal fistula and preoperative mechanical ventilation. *Aust N Z J Surg* 1990; 60: 525–7.

Randolph JG, Neuman KD, Anderson KD. Current results in repair of esophageal atresia with tracheoesophageal fistula using physiological status as a guide to therapy. *Ann Surg* 1989; 209: 526–31.

Spitz L, Kiely E, Brereton RJ. Esophageal atresia: five-year experience with 148 cases. *J Pediatr Surg* 1987; 22: 103–8.

Spitz L, Kiely E, Brereton RJ, Drake D. Management of esophageal atresia. *World J Surg* 1993; 17: 296–300.

Spitz L, Kiely E, Moorcraft JA, Drake DP. At risk groups in oesophageal atresia. *J Pediatr Surg* 1994; 29: 723–5.

Illustrations by Marks Creative Consultants

Cervical esophagostomy

Lewis Spitz PhD, FRCS, FRCS(Ed), FAAP(Hon)
Nuffield Professor of Paediatric Surgery, Institute of Child Health, University of London, and Consultant Paediatric Surgeon, Great Ormond Street Hospital for Children, London, UK

Principles and justification

Although this procedure is relatively seldom performed, it should still form part of the repertoire of the pediatric surgeon.

Indications

The principal indication is long-gap esophageal atresia, where the atretic segment extends beyond six or eight thoracic vertebral bodies or when attempts at delayed primary anastomosis have failed. Other indications include disruption of a previous primary repair of esophageal atresia, extensive stricture of the esophagus – caustic ingestion or peptic esophagitis – with chronic aspiration, and foreign body perforation of the esophagus.

In general, performing a cervical esophagostomy commits the surgeon to carrying out an eventual esophageal replacement.

Operation

Position of patient and incision

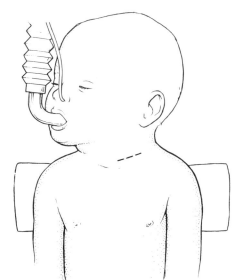

1 The patient is positioned supine on the operating table under general endotracheal anesthesia. A large-bore nasogastric tube is placed as far distally as possible in the esophagus. A rolled towel is placed under the shoulders and the neck is moderately extended.

The esophagostomy may be sited on either side of the neck but the left side is preferred. A transverse incision is made on the left side of the neck 1 cm above and parallel to the medial third of the clavicle.

Using diathermy the incision is deepened through the subcutaneous fat and platysma muscle, ligating and dividing the anterior jugular vein.

2 The clavicular head of the sternocleidomastoid muscle is divided in the line of the incision using electrocoagulation to provide hemostasis. The sternothyroid muscle is similarly divided or retracted posteriorly to reveal the carotid sheath and its contents.

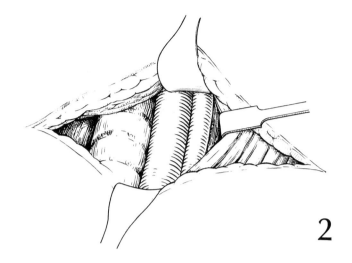

2

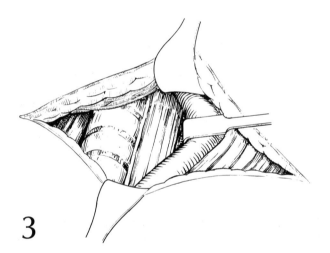

3

Preservation of recurrent laryngeal nerve

3 The carotid sheath containing the carotid artery, vagal nerve and internal jugular vein is retracted laterally. This exposes the cartilaginous rings of the trachea anteromedially and the closely applied esophagus lying on its posterior surface. It is important to identify and preserve the left recurrent laryngeal nerve which runs in the groove between the trachea and esophagus.

The esophagus is clearly identified by palpating the nasogastric tube within its lumen.

Mobilization of the esophagus

4 The esophagus is carefully separated from the posterior surface of the trachea by blunt dissection, and, remaining close to the esophageal wall, the dissection is continued posteriorly and to the opposite side until the esophagus has been encircled. By keeping the dissection close to the esophageal wall, the risk of traumatizing the right recurrent laryngeal nerve will be minimized.

A soft rubber sling is placed around the esophagus, and the dissection continued distally, remaining on the muscle wall.

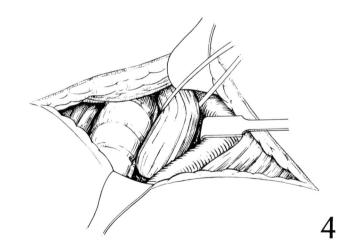

4

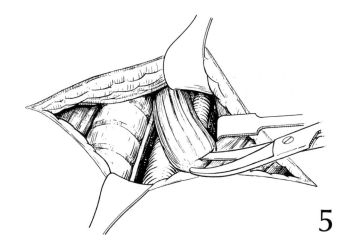

5 In isolated esophageal atresia the proximal esophageal segment is usually short and the blind end soon comes into view. In other cases, e.g. strictures, it is necessary to divide the esophagus at a convenient place, leaving sufficient proximal esophagus to reach the skin incision without tension while permitting accurate closure of the distal esophagus.

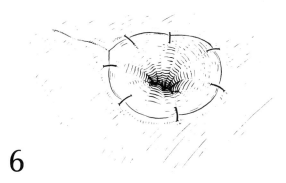

Fashioning the esophagostomy

6 The end of the esophagus is brought out of the lateral end of the incision and sutured to the skin edges with interrupted full-thickness fine absorbable sutures. There should be no tension on the suture line, and a nasogastric tube should be able to exit the stoma unimpeded.

Wound closure

The remainder of the wound is closed with interrupted sutures to the platysma muscle and subcuticular sutures to skin.

Postoperative care

The esophagostomy should be covered initially with paraffin gauze and ultimately left open to drain freely onto the surface.

An adhesive plastic bag may be applied to the skin around the esophagostomy site to collect saliva. In infants with esophageal atresia it is vitally important to practise sham feeding pending the esophageal replacement. Failure to do this will result in tremendous difficulty in establishing oral feeds when the esophageal replacement is performed.

Illustrations by Marks Creative Consultants

H-type tracheoesophageal fistula

Lewis Spitz PhD, FRCS, FRCS(Ed), FAAP(Hon)
Nuffield Professor of Paediatric Surgery, Institute of Child Health, University of London, and Consultant
Paediatric Surgeon, Great Ormond Street Hospital for Children, London, UK

Principles and justification

An isolated or H-type tracheoesophageal fistula most commonly presents during the first few days of life, when the neonate chokes on attempting to feed and/or has unexplained cyanotic episodes. The gaseous distension of the gastrointestinal tract may be sufficiently severe to mimic that of intestinal obstruction. Older infants and children are likely to present with recurrent chest infections, particularly involving the right upper lobe.

H-type tracheoesophageal fistula constitutes about 3% of tracheoesophageal anomalies.

Investigations

The most reliable method of establishing the diagnosis of an H-type fistula is by a prone tube video esophagogram. A small-caliber nasogastric tube is passed into the distal esophagus and contrast medium is gradually injected while the tube is slowly withdrawn. An H-fistula may be missed in over 50% of routine contrast swallows.

Bronchoscopy with esophagoscopy will confirm the presence of a fistula. If performed immediately before ligation of the fistula it should be possible to pass a fine tube, e.g. a ureteric catheter, through the fistula to aid subsequent identification at surgical exploration.

Having accurately identified the position of the fistula, a decision can be made on the most suitable approach. Some fistulas, including a recurrent fistula associated with a previous repair for esophageal atresia, will be best approached through the thorax, but the majority of isolated tracheoesophageal fistulas can be divided through a cervical approach with adequate neck extension.

The thoracic approach to a tracheoesophageal fistula is similar to that previously described for esophageal atresia with tracheoesophageal fistula (pp. 111–121).

Operation

Position of patient

1 The child is placed supine on the operating table with the head turned to the left. Before extending the neck, the site of the incision is drawn with a marker pen in a suitable skin crease 1 cm above and parallel to the clavicle. Failure to mark the site of the incision before extending the neck may result in a cosmetically unsatisfactory incision.

A sandbag of appropriate size placed under the shoulder ensures adequate neck extension. An approach through the right side is usually preferred. A nasogastric tube of adequate size should be passed after induction of anesthesia.

In ideal circumstances, a ureteric catheter will have been passed through the fistula under bronchoscopic control. This is invaluable in identifying the fistula site during exploration.

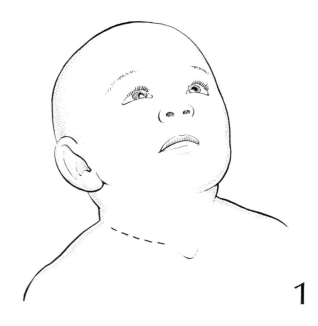

Approach to fistula

2 Having incised the skin and subcutaneous tissues, the sternocleidomastoid muscle is retracted posteriorly, dividing the sternal head of this muscle if necessary to allow adequate exposure. The plane medial to the carotid sheath is identified, and dissection allows the sheath to be retracted posteriorly. The thyroid gland, trachea and esophagus lie medially. Palpation of the endotracheal and nasogastric tubes facilitates identification of these structures. The inferior thyroid artery and middle thyroid vein are identified crossing the space between the retracted carotid sheath and the thyroid, and division of these vessels may be necessary. The plane between the trachea and esophagus is gently dissected, care being taken to identify and preserve the right recurrent laryngeal nerve.

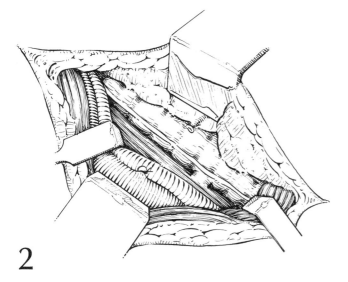

Dissection of fistula

3 Identification of the fistula requires careful dissection, and it is usually rather higher than anticipated
because of the extension of the neck. Slings positioned
around the esophagus above and below the fistula will
facilitate dissection, but extreme care is required to
preserve the left recurrent laryngeal nerve, which is
difficult to visualize.

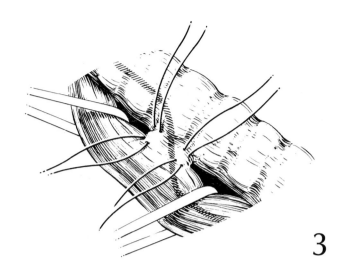

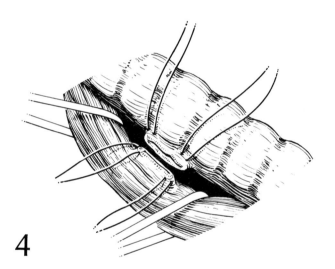

4 Having isolated the fistula, stay sutures are placed
on the esophageal side to mark its position because,
following division of the fistula, rotation and retraction
of the esophageal end may make it difficult to identify.
On the tracheal side, a 5/0 polypropylene suture is
placed at both limits of the fistula.

5 Following division of the fistula, the tracheal defect
is closed with interrupted sutures. The esophageal
end of the fistula is closed with one or two interrupted
fine polyglycolic acid sutures.

The retracted tissues will now assume a more normal
position. Some surgeons advocate interposing tissue,
e.g. fascia or muscle, between the two opposing suture
lines in order to reduce the likelihood of recurrence of
the fistulas. The wound is closed in layers with
absorbable sutures and with a subcuticular suture for
the skin.

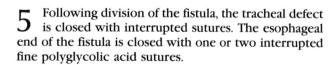

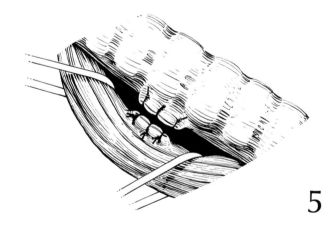

Postoperative care

Extensive dissection of the trachea and esophagus is often required during this operation. Invariably this produces some tracheal edema, which may be minimal immediately after operation but progresses in severity for up to 24 h. It is reasonable, particularly in premature infants or in those with pre-existing lung disease, to leave an endotracheal tube in position.

Following extubation, the movement of the vocal cords should be assessed. A proportion of these neonates will require intubation for some considerable time and may have a tendency to stridor, particularly when crying or coughing, for weeks or months afterwards. Feeds can be given through a nasogastric tube.

Recurrence of an H-type fistula is rare.

Further reading

Bedard P, Girvan DP, Shandling B. Congenital H-type tracheo-oesophageal fistula. *J Pediatr Surg* 1974; 9: 663–8.

Filston HC, Rankin JS, Kirks DR. The diagnosis of primary and recurrent tracheo-oesophageal fistulas: value of selective catheterization. *J Pediatr Surg* 1982; 17: 144–8.

Gans SL, Johnson RO. Diagnosis and management of 'H' type tracheo-oesophageal fistula in infants and children. *J Pediatr Surg* 1977; 12: 233–6.

Myers NA, Egami K. Congenital tracheo-oesophageal fistula. 'H' or 'N' fistula. *Pediatr Surg Int* 1987; 2: 198–211.

Illustrations by Marks Creative Consultants

Recurrent tracheoesophageal fistula

Lewis Spitz PhD, FRCS, FRCS(Ed), FAAP(Hon)
Nuffield Professor of Paediatric Surgery, Institute of Child Health, University of London, and Consultant
Paediatric Surgeon, Great Ormond Street Hospital for Children, London, UK

Principles and justification

The incidence of recurrent tracheoesophageal fistula ranges from 5% to 10%. Infants who develop respiratory symptoms following repair of an esophageal atresia, e.g. gagging, coughing, apneic or cyanotic spells during feeding, or suffer from recurrent chest infections should be suspected of having a recurrent fistula.

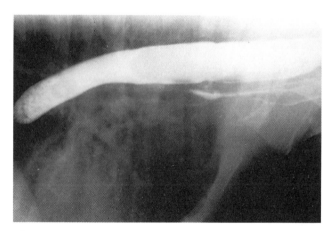

1

Preoperative

Diagnosis

Radiographs of the chest and abdomen may show an air esophagogram or an excessive amount of gas in the gastrointestinal tract. Routine contrast swallows will only detect about 50% of recurrent fistulas. Esophagoscopy carries a low diagnostic rate.

1 Cine (tube) esophagography performed in the prone position is the most reliable method of establishing the diagnosis.

Bronchoscopy with cannulation of the fistula is also a reliable diagnostic method and is invaluable in locating the fistula during the operative procedure.

Anesthesia

Anesthesia for repair of recurrent fistula is fraught with danger. Lung function may be compromised by chronic aspiration, and vascular access may have been compromised by previous surgery or the use of parenteral nutrition. Intraoperative ventilation may be difficult because of gaseous escape through a large fistula. Meticulous intraoperative monitoring is mandatory and should include pulse oximetry. Hand ventilation with high gas flow rates may be necessary because of changes in pulmonary compliance. Because of pleural adhesions following previous surgery, blood loss may be considerable and requires rapid replacement. Postoperative ventilation and intensive care are often necessary, particularly in young infants.

Operation

Bronchoscopy and cannulation of fistula

2 A rigid Storz bronchoscope of suitable size for the child's age (2.5–3.0-Fr for infants) is passed and the fistulous opening in the posterior wall of the trachea at or just above the carina identified. A fine (4–6-Fr) ureteric catheter is passed through the suction channel of the bronchoscope, through the fistula into the esophagus, advanced well down into the esophagus and left *in situ*.

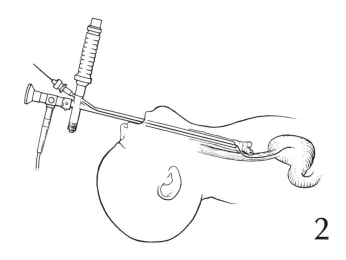

2

Incision

A posterolateral thoracotomy via the previous incision is the preferred approach. The fourth or fifth intercostal space is opened in the length of the incision and a small rib spreader used to widen the thoracotomy. Access to the mediastinum is via a transpleural route as the extrapleural approach is not an option having been used in the repair of the esophageal atresia.

3

Mediastinal dissection and mobilization of esophagus

3 The mediastinal pleura is opened longitudinally over the esophagus, exposing its lateral wall proximal and distal to the fistulous site. The esophagus proximal and distal to the fistula (identified by palpating the ureteric catheter within its lumen) is carefully mobilized from the surrounding tissue and rubber slings are passed around it above and below the fistula.

Dissection of fistula

4 Having identified and isolated the fistula, stay sutures of 5/0 polypropylene (Prolene) are inserted in the upper and lower walls of the fistula on both the tracheal and esophageal ends. These sutures are invaluable in facilitating accurate closure of the defects following division of the fistula.

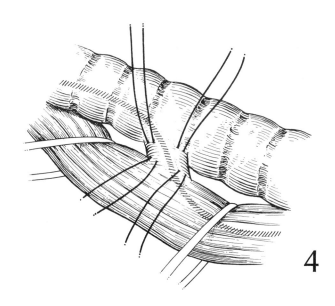

4

Division of fistula

5 The fistula is now opened. The ureteric catheter should be positively visualized traversing the fistula before being withdrawn through the mouth to allow complete division of the fistula.

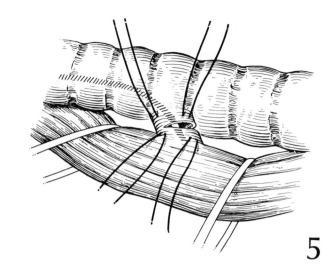

5

Closure of fistulous openings

6 The tracheal and esophageal orifices of the fistula are securely closed with interrupted 5/0 polypropylene sutures.

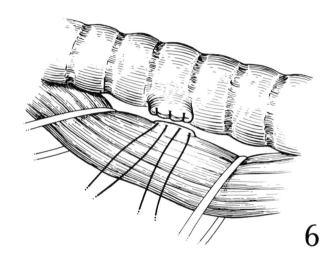

6

Separation of the suture lines

To prevent the two contiguous suture lines becoming adherent and to prevent refistulization, mediastinal pleura, intercostal muscle or a flap of pericardium is interposed between the esophagus and trachea. An intercostal drain is inserted with the tip some distance away from the area of repair.

Wound closure

The thoracotomy wound is closed with pericostal 3/0 polyglycolic acid sutures and the muscles of the chest wall approximated with continuous 4/0 polyglycolic acid sutures. The skin is closed with a subcuticular suture.

Postoperative care

Endotracheal intubation and elective mechanical ventilation are usually required for 48–72 h after operation due to tracheal edema. A contrast swallow is performed on the seventh day after operation and the chest drain removed following confirmation that there is no leak from the esophageal repair.

Complications

These include pneumothorax and esophageal leak with consequent empyema. There is a 10–20% risk of fistula recurrence.

Further reading

Ein SH, Stringer DA, Stephens CA, Shandling B, Simpson J, Filler RM. Recurrent tracheoesophageal fistulas seventeen-year review. *J Pediatr Surg* 1983; 18: 436–41.

Filston HC, Rankin JC, Kirks DR. The diagnosis of primary and recurrent tracheoesophageal fistulas: value of selective catheterization. *J Pediatr Surg* 1982; 17: 144–8.

Ghandour KE, Spitz L, Brereton RJ, Kiely EM. Recurrent tracheooesophageal fistula: experience with 24 patients. *J Paediatr Child Health* 1990; 26: 89–91.

Aortopexy

E. M. Kiely FRCSI, FRCS
Consultant Paediatric Surgeon, Great Ormond Street Hospital for Children, London, UK

Principles and justification

Tracheomalacia is suspected when an infant develops expiratory stridor on exertion. Increasing difficulty with expiration leads to difficulty with feeding, cyanotic spells and, in extreme cases, to collapse and apnea. The symptom complex has similarities with severe gastro-esophageal reflux and recurrent or missed tracheo-esophageal fistula. The three conditions may coexist.

Diagnosis

1a, b The diagnosis is confirmed endoscopically when expiratory collapse of the trachea is seen during quiet respiration. Complete obliteration of the lumen is common. The segment of collapse in infants previously treated for esophageal atresia and distal tracheoesophageal fistula is above the site of entry of the original fistula. Severe symptoms are unusual when more than 20% of the lumen remains open.

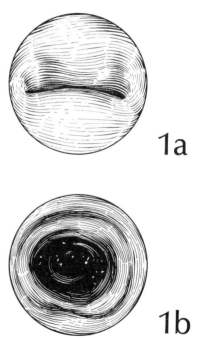

1a

1b

Operation

Position of patient

The infant is positioned supine with a small roll behind the shoulders and the left arm abducted.

Incision

2 The chest is entered through a left anterior thoracotomy incision placed over the third rib. Pectoral muscles are incised medially and split towards the lateral end of the incision.

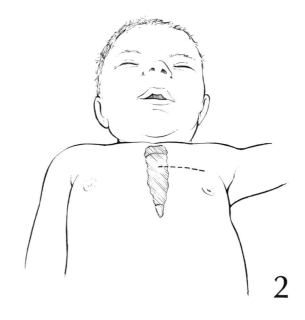

2

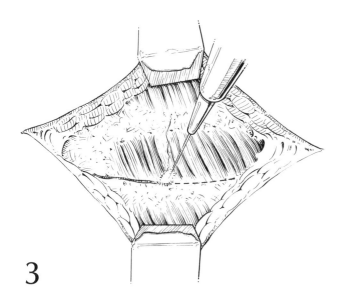

3

3 The chest may be entered through the bed of the third rib or the third intercostal space. The internal mammary vessels at the medial end of the incision should be divided.

4 The thoracotomy is held open by means of an infant-sized Finochietto retractor. The left lung is retracted laterally by means of a moist gauze and a malleable retractor.

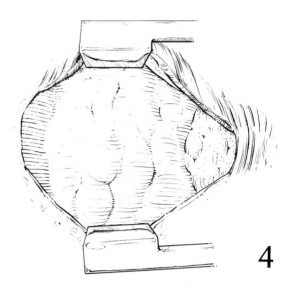

5 The pleura is incised longitudinally over the left lobe of the thymus.

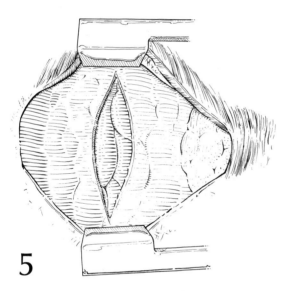

6 The left lobe of the thymus is then excised with care to preserve the phrenic nerve. The thymic vein which enters the innominate vein is identified, coagulated and divided. The great vessels are then in view.

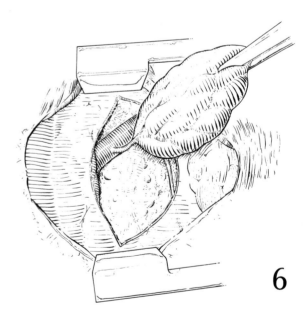

7 The roots of the great vessels are within the pericardium which is now incised transversely, close to its reflection on the aorta.

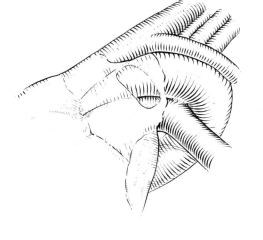

7

8 Three 4/0 polypropylene sutures are usually sufficient to perform the aortopexy. Several bites of aortic adventitia and pericardial reflection are taken with each suture. The lumen should not be entered. The sutures are then inserted into the posterior aspect of the sternum and are left untied until all are in place.

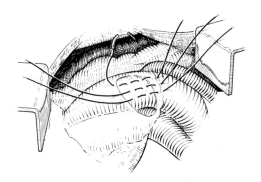

8

9 The assistant then depresses the sternum and holds this position until each has been tied.

The sternum is then released and the aorta moves forwards with it. The anterior tracheal wall also moves anteriorly to fill the potential space behind the aorta.

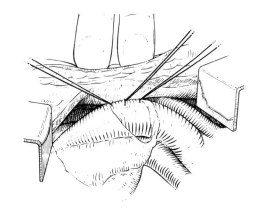

9

Wound closure

The wound is closed in the usual manner. If the operative field is dry, a chest drain is unnecessary.

Postoperative care

Oral feeding may be commenced the same day and early discharge is possible if symptoms are alleviated.

Further reading

Benjamin B, Cohen D, Glasson M. Tracheomalacia in association with congenital tracheo-oesophageal fistula. *Surgery* 1976; 79: 504–8.

Filler RM, Rossello PJ, Lebowitz RL. Life-threatening anoxic spells caused by tracheal compression after repair of esophageal atresia: correction by surgery. *J Pediatr Surg* 1976; 11: 739–48.

Keily EM, Spitz L, Brereton R. Management of tracheomalacia by aortopexy. *Pediatr Surg Int* 1987; 2: 13–15.

Malone PS, Kiely EM. Role of aortopexy in the management of primary tracheomalacia and tracheobronchomalacia. *Arch Dis Child* 1990; 65: 436–40.

Esophageal replacement with colon

H. Biemann Othersen Jr MD
Professor of Surgery and Pediatrics, and Chief, Pediatric Surgery, Children's Hospital, Medical University of South Carolina, Charleston, South Carolina, USA

C. D. Smith MD
Associate Professor of Pediatric Surgery, Children's Hospital, Medical University of South Carolina, Charleston, South Carolina, USA

Edward P. Tagge MD
Assistant Professor of Pediatric Surgery, Children's Hospital, Medical University of South Carolina, Charleston, South Carolina, USA

History

There is no ideal esophageal substitute. The best contenders at present are the colon and the stomach.

Table 1 summarizes the relative advantages of intrathoracic esophageal substitutes.

Table 1 Intrathoracic esophageal substitutes

Technique	Advantages	Disadvantages
Small intestine	Large amount of intestine available	Blood supply lacks a marginal artery; difficult to obtain a straight conduit with good blood supply
Gastric tube	Stapling devices have simplified construction of the tube	Long suture line; may not be able to reach high in the neck; difficult to place in the posterior mediastinum; Barrett's epithelium may develop in proximal esophagus
Colon	Acts as a conduit when placed either anti- or isoperistaltically; good blood supply with marginal artery and can reach high in the neck; can be placed in the posterior mediastinum in the esophageal bed	Long-term growth retardation; late redundancy and stasis; late strictures in the cologastric anastomosis
Entire stomach	Readily available and easy to mobilize	Blood supply may not allow it to reach high in the neck; large bulk may cause space problems when brought up intrathoracically; Barrett's epithelium may develop in proximal esophagus
Colonic patch	Can be tailored to the individual esophageal defect; good blood supply to reach high in the neck; does not require esophageal resection; esophageal continuity intact	Long suture line; cannot be used when entire esophagus is densely scarred; the scarred esophagus is left in place
Free patch of intestine	Only short portion of gut used – no useful intestine discarded; can be tailored to the individual area	Requires microsurgical anastomosis with threat of thrombosis and gangrene
Free or pedicled patch of pericardium	Readily available material and does not require vascular pedicle	Contracts and stricture may recur

Principles and justification

Indications

Indications in children include esophageal atresia with inadequate length for primary repair; esophageal strictures that are too long for resection and anastomosis; or extensive Barrett's epithelium in the distal esophagus.

The colon can be placed substernally or in the posterior mediastinum and the right, transverse, or left colon may be used. Right thoracotomy is preferred, since the thoracic esophagus is situated more to the right than to the left. Thus, in esophageal atresia, the cervical esophagostomy is placed in the right side of the neck.

Preoperative

Assessment

In esophageal atresia with inadequate length (such as esophageal atresia without a fistula) the proximal esophagus is left in place with sump drainage for 6–12 weeks while the child is fed via a gastrostomy. Enough growth may occur to allow primary esophagoesophagostomy. If the length is still not sufficient, a right cervical esophagostomy is performed and the child is maintained by gastrostomy feeding until 6–8 months of age. The parents must understand the importance of oral feeding just before gastrostomy feeding so that the child can learn to chew and swallow.

Bowel preparation

Clear liquids are given for 24 h before admission (the day before operation). A polyethylene glycol electrolyte solution is then administered in a dose of 25–40 ml/kg/h, usually via a nasogastric tube until stools are clear.

Chemical preparation of the colon is achieved with neomycin, 50 mg/kg, and erythromycin, 60 mg/kg, given in three divided doses. The first two doses are given 1 h apart, and the last dose at midnight before making the patient nil by mouth.

Anesthesia

General endotracheal anesthesia is used with the patient positioned to allow access to the neck, thorax and abdomen.

Operations

ESOPHAGEAL REPLACEMENT WITH COLON

Position of patient and incisions

1a, b The patient is placed in the left lateral decubitus position with the right arm prepared and draped. The arm is raised for the thoracic incision and lowered for the neck and abdominal approach. The table can be tilted laterally to improve exposures.

An oblique (or transverse) incision is made in the neck and a thoracic incision through the sixth intercostal space. The abdominal incision is made along the midline. The thoracic posterolateral incision is made first. The latissimus dorsi muscle can be retracted laterally and the interspace entered without cutting that muscle. An entrapleural approach is made by resecting the sixth rib subperiosteally and incising the posterior periosteum (rib bed); the pleura is dissected away as the rib bed is divided. If there are too many adhesions a transpleural approach is used. The esophagus is identified by the anesthetist passing a tube into it. The mediastinal pleura is incised and the esophagus dissected upwards. When the thoracic dissection is completed the abdominal incision is made. The neck approach is last.

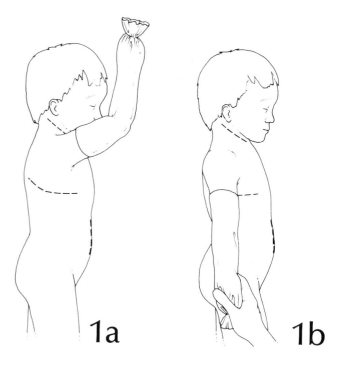

1a   **1b**

Selection of vascular pedicle

2 A length of umbilical tape is passed through the esophageal hiatus and one end is placed at the desired location of the proximal esophageal segment. The other end is passed to the vessel in the colonic mesentery which will serve as the vascular pedicle. This piece of tape is used to determine the length needed. By placing this tape on the colon, the vessels that require division are examined. By placing small vascular clamps on the vessels to be divided, the remaining blood supply can be assessed.

Passage through hiatus into chest

The intestinal segment is passed behind the stomach and up through the esophageal hiatus. The colon can be situated in either an isoperistaltic or antiperistaltic orientation.

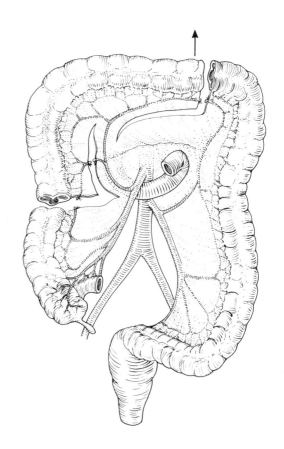

2

Examples of various techniques

3a—e There are various ways of arranging the colonic interposition. All of these, whether isoperistaltic or antiperistaltic, and whether in the posterior mediastinum or in the substernal space, function as conduits and empty by gravity.

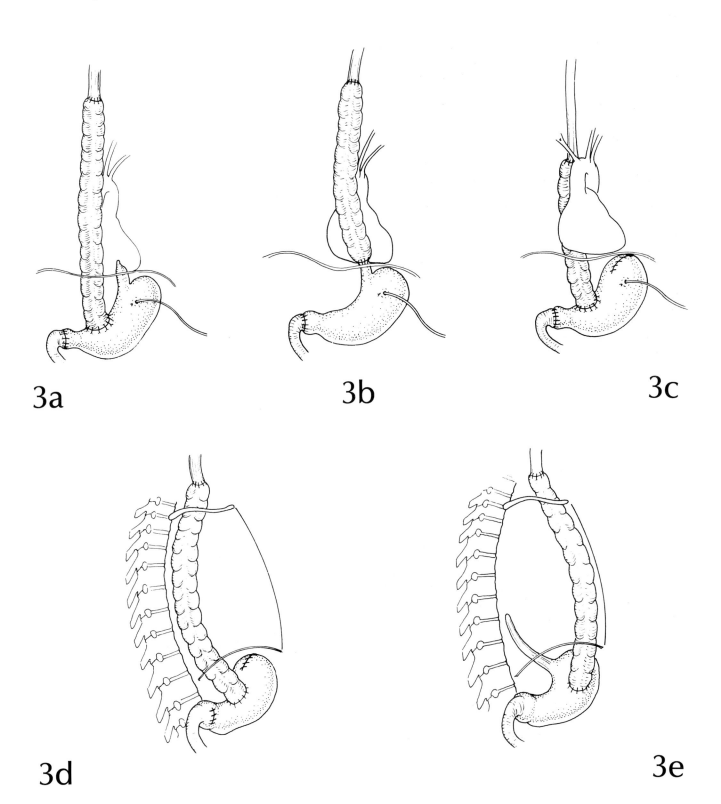

3a

3b

3c

3d

3e

Anastomosis

4 The proximal anastomosis in the chest or neck is fashioned with two layers of absorbable sutures. Distally the anastomosis is made with the anterior wall of the stomach. When the vagus nerves have been divided during esophagectomy, a pyloroplasty is performed. A temporary gastrostomy allows for gastric decompression. In this illustration the transverse and descending colonic segment is supplied by the middle colonic vessels and the vascular pedicle passes posterior to the stomach. Colocolostomy is the final anastomosis.

Extrapleural or intrapleural catheters to an underwater seal are the only drains necessary. The catheters are placed near, but not adjacent, to the suture line.

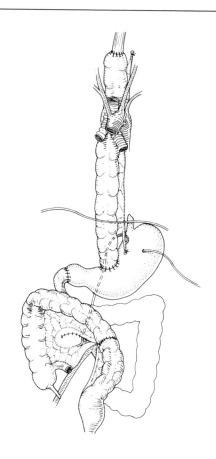

4

ESOPHAGEAL PATCHING WITH COLON (COLONIC PATCH ESOPHAGOPLASTY)

Technique

5a–d This new technique, developed by Hecker and Hollmann[1], can be used as an alternative to esophageal replacement.

Various modifications are possible. Either an intra- or extrapleural approach may be made. The vascular pedicle is measured carefully as in performing a colonic replacement procedure. The segment of colon needed to cover the esophageal defect is measured and the extra bowel removed and discarded. Care is taken to divide vessels close to the bowel wall so as to protect the vascular pedicle. When that dissection has been completed, a template is made of the esophageal defect, the colon is opened and the excessive portion of bowel is removed. The completed patch can then be passed posterior to the stomach. If the patch is too large, a pseudodiverticulum may develop. A continuous polyglycolic acid suture (3/0 or 4/0) in a single layer is used.

The anesthetist should inject saline through an esophageal catheter to check the suture line for leaks. Chest drainage is similar to that described for colonic replacement procedure.

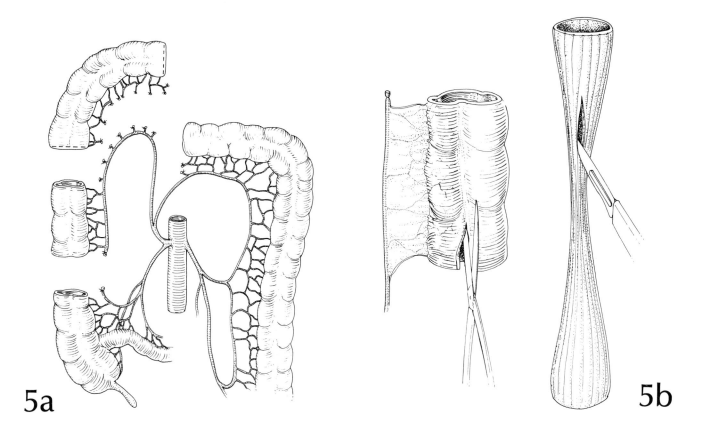

5a

5b

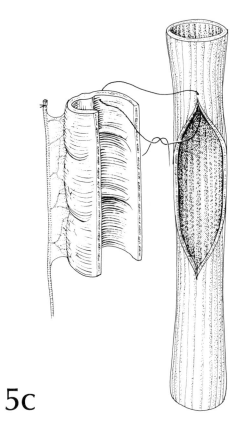

5c

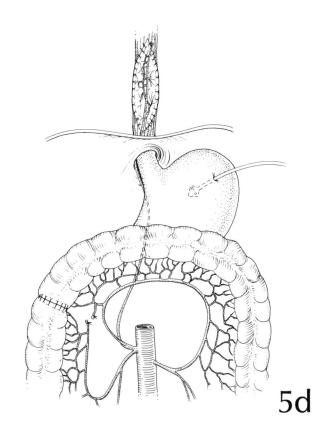

5d

Postoperative care

A contrast swallow should be obtained on the seventh postoperative day. Oral feeding may then be commenced.

Outcome

The colon appears to be the most satisfactory replacement for the esophagus in children. However, there are significant long-term complications. The advantages of the colon include a good vascular supply through the marginal artery, adequate length, appropriate size for anastomosis to the esophagus, and no acid production to erode the esophagus. The disadvantages of using the colon to replace the esophagus are a tendency to redundancy as the child grows, obstruction of the colonic conduit from excessive redundancy, lack of normal growth of the child in some cases, which may not be specific to colonic replacement.

The advantages of a colonic patch are that it retains continuity of the esophagus, it causes less injury to the vagus nerves, permits re-epithelialization and scar regression in the surrounding esophagus, is amenable to anastomosis of the vascular supply to local vessels, and causes less redundancy and difficulty with emptying. The disadvantages of a colonic patch are that it may form a pseudodiverticulum if redundant, a long intrathoracic suture line is necessary which offers the opportunity for leakage, and it is difficult to carry an anastomosis into the neck.

At the Medical University of South Carolina Children's Hospital 12 children have had colonic patch esophagoplasty since 1976. Long-term follow-up has shown no serious complications and all are eating a normal diet. A barium esophagogram showed a slight pseudodiverticulum in the early cases, but there has been no functional impairment.

Reference

1. Hecker WC, Hollmann G. Correction of long segment oesophageal stenoses by a colonic patch. *Prog Pediatr Surg* 1975; 8: 81–95.

Further reading

Othersen HB Jr, Smith CD. Colon-patch esophagoplasty in children: an alternative to esophageal replacement. *J Pediatr Surg* 1986; 21: 224–6.

Othersen HB Jr, Parker EF, Smith CD. The surgical management of esophageal stricture in children: a century of progress. *Ann Surg* 1988; 207: 590–6.

Tuggle DW, Hoelzer DJ, Tunell WP, Smith EI. The safety and cost-effectiveness of polyethylene glycol electrolyte solution bowel preparation in infants and children. *J Pediatr Surg* 1987; 22: 513–15.

Gastric tube

Sigmund H. Ein MDCM, FRCS(C), FACS, FAAP
Associate Professor, Department of Surgery, Faculty of Medicine, University of Toronto; Staff Surgeon, Division of General Surgery, Hospital for Sick Children; Consultant Staff, Division of Pediatrics, Women's College Hospital; and Associate Staff, Department of Surgery, Mount Sinai Hospital, Toronto, Ontario, Canada

History

Although Gavriliu (1951) is reputed to be the 'father of the gastric tube' and Heimlich (1961) the person who popularized it, Beck (1905) appears to have been the first to construct a gastric tube for esophageal substitution[1]. Swenson and Magruder (1944) replaced part or all of the esophagus in dogs with a gastric tube.

Gavriliu performed the first pediatric gastric tube procedure in a 15-year-old boy in 1951. In 1975 he reported the result of 542 gastric tube operations which had mostly been performed in adults[2]. His large series demonstrated the safety and versatility of these tubes in total or partial replacement of the esophagus in adults requiring esophagectomy or bypass for cancer or stricture.

Heimlich carried out his first gastric tube operation in 1957 and continued to popularize the operation. In 1972 he described his 15-year experience with 53 patients ranging in age from 14 to 70 years. He showed that the tube could be brought up to the pharynx if necessary.

Apart from Gavriliu's first case, there was no further mention of pediatric cases until 10 years later when Sanders (1962) reported a single case of gastric tube replacement in a 4-year-old boy with bleeding esophageal varices in whom a portosystemic shunt had thrombosed. The Toronto experience in 1994 totals 40 cases over a 30-year period[3]. Other proponents of the gastric tube are Cohen[4], Anderson[5] and Lindahl[6].

Principles and justification

The teaching that 'any esophagus no matter how poorly it functions is infinitely better than any substitute' remains the gold standard of pediatric surgeons. The decision to replace the esophagus of a child should therefore be taken only after very careful consideration.

The ideal esophageal replacement should have several attributes:

1. Construction of the replacement should be easy to perform with several options and variations.
2. It must be adaptable to infants and children.
3. Respiration should not be interfered with by the replacement (regardless of its position in the chest or mediastinum).
4. There should be no external evidence of the new esophagus other than a cervical scar.
5. It should remain straight and not become tortuous.
6. It must function as an efficient conduit from mouth to stomach.
7. Gastric acid reflux must be minimal and relatively harmless to the substitute.
8. The esophageal replacement should grow with the infant into adult life without added medical risks.

The gastric tube is the favored method of esophageal replacement in the Hospital for Sick Children, Toronto. It has the following advantages: it has a favorable anatomic location in the upper abdomen, and it is easy to fashion. Several variations to its construction are possible and it can reach the pharynx. It has an excellent blood supply, requires fewer anastomoses and there is no need for a pyloroplasty. The colon is untouched in case the infant has an associated anorectal anomaly. The gastric tube is a straight tube which does not become dilated, tortuous, redundant and/or elongated over the course of time. Finally, it tolerates its own secretions.

Indications

The most common indications for esophageal replacement in pediatric patients are long-gap esophageal atresia (where delayed primary anastomosis cannot be achieved), intractable and caustic esophageal stricture. The gastric tube procedure in an infant with esophageal atresia is carried out within the first year of life. There is no indication for reconstructing the esophagus in the neonatal period or for having an infant less than 6 months old swallowing into an aperistaltic tube which is no more than a conduit that will not effectively propel fluids and/or food unless the infant is in an upright position. The small stomach of a neonate with pure atresia is barely large enough to accommodate a gastrostomy. The main advantage of waiting for at least 6 months is to allow the stomach to enlarge so that a long enough gastric tube can be fashioned without compromising the size of the gastric remnant.

In the one-stage procedure, the choice of the abdominothoracic approach depends on the original esophageal pathology. If the esophageal anastomosis is to be above the aortic arch, the abdominal incision (a left subcostal incision may be best) is closed after the gastric tube has been completed and passed through the esophageal hiatus in the diaphragm, and the procedure is completed through a separate right fourth interspace posterolateral thoracotomy. The disadvantage of the approach is that the gastric tube does not have a lumen for several months and the gastroesophageal tube anastomosis will inevitably leak. A chest tube in such instances is absolutely essential. These one-stage gastric tube procedures are carried out because only the distal part of the esophagus is replaced, e.g. in pure esophageal atresia, and of necessity the gastroesophageal tube anastomosis has to be performed in the chest, or because the caustic esophageal stricture extends so far proximally that the normal esophagus cannot be brought to the surface of the neck for the usual staging. One way to avoid this predicament of not being able to bring the scarred cervical esophagus to the neck surface for staging is to construct the gastric tube at the first stage and leave the esophagus alone. At the second stage (several months later) the esophagus can be divided as high as is necessary and the cervical gastroesophageal tube anastomosis performed immediately in the usual safe, staged fashion. The rare gastric tube that has to be passed subcutaneously can be staged as above; the only indication for this is if the mediastinum and both pleural cavities are scarred from previous operations and infections.

Children needing gastric tubes for caustic strictures undergo the procedure as required, usually at an older age after multiple dilatations have failed. These children will have been fed for a number of months or years by gastrostomy, so that the size of the stomach is not a problem. In contrast, neonates with a congenitally irreparable esophagus will have received an esophagostomy at a very early age in anticipation of a later esophageal replacement. In these cases simultaneous sham feedings by mouth (at the same time as gastrostomy feeds) facilitate postoperative management of oral feeding after the reconstruction.

Preoperative

Assessment and preparation

Few specific investigations and little preoperative preparation are needed for the creation of a gastric tube. This is always an elective operation and the damaged esophagus will have been evaluated on several occasions with radiopaque contrast medium, which will usually show the size of the stomach. The stomach will have been used for gastrostomy feeds and its size should not be a problem. The operation will last at least 3 h and blood for replacement must be available. Preoperative prophylactic antibiotics (cephazolin) should be given.

If the gastric tube operation is staged, before the cervical anastomosis between the esophagus and upper end of the gastric tube is embarked upon, it is essential that the newly created gastric tube and gastric remnant be evaluated radiologically with a water-soluble, radiopaque, substance to ensure that healing has occurred without leak and/or stricture.

Anesthesia

The anesthetic for this operation should be delivered by an anesthetist familiar with pediatric patients and their specific problems. Endotracheal intubation and muscle relaxation are required, without nitrous oxide to avoid any gastrointestinal distension. Blood may occasionally be needed. Blood gas determinations during this potentially lengthy operation may be indicated, and it is advisable to give prophylactic cephazolin at least every 6 h.

The patient can usually be successfully extubated after the standard gastric tube operation. Epidural or spinal narcotics may be used to augment the general anesthetic and aid in postoperative pain management. Alternatively, a continuous intravenous morphine infusion or patient-controlled analgesia may be used for at least 48 h. If the procedure is lengthy and involves both laparotomy and thoracotomy, postoperative ventilation should be considered.

Operation

Patient position and incision

A rolled towel or sandbag is placed under the shoulders with the head turned to the side opposite the previously created esophagostomy. The left neck offers easier access to the cervical esophagus. The abdomen, chest and neck are prepared and draped in one operative field.

The abdomen is opened through an upper midline, high left paramedian or left subcostal incision. The incision should be of adequate length and extend up to and beside the xiphisternum.

Reversed antiperistaltic tube

A gastric tube can be created in several ways . The most common type is the reversed antiperistaltic tube.

1   The gastrostomy (if present) is revised and the defect in the stomach closed. Even if the original gastrostomy was placed along the greater curvature, it does not prevent the creation of a gastric tube, because the scarred stoma can be excised, the hole closed, and the tube constructed wider in that area so as not to create a tube stricture. The blood supply of the gastric tube arises from the gastroepiploic arcade in the omentum. The first step is to divide the greater omentum as far away as possible from the greater curvature to avoid interfering with the gastroepiploic blood supply. There may be a gap in the gastroepiploic arcade, but this should not devascularize the distal tube. Meticulous care must be exercised in ligating and dividing the short gastric vessels to preserve the vascularity of the spleen. The reversed antiperistaltic tube is proximally based and therefore the right gastroepiploic artery is divided about 2 cm proximal to the pylorus.

Pyloroplasty is unnecessary and its siting close to the gastric remnant suture line in the antrum could create an obstructive problem.

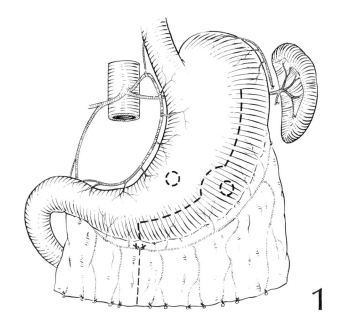

2   The proximally based reversed antiperistaltic gastric tube is started by making a 1-cm incision into the antrum of the stomach at right angles to the greater curvature 2 cm proximal to the pylorus. A 20–26-Fr catheter, depending on the size of the infant or child, is introduced into the stomach through this incision and held in position along the greater curvature by several large Babcock clamps. Care must be taken to avoid damaging the gastroepiploic vascular arcade in the neck of these clamps.

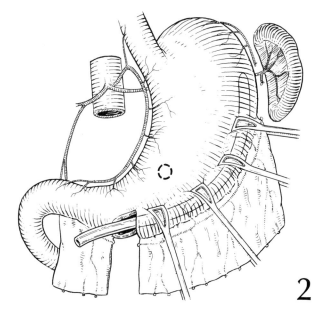

3 The gastric tube (from the greater curvature) can be cut using the catheter as a guide. The tube should not be cut freehand as areas of narrowing and/or widening are inevitable. The best gastric tubes (clinically and radiologically) have been made more narrow than wide with the aid of the catheter stent. Gavriliu recommended a narrow gastric tube to discourage reflux. Narrow gastric tubes do not become dilated, tortuous, or strictured. To minimize the blood loss, only a few centimeters of stomach are dissected at a time. Dissection can be done by cautery or scissors with bowel (Glassman) clamps applied on the stomach side, or with a GIA stapler (if the stomach is large enough). The tube and stomach can be closed in one or two layers with absorbable and/or non-absorbable sutures running, running and locking and/or interrupted. If the tube is made with staples, the suture line should be reinforced with a layer of sutures.

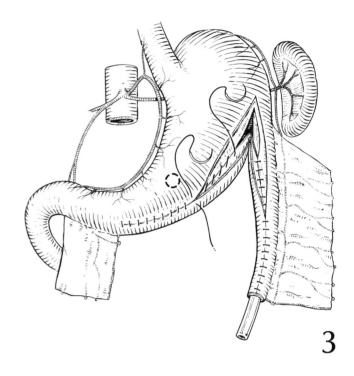

3

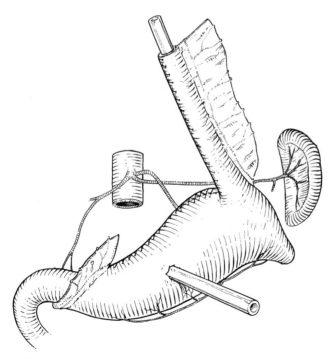

4

4 A new gastrostomy is sited on the anterior wall of the gastric remnant, and the tube is rolled upwards ready to be delivered into the neck.

Isoperistaltic tube

5 The proximally based reversed antiperistaltic tube has been the one most often used in the past, but recently the author has increasingly favored the ease of construction and greater length obtained by creating a distally based isoperistaltic tube. With this type of gastric tube, the tube is supplied by the usually larger right gastroepiploic artery. The tube is started by ligating the left gastroepiploic artery at its origin from the splenic artery. At this point (or a little more proximally along the greater curvature of the stomach) the construction of the tube is begun in a similar fashion to that described for the reversed gastric tube. In infants with pure atresia, even the small distal esophagus can be mobilized and used as the top of the isoperistaltic gastric tube. The tube can be constructed distally to within 2 cm of the pylorus. The isoperistaltic tube must not extend too far distally, however, to avoid obstructing the pylorus.

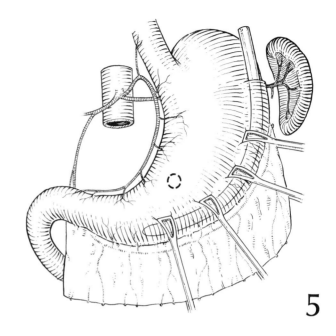

5

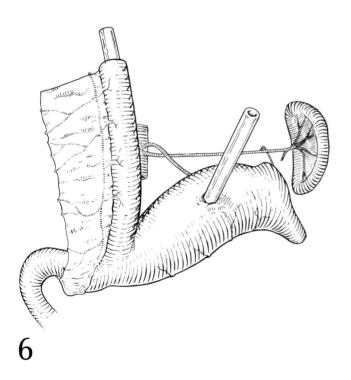

6

6 The new gastrostomy is placed on the posterior wall of the stomach, which becomes rotated anteriorly as the tube is placed retrosternally. By mobilizing the spleen and distal half of the pancreas, the entire tube and stomach remnant can roll upwards (cephalad), allowing less tube to remain in the abdomen (in front of the left lobe of the liver as it heads towards the retrosternal area) and giving more 'length' to the tube itself. This in turn allows a higher, tension-free cervical anastomosis between the cervical esophagus and the proximal gastric tube. It also avoids the necessity of passing the tube through a hole in the posteromedial aspect of the left hemidiaphragm, through the left pleural cavity in front of (or behind) the root of the left lung, and up behind the left clavicle into the neck. This is reputed to be the straightest and most direct route to the neck, but it has the disadvantages of having to go through the left hemidiaphragm and requiring a left sixth interspace thoracotomy. The diaphragmatic opening must be large enough to prevent obstruction of the vascular pedicle, but not too large to avoid herniation of abdominal contents into the chest. Phrenic nerve damage must also be avoided.

7   Whichever way the gastric tube is constructed, the author's preference is still to pass it retrosternally in preparation for a later (staged) neck anastomosis. The first incision in the neck is a 2.5–5-cm transverse incision just above the manubrium. No damage (bleeding, pneumothorax) to any mediastinal structure will ensue if the blunt dissection is carried out with the fingers hugging the posterior wall of the sternum. In most instances the surgeon's two index fingers from above and below (or a long Kelly clamp from below in older children) will meet behind the sternum to complete the tunnel. The only areas of narrowing for passage of the gastric tube are at the xiphoid process and manubrium, but provided that an opening is made wide enough to allow passage of the tube and its accompanying omental blood supply no harm can come to the tube.

The suture line of the tube should be wrapped with the omentum (held in place with a few sutures) before bringing it up into the neck. The tube is then passed retrosternally by passing it anterior to the left lobe of the liver and posterior to the xiphisternum. There is some experimental evidence to show that if at least 5–6 cm of tube remains in the abdomen potentially serious reflux of gastric contents up the gastric tube will be prevented. Leaving 5–6 cm of gastric tube within the abdomen, however, removes that portion from the overall length of the tube reaching the cervical esophagus. A few absorbable sutures are placed to fix the top of the tube in the neck as close as possible to the left esophagostomy, if present. If possible, a portion of the omentum should extend above the top of the gastric tube into the neck so that it may be used to cover the gastroesophageal tube anastomosis. No matter how long the tube is made (and how much tube is left protruding from the neck), none of it should be removed. If necessary the 'excess' tube should be tunneled sub-cutaneously and brought out higher up on the left side of the neck as a flush stoma.

    The need to remove the native (original) esophagus is a matter of some debate. It is difficult and bloody and not worth the effort to avoid the exceedingly rare occurrence of a blind loop or carcinoma in the intrathoracic esophageal remnant.

Abdominal wound closure

The abdomen is closed (without drainage) after the new gastrostomy is fashioned.

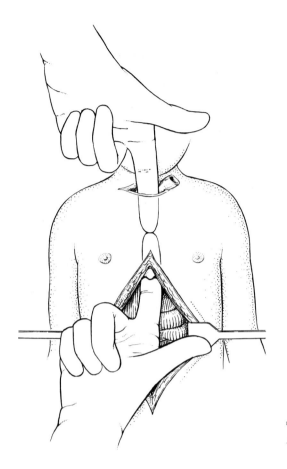

7

Postoperative nutrition was originally maintained by gastrostomy feeds, started in small amounts after 1 week when ileus had resolved. This created excoriation of the skin of the neck in almost all the patients because of reflux of gastric contents up the new gastric tube. This reflux sometimes prevented sufficient calories from being delivered by gastrostomy and also prompted earlier than ideal closure of the neck anastomosis to stop the reflux.

    To avoid these reflux problems, a no. 10–12 feeding jejunostomy tube can be placed alongside the newly created gastrostomy for elemental feeds. With the advent of more refined elemental products, the concern about lack of adequate caloric intake, hypertonic dumping, diarrhea and mechanical plugging of the small jejunostomy feeding tube has been minimized. If the jejunostomy tube is dislodged or plugged, it can be replaced after 3–4 weeks under radiological control. Any feeding tube must not be removed until it has been unused for at least 3 months.

Esophagogastric tube anastomosis

While most of the earlier gastric tubes were anastomosed to the cervical esophagus at a second stage after 2 weeks, the narrow tube always seemed to create a problem because it seldom had a visible lumen to anastomose to the esophagus. This was even more of a problem with a primary tube anastomosis. In an attempt to alleviate this problem, the upper part of the gastric tube can be made wider for an easier anastomosis. This requires more stomach, however, and may narrow either the entrance or exit of the stomach depending on whether the tube is distally (isoperistaltic) or proximally (reversed antiperistaltic) based. It is best, therefore, to avoid a primary anastomosis and to perform the second stage at least 3 months later, when the gastric tube has a good lumen and will not unravel as its upper part is mobilized before the anastomosis.

In children with long esophageal strictures that require the construction of a gastric tube, the cervical esophagostomy is usually made at the same time as the gastric tube. After the gastric tube has been delivered into the neck, the cervical esophagus is identified and divided as low as possible, and the distal end is closed and allowed to fall into the upper mediastinum, while the proximal end is brought out as a cervical esophagostomy. If the caustic stricture involves the high cervical esophagus, it may be impossible to fashion an esophagostomy. The native esophagus should be left intact until the gastric tube is ready for its cervical anastomosis to the proximal esophagus.

If the gastric tube reconstruction is staged, the long gastric tube and stomach remnant suture lines are totally defunctioned and safe. The cervical anastomosis is usually performed 3–4 months later. This is the easiest and safest course. The author seldom performs the gastroesophageal tube anastomosis anywhere except in the neck, because should a leak occur, there is contamination of only the local cervical area. After the second stage, only one short cervical suture line is present, which is away from the peritoneal, pleural and mediastinal spaces. As there is such a high rate of anastomotic leakage, it best occurs in the neck where its course is benign until it closes.

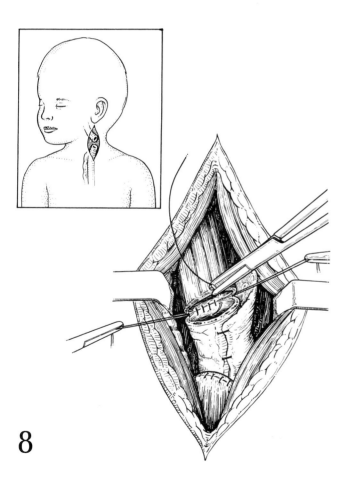

8 At operation, the best position for the cervical anastomosis is obtained by placing a small sandbag under the shoulders and turning the head to the opposite side. Both stomas are mobilized from the surrounding structures for several centimeters until the paratracheal area is identified. Care must be taken not to damage the recurrent laryngeal nerves. An end-to-end anastomosis is then made, using one or two layers of interrupted sutures. If any omentum is available in the neck from the gastric tube construction it can be wrapped around the anastomosis. If insufficient gastric tube has been brought up into the neck, the sternum will have to be split to mobilize the gastric tube to achieve a tension-free anastomosis. If the cervical anastomosis is embarked on too soon (in weeks rather than months) the gastric tube lumen may not yet be patent and/or the tube will come undone as it is mobilized; both of these problems may give rise to leaks.

Wound closure

After the anastomosis is completed, the sternocleidomastoid muscle and fascia are closed over the new anastomosis, which is drained. A nasopharyngeal suction catheter should be left in place just proximal to the anastomosis; otherwise frequent oropharyngeal suctioning of saliva will be required for 3–4 days until the anastomotic edema has decreased, the lumen is patent and the patient can swallow. Unfortunately, medication to reduce acid production does not reduce the high incidence of leaks. Nutrition is maintained by the previous gastrojejunostomy tube feedings.

8

Postoperative care

The usual postoperative care that follows any major pediatric abdominothoracic procedure should be delivered in the appropriate fashion. Postoperative pain management merges with anesthetic management during the gastric tube construction and continues during the first week.

Complications

Postoperative problems continue to be directly related to the gastroesophageal tube anastomosis and its subsequent leaking and/or stricture. Not all the leaks result in strictures, and not all strictures are preceded by leaks. It appears that the technique used in infants and children whose anastomoses were most problem-free was a meticulous two-layer, interrupted 4/0 silk anastomosis with constant proximal nasopharyngeal sump suction for 1 week. Recently, success has been achieved with a one-layer interrupted 3/0 or 4/0 polyglactin (Vicryl) anastomosis.

Most anastomotic strictures that require dilatation occur within the first few months after operation. If the stricture has not been successfully and permanently dilated after 1 year of repeated dilatations, consideration should be given to resection of the anastomosis. This may be needed in up to 25% of cases. In these cases the esophagus above the stricture and the gastric tube below it usually have a good lumen, and the anastomosis is easier to perform the second time. On a few occasions, the gastric tube cannot be mobilized as much as desired and the second anastomosis must be fashioned under some tension; the choice is either to split the sternum to mobilize the gastric tube and run the risk of a mediastinal infection, or to accept a tight anastomosis and subsequent cervical leak with minimal morbidity. The latter is the preferred choice.

Postoperative pneumonia is almost always due to aspiration following completion of the gastroesophageal tube anastomosis. These infants and children cannot, or will not, swallow their saliva immediately after the tube is connected even when the anastomosis is patent. They need constant oral suctioning and/or nasopharyngeal sump suction proximal to the anastomosis for about 1 week. Some infants have chronic swallowing problems; any method other than waiting will not overcome this type of functional dysphagia. Until such time, gastrostomy or jejunostomy feeding is the only solution.

Although all gastric tubes suffer from reflux, only a few have noticeable chronic problems from this gastroesophageal reflux, e.g. chronic night-time coughing and aspiration. This can be mostly eliminated by keeping the stomach empty for a few hours before bedtime and elevating the head of the bed. Several children develop chronic respiratory problems, but most seem to improve by 5–6 years of age. A few will require pyloroplasty to aid emptying of the stomach and gastrostomy to give them most of their fluids until the chronic chest problem improves. Attempts at operative intervention to prevent gastroesophageal reflux have not been successful, because any attempt at preventing reflux using a fundoplication tends to obstruct the primarily aperistaltic gastric tube. There have been some reports of prevention of gastroesophageal reflux without obstruction by a partial anterior wrap (Thal, Dor–Nissen) and/or 2–5 cm of intra-abdominal distal gastric tube.

Gastric tube ulcer has been reported as a rare complication.

Outcome

Since the first pediatric gastric tube procedure was carried out at the Hospital for Sick Children, Toronto, in 1964, a large enough series (about 40 patients) followed for long enough (up to 30 years) has been accumulated to allow definite conclusions to be drawn concerning the gastric tube operation and its sequelae.

Twice as many boys as girls require gastric tubes, but there is an equal ratio between congenital esophageal defects and strictures. The latter is indeed a change over the last decade, due to newer and more aggressive ways of bridging the gap between the two atretic portions of esophagus on the one hand and a greater awareness and increased popularity of antireflux procedures in treating esophageal stricture on the other. A proximally based antiperistaltic tube was constructed in most instances, but a distally based isoperistaltic tube has become the procedure of choice in the last 10 years. Most tubes were passed retrosternally, 25% through the chest, and one subcutaneously. Of these infants and children, 80% had their tube construction staged, and the remaining 20% had the entire procedure done in one stage. The spleen was removed in the early period of these gastric tube operations. There were 50% extra-tube major complications. Two-thirds of the gastric tube cervical anastomoses leaked; all but one closed spontaneously within 3 months. Gastroesophageal tube anastomotic strictures occurred in 40%, and these were dilated from one to many times; 25% required resection (usually after 1 year of repeated dilatations).

It is extremely rare for an infant or child to lose the gastric tube provided it was correctly made. It is obvious that the results depend for the most part on the status of the gastroesophageal tube anastomosis (and the necessity for dilatations) and aspiration (mostly reflux). Most of these dilatations are required within the first 3 months after the tube is functioning, and within 1 year it is apparent how successfully the gastric tube will function. In the 1990s a relatively asymptomatic endoscopic finding of cervical Barrett's esophagus (esophageal gastric metaplasia) was reported to be the result of acid reflux esophagitis. It remains to be shown whether this is similar to adult patients with Barrett's esophagus, which is associated with a high risk of esophageal adenocarcinoma. Furthermore, the treatment (positional therapy and medication) and/or investigation (lifelong periodic endoscopy) for such esophagitis has yet to be decided.

The overall outcome of the pediatric gastric tube procedure is good considering it is a substitute for the native structure (the esophagus). In deciding which patients have excellent or good results, it is difficult to be truly objective. Some infants seem not to thrive initially as well as predicted, though on contrast radiographs their gastric tube is patent and they swallow quite well. None the less, the author believes that once a patient is eating and swallowing well, does not require any dilatation and is free of chest problems, the result can be considered excellent. The children considered to have a good result do not eat as well as their peers, periodically require dilatations, and may still be troubled by some chest problems; however, 90% of the Toronto patients have been followed for more than 3 years and up to 30 years (as of 1994). By the 1990s 80% swallow normally and none require dilatation. Mild sacculation or tortuosity of the gastric tube has been encountered only once in a tube that was cut freehand.

Growth was slow in a few until school age, and two continued to aspirate so that a gastrostomy was refashioned for night-time feeds. There were four late deaths (tracheostomy complication, aspiration, gastric tube ulcer hemorrhage, bowel obstruction).

References

1. Burrington JD, Stephens CA. Esophageal replacement with a gastric tube in infants and children. *J Pediatr Surg* 1968; 3: 24–52.

2. Gavriliu D. Replacement of the esophagus by a reverse gastric tube. *Curr Probl Surg* 1975; 12: 36–64.

3. Ein SH, Shandling B, Stephens CA. Twenty-one year experience with the pediatric gastric tube. *J Pediatr Surg* 1987; 22: 77–81.

4. Cohen DH, Middleton AW, Fletcher J. Gastric tube esophagoplasty. *J Pediatr Surg* 1974; 9: 451–60.

5. Anderson KD, Randolph JG. The gastric tube for esophageal replacement in children. *J Thorac Cardiovasc Surg* 1983; 6: 333–42.

6. Lindahl H, Louhimo I, Virkola K. Colon interposition or gastric tube? Follow-up study of colon–esophagus and gastric tube–esophagus patients. *J Pediatr Surg* 1983; 18: 58–63.

Illustrations by Gillian Oliver

Gastric replacement of the esophagus

Lewis Spitz PhD, FRCS, FRCS(Ed), FAAP(Hon)
Nuffield Professor of Paediatric Surgery, Institute of Child Health, University of London, and Consultant Paediatric Surgeon, Great Ormond Street Hospital for Children, London, UK

One of the alternatives for replacing the esophagus is gastric transposition involving the whole stomach. This method has the advantage of involving only one anastomosis, which is relatively well vascularized and is associated with a low rate of leakage.

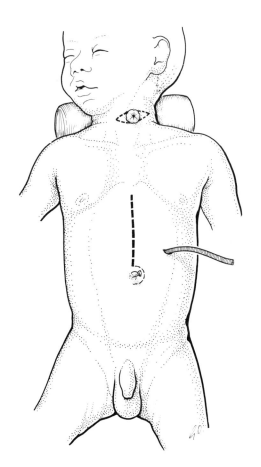

1

Operation

The procedure may be performed either by a thoraco-abdominal approach or transhiatally via the posterior mediastinum without having to resort to a thoracotomy. This latter method will be described in detail.

The importance of sham feeds before the definitive operation in simplifying the initiation of oral nutrition following the interposition should not be underestimated.

MEDIASTINAL GASTRIC TRANSPOSITION

The initial feeding gastrostomy should ideally have been sited on the anterior surface of the body of the stomach, well away from the greater curvature, in order to preserve the vascular arcades of the gastroepiploic vessels.

Incision

1 The preferred approach is via a midline upper abdominal incision extending from the xiphisternum to the umbilicus. Alternatively, a left oblique upper abdominal transverse muscle-cutting incision, which can easily be extended into a thoracoabdominal approach, may be used particularly if previous esophageal surgery renders blunt mediastinal dissection hazardous.

The gastrostomy is carefully mobilized and the defect in the stomach closed in two layers with interrupted 4/0 polyglycolic acid sutures.

Mobilizing the stomach

Adhesions between the stomach and the left lobe of the liver are released, taking care not to damage any of the major blood vessels.

2 The greater curvature of the stomach is mobilized by ligating and dividing the vessels in the gastrocolic omentum and the short gastric vessels. These vessels should be ligated well away from the stomach wall in order to preserve the vascular arcades of the right gastroepiploic vessels. Meticulous care must be exercised to avoid damaging the spleen.

The lesser curvature of the stomach is freed by dividing the lesser omentum from the pylorus to the diaphragmatic hiatus. The right gastric artery is carefully identified and preserved, while the left gastric vessels are ligated and divided close to the stomach. The lower esophagus is exposed by dividing the phrenoesophageal membrane, and the margins of the esophageal hiatus in the diaphram are defined.

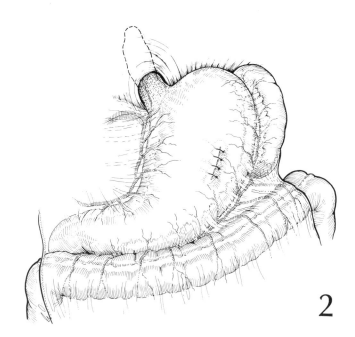

Resection of the distal esophagus

3 The inevitably short, blind-ending lower esophageal stump is dissected out of the posterior mediastinum by a combination of blunt and sharp dissection through the diaphragmatic hiatus. The vagal nerves are divided during this part of the procedure. The body and fundus of the stomach are now free from all attachments and can be delivered into the wound.

The esophagus is transected at the gastroesophageal junction and the defect closed in two layers with 4/0 polyglycolic acid sutures.

The second part of the duodenum is kocherized to obtain maximum mobility of the pylorus.

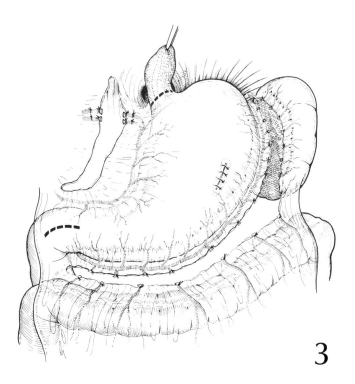

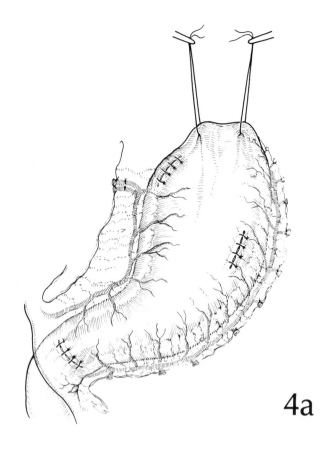

4a

Preparing for gastroesophageal anastomosis

4a, b
The highest part of the fundus of the stomach is identified and stay sutures of different material are inserted to the left and the right of the area selected for the anastomosis. These sutures help to avoid torsion of the stomach as it is pulled through the posterior mediastinum into the neck.

Pyloroplasty

A short Heinecke–Mikulicz pyloroplasty is performed, the transverse incision being closed horizontally with interrupted fine polyglycolic acid sutures.

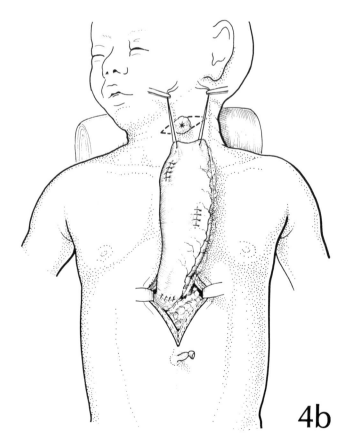

4b

Mobilization of the cervical esophagus

5 Attention is now turned to the neck, where the previously constructed cervical esophagostomy (preferably performed on the left side) is mobilized via a 3–4-cm transverse incision, taking care not to damage the muscular coat of the esophagus. The recurrent laryngeal nerve coursing upwards on the posterolateral surface of the trachea is identified and preserved.

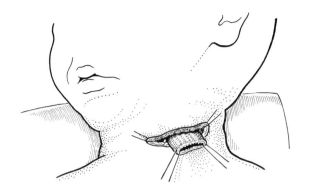

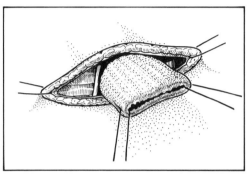

5

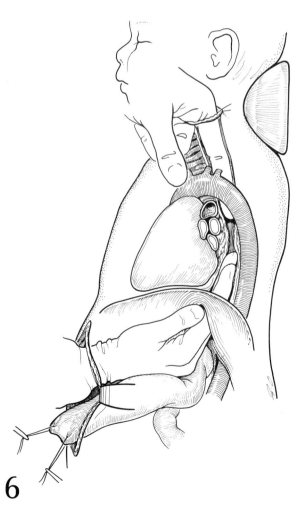

6

Preparing the posterior mediastinal tunnel

6 A plane of dissection between the membranous posterior surface of the trachea and the prevertebral fascia is established, and by blunt dissection immediately in the midline a tunnel is created into the superior mediastinum.

A similar tunnel is fashioned from below in the line of the normal esophageal route, by means of blunt dissection through the esophageal hiatus in the tissue posterior to the heart and anterior to the prevertebral fascia.

When continuity of the superior and inferior posterior mediastinal tunnels has been established, the space to be occupied by the stomach is developed into a tunnel of 2–3 fingers' breadth.

Transposing the stomach

7a, b A long, blunt hemostat is passed through the posterior mediastinal tunnel from the cervical incision, and the two stay sutures on the fundus of the stomach are grasped. The hemostat is gently withdrawn, drawing the stomach up through the esophageal hiatus and the posterior mediastinal tunnel into the cervical incision. Orientation of the fundus is checked by realigning the stay sutures in their correct position.

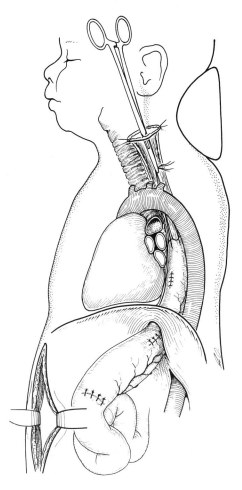

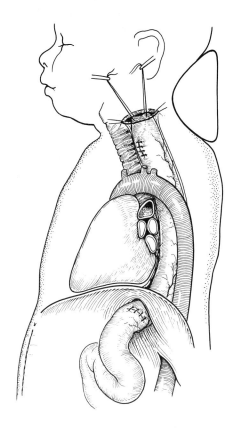

7a

7b

Gastroesophageal anastomosis

8 The end of the esophagus is anastomosed to the highest part of the stomach using a single layer of interrupted 4/0 polyglycolic acid sutures.

A large-caliber (10-gauge) nasogastric tube is inserted into the stomach through the gastroesophageal anastomosis. This is left on free drainage and aspirated at regular intervals to prevent acute gastric dilatation in the early postoperative period.

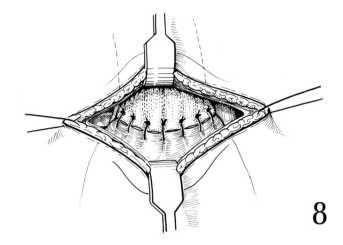

8

Wound closure

A soft rubber drain is placed at the site of the anastomosis and the wound is closed in layers.

The margins of the diaphragmatic hiatus are sutured to the antrum of the stomach with a few interrupted sutures (4/0 polyglycolic acid or braided polyamide (Nurolon)), so that the pylorus lies just below the diaphragm.

A fine-bore feeding jejunostomy has been found to be of considerable value in providing enteral nutrition in the first few weeks following the gastric transposition, before full oral nutrition is established.

The abdominal incision is closed *en masse* or in layers.

Final anatomy

9 The gastroesophageal anastomosis is protected with a nasogastric tube passing into the thoracic stomach. The pyloroplasty is below the diaphragm and a feeding jejunostomy tube is inserted for postoperative feeding.

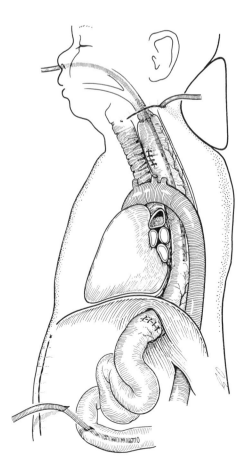

9

Postoperative care

Careful monitoring of vital functions is essential in the early postoperative period. There has been a fairly extensive dissection in the tissues posterior to the trachea, and edema may produce respiratory embarrassment. Elective nasotracheal intubation with assisted ventilation for a few days will simplify the postoperative course and reduce the incidence of respiratory problems.

Jejunal feeds are instituted on the second or third day after operation. The safest method of delivery of these feeds is by a slow continuous infusion rather than as a bolus, which can provoke a 'dumping' effect. A contrast swallow is performed 5–7 days after surgery, and if no leak is identified at the anastomosis oral feeding may be commenced. The cervical drain is removed when the integrity of the anastomosis has been demonstrated.

Complications

A 9% mortality rate has occurred in 72 patients. All deaths occurred in children who had undergone repeated previous attempts at restoring esophageal continuity. Other complications included leakage at the gastroesophageal anastomosis (12%) and stricture of the gastroesophageal anastomosis (9%) – all of these last patients responded to dilatation alone. Delayed gastric emptying and dumping syndrome also occurred in some patients. Feeding problems and recurrent vomiting are commonly encountered in the early postoperative period, but are generally transient.

Outcome

Good to excellent results are achieved in 88% of patients. Growth and development do not appear to be affected, and respiratory function is not impaired.

Further reading

Orringer HB, Sloan H. Esophagectomy without thoracotomy. *J Thorac Cardiovasc Surg* 1978; 76: 643–54.

Spitz L. Gastric transposition via the mediastinal route for infants with long-gap esophageal atresia. *J Pediatr Surg* 1984; 19: 149–54.

Spitz L. Gastric transposition for esophageal substitution in children. *J Pediatr Surg* 1992; 27: 252–9.

Spitz L, Kiely E, Sparnon T. Gastric transposition for esophageal replacement in children. *Ann Surg* 1987; 206: 69–73.

Illustrations by Marks Creative Consultants

Congenital diaphragmatic hernia

Charles J. H. Stolar MD
Professor of Surgery, Columbia University, College of Physicians and Surgeons, and Attending Surgeon, Babies' Hospital and Children's Hospital of New York, Columbia-Presbyterian Medical Center, New York City, New York, USA

History, etiology and pathophysiology

Although the earliest descriptions of congenital diaphragmatic hernia were by Paré, the concept of an embryologic etiology was first discussed by Bochdalek in 1848. He erroneously thought that the diaphragm ruptured after formation.

1 Current ideas view the defect to be an inherent abnormality of the lungs which results in a secondary abnormality of the diaphragm, or as a failure of the diaphragm to separate the pleuroperitoneal canal into the thorax and abdomen before the midgut returns from the umbilicus. Alternatively, the midgut may return too soon. As a consequence, translocation of abdominal viscera into the chest occurs in the first trimester when the lungs are at a very vulnerable lung bud/glandular stage.

The resultant abnormality leads to disordered lung growth. Both lungs are affected, the ipsilateral more so than the contralateral lung. The consequent structural abnormality features compromised bronchiolar and pulmonary arterial divisions, muscular hypertrophy of the intra-acinar arterioles, and a decreased surface available for gas exchange. Affected infants are born with a complex interface of pulmonary hypoplasia and pulmonary hypertension. Pulmonary hypoplasia can be severe enough to preclude life outside the womb, while successful management of pulmonary hypertension can lead to a fruitful life.

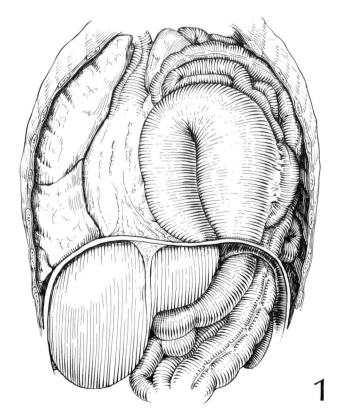

1

Diagnosis

2a–c The typical infant with congenital diaphragmatic hernia presents immediately after birth with the stigmata of respiratory distress: tachypnea, grunting and cyanosis. The infant has usually reached full term, and has a scaphoid abdomen and barrel chest. With increasing frequency, the diagnosis of this condition is made with prenatal ultrasound.

Ultrasound examination shows a fetus with mediastinal shift, bowel and/or liver in the chest, no intra-abdominal stomach, or the heart and stomach in the same plane. At birth, the diagnosis is confirmed by a chest radiograph. This will show multiple gas-filled loops of bowel and contralateral shifting of the mediastinum. There is an absence of bowel gas in the abdomen.

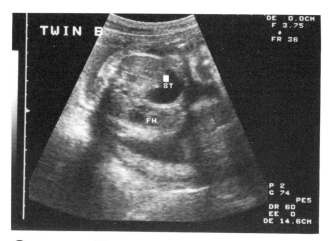

2a   ST = stomach; FH = fetal heart

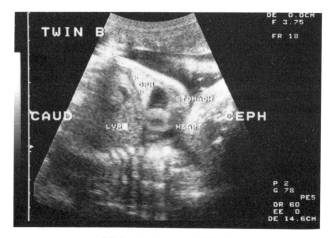

2b   DPH = diaphragm; LVR = liver

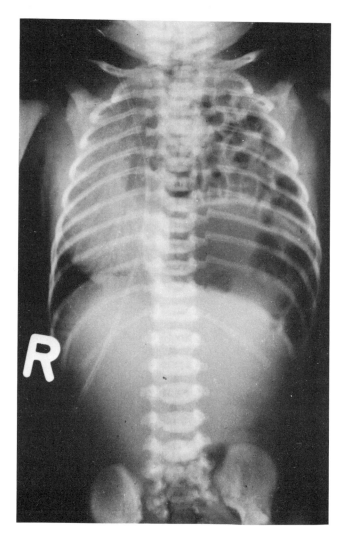

2c

Preoperative

Resuscitation

When the condition is diagnosed before birth, the mother is transferred to a level III neonatal center capable of appropriate neonatal, surgical and extracorporeal membrane oxygenation (ECMO) care. If diagnosed after birth, the infant is stabilized and then transferred to the same sort of center before operation.

Traditionally, diagnosis of congenital diaphragmatic hernia made emergency operation mandatory. Recent experience, however, has clearly demonstrated that most infants with this condition can be stabilized over several days and undergo elective surgery. Infants who cannot be stabilized may have pulmonary hypoplasia to a degree incompatible with life, but may be considered for resuscitation with ECMO. The resuscitation strategy is based on prompt intubation, nasogastric decompression, and arterial and venous vascular access. Respiratory care should preclude muscle paralysis and allow spontaneous respiration to minimize barotrauma. Ventilator settings range from low rates and modest peak airway pressure to higher rates with lower peak airway pressures, and to oscillating ventilation. Pharmacologic support may consist of pulmonary vasodilators such as dobutamine, tolazoline or nitric oxide. An umbilical artery catheter is placed for blood pressure monitoring and blood sampling, and preductal and postductal (Sa_{O_2}) cutaneous monitors are attached. Placement of a preductal arterial catheter is frequently critical. Because most of these infants have significant right-to-left shunting at the ductus arteriosus level, blood gas monitoring from the umbilical artery is often misleading and can lead to premature surgery or inordinate use of ECMO. Assessment of P_{O_2} and P_{CO_2} in the preductal location is a more accurate assessment of the lungs' ability for meaningful gas exchange. ECMO is useful in the preoperative infant who has already demonstrated evidence of adequate lung function but who then deteriorates because of pulmonary hypertension. Such an infant is unlikely to tolerate surgery easily.

Anesthesia

The airway is controlled with an appropriately sized orotracheal or nasotracheal tube (a nasotracheal tube is preferred because of the potentially lower incidence of airway complications). Volatile anesthesia is administered as needed and is complemented by muscle paralysis and narcotics. Mechanical ventilation is controlled throughout surgery with a pressure-cycled infant ventilator rather than the conventional anesthesia machine. Continuous Sa_{O_2} monitoring, both preductal and postductal, is critical.

Operation

Position of patient

The infant is positioned supine on a heating mattress with a small elevating pad beneath the thoracolumbar spine. The extremities and head are wrapped to minimize heat loss. Both the upper abdomen and chest are prepared as the operating fields. The entire operation is performed as much as possible with electrocautery because of the potential need for ECMO and heparin.

Incision

A subcostal incision is made on the side of the hernia.

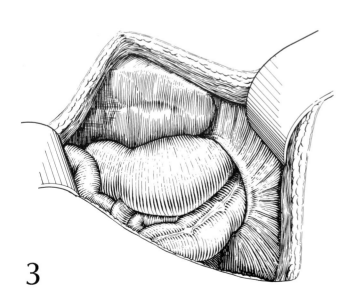

3 The cephalad portion of the incision and the anterior rim of the diaphragm are elevated to expose the defect.

Suction of the stomach is performed via the nasogastric tube and the viscera are carefully reduced. The unfixed spleen and its tenuous attachments to the colon and pancreas are especially vulnerable. Reduction of the liver may be equally challenging.

4a–c

Once the hernia has been reduced the viscera are allowed to lie on the abdominal wall. If a true hernia sac is found, it must be excised to ensure proper healing of the defect. The posterior rim can be found by tracing the anterior rim around medially. Its mesothelial covering is sharply incised and carefully mobilized. If primary closure is possible it is worth pursuing the posterior rim. If a prosthetic patch is required, dissection should be kept to a minimum. Primary repair is accomplished with interrupted simple sutures of a non-absorbable material.

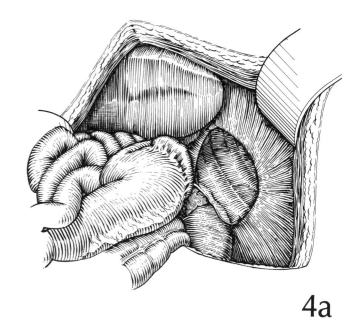

4a

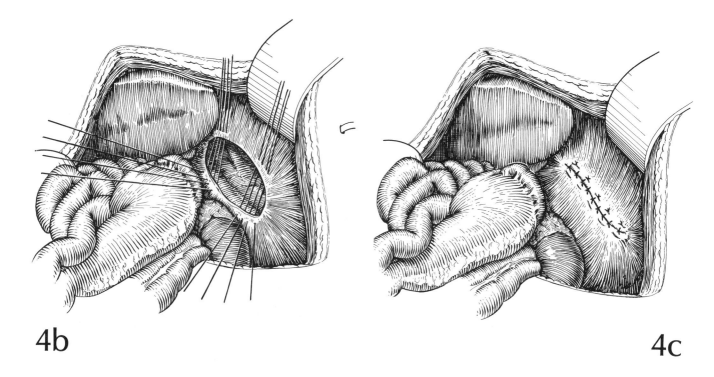

4b

4c

5 A prosthetic patch can be constructed using 1-mm thick Gore-Tex which is tailored to size and secured with interrupted sutures. Laterally the patch can be anchored to the ribs. A paucity of medial tissue requires the surgeon to be creative.

Once the diaphragm is constructed an ipsilateral tube thoracostomy is not needed unless there is bleeding or pneumothorax. It is not required for prophylaxis.

Correction of the unrotated midgut by division of Ladd's bands with or without inversion appendicectomy should be discouraged if ECMO is contemplated or in use unless mechanical obstruction is already present. Postoperative volvulus is rare, but significant bleeding after heparinization may be a major problem.

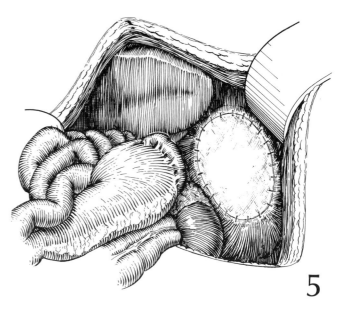

5

Wound closure

Closure of the abdominal wall can be challenging because of loss of abdominal domain. Vigorous stretching of the abdominal wall is discouraged. If the abdomen cannot be closed safely in layers without compromising venous return a silo in the manner of omphalocele management is preferred with subsequent reduction over several days.

Postoperative care

The therapeutic strategy used in the preoperative period is reinstituted in the postoperative period. Muscle paralysis is discontinued to allow spontaneous respiration. Adequate analgesia with narcotics is mandatory. Sufficient intravenous fluids are given to maintain adequate circulating blood volume and hemoglobin for oxygen delivery. As the infant recovers it is weaned from a mechanical respirator to nasal prong continuous positive airway pressure. A prolonged recovery will need to be complemented by parenteral nutrition.

Extracorporeal membrane oxygenation (ECMO)

Although this therapy is discussed in detail in the chapter on pp. 164–167, there are some special considerations for ECMO in the infant with congenital diaphragmatic hernia. Because ECMO may be appropri-

ate both before and after operation, these infants should be transferred to an ECMO center as soon as possible after diagnosis and the infant (or fetus) is stable enough for transport. It must be remembered that ECMO requires heparin and that any dissected or stretched surface may bleed.

Occasionally an infant with congenital diaphragmatic hernia will need ECMO as part of the preoperative resuscitation. In this case, surgery will be performed in the neonatal intensive care unit while ECMO is in progress. The operative technique is similar but meticulous hemostasis is critical.

Further reading

Geggel RL, Murphy JD, Langleben D, Crone RK, Vacanti JP, Reid LM. Congenital diaphragmatic hernia: arterial structural changes and persistent pulmonary hypertension after surgical repair. *J Pediatr* 1985; 107: 457–64.

Reid L. Embryology of the lung. In: de Reuck AVS, Porter R, eds. *Development of the Lung*. London: Churchill, 1967: 109–30.

Stolar CJH, Price ME, Butler MW, Lazar EL. Management of infants with congenital diaphragmatic hernia using ECMO. In: Arensman R, Cornish JD, eds. *Extracorporeal Life Support*. Boston: Blackwell Scientific Publications, 1993: 252–61.

Extracorporeal membrane oxygenation: neonatal vascular cannulation

Thomas Pranikoff MD
Lecturer in Surgery, Fellow in Extracorporeal Life Support, University of Michigan Medical School, Ann Arbor, Michigan, USA

Ronald B. Hirschl MD
Assistant Professor of Surgery, Section of Pediatric Surgery, University of Michigan Medical School, and Pediatric Surgeon, C.S. Mott Children's Hospital, Ann Arbor, Michigan, USA

History

Extracorporeal membrane oxygenation (ECMO) has been used to describe a method of extracorporeal life support (ECLS) using extrathoracic cannulation for cardiopulmonary support. ECLS is a supportive rather than a therapeutic intervention. It provides adequate perfusion and gas exchange, and so avoids deleterious effects from high oxygen concentrations and positive pressure ventilation while allowing resolution of reversible heart and lung pathology.

Principles and justification

Vascular access for ECLS in the neonate is particularly challenging due to the small vessel size. The route of access depends on the method used. Venoarterial bypass is indicated if both cardiac and pulmonary support are required, and in neonates where access for venovenous bypass cannot be obtained. Venovenous bypass is the method of choice for pulmonary support alone. Various access sites, including the umbilical, femoral and carotid/jugular vessels, have been used.

For venoarterial access, the preferred site is the right atrium via the right internal jugular vein for venous drainage and the aortic arch via the right common carotid artery for arterial infusion. The internal jugular vein and carotid artery are relatively large in the neonate and may be distally ligated with impunity.

For venovenous access, a double-lumen cannula is placed into the right atrium via the right internal jugular vein. This technique is limited by the size of the vein, because the smallest cannula currently available is 14 Fr.

Preoperative

Vascular cannulation and decannulation are performed in the neonatal intensive care unit under adequate sedation and neuromuscular blockade. Neuromuscular blockade is especially important in preventing the potentially lethal complication of an air embolus during introduction of the venous cannula. The team, instruments and sterile procedure used are identical to those used in the operating room. Heparin sodium (100 units/kg) is drawn up for subsequent administration.

Anesthesia

Local anesthesia is administered by infiltration of 1% lidocaine (lignocaine).

Operation

Position of patient

The patient is placed supine with the head turned to the left. A roll is placed transversely beneath the shoulders. The chest, neck and right side of the face are aseptically prepared and draped.

Incision

1 A transverse cervical incision approximately 2–3 cm in length is made one finger's breadth above the clavicle over the lower aspect of the right sternocleido-mastoid muscle.

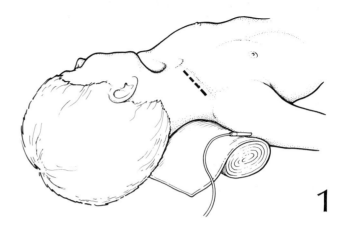

1

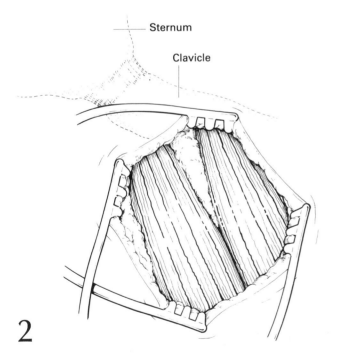

— Sternum

Clavicle

2

Exposure of the carotid sheath

2 The platysma muscle and subcutaneous tissues are divided with electrocautery and the sternocleido-mastoid muscle exposed. Dissection is continued between the sternal and clavicular heads of the muscle. The omohyoid muscle will be seen superiorly. It may be necessary to divide the omohyoid muscle tendon to expose the carotid sheath. Two alternating self-retaining retractors are placed.

Dissection of the vessels

3 The carotid sheath is opened and the internal jugular vein, common carotid artery and vagus nerve are identified and isolated. Dissection is progressed proximally and distally along the vessels, dissecting the vein first. Special care should be taken while dissecting the vein to avoid induction of spasm, which makes subsequent introduction of a large venous cannula difficult. Manipulation of the vein therefore should be minimized. There is often a branch on the medial aspect of the internal jugular vein which must be ligated. Ligatures of 2/0 silk are placed proximally and distally around the internal jugular vein. The common carotid artery lies medial and posterior and has no branches, which makes its dissection proximally and distally safe. Ligatures of 2/0 silk are also placed around the carotid artery. The vagus nerve should be identified.

Once vessel dissection is completed, heparin (100 units/kg) is administered intravenously and 3 minutes allowed for circulation. During this waiting period, papaverine is instilled into the wound to enhance vein dilatation.

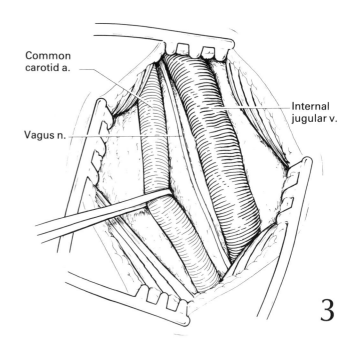

Common carotid a.

Vagus n.

Internal jugular v.

3

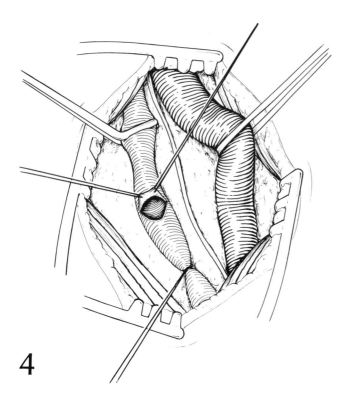

4

Arteriotomy/venotomy

4 For venoarterial bypass the arterial cannula is chosen (usually 10 Fr) and marked with a 2/0 silk ligature, left uncut, at a point that will allow the tip to lie at the ostium of the brachiocephalic artery (about 2.5 cm). The venous cannula (usually 12–14 Fr outer diameter) is similarly marked at a point equal to the distance from the venotomy to the right atrium (roughly 6 cm). An obturator is placed into the venous cannula to prevent blood flowing out through the side holes during introduction into the vessel. The common carotid artery is ligated distally. Proximal control is obtained with the use of an angled ductus clamp. A transverse arteriotomy is made near to the distal ligature. Full-thickness stay sutures of 6/0 polypropylene are placed on the proximal edge of the artery to prevent subintimal dissection during cannula insertion. Following cannulation, a venotomy is performed in similar fashion. Gentle retraction of the caudal suture around the vein precludes the need for a ductus clamp during venotomy and venous cannulation. Stay sutures are also not routinely necessary for venous cannulation.

Cannula placement

5 The cannulas are carefully placed into the artery and vein and secured using two circumferential 2/0 silk ligatures, with a small piece of plastic vessel loop inside the ligatures to protect the vessels from injury during decannulation when the ligatures are sharply divided. The ends of the marking ligatures are tied to the most distal circumferential ligature for extra security. Immediately after each cannula is secured, it is carefully debubbled via back-bleeding and filling with heparinized saline. The cannulas are then additionally secured to the skin overlying the mastoid process with two monofilament sutures. For venovenous bypass, the double-lumen cannula is placed into the venotomy and advanced 5.5 cm. It is crucial to maintain the arterial reinfusion port anteriorly during placement for proper cannula orientation to minimize recirculation of reinfused blood.

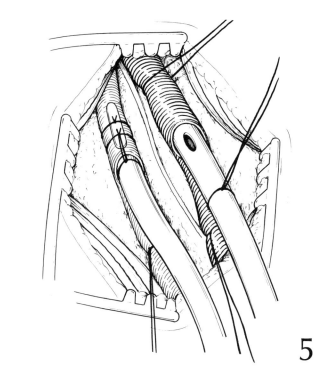

5

Wound closure

6 The wound is irrigated with saline and hemostasis obtained. The skin is closed with continuous monofilament suture. The wound is dressed with gauze secured with cotton umbilical tape around the neck. Special attention should be directed to affixing the cannulas securely to the bed.

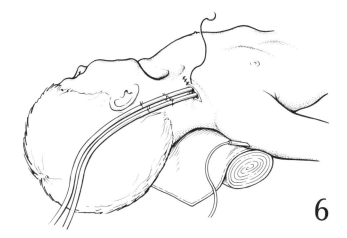

6

Postoperative care

The cannulas are connected to the extracorporeal bypass circuit, assuring that no air bubbles are present, and bypass is initiated. Dopamine infusion into the ECLS circuit reinfusion connector is often necessary for inotropic support with the initiation of venovenous bypass. Chest radiographs should be obtained following the procedure to verify optimal cannula placement in the aortic arch (arterial cannula) and inferior aspect of the right atrium (venous cannulas). Bleeding from the wound is controlled by lowering activated clotting times, platelet transfusions, administration of fresh frozen plasma and local instillation of fibrin glue. Bleeding not controlled by these maneuvers should be investigated and controlled by operative exploration.

Outcome

More than 8000 neonates have been treated since 1972, with an overall survival rate of 81%. The four most common diagnoses requiring ECLS in neonatal patients are meconium aspiration syndrome, congenital diaphragmatic hernia, pneumonia/sepsis and persistent pulmonary hypertension. Survival rates of 93%, 58%, 76% and 83%, respectively, have been achieved.

Illustrations by Peter Cox

Eventration of the diaphragm

Robert E. Cilley MD
Assistant Professor of Surgery and Pediatrics, Division of Pediatric Surgery, Department of Surgery, Pennsylvania State University College of Medicine, The Milton S. Hershey Medical Center, Hershey, Pennsylvania, USA

Arnold G. Coran MD
Professor of Surgery and Head of the Section of Pediatric Surgery, University of Michigan Medical School, and Surgeon-in-Chief, C.S. Mott Children's Hospital, Ann Arbor, Michigan, USA

History

Eventration of the diaphragm refers to the radiographic finding of an abnormally elevated hemidiaphragm. The physiologic consequences of the loss of diaphragm function are reduced lung volume, decreased tidal volume, increased work of breathing, and respiratory insufficiency which may preclude ventilator weaning. The mobility of the mediastinum of an infant may result in significant respiratory embarrassment when the normal hemidiaphragm descends during inspiration, the mediastinum shifts to the normal side and the eventration side paradoxically elevates.

The term 'diaphragm eventration' includes several distinct abnormalities. Acquired eventration (paralytic eventration) is easily understood on the basis of injury to the phrenic nerve, most commonly occurring at the time of intrathoracic surgery. Congenital eventration of the diaphragm is less well understood and probably includes a number of different entities. Phrenic nerve injury from birth trauma is similar to operative injury in that the diaphragm is developmentally normal, with a normal distribution of muscle and a normal central tendinous area. Other congenital eventrations (non-paralytic eventration) of the diaphragm are associated with anatomic abnormalities of the diaphragm. The diaphragm muscle is thinned and may be entirely absent from a portion that is normally muscular. In its most extreme forms, eventration is indistinguishable from a congenital diaphragmatic hernia with a hernia sac.

Eventration of the diaphragm was reviewed by Reed and Borden in 1935[1]. It was recognized in infants only as a post-mortem finding. The first successful surgical correction, using a form of diaphragm plication, was reported in 1947 by Bisgard[2]. Subsequently, other successful techniques were reported[3-5]. Surgical treatment is based upon removing the laxity of the abnormal diaphragm leaf to prevent paradoxical motion of a portion of the diaphragm with closure of the resultant defect, suture of a portion of the diaphragm to the chest wall, or pleating of the lax muscle to create a taut diaphragm[6,7].

Priniciples and justification

No rigid criteria exist for recommending repair of eventrations. Small eventrations with minimal compromise of lung volume may be followed by serial radiographs. A pneumonia responding to antibiotic therapy or mild respiratory distress that responds to supportive care such as chest physiotherapy and supplemental oxygen administration in association with eventration need not be treated surgically if there is complete symptomatic resolution. Recurrent symptoms or respiratory distress that requires mechanical ventilation are indications for surgical correction. When the possibility of reversible phrenic nerve injury exists, such as that due to birth trauma or operative injury, a period of observation is indicated. If there is no improvement in diaphragm function after a reasonable period of observation (2–4 weeks), diaphragm plication is performed. If function has not returned in that period of time, it is likely that prolonged mechanical ventilation will be required and surgical correction will be beneficial, allowing discontinuation of mechanical ventilation. Some function may eventually return to the previously paralyzed diaphragm, but this may require many months. Operative plication does not preclude some recovery of diaphragm function.

Several techniques have been described for correction of eventration, including transabdominal and transthoracic approaches. The excess length of diaphragm has been handled by excision and various methods of 'gathering' the excess tissue with sutures. All of these procedures have in common the creation of a taut diaphragm that is mechanically resistant to elevation when negative intrathoracic pressure is created during spontaneous breathing. Specific abnormalities lend themselves to repair by the different methods.

When concurrent abdominal pathology that requires operative correction such as malrotation is present, the transabdominal approach is used. A single abdominal incision allows correction of both problems. Likewise, the rare bilateral eventration may be approached through a single incision. The transthoracic approach is used for isolated unilateral eventration. It allows better visualization of the course of the phrenic nerve. For right-sided eventrations, the transthoracic approach avoids the need to mobilize the liver for visualization of the diaphragm.

No portion of the diaphragm needs to be excised in cases of acquired eventration. The musclar diaphragm may ultimately regain some function and excision only increases the risk of additional injury to the intra-diaphragmatic portion of the phrenic nerve. In congenital eventrations with muscular aplasia or atrophy, the thinned portion of the diaphragm may be excised when the thoracic approach is used and the course of the phrenic nerve is visualized. This allows the edges that will be brought together to be precisely visualized. Full-thickness sutures may be placed without fear of injury to intra-abdominal organs. Pledgets and non-absorbable sutures provide the most secure closure. Since diaphragmatic defects come in all shapes and sizes, the precise orientation of the plication procedure and the decision to excise some or all of the eventration must be assessed on an individual basis.

Preoperative

Assessment and preparation

Diaphragm eventration may be discovered incidentally as an elevated hemidiaphragm on a chest radiograph obtained for other reasons, or it may be the cause of respiratory failure or pneumonia. The most common presentation of eventration is postoperative respiratory failure after an intrathoracic operation as a result of phrenic nerve injury.

Unilateral eventration is suspected when the right hemidiaphragm is greater than two rib levels higher than the left, or the left hemidiaphragm is more than one rib level higher than the right. A rare bilateral eventration is suspected when respiratory failure is present in association with radiographic demonstration of bilateral diaphragm elevation. Chest radiographs may be misleading in the patient on positive pressure mechanical ventilation. A non-functioning diaphragm may not be elevated. The most convincing diagnostic tests are those that allow dynamic visualization of diaphragm function during spontaneous respiration. These include fluoroscopy and ultrasonographic imaging. Ultrasonography has the advantage that it can be performed easily at the patient's bedside in the intensive care unit. Absent or paradoxic elevation of the hemidiaphragm during spontaneous inspiratory effort is diagnostic.

Preoperative evaluation includes physical examination to determine the presence of other anomalies or stigmata of chromosomal abnormalities. An echocardiogram should be performed in the presence of congenital eventration to rule out associated structural cardiac abnormalities. An upper gastrointestinal contrast study is obtained specifically to determine if malrotation is present, since this will determine what operative approach will be used[8].

Anesthesia

General endotracheal anesthesia is used. Unilateral intubation improves exposure but, if difficult to perform or not well tolerated, it is not mandatory since the lung is easily retracted. Intraoperative orogastric intubation with regular gastric aspiration is of critical importance since a dilated stomach is at risk of injury when diaphragmatic sutures are passed. An epidural catheter for intraoperative anesthesia and postoperative analgesia may be helpful.

Operations

Incision

1 A transverse upper abdominal incision is used for bilateral eventration or in cases of unilateral eventration with malrotation. A seventh intercostal space thoracotomy is used for isolated left or right eventration.

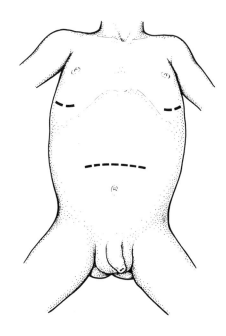

1

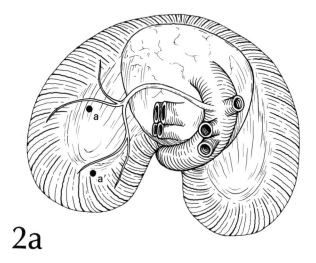

2a

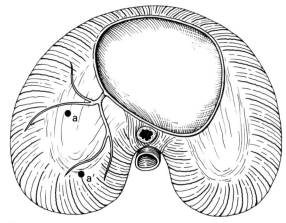

2b

TRANSTHORACIC REPAIR OF LEFT-SIDED ACQUIRED EVENTRATION

2a, b The main phrenic nerve on each side divides into an anterior and posterior division. Subsequent divisions usually include a sternal branch immediately off the anterior division and a bifurcation of the posterior division. The branches run in a medial to lateral orientation, allowing sutures to be placed to minimize the risk of injury to the muscular branches of the nerve.

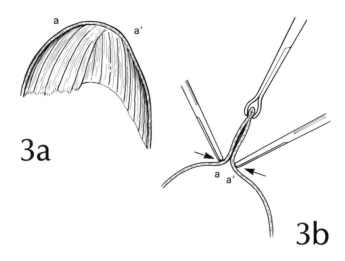

3a, b The diaphragm is grasped and manipulated to determine the amount that must be included in the plication to create a taut closure. This is conveniently performed by grasping the center of the diaphragm with a non-crushing clamp (Babcock). The extent of the plication, determined by manipulations with the two forceps, is marked with a surgical marker.

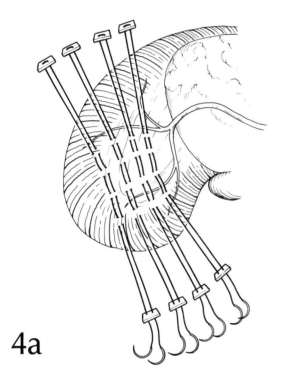

4a, b Several non-absorbable sutures are placed to bring the marked portions of the diaphragm together. The sutures are passed through the intervening diaphragm muscle three or four times. This maneuver has been referred to as gathering, reefing or pleating. The authors prefer to use pledgeted mattress sutures as shown. Care must be taken that the sutures are passed adequately through muscle but not deeply enough to penetrate adjacent abdominal viscera.

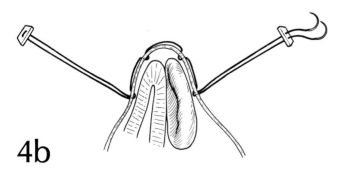

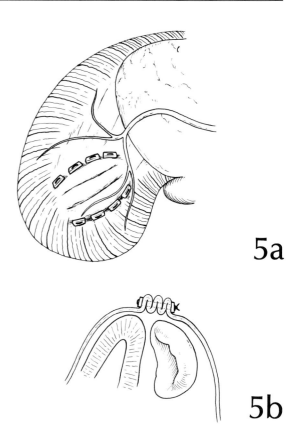

5a, b The final result of the plication creates a taut diaphragm.

5a

5b

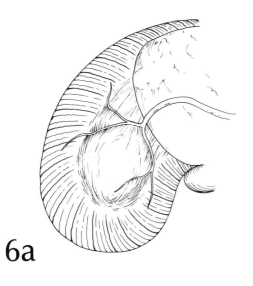

6a

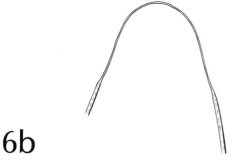

6b

TRANSTHORACIC REPAIR OF LEFT-SIDED CONGENITAL EVENTRATION

6a, b In this condition the central portion of the diaphragm is 'thinned out'. Although the diaphragm may be 'gathered' in a fashion similar to the repair of an acquired eventration, excising the thin central portion of the diaphragm allows the edges to be clearly visualized so that sutures may be placed in normal muscularized tissue and the abdominal viscera avoided.

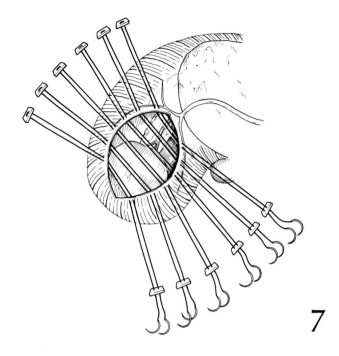

7 Non-absorbable, pledgeted mattress sutures are placed and oriented to close the defect in a transverse fashion.

7

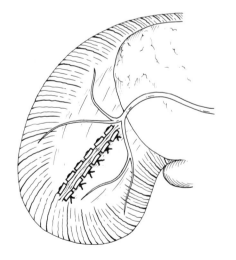

8 The final result brings muscularized diaphragm together. If excessive tension is required to bring the tissues together, some surgeons recommend the use of a prosthetic patch to close the defect. This has not been necessary in the authors' experience.

8

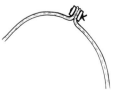

TRANSABDOMINAL REPAIR OF BILATERAL EVENTRATION

Rotational abnormalities of the intestine are addressed if present.

9 The undersurface of the diaphragm is exposed on the left by mobilizing the liver as necessary. The stomach and spleen are retracted and mobilized to give complete exposure. The right lobe of the liver is mobilized if needed. Congenital eventration with thinning of the diaphragm will require little moblization.

Plicating sutures are arranged to avoid the phrenic nerve based on its expected location. The plication is oriented anteromedial to posterolateral, identical to the transthoracic approach.

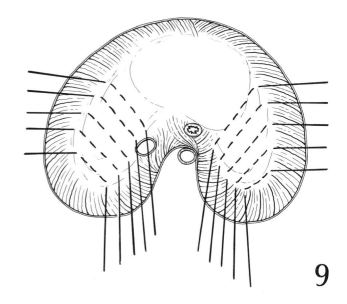

9

Postoperative care

Endotracheal intubation is maintained after surgery. Slow ventilator weaning is performed and extubation usually accomplished within 1 week. Intrapleural drainage is used briefly after surgery and the drainage tube usually removed within 2–3 days.

Outcome

Although death may result from chronic respiratory failure and pneumonia, the outcome is largely dependent upon the presence of associated conditions such as pulmonary hypoplasia or congenital heart disease. Long-term survival is variably reported as 69% to 100%[9, 10]. Children with bilateral eventration fare less well. Surgical correction is durable and recurrence requiring repeat plication has rarely been needed[11]. Many patients examined years after diaphragm plication will have evidence of appropriate although diminished movement of the involved side[12, 13].

References

1. Reed JA, Borden DL. Eventration of the diaphragm with a report of two cases. *Arch Surg* 1935, 31: 30–64.

2. Bisgard JD. Congenital eventration of the diaphragm. *J Thorac Surg* 1947; 16: 484–91.

3. State D. The surgical correction of congenital eventration of the diaphragm in infancy. *Surgery* 1949; 25: 461–8.

4. Bingham JAW. Two cases of unilateral paralysis of the diaphragm in the newborn treated surgically. *Thorax* 1954; 9: 248–52.

5. Bishop HC, Koop CE. Acquired eventration of the diaphragm in infancy. *Pediatrics* 1958; 22: 1088–96.

6. Schwartz MZ, Filler RM. Plication of the diaphragm for symptomatic phrenic nerve paralysis. *J Pediatr Surg* 1978; 13: 259–63.

7. Langer JC. Phrenic nerve palsy. In: Fallis JC, Filler RM, Lemoine G, eds. *Pediatric Thoracic Surgery*. New York: Elsevier, 1991: 210–14.

8. Malone PS, Brain AJ, Kiely EM, Spitz L. Congenital diaphragmatic defects that present late. *Arch Dis Child* 1989; 64: 1542–4.

9. Ribet M, Linder JL. Plication of the diaphragm for unilateral eventration or paralysis. *Eur J Cardiothorac Surg* 1992; 6: 357–60.

10. Jawad AJ, al-Sammarai AY, al-Rabeeah A. Eventration of the diaphragm in children. *J R Coll Surg Edinb* 1991; 36: 222–4.

11. Langer JC, Filler RM, Coles J, Edmonds JF, Plication of the diaphragm for infants and young children with phrenic nerve palsy. *J Pediatr Surg* 1988; 23: 749–51.

12. Stone KS, Brown JW, Canal DF, King H. Long-term fate of the diaphragm surgically plicated during infancy and early childhood. *Ann Thorac Surg* 1987; 44: 62–5.

13. Kizilcan F, Tanyel FC, Hiçsönmez A, Büyükpamukçu N. The long-term results of diaphragmatic plication. *J Pediatr Surg* 1993; 28: 42–4.

Illustrations by Marks Creative Consultants

Lung surgery

James A. O'Neill Jr MD
Surgeon-in-Chief, The Children's Hospital of Philadelphia, and C. E. Koop Professor of Surgery, The University of Pennsylvania School of Medicine, Philadelphia, Pennsylvania, USA

Principles and justification

Pulmonary resection in infants and children is required infrequently since they have fewer acquired lesions than adults. Conditions requiring pulmonary resection in infancy include congenital lobar emphysema, some types of lung cysts and a few rare pulmonary tumors. Childhood entities which lead to a need for lung resection include congenital and acquired cystic disease, sequestration, pulmonary infection with bronchiectasis and rare tumors.

The general principles of thoracotomy and pulmonary resection are common to both children and adults. The main differences in technical considerations between the two age groups are primarily related to growth and development. These will be outlined below. In addition, there are additional considerations related to specific anomalies such as sequestration.

Principles of pulmonary resection

Pulmonary resection may be performed with the patient in one of three positions. The first is anterolateral thoracotomy which is generally used for lung biopsy. The second, which is by far the most common approach to virtually all lesions requiring pulmonary resection in childhood, is the standard posterolateral thoracotomy performed with the patient in the lateral decubitus position. The third is the prone position, an approach that has been used to avoid spillage of infected pulmonary secretions; however, that complication is better prevented by lung isolation with the use of special endotracheal tubes, so this position is no longer used routinely.

For anterolateral thoracotomy, the patient is elevated 30–45° from the horizontal plane of the operating table with the ipsilateral arm either elevated above the chest or allowed to fall backward alongside the patient. A wide antiseptic preparation of the skin and draping is performed with the entire anterior and lateral chest exposed. A slightly curved incision conforming to the direction of the intercostal space is performed from below the level of the nipple, at a level to avoid damage to any underdeveloped breast tissue, and extending toward the axilla. Only the pectoralis muscles and the intercostals are divided, entering the fourth or fifth intercostal space as desired depending upon the segment of lung to be exposed. This approach is mostly used for lung biopsy or for limited segmental resection or well-defined lesions. A chest tube which will accommodate to the size of the intercostal space is brought in approximately two interspaces below the incision and placed at the apex of the chest. The chest tube is sutured in place, and the incision closed first with large absorbable pericostal sutures and then by approximation of the thoracic wall muscles with a continuous suture of absorbable material. After subcutaneous closure, a subcuticular closure of the skin with absorbable suture is usually appropriate.

1 For posterolateral thoracotomy, the patient is placed in either the right or left lateral decubitus position with the body at right angles to the operating table (*see* chapter on pp. 103–110). A small rolled towel or sheet is placed under the patient's axilla to protect the dependent shoulder and arm from being excessively stretched. The arm and shoulder on the upright side of the chest which is to be operated upon are elevated toward the head but supported in order to avoid excessive stretch on the brachial plexus. Antiseptic preparation of the skin and draping is performed with the chest exposed from the level of the axilla to below the rib cage and also from the vertebral column behind to the sternum anteriorly after selecting the appropriate interspace for the incision. A gently curved thoracotomy incision is made. For exposure of posterior mediastinal structures, a straight incision over the interspace selected may be made from the anterior axillary line as far posteriorly as necessary. For wide exposure of the entire chest, the incision is started below the level of the breast and carried straight posteriorly. This is different from the usual approach in the adult in that every effort is made to divide only the pectoralis, serratus anterior and latissimus muscles, and to avoid division of the trapezius and rhomboid muscles so that late scoliosis is avoided. Additionally, as the muscles of the chest wall are divided over the ribs, the paraspinal muscles are freed up longitudinally to expose the interspace but not divided. This measure also helps to avoid postural deformities which may occur with subsequent growth. Following performance of the intrathoracic portion of the procedure and ensuring of hemostasis, a chest tube is inserted at the apex of the chest and brought out two interspaces or more below the incision and carefully sutured in place. Closure of the chest wall is as described above.

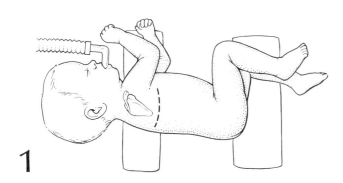

1

Lobar emphysema

Lobar emphysema may be either congenital or acquired. In most instances acquired lobar emphysema is either the result of mucus plugging in patients on ventilators or the result of accumulation of interstitial air in immature infants with severe respiratory distress syndrome. In congenital lobar emphysema, pathology is either based on absence of a bronchial cartilage resulting in a ball valve mechanism of obstruction or, in a few instances, trapping of air distally at the alveolar level. Progressive air trapping will result in overdistension of an individual lobe, marked mediastinal shift and diminished venous return with circulatory compromise, primarily in small infants. Most cases occur during the first 6 months of life. The left upper lobe is involved most commonly followed by the right upper and middle lobes. Appropriate treatment is emergency lobectomy.

2a, b The diagnosis is generally suspected on the basis of an infant presenting with marked respiratory distress in whom breath sounds are diminished over the involved portion of the chest wall, and there is evidence of marked mediastinal shift toward the contralateral side. Anteroposterior and lateral chest radiographs are generally diagnostic demonstrating typical findings of hyperlucency of the involved thorax associated with evidence of a collapse of the remaining lobe or lobes on that side and shift of the heart toward the opposite side. The illustrated case shows overexpansion of the left upper lobe and marked mediastinal shift. Fine vascular markings can ordinarily be distinguished within the cystic lobe. A ventilation/perfusion scan will usually demonstrate matched decreases in ventilation and perfusion, but such scans are difficult to interpret because of the degree of herniation of the overdistended lobe into the opposite thorax. Bronchoscopy may demonstrate a collapsed bronchus which is missing a segment of cartilage. Patent ductus arteriosus is a common accompaniment of congenital lobar emphysema.

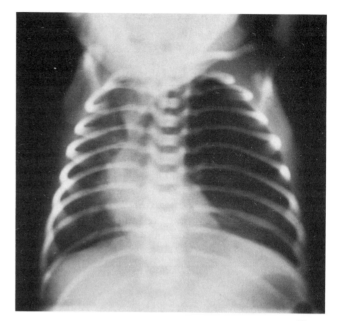

2a

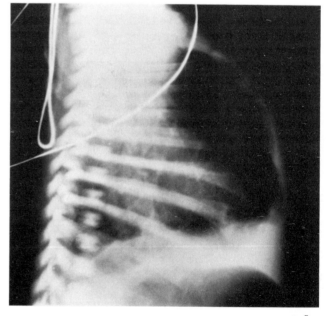

2b

Sequestration

The most common form of sequestration is intralobar, but rarely extralobar sequestration will be encountered. Extralobar sequestration usually occurs in infants with posterolateral diaphragmatic hernias, congenital heart disease or duplication cysts.

3 Whether intralobar (left) or extralobar (right), a sequestered portion of the lung is non-functional and has poor drainage. Intralobar sequestrations are susceptible to chronic infection whereas extralobar sequestrations are usually asymptomatic. Sequestrations characteristically receive blood supply from a systemic vessel and, since most are inferior in the chest, the systemic vessel ordinarily comes from the abdominal aorta through the inferior pulmonary ligament or secondarily as one or more vessels coming laterally off the thoracic aorta. Pulmonary venous drainage is usually normal to the left atrium, but occasionally empties into a systemic vein or the portal vein.

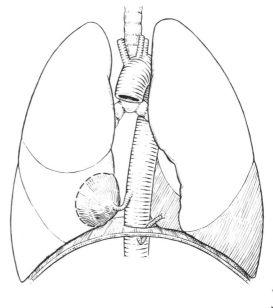

3

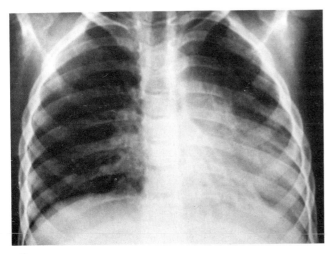

4

4 A history of recurrent infections in the same location on the chest radiograph is the classic indication that a sequestration is present. Most occur in the left lower lobe and secondly in the right lower lobe in posterior basal locations. The case illustrated shows chronic infiltrate in the left lower lobe. This child had repeated episodes of pneumonia typical of intralobar sequestration.

5 The diagnosis is suspected on serial chest radiography and may be confirmed on computed tomographic scanning using intravenous contrast.

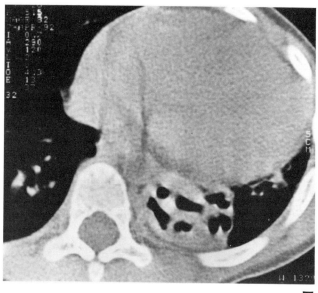

5

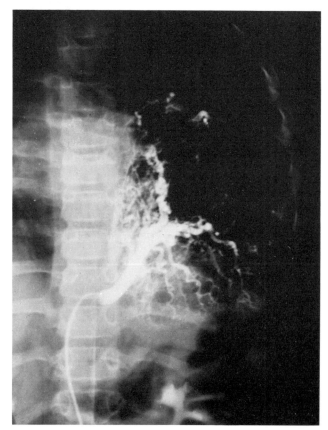

6

6 While aortography is diagnostic, it is usually not required to make the diagnosis. This angiogram demonstrates the classic appearance of the abnormal systemic vessel.

Cystic adenomatoid malformation and lung cysts

Pulmonary cysts may either be single or multiple. The most common form of this type of anomaly in the neonate is cystic adenomatoid malformation which probably results from failure of a portion of the lung to develop. Characteristically, the gross pathology demonstrates a mixture of solid adenomatous portions of the involved lobe associated with multiple cysts of varying sizes. This may result in marked overdistension of that part of the lung resulting in much the same pathology as congenital lobar emphysema. Lower lobes are frequently involved, and the clinical picture is often confused with congenital posterolateral diaphragmatic hernia. These multilocular cysts are lined with respiratory epithelium so both mucus and air are present within these cysts. In older children, respiratory distress is rarely present but recurrent infection is the problem.

7, 8 Routine chest radiography will demonstrate hyperlucency of the involved portion of the lung, usually associated with marked mediastinal shift. While there is some similarity to the appearance of loops of intestine in the chest, it is usually possible to distinguish these two entities as more solid elements are present in the patients with cystic adenomatoid malformation or congenital cystic disease. The radiograph illustrated shows cystic adenomatoid malformation of the right middle lobe. It is understandable how this might be confused with a diaphragmatic hernia. *Illustration 8* shows the gross appearance of this case at operation.

Computed tomographic scanning may be useful in older patients to delineate the pathology more clearly before operation. Air-fluid levels may be seen in older patients within a cystic malformation.

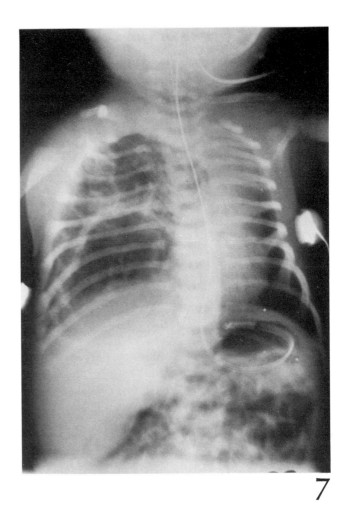

7

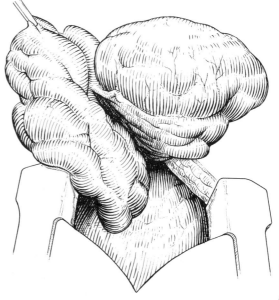

8

Indications

Lung biopsy

A number of conditions may require lung biopsy material for appropriate management including chronic pulmonary infiltrates related to infection, immune suppression, autoimmune disease and a variety of other acquired conditions in which the pattern of disease is not characteristic of a single disorder. In many instances lung biopsy results are required before initiating potentially toxic therapy for presumed chronic infection of unknown type. In addition, single or multiple small metastatic tumors may require resection. In the latter instance, if the tumors are distributed widely bilaterally, midline sternotomy may be appropriate to gain access to both thoracic cavities (*see* chapter on pp. 103–110). In most instances lung biopsy will be performed for generalized, bilateral pulmonary infiltrates, and lingular biopsy is usually the simplest approach.

Lobectomy

Lobectomy is ordinarily indicated in cases of congenital lobar emphysema, sequestration, large lung cysts which are either congenital or acquired, large pulmonary tumors or for injuries. On rare occasions pneumonectomy is necessary, but it should be avoided if at all possible. Pneumonectomy in children is associated with severe long-term complications which lead to shortening of the life span of the child. The problems encountered are overexpansion of the contralateral lung, severe scoliosis and tracheal obstruction by rotation of the intrathoracic vasculature. These problems have led to the use of plombage techniques such as the placement of a variety of materials including gradually expandable prostheses. However, there are complications attendant on the use of these devices, and the long-term results are not clear, so pneumonectomy is best avoided if at all possible.

Lobar emphysema

When respiratory distress from lobar emphysema is sufficiently severe and the radiographic findings are characteristic, immediate operation is indicated. When lobar emphysema involves the right side, occasionally both the upper and middle lobes will be affected. In cases where lobar emphysema is associated with very mild symptoms, operation may not be required as patients improve. However, patients of this nature must be observed very carefully since symptoms may worsen rapidly.

Sequestration

Once a sequestration has been diagnosed, elective removal should be performed since recurrent infection and potentially empyema are inevitable.

Cystic adenomatoid malformation and lung cysts

Respiratory distress in the neonate associated with a space-occupying pulmonary lesion due to cystic adenomatoid malformation or congenital cystic disease is an indication for operation. In older patients, chronic infection is an indication for operation, but even asymptomatic patients with cystic disease should have elective removal.

Other indications

Patients with empyema are usually treatable by simple tube thoracostomy drainage or endoscopic or operative decortication with tube thoracostomy drainage. At times, empyema is associated with a necrotic lobe of the lung in which case lobectomy is indicated as well.

Lobectomy, or occasionally segmental resection, is indicated in patients who have irreversible bronchiectasis of the sacular type either with or without associated lung abscess. In the latter types of patients, it is usually best to perform bronchoscopy immediately before thoracotomy in order to drain the lung as much as possible. Also, the tracheobronchial tree should be isolated with a double-lumen endotracheal tube to prevent spillage of infected secretions into the contralateral lung.

Metastatic tumors of the lung can generally be treated by wedge resection using a TA-55 or GIA stapler or suture with overlapping horizontal mattress sutures of non-absorbable material. In the case of bronchial adenomas or inflammatory tumors of the lung, lobectomy is usually the best approach. Bronchoscopy may be extremely useful in cases of bronchial adenoma in order to map the full extent of bronchial involvement. Another rare entity encountered in childhood is arteriovenous malformation of the lung. This is frequently hereditary and usually only a single lobe is involved. Routine chest radiography is generally sufficient to make the diagnosis, but occasionally computed tomographic scanning with intravenous contrast medium is necessary. Pulmonary angiography may also confirm the diagnosis. Lobectomy is the most effective approach to treatment.

Preoperative

Patients who present with sequestration and infection should be treated vigorously before surgery. All patients undergoing operation for sequestration should have broad spectrum antibiotic coverage.

Anesthesia

The most critical aspect of management of lobar emphysema has to do with induction of anesthesia, which should not be performed until the surgeon is ready to open the chest. The infant should be permitted to breathe himself with minimal positive pressure assistance since that may worsen the degree of overdistension of the involved lobe and produce cardiac arrest.

Operations

LUNG BIOPSY

For routine lung biopsy of the lingula of the left upper lobe, a short submammary left anterolateral thora-cotomy is performed through the fifth interspace. The lingula is then easily brought into view. At this point either a stapler or overlapping horizontal mattress sutures of non-absorbable material may be used to seal the cut edge of the lung and the biopsy excised. After placement of a chest tube through an inferior inter-space, the incision is closed as described in the section on thoracotomy.

An alternative approach to a limited anterolateral thoracotomy for purposes of lung biopsy is endoscopic lung biopsy. This requires one anterior opening in the chest wall for placement of the telescope and a second opening for placement of a port which would be used to pass a stapler into the chest for lung biopsy. At times, a third opening is necessary for introduction of a ring forceps which is used to manipulate the lung if adhesions are present. Endoscopic lung biopsy requires temporary collapse of the lung undergoing biopsy, and many patients are unable to tolerate this maneuver. Consequently, open lung biopsy which permits full pulmonary expansion may be necessary in patients with respiratory compromise.

LOBECTOMY

Whether one is dealing with the right or the left chest, any pulmonary resection can ordinarily be performed via a posterolateral thoracotomy incision through the fifth intercostal space. At times the fourth or sixth intercostal spaces should be used when a particular anomaly dictates. For example, with intralobar seque-stration in the left lower lobe, use of the sixth intercostal space may permit better visualization of the anomalous vessel usually encountered in the inferior pulmonary ligament.

The principles of lobectomy are the same in children as in adults. The basic principle is adequate exposure with good visualization of the pulmonary arterial and venous branches going to the involved lobe as well as the lobar bronchi. In most instances it is advantageous to dissect and divide the pulmonary arterial branches first, the venous drainage second and the bronchus last. At times, bronchial dissection may be necessary as a first maneuver, particularly when the lobe to be resected is severely infected.

Although certain lobes are involved more commonly with particular conditions such as the left upper lobe in congenital lobar emphysema, all lobes of both lungs may require resection in the pediatric age group.

Right upper lobectomy

9a, b The patient is positioned in the left lateral decubitus position and a right postero-lateral thoracotomy incision is made via the fifth intercostal space. The lung is retracted posteriorly and the pleura covering the hilum of the right lung is opened from below the level of the superior pulmonary vein to the level of the azygos vein and around the hilus superiorly and posteriorly to a level below the right mainstem bronchus (*Illustration 9a*). Care is taken to avoid injury to the right phrenic nerve. It should be noted that considerable variation in vascular anatomy occurs, but the usual pattern is shown in the illustration. Bronchial anatomy is more standard. There are usually three segmental pulmonary artery branches demonstrable in the anterior portion of the hilus of the right upper lobe, and these are divided first. The oblique fissure is then opened between the superior surface of the right middle lobe and between the upper and lower lobes (*Illustration 9b*). This permits the dissection and isolation of the posterior ascending segmental pulmonary arterial branch which ordinarily comes off the pulmonary artery after the middle lobe branches. All vessels are best managed by double ligation with non-absorbable suture as well as suture ligation on the side of the main pulmonary artery.

There are usually three veins draining the right upper lobe which should be ligated just before their junction with the superior pulmonary vein. These are best visualized by retraction of the lung posteriorly in order to give wide exposure to the anterior hilum.

After the division of the arterial and venous branches related to the right upper lobe, nodal and adventitial tissues surrounding the bronchus supplying the right upper lobe are cleared away. The bronchus only needs to be dissected out enough to identify its origin since removal of all adventitial tissue may compromise blood supply to the bronchus and result in delayed healing of the bronchial stump. Stay sutures of non-absorbable material are placed on either edge of the right upper lobe bronchus in such a fashion that a long stump which might permit accumulation of secretions is avoided. A bronchus clamp is then placed distally toward the upper lobe and the bronchus is divided with a scalpel. After removal of the lobe, the bronchial stump is suctioned clean, and the stump closed with interrupted sutures. Sufficient sutures are used to close the stump without

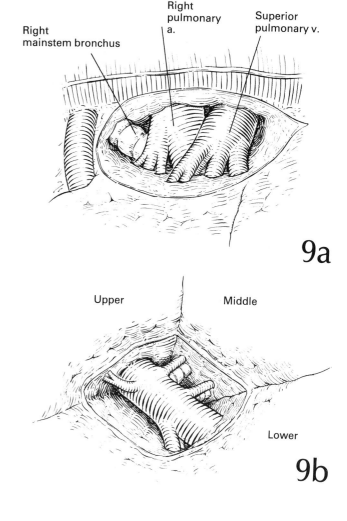

Right mainstem bronchus

Right pulmonary a.

Superior pulmonary v.

9a

Upper   Middle

Lower

9b

devascularizing it. Saline is then placed in the chest, and the lung expanded to $40\,cmH_2O$ pressure to ensure airtight closure. The surrounding pleura is used to reinforce the bronchial closure and to promote healing. These maneuvers are common to all bronchial closures.

After ensuring that bleeding has been controlled, a chest tube is placed in the apex of the chest and brought out through an inferior interspace and routine closure of the chest performed. Depending upon the age and size of the child, the chest tube should be connected to an underwater seal with positive/negative suction pressure of $10-20/2-4\,cmH_2O$. The lower range is appropriate for neonates and the higher range for older children.

Right middle lobectomy

10 The arteries to the right middle lobe are best exposed through the oblique fissure between the upper, middle and lower lobes. After development of the interlobar fissure, one or two middle lobe arteries are ordinarily encountered which are doubly tied and suture ligated (*see Illustration 9b*). The lung is retracted posteriorly to expose the anterior hilum which is also fully dissected and one or two right middle lobe veins are ordinarily encountered joining the right superior pulmonary vein. At times the interlobar fissure is incomplete and dissection down to the vasculature must be performed by dividing pulmonary tissue between clamps. Once the middle lobe has been separated from the upper lobe and both arterial and venous branches divided, the middle lobe is retracted anteriorly and the bronchus divided. In most cases the middle lobe bronchus bifurcates into lateral and medial segmental branches. The middle lobe bronchus is divided and sutured at its base as described above.

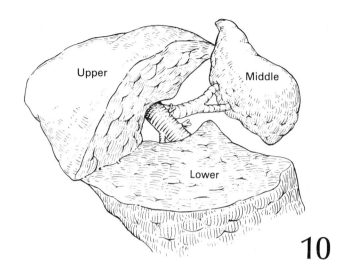

10

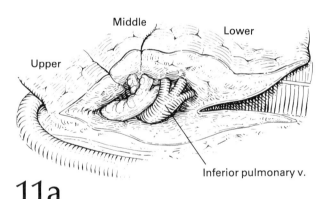

11a

Inferior pulmonary v.

11b

Superior pulmonary v.   Left pulmonary a.

Right lower lobectomy

11a, b For right lower lobectomy either the fifth or sixth intercostal spaces may be used. The interlobar fissure is exposed by retraction of the upper and middle lobes superiorly and the lower lobe inferiorly. The branches of the interlobar portion of the right pulmonary artery are exposed and identified. Just beyond the middle lobe arterial branches and opposite, one or two superior segmental arteries supplying the superior segment of the lower lobe are encountered. These are divided following ligation. The remaining artery to the basilar segments is divided. The right lower lobe is then retracted anteriorly to fully expose the posterior hilum. The inferior pulmonary vein is best exposed posteriorly by first dividing the inferior pulmonary ligament and carrying the pleural dissection upward which then allows isolation and ligation of the inferior pulmonary vein. After all of the vasculature is divided, this allows identification and dissection of the right lower lobe bronchus. Again, care is taken to divide and suture this bronchus leaving a minimum of stump so that secretions will not accumulate and promote a bronchopleural fistula.

Left upper lobectomy

12a, b For left thoracotomy, the patient is positioned in the right lateral decubitus position and a posterolateral thoracotomy is performed as described previously. The fifth interspace is used to expose the thoracic cavity. As with the right lung, the pleura overlying the hilus of the lung anteriorly is incised and carried superiorly and posteriorly below the level of the left mainstem bronchus. The left pulmonary ary artery is best identified anteriorly first, and then visualized as it courses superiorly and posteriorly to the left upper lobe bronchus. Anywhere from four to six branches of the left pulmonary artery to the upper lobe may be encountered. Anteriorly, anterior, apical and posterior segmental arteries may be seen. The apical segmental artery may be encountered superiorly and an anterior segmental and lingular segmental branches are usually seen in the interlobar fissure. After ligation of all of these arteries at their origin, the lung is retracted posteriorly and the left superior pulmonary vein ligated just before it divides. At times the left superior and inferior pulmonary veins unite to form a common vein, so before ligation of the superior pulmonary vein on the left side the inferior pulmonary vein should be identified. With the left upper lobe retracted anteriorly, it is then possible to visualize and isolate the bronchus to the left upper lobe and lingula and to divide it and close it at its origin.

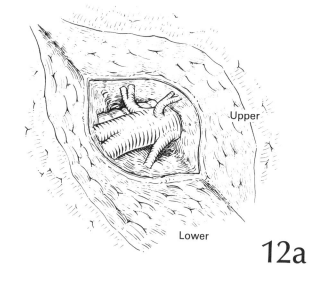

12a

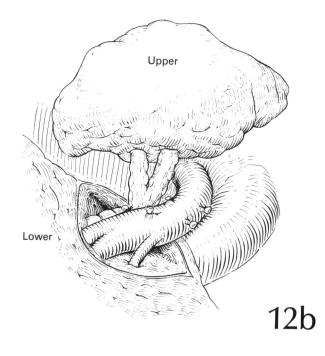

12b

Left lower lobectomy

13 Either the fifth or sixth intercostal space may be used to perform left lower lobe resection. The arteries are visualized first by retracting the left upper lobe anteriorly to expose the interlobar fissure. One or two arteries ordinarily supply the superior segment of the left lower lobe, but care must be taken in this dissection since the superior segmental artery frequently arises proximal to the lingular vessels. Thus the lingular arteries must be identified in the course of this dissection. Following ligation of the arterial supply to the superior segment of the lower lobe, the basilar portion of the pulmonary artery may be divided just distal to the origin of the lingular arteries to the upper lobe. After this, the lung is retracted anteriorly to expose the posterior hilum. The inferior pulmonary ligament is divided to a level above the inferior pulmonary vein. This vein is divided as described above taking care to be certain that there is adequate drainage of the superior pulmonary vein. After division of the vasculature to the lower lobe, the lobe is retracted posteriorly and the bronchus isolated and divided as described above.

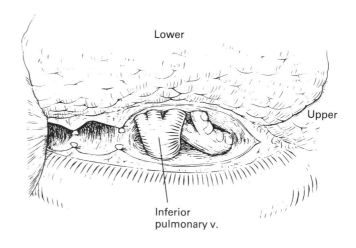

Lower

Upper

Inferior
pulmonary v.

13

RESECTION OF SEQUESTRATION

Since extralobar sequestrations are usually asymptomatic and have not been complicated by infection, their removal is straightforward. Following isolation and division of the feeding and draining vessels, an extralobar sequestration is simply resected.

On the other hand, management of an intralobar sequestration presents more of a challenge, particularly when the patient has suffered repeated bouts of infection which may produce dense, vascular adhesions and obliterate normal tissue planes. The phrenic and vagus nerves and the esophagus may be in jeopardy, so careful dissection is critical. Lobectomy is the best approach even when the intralobar sequestration appears as if it might be easily dissected from the remaining normal appearing lung. It is no longer felt to be necessary to have all of the systemic blood supply demonstrated ahead of time on angiography since the possible locations of these systemic vessels occur in a fairly standard fashion. The most common pattern of systemic arterial supply is a single large vessel coming off the upper part of the abdominal aorta traversing the diaphragm and running in the inferior pulmonary ligament to supply the posterior basal sequestration. These vessels are quite friable and have the consistency of a ductus arteriosus so extreme care must be taken in dissection, isolation and ligation of these vessels. There may also be multiple vessels coming off the aorta medial to the lower lobe, and these should be handled individually. The remainder of the lobectomy is handled in standard fashion.

LOBECTOMY FOR CYSTIC ADENOMATOID MALFORMATION AND LUNG CYSTS

Lobectomy is preferable to limited resection for cystic adenomatoid malformations or multiloculated cystic disease because of the high incidence of recurrence and persistent air leak in patients in whom segmental resections have been performed. Older patients with solitary cysts are occasionally encountered in whom limited resection may be performed with careful ligation of any air leaks.

Acquired lung cysts may be the result of trauma, infection or parasitic disease. Patients with pneumatoceles related to staphylococcal infection should be observed for several months since most of these cysts resolve without the need for intervention. The same is true for the majority of patients with traumatic lung cysts, but some of these will require segmental resection when infection becomes a problem. In the case of echinococcal cysts, resection is preferred when the diagnosis is either suspected or proven on serologic testing.

Echinococcal cysts may usually be enucleated from the surrounding normal lung after incising the fibrous capsule around the cyst.

Postoperative care

The cardinal principles of management after thoracotomy include promotion of full pulmonary expansion, avoidance of infection and aggressive pulmonary toilet. The chest tube must be managed in an appropriate fashion to be sure that it remains patent so that it may function both as a monitor of blood and fluid loss as well as a tool to evacuate the thoracic space so that the lung may be fully expanded. It must be remembered that the presence of a chest tube is painful and that it should be removed as soon as it is no longer necessary for evacuation of blood, serum or air.

In the early postoperative period, particularly while the chest tube is in place, if patients are not able to cough adequately on their own, aggressive endotracheal suction should be used. This is particularly important in infants who have undergone thoracotomy and whose respiratory efforts are expected to be weak. Pulmonary toilet may require maintenance of an endotracheal tube and assisted ventilation. Judicious use of antibiotics is also appropriate. Precautions must be taken to prevent overhydration in patients with diminished cardiopulmonary function, particularly infants. In addition, gastric retention and acute gastric dilatation are common during the first 24 h after thoracotomy so feeds are delayed for that period and appropriate measures taken to avoid accumulation of air in the stomach.

Outcome

Operative mortality for lobar emphysema should be minimal. In our experience, the only mortality has occurred in infants with associated complex congenital heart disease or those who have had areas of cartilaginous bronchial deficiency in multiple lobes.

Using the procedure described for resection of sequestrations, morbidity and mortality should be minimized.

Further reading

Andrassy RJ, Feldtman RW, Stanford W. Bronchial carcinoid tumours in children and adolescents. *J Pediatr Surg* 1977; 12: 513–17.

Buntain WL, Isaacs H, Payne VC, Lindesmith GG, Rosenkrantz JG. Lobar emphysema, cystic adenomatoid malformation, pulmonary sequestration, and bronchogenic cyst in infancy and childhood: a clinical group. *J Pediatr Surg* 1974; 9: 85–93.

Clements BS, Warner JO. Pulmonary sequestration and related congenital bronchopulmonary-vascular malformations: nomenclature and classification based on anatomical and embryological considerations. *Thorax* 1987; 42: 401–8.

Johnston MR. Median sternotomy for resection of pulmonary metastases. *J Thorac Cardiovasc Surg* 1983; 85: 516–22.

Kittle CF. Thoracic incisions. In: Baue AE, ed. *Glenn's Thoracic and Cardiovascular Surgery* 5th edn. London: Prentice-Hall International, 1991: 67–82.

Luck SR, Reynolds M, Raffensperger JG. Congenital bronchopulmonary malformations. *Curr Probl Surg* 1986; 23: 245–314.

Mediastinal masses

Robert C. Shamberger MD
Associate Professor of Surgery, Harvard Medical School, Associate in Surgery, Children's Hospital, Boston, Massachusetts, USA

Principles and justification

Many lesions present as a mediastinal mass, which may appear at any age throughout infancy and childhood. The mass may be cystic or solid and of congenital or neoplastic origin. The symptoms produced by a mediastinal mass are almost as diverse as the underlying pathology of these lesions, but most are due to the 'mass effect' of the lesion compressing the airway or esophagus and, less frequently, the lung. Occasionally they present with pain from infection or perforation of a cyst or from invasion of the chest wall by a malignant tumor. Many, in fact, are found as a radiographic abnormality on a study obtained for symptoms unrelated to the mass. Respiratory symptoms of expiratory stridor, cough, dyspnea, or tachypnea require urgent investigation. Cystic lesions within the mediastinum located at the carina may produce major airway obstruction in infants. These lesions 'hidden' in the normal mediastinal shadow may not be apparent on the anterior–posterior or lateral chest radiographs. Orthopnea and venous engorgement from superior vena caval syndrome are found with extensive involvement of the anterior mediastinum. Less frequently, dysphagia from pressure on the esophagus is the presenting symptom. Neurologic symptoms from spinal cord compression or Horner's syndrome are seen with neurogenic tumors arising in the posterior mediastium.

Indications for resection

Management of these lesions is determined by the presumed diagnosis. Cystic lesions in the anterior mediastinum are generally resected. Acute enlargement in thymic cysts has been noted following viral respiratory illnesses. Teratomas, because of their possible malignant degeneration, are also resected. Lymphangiomas often secondarily involve the mediastinum (the mediastinum only is involved in <5% of cases) with the predominant component in the cervical facial area. Pericardial cysts are the most innocent of these lesions and, if they are clearly visible on scans and radiographs, often are simply followed because they rarely increase in size and are unlikely to compress any vital structures.

Primary treatment of Hodgkin's and non-Hodgkin's tumors is chemotherapy or radiotherapy; the surgeon's role is to establish the diagnosis. The primary treatment of the malignant germ cell tumors is chemotherapy; surgical resection is not generally recommended for any of these.

Teratomas or dermoids are the only neoplastic lesions which require resection as they may become secondarily infected or undergo malignant degeneration. Retrosternal thyroid goiters are resected through the neck.

Bronchogenic cysts and esophageal duplications arising in the middle mediastinum (more frequently found in the posterior mediastinum) develop in the embryo during division of the aerodigestive systems. Bronchogenic cysts are generally lined by respiratory epithelium and esophageal duplications by intestinal mucosa, but ectopic mucosa may be present. These lesions should be resected because of their potential for increasing in size with accumulation of secretions, for becoming secondarily infected, for developing malignancy, and for lesions with gastric mucosa to erode into the bronchial or esophageal lumen.

Solid tumors in the posterior mediastinum should be resected. Resection of a thoracic neuroblastoma is a major component of its treatment. The requirement for further treatment with radiation or chemotherapy will depend on the age of the child, the presence of metastatic disease and the cytogenetic findings of the tumor, particularly amplification of the *N-myc* oncogene which suggests an aggressive tumor. Ganglioneuroma, while benign, may grow locally, may erode the ribs, and may extend into the spinal canal producing neurologic symptoms. While these benign lesions often are found when asymptomatic, resection is generally recommended to establish a diagnosis and prevent local extension. A paraganglioma (extra-adrenal pheochromocytoma) should be removed to control the systemic manifestations of neuropeptide production. The patient should be well prepared for surgery with α and β blocking agents. Pulmonary sequestrations are generally resected to obtain a definitive pathologic diagnosis.

Diagnosis

The preoperative diagnosis of a mediastinal mass can be obtained quickly with only a few studies. Anterior–posterior and lateral chest radiographs will demonstrate the area of the mediastinum in which the mass arises. The location and knowledge of whether the mass is cystic or solid and the age of the patient will often allow an accurate diagnosis to be made.

1 Lesions occurring in each of the three compartments of the mediastinum are shown, grouped by their cystic or solid nature.

Further investigation is determined by the location of the lesion.

Masses in the anterior compartment

Masses in the anterior mediastinum may produce respiratory symptoms and cause compression of the trachea. Computed tomographic (CT) scanning is generally best for evaluating masses in this area; it defines the cystic or solid nature of the lesion and most accurately demonstrates the extent of tracheal compression[1]. The extent to which the trachea is compressed will determine the safety of anesthesia required for further diagnosis or resection.

The cystic lesions may be differentiated by their nature and location. A teratoma generally has both cystic and solid components, with areas of varying density that are well demonstrated on the CT scan. A lymphangioma has multiple cystic areas with very thin walls which often extend up into the neck; very few lymphangiomas are limited to the anterior mediastinum. Thymic cysts are often single, thin-walled and continuous with the thymus. Pericardial cysts arise in the inferior portion of the chest adjacent to the pericardium.

Solid anterior mediastinal lesions are also easily assessed on a CT scan. A dermoid or entirely solid teratoma has areas of varying fat and water density and often some calcification. A substernal thyroid goiter arises from the thyroid gland and extends into the neck. Thymomas are extremely rare in children. Lymphomas involve multiple nodal sites. The CT scan also defines lymph node enlargement in the pulmonary hilum and pulmonary parenchymal lesions. Germ-cell tumors are uncommon, arising primarily in teenagers or young adults. These tumors are usually diagnosed with serum markers.

Masses in the middle compartment

A bronchogenic cyst at the carina may be 'hidden' in the mediastinal shadow on the chest radiograph despite significant respiratory distress. Fluoroscopy will demonstrate compression and anterior displacement of the airway, and ingestion of barium into the esophagus will demonstrate displacement of the esophagus posteriorly and confirm a space-occupying lesion. While CT scanning and magnetic resonance (MR) imaging will demonstrate these lesions more definitively, the sedation required for these studies in infants may be dangerous if respiratory compromise is significant.

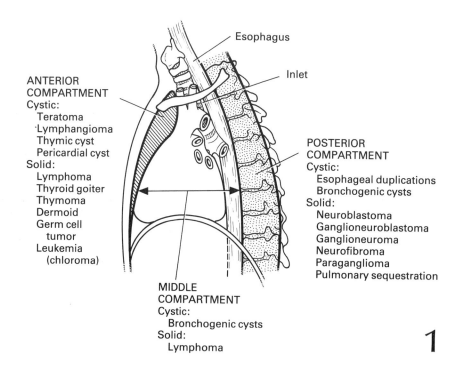

Esophagus

Inlet

ANTERIOR
COMPARTMENT
Cystic:
  Teratoma
  Lymphangioma
  Thymic cyst
  Pericardial cyst
Solid:
  Lymphoma
  Thyroid goiter
  Thymoma
  Dermoid
  Germ cell
    tumor
  Leukemia
    (chloroma)

POSTERIOR
COMPARTMENT
Cystic:
  Esophageal duplications
  Bronchogenic cysts
Solid:
  Neuroblastoma
  Ganglioneuroblastoma
  Ganglioneuroma
  Neurofibroma
  Paraganglioma
  Pulmonary sequestration

MIDDLE
COMPARTMENT
Cystic:
  Bronchogenic cysts
Solid:
  Lymphoma

1

Masses in the posterior compartment

The main cystic lesions in this area are bronchogenic cysts and esophageal duplications, which are typically ovoid in shape and may be diagnosed on routine radiography.

The solid neural tumors have a fusiform shape and are based in the posterior sulcus between the vertebral bodies and the ribs. The age of the patient will give some hint of the diagnosis: neuroblastomas and ganglioneuroblastomas arise more often in infants. Ganglioneuromas occur in older children and are generally asymptomatic, but can extend into the spinal canal and produce neurologic symptoms. Neurofibromas arise primarily in conjunction with neurofibromatosis (von Recklinghausen's disease) and are often associated with scoliosis. Paragangliomas may arise in the posterior mediastinum, although they are rare, and often present with symptoms related to catecholamine secretion – particularly paroxysmal hypertension, diaphoresis and palpitations. Extralobar pulmonary sequestrations arise in the posterior mediastinum with arterial supply from the aorta. They generally can be distinguished by their triangular shape.

MR scanning is frequently used to evaluate patients with masses in the posterior mediastinum because it provides a better definition of possible extension of the tumor into the spinal canal than CT scanning. This extension is important to identify before surgical resection. In infants and young children in whom neuroblastoma is a major diagnostic concern, evaluation of metastatic disease is also important. This should include a bone marrow biopsy, bone scan and measurement of urinary catecholamines, which are elevated in 95% of infants and children with neuroblastoma. Some children with duplication cysts (large cysts extending into the abdominal cavity and originating from the stomach, pancreas or duodenum) demonstrate abnormalities of the vertebrae, but most esophageal and bronchogenic cysts are not associated with vertebral anomalies.

Preoperative

Solid lesions require further histopathologic diagnosis. The most common solid tumor in the anterior mediastinum is Hodgkin's disease followed by non-Hodgkin's lymphoma[1]. Other areas of involvement, particularly the neck, should be sought where biopsy could be more easily performed. In those rare instances where only the mediastinum is involved, a germ cell tumor should be suspected and serum alpha fetoprotein and human chorionic gonadotropin levels should be obtained. In cases where there is no extrathoracic tumor, either a needle biopsy or a limited anterior thoracotomy may be required to obtain a tissue diagnosis. The rare chloroma of leukemia presenting as a mediastinal mass can be diagnosed with the initial complete blood count and bone marrow biopsy.

Preparation for surgery

The child should be prepared for surgery after completion of diagnostic studies. If a bronchogenic cyst is compressing the airway sufficiently to produce pneumonia or respiratory distress, no undue delay should occur. Appropriate antibiotic coverage and physiotherapy should be instituted for pneumonia. Preliminary bronchoscopy should be avoided in these patients because a tenuous airway in an infant or child will be further damaged by manipulation. Catecholamine-secreting tumors, primarily paraganglioma, require institution of α and β blocking agents. Direct involvement of the bronchus is very rare and compression of the airway can be defined most safely radiographically. In the occasional case of thymoma and associated myasthenia gravis, the neuromuscular deficit should be minimized before surgical intervention.

Anesthesia

Anesthesia is of major concern, primarily for solid lesions of the anterior compartment which often compress the airway. A cross-sectional tracheal area of less than 50% of that expected for age predicts significant risk for respiratory collapse upon induction of anesthesia[1]. These children must be limited to local anesthesia with sedation; general anesthesia (particularly paralytic agents) must be avoided at all costs. Bronchogenic cysts in the area of the carina may also cause significant airway obstruction in infants, but the endobronchial tube can generally be passed down one of the mainstem bronchi to provide adequate ventilation until the pressure is relieved. This maneuver may not be feasible in children with a solid mass compressing the airway.

Appropriate monitoring of these patients requires transcutaneous oximetry and, in those children requiring extensive resections, central venous as well as arterial pressure monitoring. Uncuffed endotracheal tubes are routinely used in younger children to avoid any injury to the airway from pressure. An 'air leak' should be present around the endotracheal tube to confirm that pressure on the subglottic mucosa, the narrowest segment of an infant's upper airway, is not excessive.

Choice of approach and applied anatomy

The approaches to these masses are based primarily on their location and nature; most may be resected through a posterolateral thoracotomy. If a teratoma or dermoid is primarily located in the midline, it may be most easily resected through a median sternotomy. Often these lesions are asymmetric and prolapse into one of the hemithoraces allowing them to be resected from that side. This is also true of a thymic cyst. Extensive lymphangiomas, if they extend into the thoracic cavity, are also best approached through a thoracotomy. Sternotomy should be avoided for suspected lympho-mas because compression of the airway can occur when the sternum is closed after biopsy of the mass. A posterolateral thoracotomy is the procedure of choice for lesions of the posterior compartment. Extension into the spinal canal from benign tumors requires a preliminary laminectomy with resection of the tumor, or a combined laminectomy and thoracotomy[2,3]. Swelling of the residual segment of tumor in the canal after resection of the thoracic component could produce neurologic sequelae.

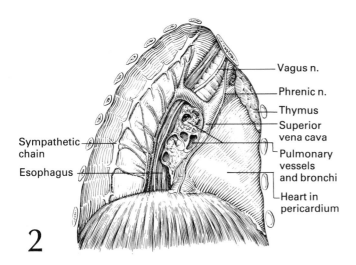

Vagus n.
Phrenic n.
Thymus
Superior vena cava
Pulmonary vessels and bronchi
Heart in pericardium
Sympathetic chain
Esophagus

2

2 The major structures of concern on the right side of the mediastinum are shown. Particular care should be taken to preserve the phrenic nerve, avoiding loss of diaphragmatic function. The upper mediastinum and carina are most readily approached from the right side because the aortic arch and its branches are on the left.

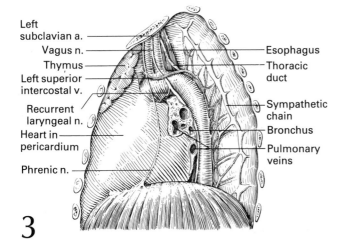

Left subclavian a.
Vagus n.
Thymus
Left superior intercostal v.
Recurrent laryngeal n.
Heart in pericardium
Phrenic n.
Esophagus
Thoracic duct
Sympathetic chain
Bronchus
Pulmonary veins

3

3 On the left side attention must be paid in the upper mediastinum to the course of the vagus nerve and the recurrent laryngeal nerve, which loops around the aortic arch to return to the larynx, in addition to the phrenic nerve.

Operation

POSTEROLATERAL THORACOTOMY

Position of patient

4 The patient's back should be perpendicular to the ground. The lower leg should be flexed, the upper leg straight and a pillow placed between them. The axilla should be padded. The uppermost arm should be angled at 90° and brought anterior to the chest. Extension to greater than this should be avoided as traction injury to the brachial plexus may occur. Adequate padding of all weight-bearing areas on the table is critical, particularly for extended procedures.

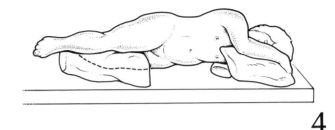

4

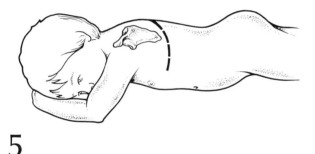

5

Incision

5 The incision curves from below the nipple in the estimated inframmammary crease to a point two finger breadths below the tip of the scapula, traveling superiorly to a point midway between the scapula and the spinous processes. This incision does not have to be extended far superiorly because of the mobility of the scapula.

The latissimus dorsi muscle is divided with electrocautery. The serratus muscles may generally be adequately mobilized anteriorly and are not divided.

The intercostal space is then entered; if the mass is in the superior mediastinum, the chest is best entered in the fourth intercostal space; if the mass is lower, the fifth intercostal space should be used. Neurogenic tumors with an inferior location near the diaphragm are approached through the sixth or seventh intercostal space. A thoracoabdominal incision is occasionally required for extensive neurogenic tumors with abdominal and thoracic components. The surgeon should take care not to be 'trapped' through too low an incision which does not allow access to the apex of the mass. It is rarely necessary to remove a rib in children for adequate exposure. The pleura is opened and the chest is entered.

6 The thoracic cavity is explored to identify the extent of the mass to be resected and its relationship with the vital intrathoracic structures. The lung is retracted anteriorly to expose the mass.

During resection of cystic lesions aspiration is unnecessary unless the airway is compressed or the lesion is too large for safe dissection. Keeping the cyst filled with secretions actually facilitates dissection around it.

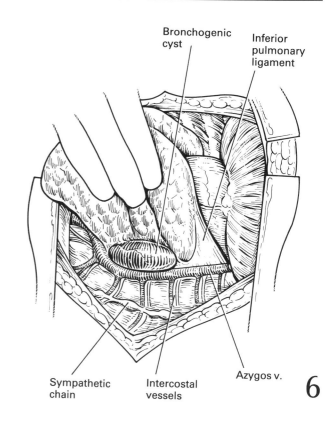

6

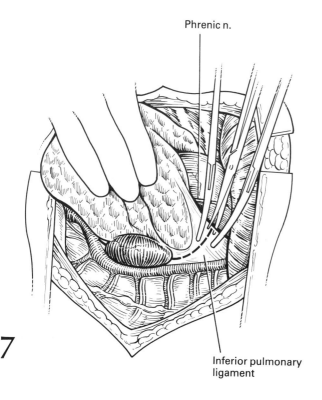

7

7 The pleura around a cystic lesion is first incised.

8 Bronchogenic cysts generally lie adjacent and posterior or lateral to the bronchus or trachea but direct communication is extremely rare. These lesions are easily dissected from surrounding structures and removed intact.

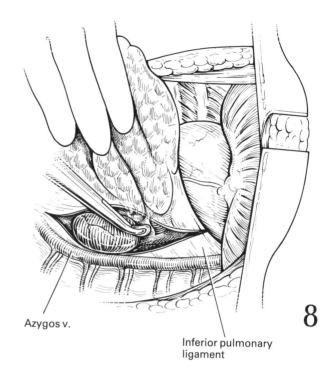

Azygos v.

Inferior pulmonary
ligament

8

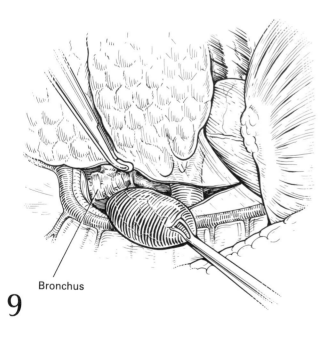

Bronchus

9

9 Cysts associated with the right bronchus, carina and central left bronchus are best approached through the right side of the chest; only more peripheral lesions of the left bronchus lateral to the aortic arch are resected through the left chest.

Inflammatory reaction around the cyst suggests ectopic gastric mucosa within the cyst or secondary infection of the cyst. Only rarely, when acid produced by the gastric mucosa has eroded through the cyst wall, will it densely adhere to either the bronchus or the esophagus. Significant hemorrhage or pulmonary reaction can occur in this situation. Cysts with gastric mucosa eroding into the bronchus or the esophagus may present with hemoptysis, hematemesis or pain.

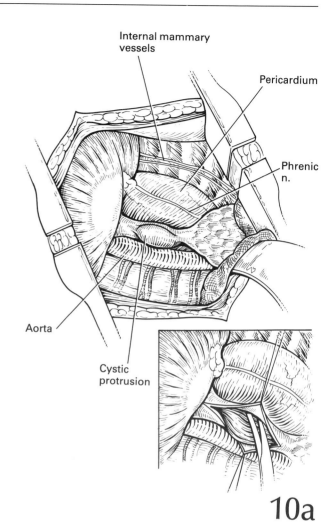

Internal mammary vessels

Pericardium

Phrenic n.

Aorta

Cystic protrusion

10a

10a, b Esophageal duplications are often surrounded by esophageal muscle. They are best approached through the thorax, into which they protrude. The pleura is first incised over the esophagus and then the muscle overlying the cystic lesion is opened longitudinally. It is particularly helpful to keep the cyst intact in these patients.

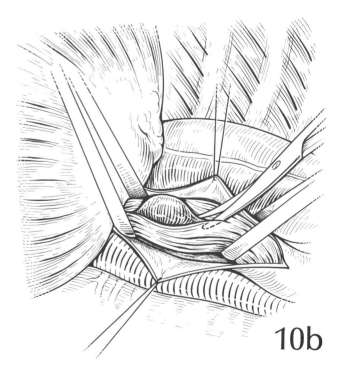

10b

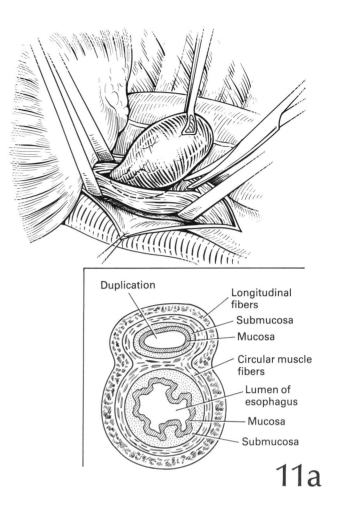

11a

11a, b Submucosal dissection of the cyst from the eosphagus will avoid an untoward entrance into the esophageal lumen, as a single muscular layer comprises the wall between the esophagus and the duplication.

Bronchogenic cysts and esophageal duplications should be removed in their entirety because any remaining mucosa may cause the cyst to recur. Aspiration or sclerosis of these lesions is not recommended because the mucosal surface will regenerate and produce a recurrent mass. The risk of development of malignancy must always be considered.

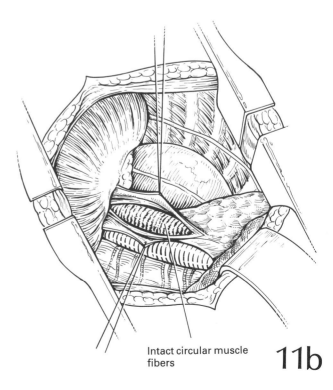

Intact circular muscle fibers   11b

12 Solid posterior mediastinal lesions are broad-based and adhere to the ribs, intercostal muscles and sulcus of the vertebral bodies. They commonly arise from the sympathetic chain and may involve the stellate ganglion. Resection of this ganglion with an apical tumor will produce Horner's syndrome with apparent ptosis, miosis and anhidrosis. The family and child should be forewarned of this possibility.

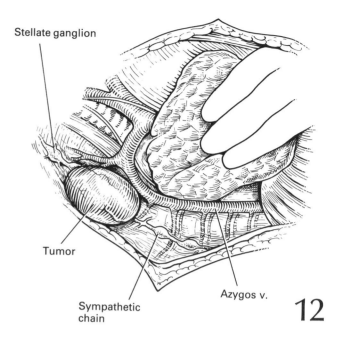

12

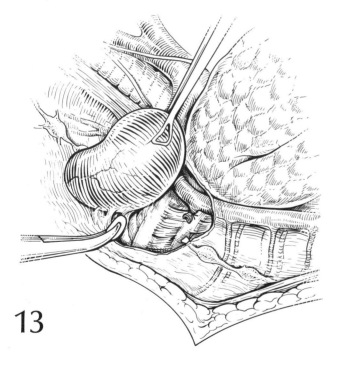

13

13 After incision of the pleura around the periphery, blunt dissection is used to elevate the tumor off the ribs. This will facilitate identification of the plane between the tumor and the intercostal muscles.

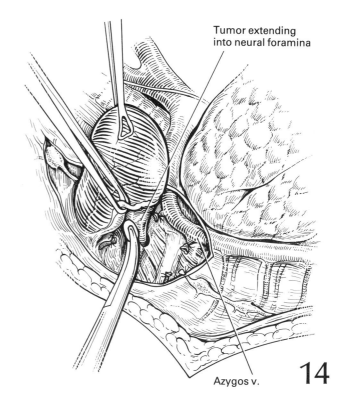

Tumor extending
into neural foramina

Azygos v.

14

14 The difficult part of this dissection occurs at the sulcus, where the tumor may extend into the neural foramina. An artery and vein accompany the nerve from each foramen. The use of bipolar cautery in this area avoids the risk of conduction of current to the spinal cord. The aorta and esophagus, when involved, can generally be dissected from the anterior aspect of the tumor easily as direct involvement of the tumor is rare. As the aorta is dissected forward, each intercostal artery should be controlled and ligated. The tumor rarely extends through the periosteum of the vertebral bodies. A combination of blunt and cautery dissection is utilized to mobilize the tumor off each of the vertebral bodies.

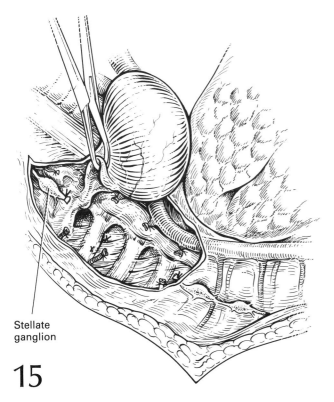

Stellate
ganglion

15

15 Dissection progresses around the mass, working where progress can most readily be achieved. The sympathetic chain is divided superior and inferior to the tumor. The stellate ganglion should be preserved if possible to avoid Horner's syndrome.

Ganglioneuromas and neurofibromas do not have an extensive blood supply and are firm and fibrous and easy to keep intact during dissection. The neuroblastomas are much softer and more vascular and rupture should be avoided. If preliminary chemotherapy has been administered, the neuroblastomas are much firmer and fibrotic and less vascular. A nasogastric tube in the esophagus will facilitate its identification and dissection from a large tumor.

Once the mass, whether cystic or solid, has been completely removed the area should be inspected for any bleeding or evidence of lymphatic leak in the posterior lesions. These should be controlled and an intercostal chest tube inserted.

The bed of a resected neuroblastoma should be marked with radio-opaque tantalum clips to facilitate radiation therapy if required, particularly if gross residual tumor is present (this should be rare in the mediastinum except for tumor extending through the neural foramina).

Wound closure

It is rarely possible to cover the defect with pleura, particularly in the solid tumors where a significant amount of pleura is resected with the tumor. A chest tube is placed in the midaxillary line two intercostal spaces below the incision so it can be brought out through the muscle in a superior trajectory. It is secured with non-absorbable sutures. The ribs are then approximated with pericostal sutures and the musculofascial layers reapproximated with absorbable sutures. Subcuticular polyglycolic acid absorbable sutures are used to reapproximate the skin edges.

Postoperative care

Management of the airway

Most children can be extubated following surgery unless the procedure has been particularly long or has required significant volume replacement. Infants and young children will often tolerate a humidified oxygen tent better than a face mask. In very young infants a short period of postoperative ventilation will allow equilibration and progressive withdrawal of respiratory support. If a child is to remain intubated an 'air leak' must exist around the endotracheal tube; this confirms that the uncuffed tube is not producing undue pressure on the tracheal or subglottic mucosa with a risk of developing a postoperative stricture.

Intercostal drainage

Suction is employed for 48 h and if drainage is insignificant the tube may be removed. Air leakage is rare following this sort of resection. The intercostal tube is removed once the lung is fully expanded with no air leak. Serous drainage occurs frequently but does not usually require extended intercostal drainage. A chest radiograph should be obtained once the drain is removed to document continued full expansion of the lung.

Analgesia and sedation

Young children often need analgesia for the first few days; infants require a shorter duration. Sedation is also necessary in all infants and children during mechanical ventilation.

References

1. Shamberger RC, Holzman RS, Griscom NT, Tarbell NJ, Weinstein HJ. CT quantitation of tracheal cross-sectional area as a guide to the surgical and anesthetic management of children with anterior mediastinal masses. *J Pediatr Surg* 1991; 26: 138–42.

2. Saenz NC, Schnitzer JJ, Eraklis AE *et al*. Posterior mediastinal masses. *J Pediatr Surg* 1993; 28: 172–6.

3. Grillo HC, Ojemann RG, Scannell JG, Zervas NT. Combined approach to 'dumbbell' intrathoracic and intraspinal tumors. *Ann Thorac Surg* 1983; 36: 402–7.

Surgical treatment of chest wall deformities in children

J. Stark MD, FRCS
Consultant Cardiothoracic Surgeon, Cardiothoracic Unit, Great Ormond Street Hospital for Children, London, UK

T. R. Karl MD
Consultant Cardiac Surgeon, Royal Children's Hospital, Melbourne, Victoria, Australia

Pectus excavatum

Principles and justification

Pectus excavatum is the most common of the chest wall deformities. Its incidence is 7.9 per 1000 births, with a male preponderance[1]. The deformity is caused by unbalanced growth of the costochondral region which results in sharp posterior curvature of the sternal body. The lower costal cartilages are bent dorsally and form a depression with sharply angled lateral borders. Sometimes the sternum is rotated towards one side and the deformity becomes asymmetrical. Pectus excavatum is usually present at birth and may be progressive.

Indications

Ravitch[2], Wada[3, 4] and others reported patients with respiratory symptoms, arrhythmias and decreased exercise tolerance. Although such symptoms can occur, the authors have not encountered them and find, instead, that psychologic and social problems usually dominate the picture. It is, therefore, important to discuss the deformity extensively with the parents and, in the case of an older child, he or she should be closely involved in the discussion. If the deformity is severe the psychologic impact may become important, especially during puberty. The authors recommend operation for severe deformities, but stress the cosmetic nature of such an operation. When the deformity is moderate to mild they are more conservative and usually recommend exercises to develop and strengthen the pectoral muscles and to improve the posture. This often improves the overall appearance. If the patient or the parents are still concerned surgery is considered even for moderate deformities.

Operations

Many operations have been recommended. The authors have experience with the sternal turnover[3,5] and with the Ravitch[2] operation. Flucloxacillin and an aminoglycoside are used as antibiotic cover. The first dose is given with premedication, and antibiotics are continued for 24 h. Standard endotracheal anesthesia is used. Satisfactory venous access for drugs and transfusion is required. The skin is prepared with povidone-iodine, and Steridrapes are used.

STERNAL TURNOVER

The operation was first described by Nissen in 1944[5]. Subsequently it has been used extensively by Wada[3,4]. The authors have used it for symmetrical deformities during the past 13 years with excellent results.

1 A submammary transverse incision gives a good exposure and is cosmetically superior to the midline incision. A scalpel is used for the skin, and all subsequent layers are cut with a diathermy needle.

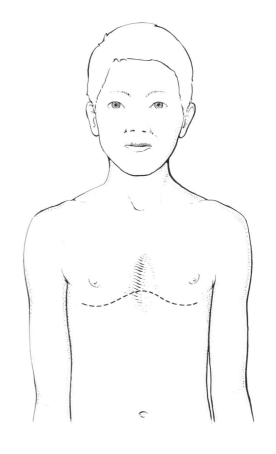

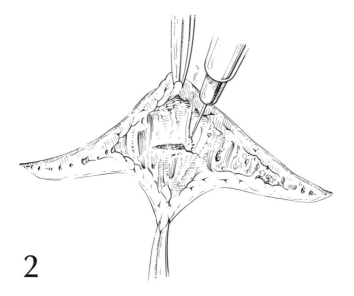

2 The skin flaps are developed superiorly to the manubrium and inferiorly to the xiphoid process and lower costal margins. Great care must be taken to avoid injury to the skin flaps. Towels are then sutured to the subcutaneous tissue. Throughout the procedure the tissues are kept moist with warm saline. Flucloxacillin and an aminoglycoside can be added to the saline.

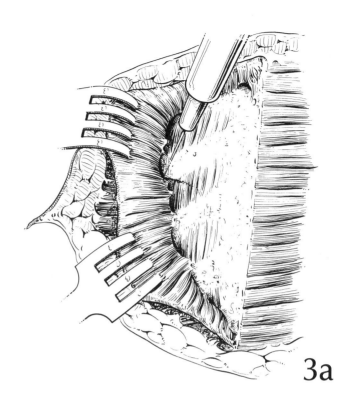

3a

Muscle mobilization

3a, b The midline incision is then carried down to the periosteum of the sternum and the pectoralis major muscles are dissected laterally to expose the costochondral junctions. Inferiorly the xiphoid process is freed and detached, retaining the insertions of the rectus abdominis muscles. It is advisable to detach the xiphoid with periosteum; reattachment at the end of the operation is then facilitated.

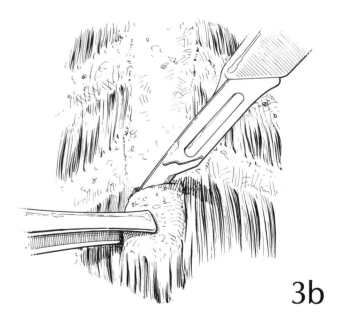

3b

Mobilization of sternum

The lower end of the sternum is grasped with Kocher forceps and elevated. The mediastinum is dissected bluntly with a finger and wet swabs. Care is taken to displace both pleural sacs laterally to avoid injury, but this is only rarely achieved. If pleural spaces are opened they should be drained. The perichondrium is then cut with a diathermy needle and the cartilage is divided with a scalpel.

4 The incision is made at the lateral border of the deformity. Intercostal vessels are identified, doubly ligated, and divided.

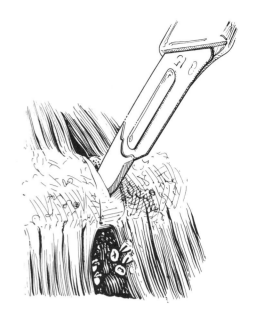

4

5a, b When all cartilages (except the first and second) have been divided on both sides, the sternum is elevated, the internal mammary vessels are ligated and the sternum is transected at the junction with the manubrium. The sternum, with all adjacent cartilages, is removed.

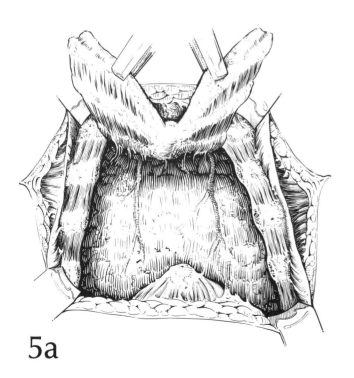

5a

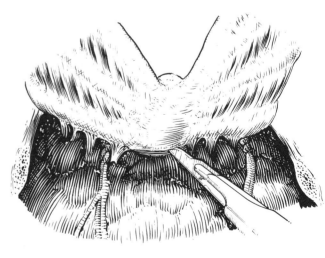

5b

Remodeling of plastron

6a–c The sternum, with the adjacent cartilages, is placed on a board and all the attached soft tissues, including intercostal muscles, are excised. Wedge resection and resuture of some of the cartilages will remodel the sternal plastron. The sternum is then turned upside down. Shortening of some of the cartilages may be required. All pieces of resected cartilage are kept in a bowl of saline to which an aminoglycoside and flucloxacillin have been added. They may be required to lengthen the shorter side of the plastron. If the sternal depression was deep, corrective wedge osteotomy of the sternum may also be required.

While the plastron is being prepared the assistant carefully controls all bleeding points, and if the pleural spaces were opened chest drains are inserted. The lateral ends of the costal cartilages may be broken and turned upwards to further remodel the thoracic cage. The whole plastron is repeatedly bathed in warm saline with antibiotics.

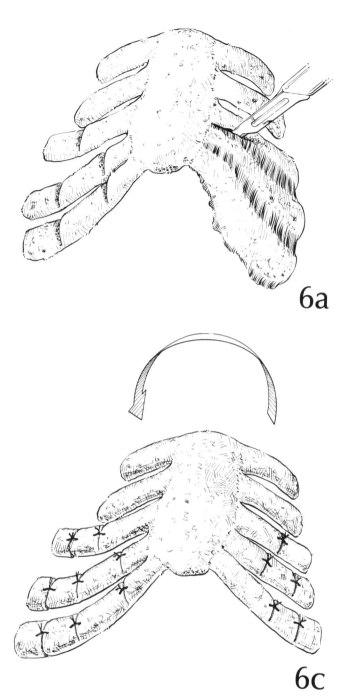

6a

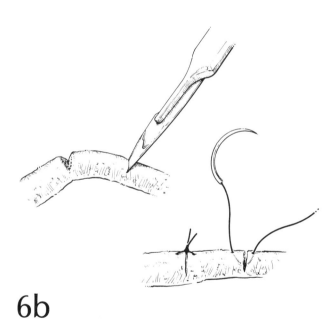

6b

6c

Reinsertion of plastron

7a–c The plastron is turned upside down and placed into the defect. The sternum is then sutured with two wires to the manubrium. The length of the cartilages is then considered. Additional resections on one side with insertion of the resection pieces on the other side is occasionally necessary. Cartilages are sutured with mattress or figure-of-eight sutures of non-absorbable material (Ethibond 2/0 or 0 depending on the size of the patient). The xiphoid process is then reattached to the lower end of the sternum with wire sutures.

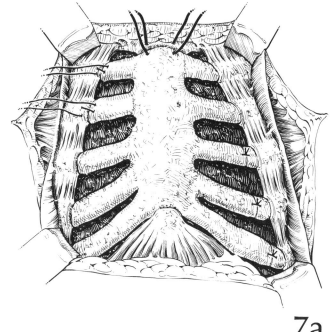

7a

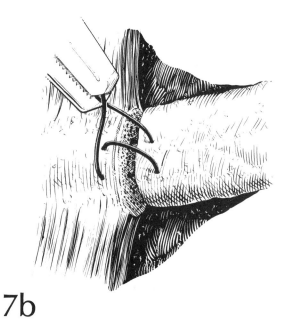

7b

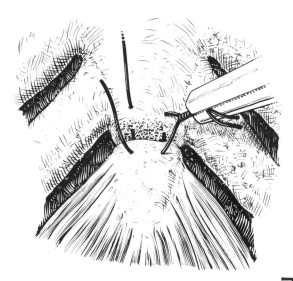

7c

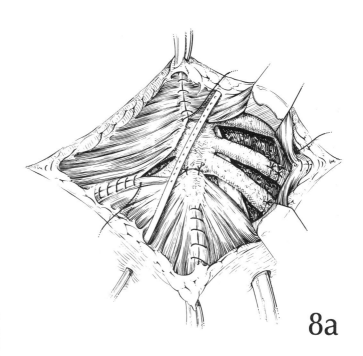

8a

Closure

8a, b Pleural spaces, if opened, are drained with Argyle drains. The pectoralis muscles are reattached in the midline, using 2/0 polyglycolic acid (Dexon). The rectus muscles are also sutured together and superiorly attached to the pectoralis muscles. Several single stitches are placed to achieve symmetrical reattachment of the skin flaps. Redivac drains are placed under the skin flaps. A running suture of 3/0 or 4/0 polyglycolic acid is used for subcutaneous tissue, and the skin is closed with intracuticular polyglycolic acid.

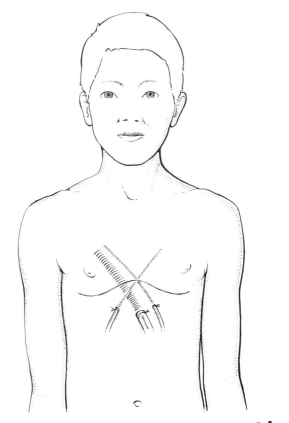

8b

RAVITCH PROCEDURE

The Ravitch[2] repair can be performed through the same type of incision as the sternal turnover. Skin flaps are raised and the muscles reflected in a similar fashion. The sternum is mobilized posteriorly, using the finger and moist swabs.

Freeing the perichondrium

9a–d
The perichondrium is incised longitudinally from the sternum to the lateral extent of the deformity, using the diathermy needle. A T incision is made at either end. A fine periosteal elevator is used to free the perichondrium from the cartilage. The edges of the perichondrium are grasped with several arterial forceps and the dissection continued. This technique causes less bleeding than a transperichondrial resection. The bone can also regenerate from the residual perichondrium, resulting in better chest wall stability. The dissection is completed with the right-angled periosteal elevator.

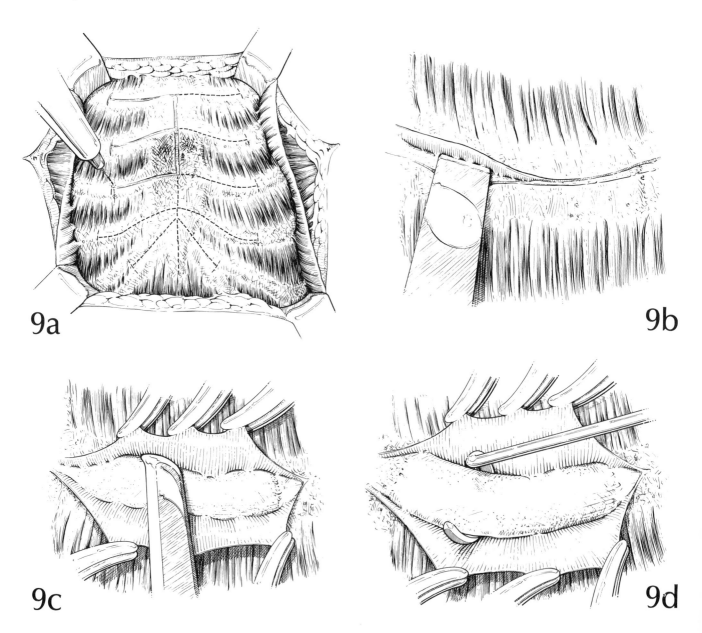

9a

9b

9c

9d

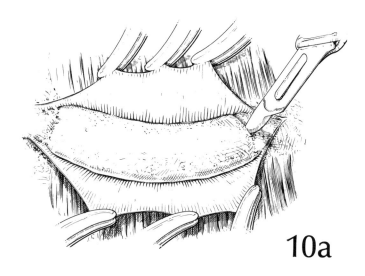

10a, b The cartilage is then transected close to the costochondral junction. The end is elevated with Kocher clamps and disarticulated at the chondrosternal junction. The extent of resection depends on the type of deformity; usually three to five cartilages are resected bilaterally.

When the cartilages have been resected the intercostal vessels are identified, doubly ligated and divided. The lowest non-deformed cartilage (usually the second or third) is then transected 1 cm lateral to its sternal articulation. The transection is made oblique to facilitate stabilization of the sternum after elevation. The incision runs from the anteromedial to posterolateral aspect. This step allows the sternum to move anteriorly, hinged in the interspace above the lowest normal cartilage, thus relieving the deformity.

10a

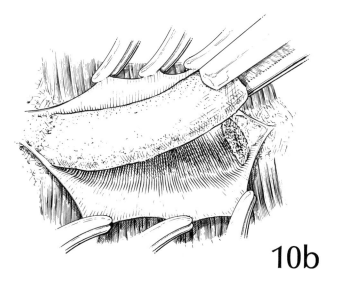

10b

Posterior osteotomy

The osteotomy can be made anteriorly or posteriorly, but the latter will give the best result. Osteotomy is performed with a Gigli saw which is passed behind the sternum. Only one cortex is broken (greenstick fracture).

Stabilizing the sternum

11 Various techniques to stabilize the sternum have been described, but the authors prefer to use a stainless steel bar. It is passed under the lower part of the sternum and attached to the ribs or cartilage on both sides. The bar is removed 6–12 months later.

Closure

Closure follows the same course as that described for the sternal turnover operation.

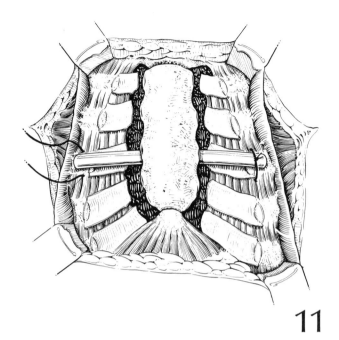

11

Postoperative care

For both the sternal turnover and Ravitch operations adequate sedation and pain relief is recommended for the first 24–48 h after surgery using a morphine drip (0.5 mg morphine/kg body weight in 50 ml 5% dextrose, given at 2 ml/h). In recent years epidural anesthesia with bupivacaine 0.25% or 0.375% has been used. Analgesia is maintained with a mixture of local anesthetic and opiate. Chest drains are usually removed the following morning, and the Redivac drains after 24–48 h. Once the chest drains have been removed the child is allowed out of bed and usually discharged after 5–7 days. The child is allowed to return to school after 4 weeks but contact sports should be avoided for a period of 3 months.

Outcome

The current operative mortality rate should approach zero. The best results are obtained in younger children with symmetric central deformities. Long-term follow-up suggests that there is continued growth of the inverted or mobilized sternum and continued improvement of the chest contour with age. Recurrence of the pectus deformity is rare after either procedure[6], but may be treated by a secondary operation if indicated.

Pectus carinatum

The carinatum deformity is about one-tenth as common as the excavatum type. It is probably caused by overgrowth of the costal cartilages, with forward displacement and secondary deformity of the sternum. There is a considerable variability in degree of asymmetry and rotation. Synostosis or complete non-segmentation of the sternum is typical but not clearly etiologically related. As with pectus excavatum, this deformity presents a cosmetic problem with associated psychologic and social complications. Lester performed the first corrective operation for this condition in 1953, employing cartilage and partial sternal resection[7]. Ravitch[8] has stressed that the pathology is in the costal cartilages and his repair, described in 1960, recommends resection of the costal cartilages and preservation of the sternum. The authors have followed Ravitch's principles.

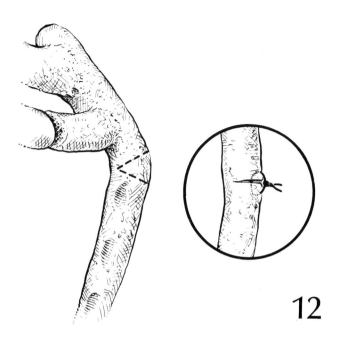

12

Operation

Indications for operation are similar to those described for pectus excavatum.

The transverse inframammary incision is used. This is performed as in the pectus excavatum repair, including raising of skin and pectoralis flaps and detachment of rectus muscles from the sternum and costal arches. The upper margin of muscle reflection usually need not be above the third cartilage.

The perichondrium is incised with a diathermy needle and freed from the cartilage, using the technique described under the Ravitch operation (*Illustration 9a*). All deformed cartilages are then resected with strong shears or a scalpel. In older children the resection may extend into the bony rib for 1–2 cm if necessary. Interrupted 2/0 Ethibond mattress sutures are used to plicate the perichondrial beds to eliminate the carinatum defect. It is usually not necessary to divide the intercostal neurovascular bundles.

12 If an osteotomy is required, it is performed as illustrated.

Closure is identical to that in the pectus excavatum repair. One or two Redivac drains are left under the skin flap for 24–48 h.

Outcome

Mortality should approach zero for this operation. The cosmetic results are very satisfactory and recurrence is rare. Growth and development of the anterior chest is normal following the operation.

Sternal cleft

Failure of fusion of the primitive sternal bars results in a cleft which may be partial or complete. Simple cleft sternum usually involves the manubrium and variable parts of the body but may extend to or through the xiphoid. The cleft can be V-shaped, or broad and U-shaped. True ectopia cordis is associated with variable degrees of cleft. Major intracardiac and other developmental abnormalities are commonly present. Cantrell's pentalogy is a complex anomaly involving lower sternal, midline abdominal, intracardiac and other severe defects[9]. The simple sternal cleft is most amenable to surgical repair and is considered here.

Principles and justification

Despite the alarming appearance of the sternal cleft, with the beating heart visible through its attenuated skin covering, patients are usually asymptomatic. The heart and great vessels are, however, vulnerable to injury. Operative correction is best undertaken in the first few months of life, as it is both safer and easier at this time. Later on the infant's cardiopulmonary system will accommodate to the size of the thorax, making closure a physiologic compromise. Furthermore, the chest wall becomes increasingly firm with age.

Preoperative

Preoperative investigation (cross-sectional echocardiography and/or cardiac catheterization and angiocardiography) should exclude any associated intracardiac defects. Endotracheal anesthesia is used.

Operation

Incision

A standard midline incision from the level of the clavicular heads to the xiphoid is used. The proximity of pericardium and heart to the skin should be kept in mind.

13 Skin flaps are developed with sharp dissection laterally to expose the entire sternum. The dissection is carried out in the plane just superficial to the sternum and pectoralis muscles. The sternal edges are mobilized from underlying mediastinal structures with blunt dissection.

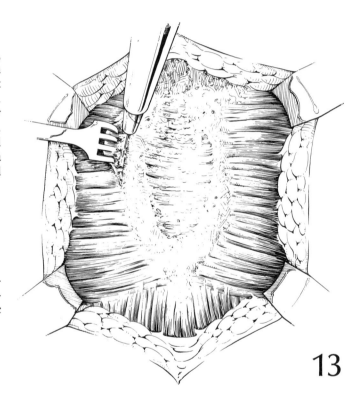

13

Approximation of sternum

14 Ethibond sutures (2/0 and 0) are passed through the manubrium and around the sternum at each interspace. With a U-shaped defect a wedge of distal sternum and xiphoid may be resected to facilitate closure. The sternal bars can be notched to straighten them and improve alignment, although in small infants this is usually unnecessary. Patients beyond early infancy may require multiple chondrotomies to attain safe closure. These can be made subperichondrially in an oblique manner to retain sternal stability. The suture holes are checked for bleeding anteriorly and posteriorly. Sutures are then crossed and a trial apposition of the sternum is made while blood pressure and ventilation are observed for any signs of a thoracic compression. If satisfactory, the sutures are tied.

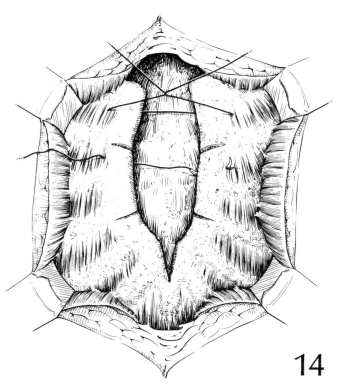

14

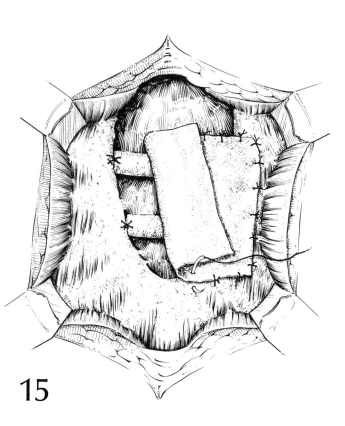

15

15 Patients who do not tolerate apposition of the sternal bars can be treated palliatively with a Marlex or Silastic mesh to bridge the sternal defect, and thus to improve protection of the underlying heart and great vessels. These may be strengthened by rib grafts placed under the mesh.

Closure

The fascia and subcutaneous tissues are closed with continuous polyglycolic acid sutures, and the skin with fine nylon interrupted mattress sutures. Redivac drains may be placed under the skin flaps. As the skin in this area is often quite attenuated, great care should be taken to avoid injuring it with forceps during the closure.

Outcome

With current techniques of neonatal anesthesia, surgery and postoperative care, excellent results can be expected. The long-term outlook is related to the severity of any coexisting defect.

Poland's syndrome

This curious syndrome was reported in 1841 by Poland[10]. Features include deficiency or absence of the pectoralis major and minor, serratus and external oblique muscles. Syndactyly and agenesis of the middle phalanges are also common. Varying numbers of ribs may be malformed, hypoplastic, or completely absent. In the latter case the deficit begins near the sternal edge. The defect extends for some distance laterally, where the ribs may fuse. The defect is commonly unilateral, and the ipsilateral breast may be hypoplastic or absent.

Principles and justification

The muscular deficit, while disfiguring, is not a severe physiologic handicap. It is, therefore, the rib anomalies that are brought to the attention of the surgeon. An extensive deficit requires operative correction in order to protect the underlying heart, lung and mediastinum. In addition, the missing segment results in a flail chest with paradoxical movement during breathing, and resulting ventilatory compromise. Repair of the deficit should be undertaken in early childhood as the ribs bordering the deformity may bow with time, thus increasing the problem.

Operation

Incision

16 The patient is placed supine and the entire anterior and lateral chest is painted with antiseptic solution. The incision is made inferior and parallel to the border of the defect. The incision should be kept over the bony portion of the chest wall and not over the defect.

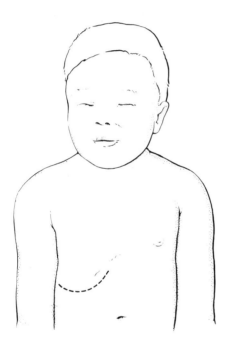

16

17 The area of the breast should be avoided in order to facilitate future mammoplasty in girls. Skin flaps are developed to expose the entire defect.

Harvesting ribs

An adequate length of rib is harvested from the contralateral chest. The rib is exposed through an incision directly over it, after retracting and splitting the interposed muscle. An adequate length of rib is scored with diathermy needle and then a periosteal elevator is used to expose the bony portion. This is excised with rib shears. The rib is split longitudinally with an oscillating saw to provide two grafts. If three grafts are required, a second donor rib is used. The donor incision is closed in layers with continuous polyglycolic acid.

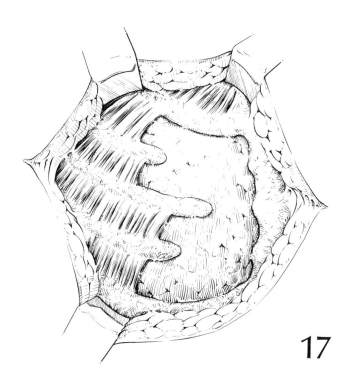

17

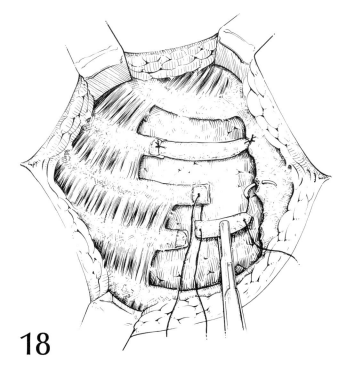

18

Placing the grafts

18 The rib end to be placed medially is sharpened with a scalpel and pressed into a recess in the lateral sternum which has been created with a Kelly clamp. This is secured with 2/0 Ethibond sutures or fine wire placed through the rib and sternum. Lateral ends are secured subperichondrally or subperiosteally to the recipient rib ends using the same suture material. The convex surfaces of the ribs should be placed facing exteriorly.

Stabilizing the grafts

19 A sheet of Marlex or Silastic mesh is cut to the shape of the deformity and sutured to the edges of the defect and to the rib grafts themselves, using 2/0 Ethibond sutures. This serves to stabilize the chest wall and to prevent rotation of the rib grafts, providing a better cosmetic and functional result.

Closure

Any fascia present, and subcutaneous tissues, are closed with continuous 3/0 polyglycolic acid sutures. A subcuticular suture completes the operation.

Postoperative care

No specific problems are anticipated.

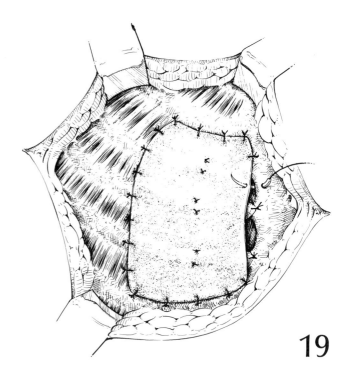

19

Outcome

This syndrome is rare and a large series is not available for review. Results in individual cases have, however, been gratifying, in terms of both chest wall stability and cosmetic appearance. Subsequent implantation mammo-plasty has been performed with good results in some female patients.

References

1. Clarke JB, Grenville-Mathers R. Pectus excavatum. *Br J Dis Chest* 1962; 56: 202–5.

2. Ravitch MM. Pectus excavatum. In: *Congenital Deformities of the Chest Wall and their Operative Correction.* Philadelphia: WB Saunders, 1977: 78–205.

3. Wada J. Surgical correction of the funnel chest 'sterno-turnover'. *West J Surg Obstet Gynecol* 1981; 69: 358–61.

4. Wada J, Ikeda K, Ishida T, Haegawa T. Results of 271 funnel chest operations. *Ann Thorac Surg* 1970; 10: 526–32.

5. Nissen R. Osteoplastic procedure for correction of funnel chest. *Am J Surg* 1944; 64: 169–74.

6. Humphreys GH, Jaretzki A. Pectus excavatum; late results with and without operation *J Thorac Cardiovasc Surg* 1980; 80: 686–95.

7. Lester CW. Pigeon breast (pectus carinatum) and other protrusion deformities of the chest of developmental origin. *Ann Surg* 1953; 137: 482–9.

8. Ravitch MM. The operative correction of pectus carinatum (pigeon breast). *Ann Surg* 1960; 151: 705–14.

9. Cantrell JR, Haller JA, Ravitch MM. A syndrome of congenital defects involving the abdominal wall, sternum, diaphragm, pericardium and heart. *Surg Gynecol Obstet* 1958; 107: 602–14.

10. Poland A. Deficiency of the pectoral muscles. *Guy's Hospital Reports* 1841; VI: 191–3.

Patent ductus arteriosus

Neil J. Sherman MD, FACS, FAAP
Associate Clinical Professor of Surgery (Pediatric), University of Southern California, Los Angeles, California, USA

Principles and justification

The ductus arteriosus of many preterm infants remains patent until after birth. Patency approaches 75% at 28–30 weeks of gestation, 45% at 31–33 weeks and 21% at 34–36 weeks. There is an 83% patency in neonates with birth weight under 1000 g; this drops to 47% in those weighing 1000–1500 g at birth and to 27% in neonates weighing more than 1500 g.

Indications

The hemodynamic significance of a patent ductus arteriosus, rather than simply its patency, determines the course of treatment. Clinical findings include increased pulmonary blood flow, collapsing pulses, cardiomegaly and a continuous murmur. Less striking findings are continuing dependency on a ventilator and an increasing or persistently high oxygen requirement. Therapeutic measures such as decreasing intravenous fluids, use of digitalis and diuretics and adding positive end expiratory pressure may modify the degree of left-to-right shunting, but do not usually expedite ductal closure.

Diagnosis is confirmed by the two-dimensional echo seen on echocardiography but, although this modality is invaluable in assessing patency and pressure, it does not accurately determine the magnitude of flow through the patent ductus arteriosus. The decision to close a patent ductus arteriosus, using medical or surgical techniques, remains a clinical one.

Non-surgical closure

The treatment of choice for non-surgical closure of a patent ductus arteriosus in most neonatal intensive care units is indomethacin. Two or three courses are usually required to effect closure, but further administration beyond this rarely improves the closure rate. Indomethacin tends to become less effective as the infant grows older. Contraindications to use of indomethacin include sepsis, necrotizing enterocolitis, azotemia and coagulation abnormalities. When these conditions exist, surgical intervention is necessary.

Operation

Position of patient

1 The infant is placed in the lateral decubitus position with the right side down. The surgeon stands on the left, facing the infant's back. A headlight provides valuable illumination of the small operative field. A lateral incision is made; it is unnecessary to divide any of the chest wall muscles to gain satisfactory exposure.

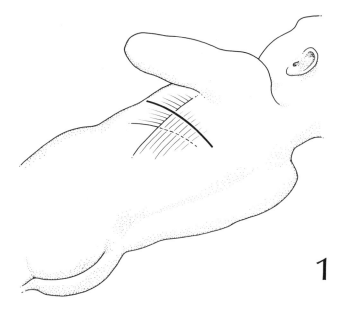

1

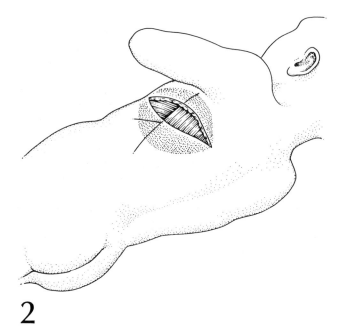

2 The subcutaneous layer is mobilized from the underlying muscles, allowing the muscle to be mobilized without cutting any of its muscle fibres.

2

3 The flimsy attachments of the anterior portion of the latissimus dorsi muscle and the inferior margin of the serratus anterior muscle are incised, thus facilitating elevation of the muscles. The third or fourth intercostal space is entered and a small self-retaining rib spreader placed and opened. A second self-retaining retractor displaces the muscles in an anterior–posterior direction.

The ductus arteriosus may be as large as, or larger than, the aorta and its exact origin varies among patients. It may arise from various anatomical sites on the ventral side of the aorta, just inferior to or more distal from the aortic arch (inset). Accurate identification of the aorta, ductus arteriosus and pulmonary artery is essential before proceeding further.

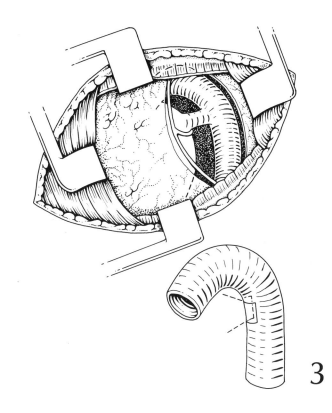

3

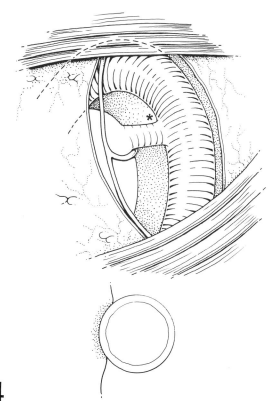

4

4 The mediastinal pleura overlying the aorta is opened; to achieve this it is often necessary to divide a superior intercostal vein. A malleable retractor keeps the lung anteriorly, out of the operative field, but in unstable infants it may be necessary to allow intermittent pulmonary expansion during the procedure. The vagus nerve and recurrent branch are prominent and should be reflected anteriorly with the mediastinal pleura.

The ductus arteriosus is usually 4–5 mm in length and is extremely friable. Adequate exposure of the ductus arteriosus may be achieved by incising and spreading transversely the tissue just superior and inferior to the ductus. The use of tenotomy scissors enhances the accuracy of this dissection. The areolar tissue above and below the ductus arteriosus can be grasped with forceps but care should be taken to avoid direct handling of the ductus arteriosus. The superior angle between the aorta and the ductus arteriosus (*) is particularly delicate and dissection at this point should be avoided.

It is not necessary to completely dissect and encircle the ductus arteriosus, and the dissection is complete once the back wall can be visualized inferiorly. The shaded area (inset) remains undissected. A small or medium hemoclip is placed closer to the aortic end of the ductus arteriosus (but not flush against the aorta).

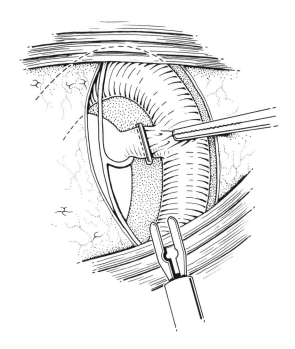

5 The adventitia of the aorta can be grasped and gently retracted towards the surgeon, if necessary, to allow accurate placement of the clip. The tip of the hemoclip must extend beyond the limit of the ductal wall to ensure complete occlusion.

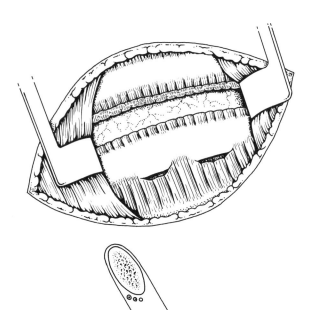

Wound closure

6 One or two absorbable pericostal sutures are placed through a periosteal window around the inferior rib to avoid ligating the intercostal nerve and vessels. A small rubber catheter is put into the pleural space, suction applied and the catheter removed once the pericostal sutures have been tied. The muscle does not need to be sutured. A very fine skin closure is performed.

Postoperative care

The operation should be completed in less than 30 minutes and, in many centers, is performed in the neonatal intensive care unit. After surgery lung re-expansion is confirmed by chest radiography. The infant should recover quickly from the short-acting intravenous anesthetic agent used. The hemodynamic response of an infant treated for a large left-to-right shunt improves almost immediately after surgery, but the pulmonary status usually improves more gradually. Intercostal infiltration of a dilute local anesthetic will alleviate any postoperative pain.

Complications

Postoperative complications are uncommon, but may include chylothorax or transient vocal cord paralysis in addition to the usual sequelae of any thoracic surgical procedure. If the left pulmonary artery or aorta have inadvertently been ligated, or if major intraoperative hemorrhage occurs, the patient invariably dies.

The incidence of retinitis of prematurity is slightly higher following surgical ligation than following indomethacin treatment, but the reason for this is unclear.

Outcome

It is difficult to compare the results of indomethacin treatment with those of surgical ligation because the patient groups are different. In addition, because ductal closure by either medical or surgical methods appears to have little influence on overall survival, comparison of the two methods of treatment is not meaningful.

Hernias in children

J. L. Grosfeld MD
Professor and Chairman, Department of Surgery, Indiana University School of Medicine, and Surgeon-in-Chief, James Whitcomb Riley Hospital for Children, Indianapolis, Indiana, USA

Inguinal hernia and hydrocele

History

The first reference to hernia repair in children is credited to Celsus who in AD25 recommended removal of the hernia sac and testes through a scrotal incision. Paré recommended treatment of childhood hernia; however, the first accurate description was made by Pott in 1756. Czerny performed high ligation of the hernia sac through the external ring in 1877. Ferguson recommended that the spermatic cord should remain undisturbed during inguinal hernia repair in 1899. In 1912, Turner documented that high ligation of the sac was the only procedure necessary in most children. Herzfield was the first advocate of outpatient surgical repair of inguinal hernia in children in 1938. Early repair in infancy was recommended by Ladd and Gross in 1941. The concept of bilateral inguinal exploration was promoted by Duckett, Rothenberg and Barnett, among others. Advances in neonatal intensive care have resulted in improved survival of premature infants who have a high incidence of hernia and an increased risk of complications. These cases have stimulated great interest into considerations regarding the timing of operation and choice of anesthesia. Recently, Puri and others have challenged the necessity of routine bilateral inguinal exploration.

Principles and justification

The occurrence of congenital inguinal hernia is related to descent of the testis which follows the gubernaculum testis as it descends from an intra-abdominal retroperitoneal position to the scrotum. Those factors affecting descent (androgenic hormonal influences for the abdominal descent phase and local hormonal influences, such as GFRH release from the genitofemoral nerve for the scrotal descent phase) are beyond the scope of this chapter. However, as the testis passes through the internal ring it drags with it a diverticulum of peritoneum on its anteromedial surface referred to as the 'processus vaginalis'. In girls the persistence of the processus vaginalis that extends into the labia majora is known as the canal of Nuck. The layers of the processus vaginalis normally fuse in >90% of full-term infants, obliterating the entrance to the inguinal canal from the peritoneal cavity. Failure of obliteration may result in a variety of inguinal–scrotal anomalies including complete persistence resulting in a scrotal hernia, distal processus obliteration and proximal hernial patency, complete patency with a narrow opening at the internal ring referred to as a communicating hydrocele, hydrocele of the canal of Nuck in girls or inguinal canal in boys, and a hydrocele of the tunica vaginalis.

Clinical presentation

The majority of inguinal hernias in infants and children are indirect hernias. Boys are more commonly affected than girls in a ratio of 9:1; 60% present on the right side due to later testicular descent and obliteration of the processus vaginalis on the right, 25% occur on the left side, and 15% are bilateral. The diagnosis is often apparent as a bulge and can be observed in the groin with crying or straining. Scrotal enlargement and frequent change in scrotal size resulting from transfer of fluid between the peritoneal cavity and the sac may be noted. Physical examination will often confirm these observations: however, diagnosis may depend on visualization of these events by the referring pediatrician or parent.

Inguinal hernia is a high-risk hernia as it is frequently complicated by incarceration, occasionally leading to strangulation and obstruction. In young infants with undescended testes and associated hernia the testis is sometimes at risk of torsion or atrophy caused by compression of the vascular supply by a hernia sac filled with bowel compressing the testicular vessels at the level of the internal inguinal ring. The incidence of incarceration is highest in the youngest patients, particularly premature infants and infants under the age of 1 year where an incarceration rate of 31% has been reported. The incarceration rate in children up to 18 years of age is 12–15%.

Indications

Because of the high rate of complications associated with inguinal hernia there is no place for conservative management except in instances of an isolated hydrocele of the tunica vaginalis. The natural history of this particular abnormality is often associated with spontaneous involution at 6–12 months of age. As long as the hydrocele does not change in size, this can be watched. All other inguinal scrotal anomalies require surgical intervention. In addition to instances of incarceration seen in boys, girls can present with a mass in the labia majora due to a sliding hernia of the ovary and fallopian tube. This may be associated with a risk of torsion of the ovary in the hernia sac.

The operation is usually performed shortly after the diagnosis is made. Attempts to reduce an incarcerated hernia using sedation and manual reduction are successful in more than 80% of cases. An elective operation is then carried out within 24 h of the reduction. In the case of hernias in small premature infants already hospitalized in the neonatal intensive care unit because of other illnesses, elective repair is carried out just before discharge. For infants diagnosed after discharge from the hospital who require ventilatory support or experience episodes of apnea and/or bradycardia in the neonatal period, elective repair is usually delayed until 44–60 weeks of corrected conceptional age. Although most infants and children can be managed in an ambulatory setting, infants with bronchopulmonary dysplasia or those who required ventilator support at the time of birth should be observed after surgery in an extended observation (23-h) center and monitored for episodes of apnea and bradycardia.

Preoperative

The operation is usually performed under general anesthesia, although some surgeons prefer spinal anesthesia in very premature infants.

The lower abdomen, inguinal scrotal area, perineum and thighs are prepared with iodophor solution and draped appropriately for herniorrhaphy.

Operation

1 A transverse incision is made in the lowest right inguinal crease above the external inguinal ring. Scarpa's fascia is incised and the external oblique fascia identified. The inguinal ligament is located and traced down to expose the external inguinal ring.

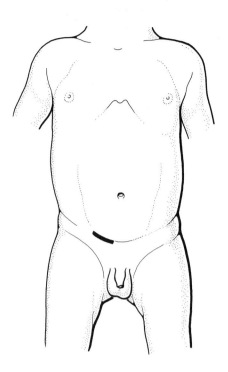

1

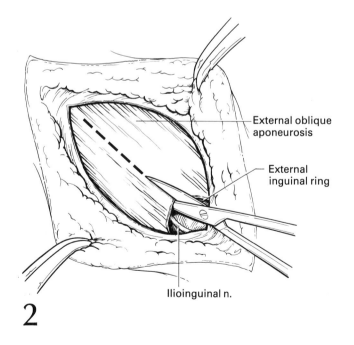

External oblique aponeurosis

External inguinal ring

Ilioinguinal n.

2

2 The external oblique fascia is opened along the axis of its fibers, perpendicular to the external inguinal ring, for 1–2 cm.

3 The spermatic fascia covers the cord structures. The ilioinguinal nerve can be seen on the outer vestment of the fascia. The cremasteric muscle is teased open by blunt dissection on the anteromedial surface of the cord, exposing the glistening hernia sac.

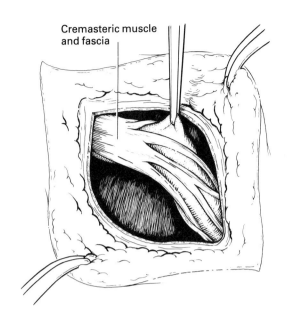

4 The sac is elevated anteromedially and the vas deferens and spermatic vessels are carefully dissected free from the diverticular structure of the inguinal hernia sac. The vas deferens should never be grasped with a forceps or a clamp as this can result in an injury.

The hernia sac often extends to the testicular area. Once the vital structures are identified and mobilized laterally, the sac can be divided between clamps and the upper end dissected superiorly to the level of the internal inguinal ring. The extent of the superior dissection is identified by the presence of retroperitoneal fat at the neck of the sac.

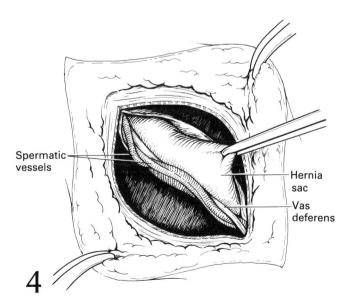

5 The contents of the sac should be reduced and a clamp placed on the sac which is twisted in a clockwise manner to ensure that all of the contents are reduced. A pair of DeBakey forceps is placed at the base of the sac to protect the cord structures. The neck of the sac is transfixed with a 4/0 (in small infants) or 3/0 non-absorbable suture ligature. A free tie should never be used as distension of the abdomen may push the tie off the peritoneum.

The distal end of the hernia sac is opened on its anterior surface. If a separate hydrocele is present, this should be excised at the same time. If the internal ring is excessively large, this can be snugged (made smaller) inferior to the cord vessels with an interrupted 3/0 silk suture. The floor of the canal usually requires no specific therapy and, during the dissection, the surgeon should avoid any injury to the transversalis fascia. High ligation of an infant hernia is usually all that is required. In rare cases where there is an associated direct hernia, this can be repaired by inserting two or three sutures between the conjoined tendon and Poupart's or Cooper's ligament. The testis should be returned to a normal intrascrotal location at the end of the procedure. Administration of a local anesthetic (e.g. bupivacaine) along the ilioinguinal and hypogastric nerves will reduce postoperative pain.

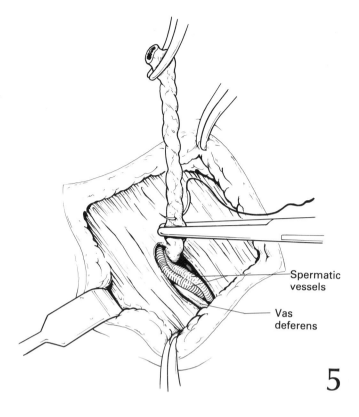

Spermatic vessels

Vas deferens

5

6 Wound closure is accomplished with interrupted 4/0 silk or polyglactin (Vicryl) sutures on the external oblique fascia.

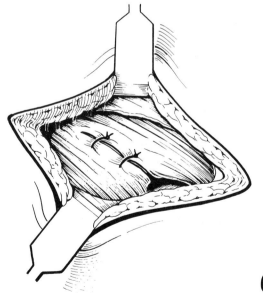

6

7 Scarpa's fascia is closed with one or two interrupted 4/0 polyglactin sutures, burying the knot. The skin edges are opposed with interrupted 4/0 or 5/0 plain gut or polyglactin subcuticular sutures. The skin edges are opposed with a collodion dressing in infants before they are toilet-trained or with sterile skin closure strips (e.g. Steristrips) and a semipermeable adhesive film dressing (e.g. Opsite) in older children.

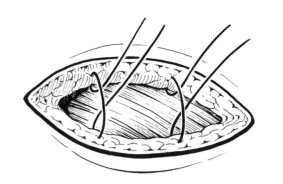

7

The author routinely explores the contralateral side in some cases, particularly those infants younger than 1 year, girls less than 5 years, and in selected patients with a clinically apparent left inguinal hernia. Contralateral exploration is reasonable if the operator is experienced and skilled in performing inguinal hernial repairs in infants, if the anesthetist has considerable expertise in administering anesthesia to young infants, and if the patient has no serious underlying condition that increases the risk of an operation. An operation is always performed first on the side with the clinically obvious hernia.

Postoperative care

With the exception of infants who require extended observation, most patients are discharged from the day surgery room within 2 h after operative repair. Oral intake may be resumed when the child awakens. Tylenol with codeine is used for analgesia for 48 h following the procedure. Baths can be resumed on the third postoperative day. There are no activity restrictions for infants but older children should refrain from bicycle riding or other vigorous physical activity for one month.

Complications

Injury to the spermatic vessels or vas deferens is unusual. If the vas deferens is divided it should be repaired with interrupted 7/0 or 8/0 monofilament sutures. The use of magnifying loupes or an operating microscope will make the repair more precise.

Intraoperative bleeding is also an unusual complication unless the floor of the canal is weakened and requires repair. Needle-hole injury to the epigastric vessels or the femoral vein can usually be controlled by withdrawal of the suture and direct pressure.

Postoperative complications include wound infection, scrotal hematoma, postoperative hydrocele and recurrent inguinal hernia. The wound infection rate at most major pediatric centers is quite low (1–2%). An increased incidence of infection might be expected in incarcerated hernias.

Recurrent inguinal hernia is a relatively uncommon complication in children with recurrence rates of less than 1% having been reported by experienced pediatric surgeons. Of these, 80% are noted within the first postoperative year. The major causes of recurrent inguinal hernia in children include: (1) a missed hernial sac or unrecognized peritoneal tear; (2) a broken suture ligature at the neck of the sac; (3) failure to repair (snug) a large internal inguinal ring; (4) injury to the floor of the inguinal canal, resulting in a direct inguinal hernia; (5) severe infection; (6) increased intra-abdominal pressure; and (7) connective tissue disorders.

Postoperative hydrocele may rarely occur after high ligation of the proximal hernial sac and incomplete excision of the distal portion. To avoid this complication the anterior surface of the distal hernial sac can be split and the anterior and lateral aspects of the sac partially resected. The postoperative hydrocele often resolves spontaneously. Rarely, long-term persistence of the hydrocele may require a formal hydrocelectomy.

Testicular atrophy has been observed after incarcerated hernias and acute tense hydroceles in young infants.

Femoral hernias

Principles and justification

Femoral hernia is the least common hernia occurring in the inguinal region in infants and children. The diagnosis, however, must be considered when examining a swelling in the inguinal region, especially if the bulge or mass presents inferior to the inguinal ligament. Femoral hernia may occasionally be confused with an enlarged swollen infected lymph node near the saphenofemoral junction (lymph node of Cloquet) just inferior to the inguinal ligament. Careful examination for a lower extremity focus of infection should be performed. Femoral hernias are most common in girls of 5–10 years. Occasionally, a femoral hernia may be noted shortly after an ipsilateral inguinal hernia repair. This may represent either a missed femoral hernia or operative damage involving the femoral canal.

Indications

The presence of a femoral hernia is an indication for operation. Conservative management is contraindicated because of the risk of incarceration and strangulation. The fixed margins of the femoral ring result in early compression of swollen tissues and increase the risk of visceral compromise when incarceration occurs.

Choice of procedure

There are three possible approaches for repairing a femoral hernia: (1) the lower infrainguinal ligament procedure of Langenbeck, (2) transinguinal Cooper's ligament repair (McVay procedure), and (3) an abdominal extraperitoneal repair (Cheatle–Henry). Although femoral hernia repair has also been performed using endoscopic techniques through the laparoscope in adults, the author has not used this technique in children. It may have a role in instances of recurrence in older children.

An inguinal or extraperitoneal approach should be used in instances of strangulated obstruction; however, since this is rarely seen in infants and young children, the low infrainguinal repair is preferred. If a concomitant inguinal hernia is present, an inguinal incision and McVay repair is recommended.

Preoperative

In elective cases, the infant or child is kept without oral intake for 4–6 h before the anticipated procedure. An outpatient operation may safely be carried out. Mild sedation is administered preoperatively and general endotracheal anesthesia is employed.

Following appropriate skin cleansing of the lower abdomen, inguinoscrotal (or labial) area, thigh and perineum, sterile drapes are applied.

Operation

The infrainguinal (Langenbeck) repair will be described as the other approaches are dealt with in the section on inguinal hernia.

INFRAINGUINAL (LANGENBECK) REPAIR

8 A transverse incision is made in a skin crease over the mass from a point just inferior to the pubic tubercle medially, extending laterally just past the palpable pulsation of the femoral artery.

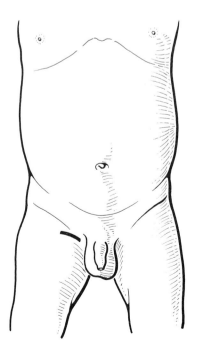

8

9 Hemostasis is effected with an electrocoagulator and the wound is deepened to expose the hernia sac bulge. The sac is covered by cribriform fascia and groin fat and may overlie the femoral vein and extend upwards over the inguinal ligament.

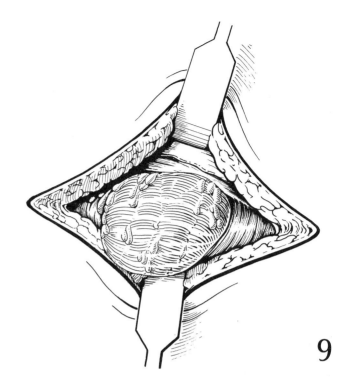

9

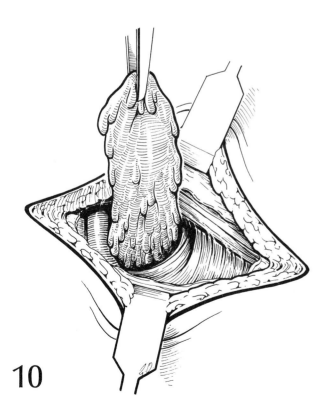

10

10 The cribriform fascia and fat layers are incised, exposing the femoral hernia sac. The sac should be carefully palpated for visceral contents which should be gently reduced through the defect. Occasionally, when incarceration is present and reduction is difficult, a small incision anteriorly in the inguinal ligament will allow safe reduction of the sac contents. The sac is then traced to the ring margins: the lacunar ligament medially, the femoral vein laterally, the inguinal ligament anteriorly, and Cooper's ligament covering the pectineus fascia and pubic ramus posteriorly.

11a, b The peritoneal sac is frequently small; however, it may have a considerable amount of retroperitoneal fatty tissue at its base. The sac can be opened (to ensure reduction of contents) if there is any question of a complete reduction. High ligation of the sac similar to an inguinal hernia is possible when an elongated sac is present. This is accomplished with 3/0 non-absorbable suture ligatures. The sac may be bulky, however, and an alternative method of sac closure is inversion and reduction of the intact sac, placing one or two 3/0 non-absorbable purse-string sutures at a level just above the femoral defect.

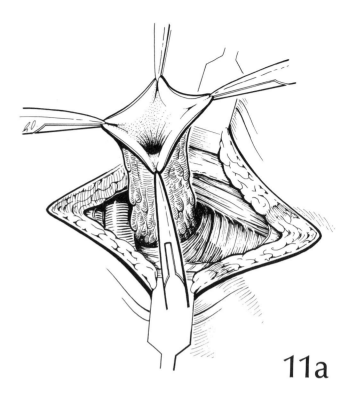

11a

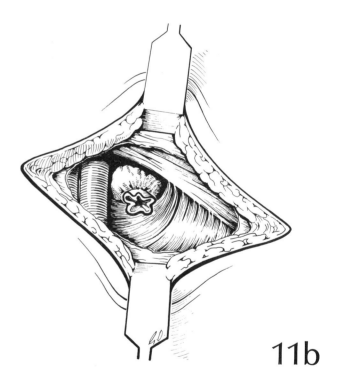

11b

12 Repair of the femoral defect is facilitated by placing a small retractor to raise the inguinal ligament superiorly in order to expose the pectineus fascia and Cooper's ligament. All sutures are placed between Cooper's ligament and the inguinal ligament under direct vision before tying. The author uses interrupted 3/0 non-absorbable material in infants and 2/0 non-absorbable material in older children. Special attention is given to avoid either injury to the femoral vein by the needle or its compression when the sutures are tied. Gentle lateral retraction of the vein during suture insertion is useful.

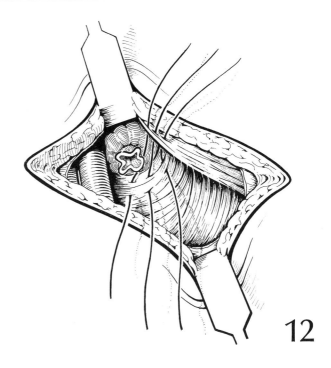

13 Wound closure is accomplished with a few interrupted inverting 4/0 absorbable polyglactin (Vicryl) sutures, burying the knots. The wound edges are approximated with 5/0 subcuticular absorbable suture material and the wound sealed with Steristrips and a semipermeable adhesive film dressing (e.g. Opsite) in children or with collodion in infants who are not toilet-trained.

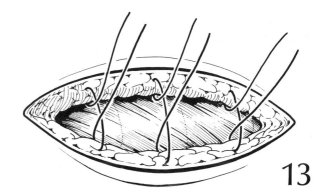

Postoperative care

Oral intake may be resumed when the infant is alert. Acetaminophen (paracetamol) with codeine may be used for pain control for 24–48 h. Most young children return to normal activity within a few days. In older children or teenagers, avoidance of competitive athletics and bicycle riding is advised for 30 days.

Complications

In most cases recovery from elective femoral hernia repair is uncomplicated. A superficial wound infection may develop in 1% of cases and should be recognized promptly and drained early to avoid possible extension of a closed infection to the deeper tissues. A wound hematoma is rarely observed and may be caused by an unrecognized tear in a saphenous/femoral venous branch.

Pain and ipsilateral leg swelling may be the result of compression of the iliac or femoral vein.

Since femoral hernia is relatively rare in children, data concerning recurrence are not available. A recurrence rate of 1–2% in children might be expected.

Umbilical hernia

Principles and justification

An umbilical hernia is a common occurrence in infants and young children. The hernia sac protrudes through a defect in the umbilical ring due to a failure of complete obliteration at the site where the fetal umbilical vessels (umbilical vein and the two umbilical arteries) are joined to the placenta during gestation.

Approximately 20% of full-term neonates may have an incomplete closure of the umbilical ring at birth. However, 75–80% of premature infants weighing between 1.0 kg and 1.5 kg may show evidence of an umbilical hernia at birth. Umbilical hernia is more common in girls than boys. Black children have a higher incidence than white children.

The umbilical bulge becomes more apparent during episodes of crying, straining, or even during defecation, and may result in considerable protrusion of the sac and, at times, visceral content through the ring. The hernial protrusion is composed of peritoneum adherent to the undersurface of the umbilical skin. The hernia often causes considerable parental anxiety and frequent requests for operative repair in early infancy.

Although rupture or incarceration of an umbilical hernia occurs, this is an exceptionally rare event in the author's experience (three cases during the past 22 years). The hernia is rarely a cause of pain or other symptoms. Almost 80% of umbilical hernias will decrease in size and close spontaneously by 5–6 years of age. Careful counseling will usually allay unnecessary parental anxiety and fear.

Indications

As the majority of these very low-risk hernias will close spontaneously, it is safe to wait until the child is 5 years of age (particularly if the umbilical ring is less than 1.5 cm in diameter) before attempting repair. In contrast, defects of more than 2.0 cm diameter rarely close spontaneously. Since there is a significant risk of complications including incarceration and strangulation in adults with umbilical hernia, those hernia defects that do not close by 5 years of age should be electively repaired. The umbilical defect can also be repaired in children under 5 years of age with a ring of more than 2.0 cm in whom a general anesthetic is anticipated for another condition (including repair of an inguinal hernia).

Preoperative

The child is kept without oral intake for 6 h before the anticipated time of the procedure. The operation can safely be carried out on an outpatient basis.

Careful preparation of the skin is essential as the umbilicus is often a repository of surface debris, lint, etc. and is not always kept immaculate. Preoperative cleansing with cotton applicator sticks may be useful.

Anesthesia

After administration of mild preoperative sedation, the procedure is carried out under general endotracheal anesthesia.

Operation

14 After appropriate skin preparation and application of sterile linen drapes, a curved ('smile') incision is made in a natural skin crease immediately below the umbilicus. A supraumbilical incision is also acceptable, especially if a supraumbilical defect is encountered. Placement of four-quadrant traction by the assistant on the abdominal wall and slight upward traction of the defect allows selection of the site of the incision. The curved incision should not extend beyond 180°.

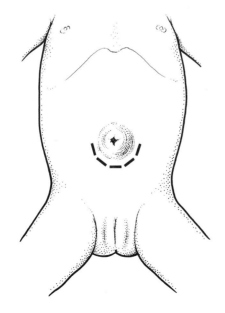

14

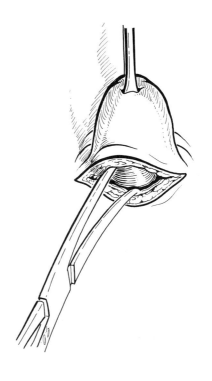

15a

15a, b The subcutaneous tissue is incised and bleeding points controlled with a fine tip electrocoagulator. With upward traction on the inner margin of the upper lip of the incision, dissection is carried out down along the sac to the level of the anterior abdominal wall fascia. By blunt dissection with a mosquito clamp a plane is developed on either side of the sac, extending superiorly to gain control of the entire circumference of the sac. Any contents in the sac should be reduced into the peritoneal cavity. If the sac is large, the surgeon or assistant places an index finger in the skin defect to evert the sac where it is attached to the skin. The sac is dissected free from its skin attachments, preserving the umbilical skin for an umbilicoplasty. Bleeding points are controlled with an electrocoagulator. Separation of the sac may require its transection near the skin to preserve the umbilicus for cosmetic purposes.

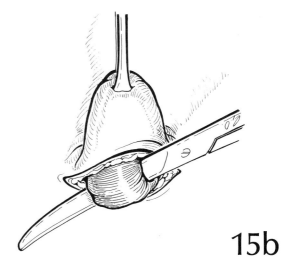

15b

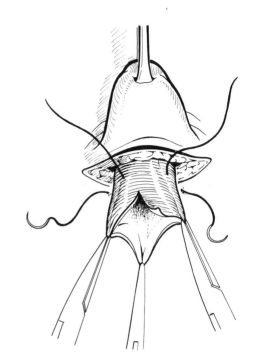

16a

16a, b

The entire sac is elevated by mosquito clamps to maintain control of the edge of the defect and to have direct visualization during placement of sutures to avoid visceral injury. The sac is opened and any contents reduced. The rim of the defect is identified and the sac incised to allow placement of sutures starting at the corner farthest from the surgeon. Interrupted 3/0 (infants and young children) or 2/0 (older children and teenagers) non-absorbable sutures are placed but not initially tied. The sutures are elevated to maintain upward traction on the abdominal wall. The sac is partially excised at the level of the abdominal wall as more sutures are placed. A traction suture is also placed at the corner of the transverse wound closest to the operating surgeon, and the remaining sac is excised. All of the sutures are then tied. If a lot of redundant tissue is present or the initial tissue layer seems sparse, a layer of fascia can be imbricated over the initial line of repair with interrupted non-absorbable sutures.

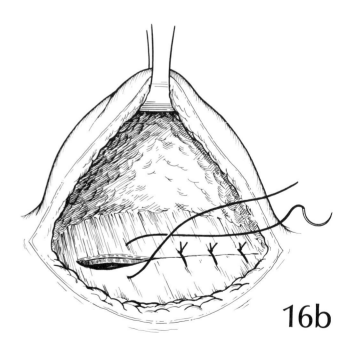

16b

17a, b An umbilicoplasty is performed for cosmetic purposes by inverting the undersurface of the redundant umbilical skin to the anterior abdominal wall fascia with one or two interrupted 4/0 absorbable sutures. Any remnant of the peritoneum on the umbilical sac that is adherent to the skin may be safely left behind.

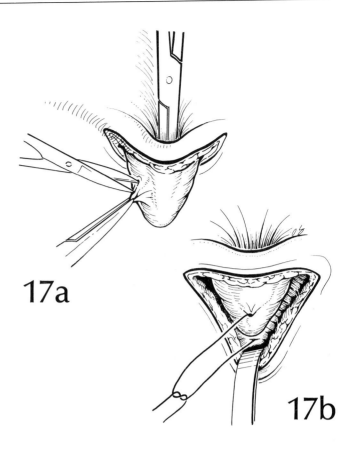

17a

17b

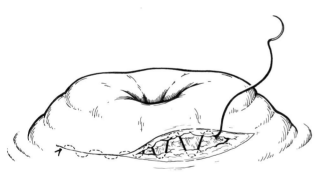

18

18 The wound is closed by a few interrupted inverted 4/0 polyglactin sutures in the subcutaneous fascia. The skin edges are opposed with a collodion dressing. No skin sutures are placed. When the collodion dries, a pressure dressing is applied to obliterate any dead space and prevent hematoma formation.

Postoperative care

Oral fluids can be offered when the infant is alert. Acetaminophen with codeine may be used for pain control for 24–48 h. Postoperative activity restrictions are the same as for inguinal hernia repair.

Complications

Complications are unusual and are limited to a wound infection (1%) or an occasional wound hematoma. Recurrence is rare, the only recurrence observed by the author being in a child with renal failure on long-term continuous ambulatory peritoneal dialysis.

Supraumbilical and epigastric hernias

Principles and justification

A number of defects may be observed along the linea alba between the xiphoid process and the umbilicus. Failure of fixation of the medial borders of the rectus abdominis muscles at the linea alba results in a large, bulging defect – a diastasis recti – which is virtually of no consequence and resolves spontaneously as the linea alba becomes a firm structure.

Epigastric hernias usually occur in the mid-epigastrium. The actual defect may be small; however, it is often symptomatic. Fat from the falciform ligament or the omentum can incarcerate and cause pain. In some cases a tender mass of incarcerated fatty tissue can be palpated in the defect. Since epigastric hernias do not spontaneously close and are often symptomatic, they should be repaired. As the hernial defect may be small, it is wise to mark the skin over the exact site before surgery with the child awake in a standing position.

Preoperative

Repair can be performed on an outpatient basis. General anesthesia is required. The abdomen is prepared with an iodophor solution and draped appropriately.

Operation

19 A transverse incision is made directly over the premarked area identifying the site of the hernia defect.

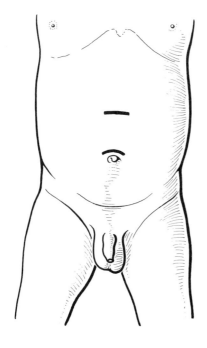

19

20a, b Hemostasis is effected with an electro-coagulator. There is often no peritoneal sac identified in instances of epigastric hernia. A fatty mass protruding through the defect in the linea alba is observed and may be suture ligated and excised *or* inverted and reduced into the peritoneal cavity.

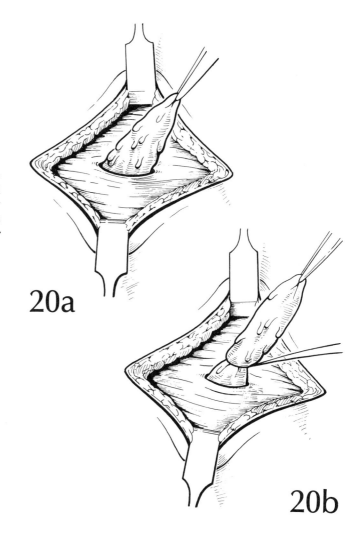

20a

20b

21a

21b

21a, b The small defect is repaired with interrupted 3/0 non-absorbable sutures. Wound closure is accomplished with subcuticular sutures of 5/0 polyglactin and either Steristrips or a collodion dressing.

Postoperative care

Postoperative care is similar to that described for umbilical hernias.

Further reading

Askar OM. Aponeurotic hernias: recent observations upon paraumbilical and epigastric hernias. *Surg Clin North Am* 1984; 64: 315–33.

Blumberg NA. Infantile umbilical hernia. *Surg Gynecol Obstet* 1980; 150: 187–92.

Brandt CP, Gauderer MWL. Umbilical hernia in infants and children. In: Grosfeld JL, ed. *Common Problems in Pediatric Surgery*. Chicago: Year Book Publishers, 1991: 36–59.

Fonkalsrud EW, de Lorimer AA, Clatworthy HW. Femoral and direct inguinal hernias in infants and children. *JAMA* 1965; 192: 597–9.

Grosfeld JL. Current concepts in inguinal hernia in infants and children. *World J Surg* 1989; 13: 506–15.

Grosfeld JL. Groin hernia in infants and children. In: Nyhus LM, Condon RE, eds. *Hernia*. 3rd edn. Philadelphia: JP Lippincott, 1989; 81–98.

Grosfeld JL. Inguinal hernia in the premature neonate, In: Grosfeld JL, ed. *Common Problems in Pediatric Surgery*. Chicago: Year Book Publishers, 1991: 3–8.

Grosfeld JL, Minnick K, Shedd F, West KW, Rescorla FJ, Vane DW. Inguinal hernia in children: factors affecting recurrence in 62 cases. *J Pediatr Surg* 1991; 26: 283–7.

Lassaletta L, Fonkalsrud EW, Tovar JA *et al.* The management of umbilical hernias in infancy and childhood. *J Pediatr Surg* 1975; 10: 405–9.

Melone JH, Schwartz MZ, Tyson KR *et al.* Outpatient inguinal herniorrhaphy in premature infants: is it safe? *J Pediatr Surg* 1992; 27: 203–8.

Neblett WW III, Holcomb GW III. Umbilical and other abdominal wall hernias. In Ashcraft KW, Holder TM, eds. *Pediatric Surgery*, 2nd edn. Philadelphia: WB Saunders, 1993: 557–61.

Scherer LR, Grosfeld JL. Inguinal hernia and umbilical anomalies. *Pediatr Clin North Am* 1993; 40: 1121–31.

Skinner MA, Grosfeld JL. Inguinal and umbilical hernia repair in infants and children. *Surg Clin North Am* 1993; 73: 439–49.

Surana R, Puri P. Is contralateral exploration necessary in infants with unilateral inguinal hernia? *J Pediatr Surg* 1993; 28: 1026–7.

Illustrations by Gillian Oliver

Omphalocele/exomphalos

Thomas R. Weber MD
Professor of Pediatric Surgery, St Louis University and Director, Department of Pediatric Surgery, Cardinal Glennon Children's Hospital, St Louis, Missouri, USA

History

Ambrose Paré, the famous French surgeon, first described an infant with omphalocele in 1634, while gastroschisis was first described by Calder in 1733[1]. Although small omphaloceles were subsequently successfully repaired, there were few reported survivors of larger abdominal wall defects until the 1940s when Gross described a two-stage closure of an omphalocele using skin flaps followed by ventral hernia repair. Further advancement in the treatment of massive omphalocele and irreducible gastroschisis defects occurred when Schuster devised an extracoelomic 'pouch' to temporarily house eviscerated bowel[2]. This was later modified by Allen and Wrenn who devised the additional innovation of staged reduction of abdominal contents to allow gradual enlargement of the abdominal cavity[3]. The development of total parenteral nutrition in the 1960s allowed vigorous nutritional support of infants with gastroschisis, in whom a period of 1–3 weeks of intestinal dysfunction is expected after the operation. The basic principles of occasional non-operative therapy, primary closure when possible, and staged reduction with a temporary Silastic pouch, remain the mainstays of contemporary therapy for these common congenital defects.

Embryology

Although controversy continues regarding the similarities, relationships and embryological events surrounding omphalocele and gastroschisis, it is probably most reasonable to consider these as separate entities. Omphalocele is basically a persistence of the body stalk in the midline, where somatopleure normally develops. Failure of return of the normally herniated midgut at the 12th fetal week either causes or aggravates the condition. Unless ruptured, omphaloceles are covered with a sac consisting of inner peritoneum and outer amnion. Infants with omphalocele frequently have associated anomalies (cardiac, renal), chromosome abnormalities (trisomy 13–15, 16–18), or recognizable syndrome associations (Beckwith–Wiedemann, Cantrell's pentalogy).

A gastroschisis defect is a full-thickness hole in the abdominal wall, usually to the right of the umbilical cord. A bridge of skin frequently separates the defect from the cord. The defect is probably a result of involution of the right umbilical vein producing a weakened area of abdominal wall, or a rupture of paraumbilical somatopleure[4]. There is no sac covering a gastroschisis, and virtually no association with anomalies, chromosome abnormalities, or syndromes.

Principles and justification

Omphalocele

Because of the possibility of serious, life-threatening or even lethal associated anomalies, infants with omphalocele are occasionally treated non-operatively. Painting the sac with agents designed to induce eschar formation, followed by gradual epithelialization from the base of the defect upwards, will eventually produce a covered ventral hernia. Early use of alcohol, iodine and mercury-containing compounds produced toxicity due to systemic absorption of these compounds, and these therefore have been largely replaced by silver nitrate solution or silver sulfadiazine cream. Such non-operative treatment is never appropriate management in infants with gastroschisis.

The operative treatment of choice for small to medium sized omphaloceles is excision of the sac, with primary closure of fascia and skin. If fascia closure increases intra-abdominal pressure sufficiently to cause respiratory embarrassment, skin closure alone, with later repair of the ventral hernia, is advisable. For giant omphaloceles, frequently containing liver as well as bowel, attaching a Silastic 'pouch' to the fascia allows gradual (10–14 days) reduction of the contents into the abdominal cavity, with eventual skin flap closure. Occasionally a prosthetic patch is needed to close the fascial defect in this setting, but skin must be mobilized sufficiently to cover the prosthesis.

Gastroschisis

The surgical choices for gastroschisis are considerably more straightforward. Since the eviscerated bowel is uncovered, non-operative treatment is not an option. The majority of gastroschisis defects can be closed primarily, after reduction of the edematous, matted gut is accomplished. 'Milking' intestinal contents proximally or distally may allow easier reduction, but the bowel must be handled gently during this maneuver. The presence of necrosis or atresia in the herniated bowel usually requires the construction of an ostomy at the time of repair, as anastomosis of the very edematous gut is difficult and is associated with a significant failure rate. Large, irreducible gastroschises are generally treated with a Silastic pouch, which allows resolution of much of the bowel edema and gradual reduction of the gut into the enlarging abdominal cavity.

Preoperative

Assessment and preparation

Newborn infants with either omphalocele or gastroschisis must be placed immediately in a warm, aseptic environment to prevent evaporative fluid loss, hypothermia and infection. Warm soaked sterile gauze can be placed on the defect, covered by transparent plastic wrap. Alternatively a transparent plastic drawstring 'bowel bag' may be used which can be kept sterile in the delivery room. The lower two-thirds (to the axillae) of the neonate can be placed within the bag.

Intravenous access must be established soon after birth to replace evaporative fluid loss and administer broad-spectrum antibiotics. Placement of the intravenous line above the diaphragm is preferable, because of the possibility of inferior cava compression and partial obstruction as the eviscerated bowel and/or liver are reduced. An oral gastric or nasogastric tube should be placed to prevent gastric distension. Preoperative endotracheal intubation is reserved for premature infants or those with significant respiratory distress. All infants with omphalocele should undergo complete cardiac and renal evaluation before they are subjected to operative repair[5].

Anesthesia

General, endotracheal anesthesia with complete muscle paralysis is recommended for all infants with either omphalocele or gastroschisis. As stated above, infants with omphalocele who have serious or life-threatening associated anomalies, especially cardiac, should probably be treated non-operatively with application of escharotic agents to the sac.

Operations

SMALL TO MODERATE SIZED OMPHALOCELE

1 A small ('hernia into cord') or moderate omphalocele, which may contain a small portion of liver, has the umbilical cord inserted into the top of the sac.

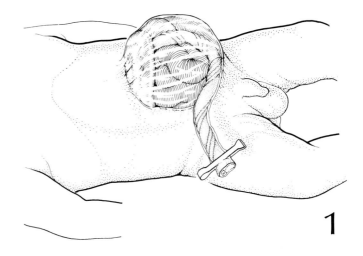

1

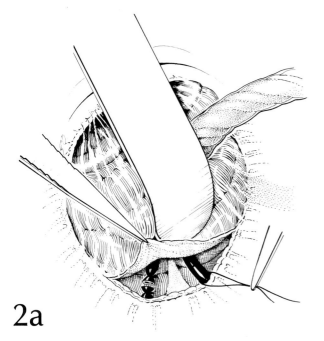

2a

2a, b Although some surgeons advocate leaving the sac intact and repairing the fascia and skin over it, most surgeons favor excision of the sac to allow complete intra-abdominal exploration. The sac is sharply removed at the skin/fascia edge, with careful identification and ligation of the umbilical vessels.

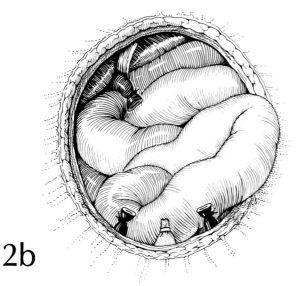

2b

3 The abdominal cavity can be enlarged by manual stretching.

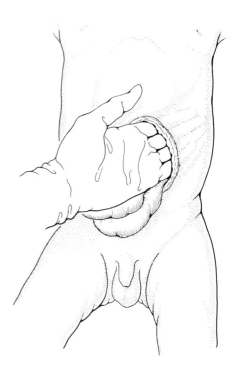

3

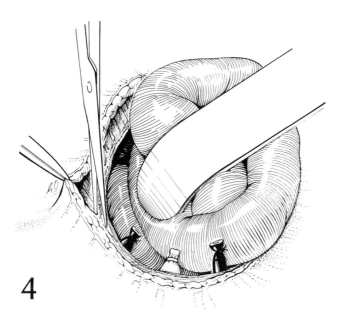

4

4 The skin is carefully 'undermined', separating it from the deep fascia layers.

5 The fascia is closed with running or interrupted absorbable sutures (polyglactin or polydioxanone) and the umbilicus reconstructed.

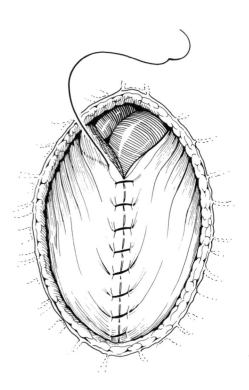

5

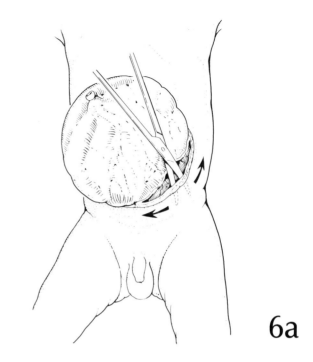

6a

LARGE OMPHALOCELE: STAGED REPAIR

6a–c Large omphaloceles, frequently containing most of the liver, are usually not fully reducible at the first operation and staged repair is necessary. After undermining the skin, the skin is closed over the abdominal viscera, producing a ventral hernia that can be repaired 6–12 months later.

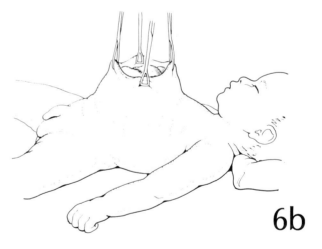

6b

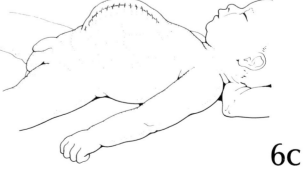

6c

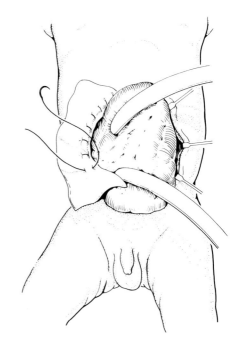

7a

7a, b An alternative approach utilizes prosthetic closure of the fascia defect over polyethylene or Silastic sheeting to prevent adhesion of the viscera to the prosthetic material. The skin is closed over the fascia prosthesis.

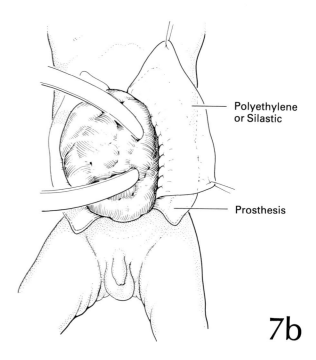

Polyethylene
or Silastic

Prosthesis

7b

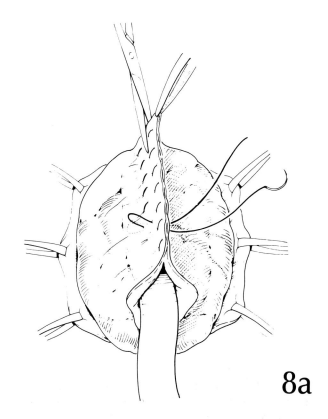

8a

8a, b At 2–4 week intervals the wound can be reopened and the skin dissected from the prosthesis. The central portion of the prosthesis and sheeting are resected and resutured to pull the fascia together. Eventually the fascia can be closed without the prosthesis.

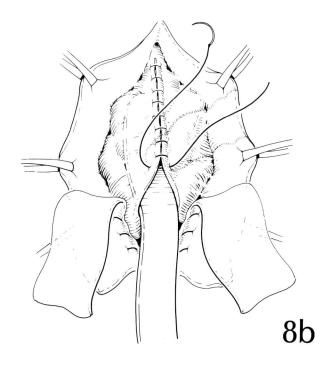

8b

GASTROSCHISIS

9 The eviscerated bowel in a gastroschisis defect is usually thickened, foreshortened, edematous and distended with intraluminal contents. If the gut can be reduced primarily without undue respiratory compression or inferior vena cava compression, then primary closure of the fascia and skin (as shown in *Illustration 5*) is the preferred treatment.

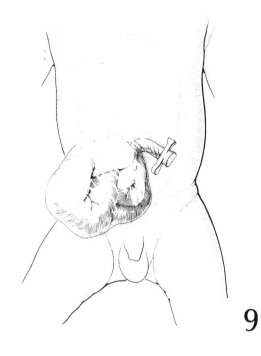

9

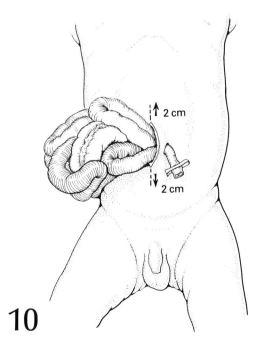

10

10 In instances where the gut cannot be reduced primarily, the use of a Silastic pouch is an excellent alternative. The incision is enlarged 1–2 cm superiorly and inferiorly.

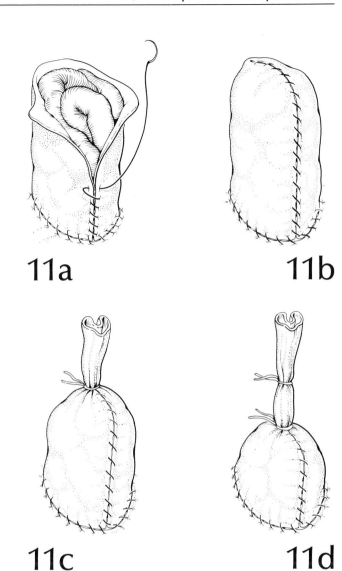

11a

11b

11c

11d

11a–d A Dacron reinforced Silastic sheet is attached to the abdominal wall with a running non-absorbable suture, and fashioned into a pouch using the same suture.

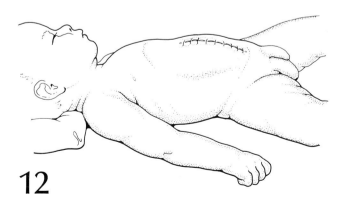

12

12 The viscera are gradually reduced into the abdominal cavity using gentle squeezing pressure on the top of the pouch, which is then occluded by umbilical tape tie or suture to maintain reduction. This is usualiy performed without anesthesia every other day over a 7–10 day period, until the gut is fully reduced.

The infant is then returned to the operating room for removal of the pouch and fascia and skin closure. In cases of associated bowel atresia ostomy can be formed, if necessary, at the time of complete closure.

Postoperative care

All infants should be maintained on systemic antibiotics for 5–7 days or until the prostheses are removed. Intravenous nutrition should be initiated as soon as possible, and continued until bowel function returns. In infants with omphalocele this may be a period of several days, while infants with gastroschisis typically take 2–3 weeks or longer before they are able to tolerate oral feeding. Aggressive ventilator management is a mainstay of therapy in these infants.

Respiratory compromise is common after primary repair, or during staged reduction of either omphalocele or gastroschisis, and the use of endotracheal intubation, ventilators, sedation and, occasionally, muscle relaxants are common interventions in these infants in the early postoperative period.

Outcome

The outcome in these infants depends on the presence and degree of prematurity, associated anomalies and, especially in the case of gastroschisis, the loss of bowel length due to atresia or gut infarction from mesenteric vascular compromise.

Neonates with omphalocele have a high (50–60%) incidence of associated anomalies and chromosome abnormalities which precludes long-term survival in 20–30% of cases. Severe cardiac defects are particularly troublesome in these infants. The survival for babies with gastroschisis, on the other hand, exceeds 90% in most series, even when intestinal atresia or gut infarction is present and multiple operative procedures are necessary[6]. Modern neonatal intensive care and intravenous nutrition have undoubtedly been responsible for the continued improvement in survival for these critically ill infants.

References

1. Grosfeld JL, Weber TR. Congenital abdominal wall defects: gastroschisis and omphalocele. *Curr Probl Surg* 1982; 19: 159–213.

2. Schuster SR. A new method for the staged repair of large omphaloceles. *Surg Gynecol Obstet* 1967; 125: 837–50.

3. Allen RG, Wrenn EL. Silon as a sac in the treatment of omphalocele and gastroschisis. *J Pediatr Surg* 1969; 4: 3–8.

4. deVries PA. The pathogenesis of gastroschisis and omphalocele. *J Pediatr Surg* 1980; 15: 245–51.

5. Knight PJ, Buckner D, Vassy LE. Omphalocele: treatment options. *Surgery* 1981; 89: 332–6.

6. Grosfeld JL, Dawes L, Weber TR. Congenital abdominal wall defects: current management and survival. *Surg Clin North Am* 1981; 61: 1037–49.

Gastroschisis

Marshall Z. Schwartz MD

Chairman, Department of Surgery, Surgeon-in-Chief, Children's National Medical Center, Professor of Surgery and Pediatrics, George Washington University School of Medicine, Washington DC, USA

Principles and justification

1 Gastroschisis is an anterior abdominal wall defect that occurs *in utero* and through which there is herniation of intra-abdominal viscera into the amniotic sac. The embryologic cause for this abdominal wall defect is controversial[1]. It has been postulated that gastroschisis is an *in utero* rupture of an omphalocele or hernia of the umbilical cord.

Most infants with gastroschisis are born prematurely (35–37 weeks' gestation) weighing 2000–2500 g. The defect is almost always to the right of the umbilicus and generally measures 2–3 cm in diameter. All or a portion of the midgut is usually herniated through the defect. In addition, the stomach, urinary bladder and, in females, the fallopian tubes and ovaries may also be extra-coelomic.

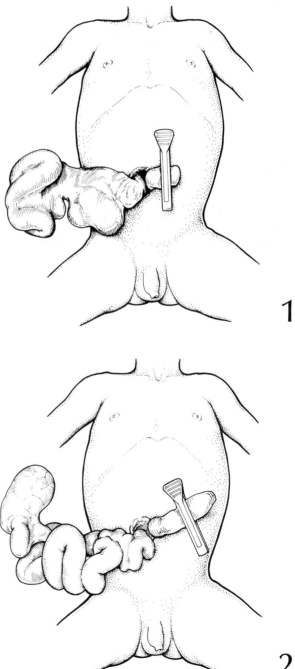

2 The intestine is foreshortened, edematous and generally has a fibrin coating. Atresia of the small and large intestine is more frequent (approximately 14%) than in patients with omphalocele (1%). The most striking difference between omphalocele and gastroschisis is the absence of a sac or membrane covering the herniated contents in gastroschisis. Continuous contact of the herniated contents with amniotic fluid has been proposed as the reason for the thickened, foreshortened and edematous bowel. There is also increasing evidence that the fascial defect begins to decrease in diameter near the end of the third trimester which could lead to venous congestion of the midgut and contribute to the abnormal appearance of the bowel.

Preoperative

Gastroschisis requires prompt surgical intervention. Delays in surgical management should only be incurred as a result of transport of the infant to a pediatric surgical center or the need for prolonged preoperative stabilization. Other life threatening anomalies, which are rare, may delay surgery to allow for evaluation. Appropriate preoperative preparation is essential to ensure a good outcome.

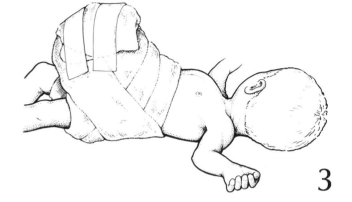

3 Maintenance of the infant's temperature within the normal range is critical. Heat loss can be reduced by using a damp roll of gauze wrapped around the herniated contents followed by one or two dry gauze rolls wrapped around the patient's abdomen. The rolls of gauze help to stabilize the bowel and, therefore, diminish the risk of compromising its blood supply at the fascial ring. Thin plastic wrap has also been used to maintain temperature and diminish evaporative fluid loss. The infant should be in a warming isolette or under an overhead radiant warmer to help maintain normothermia.

Most infants with gastroschisis are dehydrated at birth and require at least 125% of normal maintenance fluids to regain normovolemia[2]. It is appropriate to give broad-spectrum antibiotics during the perioperative period because of exposure of the bowel and peritoneal cavity to bacterial contamination. A nasogastric tube is necessary for gastrointestinal decompression because of the bowel inflammation and resulting ileus.

Thus, before surgery, the infant with gastroschisis should be normothermic and hemodynamically stable following adequate fluid resuscitation.

Anesthesia

General anesthesia is required for appropriate operative management of gastroschisis. The choice of anesthetic agents should be made by the anesthetist but two points should be emphasized: first, muscle paralysis is useful in optimizing the chances for complete reduction of the herniated bowel and primary abdominal wall closure, and second, nitrous oxide should not be used as it would diffuse into the lumen of the bowel causing distension and compromising the likely success of primary abdominal wall repair.

Operation

The operation should be performed under an overhead radiant warmer. Alternatively, warming lights, a safe warming blanket or increasing the temperature of the operating room should be used to maintain the infant's temperature in the normal range during the procedure. After induction of general anesthesia, the dressing previously placed over the herniated contents should be removed. The bowel should be handled with sterile gloves. The umbilical cord, which has usually been left long, should be clamped 2–3 cm above the abdominal wall and the excess cord then removed. Holding the bowel and clamp on the umbilical cord in one hand, the bowel should be prepared using gauze sponges soaked in a 50:50 mixture of povidone-iodine solution and saline. The antiseptic solution should be warm to the touch in an effort to minimize heat loss. After gently washing the bowel and the anterior and lateral abdominal wall, drapes are appropriately placed and the herniated contents are laid on the drapes. The surgeon should then scrub and put on gown and gloves. Next the herniated intestine should be carefully inspected for areas of perforation or sites of atresia, although no effort should be made to dissect matted loops of intestine.

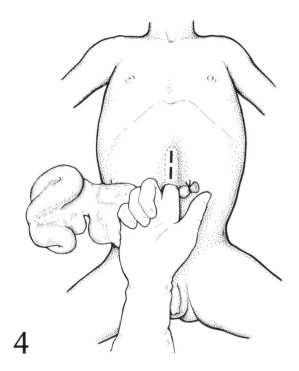

4

4 It is almost always necessary to extend the abdominal wall defect to facilitate reduction of the herniated bowel. This is generally done by extending the defect superiorly in the midline by 2–4 cm, the length of this incision depending on the size of the original defect and the bulkiness of the herniated bowel.

The herniated intestine is reduced into the peritoneal cavity as much as possible, distributing the bowel to all quadrants of the peritoneal cavity. Two techniques have been described to facilitate complete bowel reduction and abdominal wall closure: (1) stretching of the anterior abdominal wall and (2) 'milking' the intestinal contents into the stomach where they can be aspirated through the nasogastric tube. Although gentle stretching of the anterior abdominal wall can be useful, the author is opposed to vigorous stretching because this can lead to rectus muscle hemorrhage and abdominal wall edema after the operation, resulting in ventilation difficulties and wound-related problems. Neither does the author advocate manipulating the intestine to 'milk' the intestinal contents into the stomach, believing that this can cause further damage to the bowel wall resulting in increased bowel wall thickening and additional delay in bowel recovery.

5 After reduction of the herniated intestine, the abdominal wall is assessed for primary closure; if it can be closed without undue tension, 3/0 absorbable, monofilament sutures are used. These sutures are placed in a figure-of-eight fashion, allowing the suture to 'stretch' without breaking or pulling through the tissue. When all the sutures have been placed, they are tied in sequence with a thin malleable retractor initially underneath the fascia to prevent a loop of intestine from becoming entrapped in the closure.

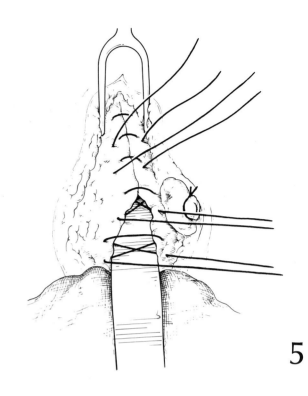

5

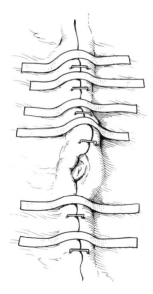

6

6 When the fascia has been closed, the skin edges are approximated using a few skin staples and sufficient sterile skin closure strips, allowing distribution of skin tension over a wider surface area thus creating less likelihood of skin disruption.

About 60–70% of infants with gastroschisis can be operatively treated in this way without creating undue intra-abdominal pressure or tension in the abdominal wall closure. Defining when primary abdominal wall closure will result in excessive intra-abdominal pressure, and thus risk of bowel infarction or difficulty with ventilation, can be very difficult. Some pediatric surgeons have found it useful to measure intra-abdominal pressure using an intragastric or intravesical pressure-sensing catheter[3].

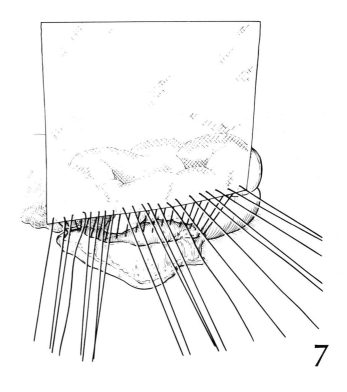

7 For patients in whom complete reduction of the herniated bowel and abdominal wall closure are not possible or appropriate, the staged reduction technique described by Schuster in 1967 has proved to be very useful[4]. Reinforced Silastic sheeting (0.8–1.0 mm thick) is sutured to the fascial edges. This is accomplished with interrupted 3/0 silk mattress sutures.

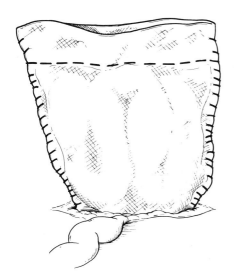

8 The cephalad and caudad edges of the Silastic sac are constructed with running 3/0 monofilament sutures. Before closing the top of the Silastic sac, as much of the bowel as possible is reduced into the peritoneal cavity by manual compression within the sac while avoiding excessive intra-abdominal pressure. The top of the sac is oversewn with a 3/0 monofilament suture placed in a running horizontal mattress fashion.

The Silastic sac is covered with povidone-iodine ointment followed by dry roll gauze to act as a protective dressing and provide support to the Silastic sac at the fascial level.

Postoperative care

Most patients with gastroschisis require parenteral nutrition via a cuffed Silastic central venous catheter for 2–6 weeks after the operation while awaiting the return of function of their intestinal tract. Appropriate energy and nutrition for normal growth and development should be provided. Nasogastric decompression is necessary until there is evidence of bowel function. Broad-spectrum antibiotics are generally continued for a minimum of 5 days. Those infants who undergo the staged approach require a longer period of antibiotic treatment (usually until 1–2 days after the sac has been removed).

9 The staged reduction technique requires daily reduction of the herniated intestine within the Silastic sac. The target for completely reducing the bowel, removing the Silastic sac and closing the abdominal wall is by 1 week of age. Any delay substantially increases the risk of fascial infection, tearing away of the Silastic sheeting from the anterior abdominal wall and failure of the technique. Daily reduction of the intestinal contents within the sac can be accomplished in the neonatal intensive care unit using sterile technique and sedation. Each time the procedure is performed the sac and anterior abdominal wall are prepared with warm povidone-iodine solution before the reduction and povidone-iodine ointment is applied followed by roll gauze after the procedure. General anesthesia is not necessary.

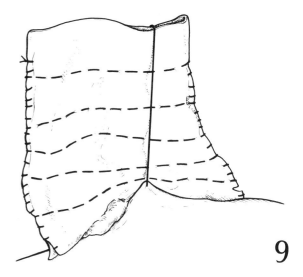

9

When the herniated bowel has been successfully reduced into the peritoneal cavity and the fascial edges brought to within 1 cm of each other the patient is ready for removal of the sac and primary abdominal wall closure in the operating room under general anesthesia.

Once there is evidence of gastrointestinal function, enteral feeding can be introduced and gradually progressed to a low-residue elemental type formula with appropriate enteral caloric intake.

Complications

10a, b Complications in infants with gastroschisis are generally related to the gastrointestinal tract or the abdominal wall closure. As noted earlier, *in utero* complications from intestinal atresia or perforation can occur. Intestinal perforation can be managed in one of several ways, depending on the specific circumstances. The options at the time of birth include suture closure, resection of the site of perforation with oversewing of the two ends of the bowel (i.e. creating 'intestinal atresia'), or creation of a stoma if primary abdominal wall closure can be accomplished.

It is generally not recommended to attempt a bowel anastomosis because of the marked thickening and inflammation of the intestinal wall. Intestinal atresia can be managed by creation of a stoma if primary abdominal wall closure is possible or leaving the atresia *in situ* if staged reduction is undertaken. A stoma can be created at the time of removal of the Silastic sac and primary wall closure. A devastating complication can be partial or complete necrosis of the midgut as a result of excessive intra-abdominal pressure or kinking of the blood supply to the bowel at the time of reduction of the herniated bowel. This complication may lead to the death of the patient or to short bowel syndrome. Additional complications associated with the abdominal wall closure are wound dehiscence and bowel fistula formation. These complications are also often associated with excessive intra-abdominal pressure. It is preferable to use the staged reduction approach when primary abdominal wall closure might result in excessive intra-abdominal pressure.

Outcome

Availability of neonatal intensive care units, parenteral nutrition, and the technique of staged reduction have resulted in significant improvement in the outcome for infants with gastroschisis over the past two decades. Survival of infants with gastroschisis has exceeded 90%[5]. Morbidity should be relatively low if attention to the details of the surgical correction are followed. In the author's experience, infants successfully treated for gastroschisis do not have significant complications during later infancy and childhood.

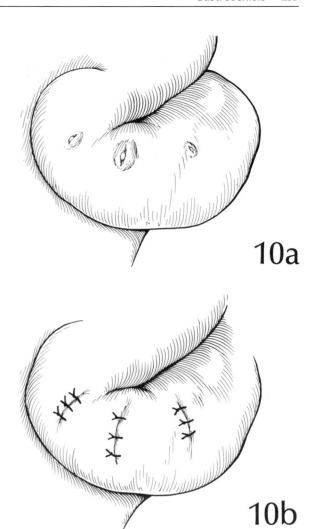

10a

10b

References

1. Schuster SR. Omphalocele and gastroschisis. In: Welch KJ, Randolph JG, Ravitch MM, O'Neill JA Jr, Rowe MI, eds. *Pediatric Surgery*, 4th edn. Chicago: Year Book Publishers, 1986, 740–63.

2. Mollitt DL, Ballantine TV, Grosfeld JL, Quinter P. A critical assessment of fluid requirements in gastroschisis. *J Pediatr Surg* 1978; 13: 217–19.

3. Wesley JR, Drongowski R, Coran AG. Intragastric pressure measurement: a guide for reduction and closure of the Silastic chimney in omphalocele and gastroschisis. *J Pediatr Surg* 1981; 16: 264–70.

4. Schuster SR. A new method for the staged repair of large omphaloceles. *Surg Gynecol Obstet* 1967; 125: 837–50.

5. Schwartz MZ, Tyson KR, Milliorn K, Lobe TE. Staged reduction using a Silastic sac is the treatment of choice for large congenital abdominal wall defects. *J Pediatr Surg* 1983; 18: 713–9.

Illustrations by Marks Creative Consultants

Abdominal surgery: general principles of access

David A. Lloyd MChir, FRCS, FACS, FCS(SA)
Professor of Paediatric Surgery, University of Liverpool, and Consultant Paediatric Surgeon, Alder Hey Children's Hospital, Liverpool, UK

Principles and justification

Anatomic considerations

1a, b There are important anatomic differences between the abdomen of the neonate and that of the older child or adult. Characteristics of the infant are: (1) the shape of the abdomen is a square compared with the rectangular shape of the older child. A transverse mid-abdominal incision in an infant will therefore provide access to the whole peritoneal cavity with the possible exception of the pelvis; (2) the compliant rib cage and wide subcostal angle facilitate access to the upper abdominal organs and diaphragm; (3) the rectus muscle is wider and extends further laterally; (4) the liver is relatively large and occupies the right upper quadrant and epigastrium; and (5) the umbilicus is relatively low and nearer the pubic symphysis, and the bladder extends up to the umbilicus. There is therefore limited space for an incision below the umbilicus.

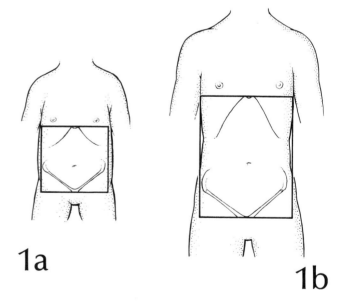

1a

1b

Site and size of incision

The surgeon must be able to see what he/she is doing. In a modern environment it is unusual to operate on a patient who is not stable, and the surgeon is able to place greater emphasis on the cosmetic aspects of the incision than was possible in the past. An incision which has been correctly sited does not need to be unduly long. Nonetheless, common reasons for a surgeon to experience difficulty are inadequate exposure due to an incision which is too small, poor retraction by the assistant, and inadequate muscle relaxation.

Blood loss must be kept to a minimum, particularly in the small infant. Except for the skin and peritoneum, electrocautery (diathermy) is used to divide the layers of the abdominal wall.

Preoperative

Skin cleansing

A variety of topical preparations are in use for removing potential pathogens from the skin in the operative field. Alcohol-based solutions evaporate rapidly, promoting heat loss, while iodine-based preparations may irritate the skin. Aqueous chlorhexidine (Hibitane) has none of these potential disadvantages and has effective antibacterial activity. In newborn infants the solution should be warmed.

Draping

Sterile towels or drapes are used to provide a sterile environment around the incision. These are covered with a large sterile adhesive plastic sheet which stabilizes the towels and also helps to keep the infant warm by reducing heat loss from the skin and by keeping the infant dry.

Operations

TRANSVERSE ABDOMINAL INCISION

The muscle-cutting transverse upper abdominal incision is suitable for most operations in infants, except when access is required to the distal colon and rectum. The incision may be limited to one side of the abdomen or can be extended across the midline, dividing both rectus muscles. For some procedures, e.g. reduction of intussusception, a transverse incision lateral to the right rectus muscle will suffice.

Position of patient and incision

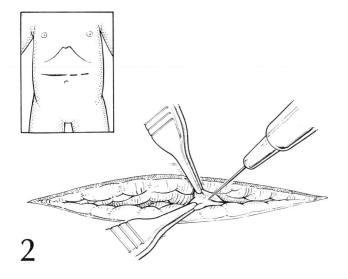

2   The patient lies supine. The skin incision starts in the midline, 1–2 cm above the umbilicus, and extends laterally across the rectus muscle. The subcutaneous fat is lifted with two pairs of fine-toothed forceps (one held by the surgeon and one by the assistant) and cut with the diathermy. Bleeding from small vessels in the skin edge will stop spontaneously with compression; larger vessels are touch-coagulated with the needle-point diathermy or picked up accurately with fine-toothed forceps and coagulated, taking care not to damage the skin.

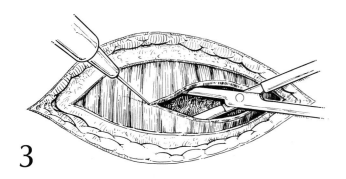

3   This exposes the anterior rectus sheath, which is incised transversely. A pair of artery forceps inserted deep to the rectus muscle is used to lift the muscle while cutting it with the diathermy. The vessels are identified and cauterized before being cut.

4 The posterior rectus sheath is picked up with two pairs of artery forceps placed about 1 cm apart, taking care not to include the underlying bowel, and a small incision is made between them. Once air has entered the peritoneal cavity, the bowel falls away (unless there are adhesions) and the incision is safely extended using scissors. In the neonate the transversalis muscle in the posterior rectus sheath is well developed and may be divided as a separate layer using the diathermy.

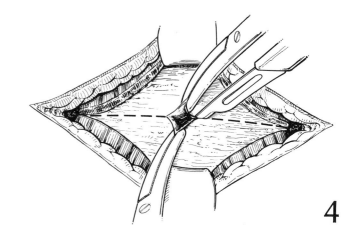

4

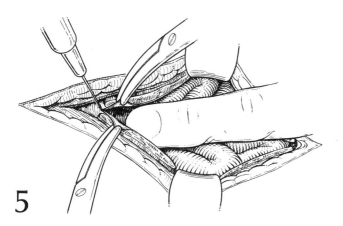

5

Extending the incision

5 The incision may be extended lateral to the rectus muscle by lifting the abdominal wall muscles with artery forceps applied to the upper and lower edges of the posterior rectus sheath, and cutting the muscle layers with the diathermy.

The underlying bowel is protected with a finger or a retractor.

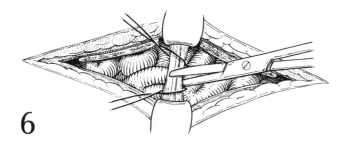

6

6 If the incision is extended medially across the midline, the falciform ligament is cut with scissors and the ligamentum teres is ligated with absorbable ligatures and divided.

Wound closure

7 The abdomen is closed in layers using absorbable sutures (4/0 or 3/0 sutures on a round-bodied needle for infants and 2/0 for children).

The margins of the peritoneum and transversalis muscle or fascia are grasped with artery forceps, elevated and approximated with a continuous absorbable suture. In the older child, if the incision divides both rectus sheaths, closure of the midline (linea alba) is reinforced with a single figure-of-eight suture. No sutures are placed in the rectus muscle, which is adherent to the rectus sheath and does not retract.

The anterior rectus sheath is also repaired using a continuous suture. Lateral to the rectus sheath, the internal and external oblique muscles are repaired in separate layers.

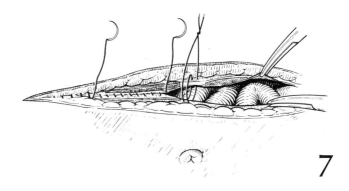

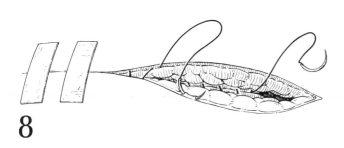

8 Before closing the skin, local anesthetic is infiltrated into the layers of the abdominal wall surrounding the incision. In most infants the subcutaneous fat falls together without the need for sutures, and the skin is approximated with adhesive strips. In older children the deep fascia is repaired with a 4/0 or 3/0 absorbable suture. This takes the tension off the skin, which is approximated with adhesive strips or a subcuticular 5/0 absorbable suture. The incision is covered with a dressing, mainly to allay the anxiety of the child.

Insertion of drain

9a–c If an abdominal drain is required, it must be placed through the abdominal wall before closing the incision. At a suitable site, often in the left or right iliac fossa, a short transverse incision is made through the skin and external oblique muscle.

With a hand in the peritoneal cavity to protect the bowel, an artery forceps is pushed through the abdominal wall into the peritoneal cavity to grasp a Penrose drain.

The drain is pulled out through the abdominal wall and sutured to the skin. A safety pin is passed through the drain to prevent it slipping into the abdomen.

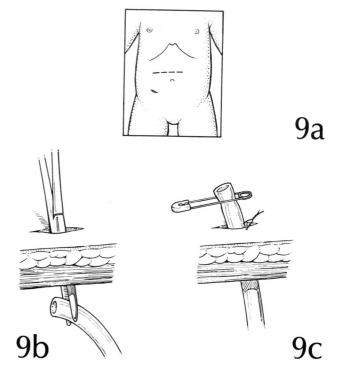

SUBCOSTAL INCISION

The left subcostal incision is useful for access to the diaphragm (congenital diaphragmatic hernia), esophagus (fundoplication) or spleen. On the right, the incision is used for operations on the gallbladder and bile ducts; if the liver is to be exposed the incision is extended to the left subcostal region (*see below*).

10 Depending on the age of the patient, the skin incision is made 1.5–3 cm below and parallel to the costal margin. It should not overlie the costal margin when sutured. In the midline the incision may be extended cranially to the xiphisternum for better access to the esophagus or diaphragm.

The layers to be divided are the same as for a transverse incision, but in an oblique direction.

Wound closure

Closure is as for a transverse incision. If a gastrostomy has been inserted, the most direct route is to bring it out through the incision. In this case the incision is closed in two halves on either side of the catheter. On each side of the gastrostomy the stomach must be securely anchored to the abdominal wall with a non-absorbable suture.

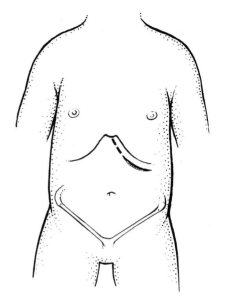

10

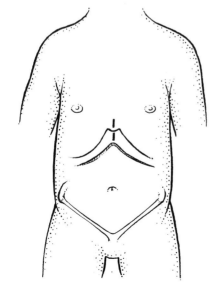

11

BILATERAL SUBCOSTAL(ROOFTOP) INCISION

This is the preferred exposure for surgery of the liver and portal structures.

11 For initial exploration of the liver a right subcostal incision is made; this is then extended to the left with a curve across the midline. A further extension may be made cranially in the midline to enter the mediastinum if necessary.

Wound closure

Closure is as for subcostal and midline incisions. A single reinforcing suture is placed in the midline.

MIDLINE ABDOMINAL INCISION

The access offered by the upper abdominal midline incision in the infant is restricted by the relatively large liver, but this disadvantage is offset by the wide costal angle and the cosmetic scar. The incision is useful for pyloromyotomy, gastrostomy and fundoplication. In the older child this is the incision of choice for blunt abdominal trauma.

12 The skin is incised from xiphisternum to umbilicus (for pyloromyotomy a shorter incision is adequate). If it is necessary to extend the incision caudally, it should be taken straight through the umbilicus and not around it. This gives a superior cosmetic result and the risk of infection is not increased if the umbilicus is properly cleaned. The subcutaneous tissues are cut with the diathermy down to the fascia.

A short incision is made in the linea alba using a scalpel, and the falciform ligament is entered. The edges of the incision are grasped with artery forceps and elevated. A plane is developed deep to the linea alba, which is incised with scissors. Near the umbilicus the peritoneum fuses with the linea alba and the peritoneal cavity will be entered as the incision is extended caudally. The left or right fold of the falciform ligament is incised, depending on the exposure required; if necessary the ligamentum teres is ligated and divided.

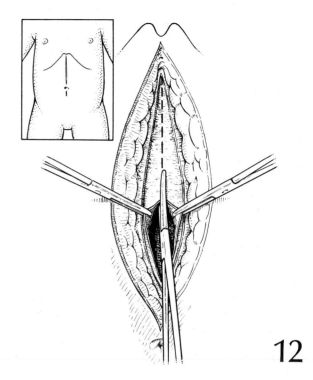

12

Wound closure

The falciform ligament/peritoneum may be repaired but this is not essential. The linea alba is approximated with a continuous strong suture of slowly absorbable material such as polydioxanone (PDS), or with a nylon suture (3/0 for infants, 2/0 or 0 gauge for children). The knot at each end should be buried to avoid an unsightly nodule. A subcutaneous suture may be required. The skin is closed with adhesive strips or a 5/0 continuous subcuticular absorbable suture.

GRID-IRON INCISION

The modified McBurney incision is the best incision for acute appendectomy in childhood.

13 The incision is centered over McBurney's point, which is one-third of the way from the anterior superior iliac spine to the umbilicus. It should be lateral to the rectus muscle which is relatively broad in a child; a common error is to make the incision too medial and too low. If a mass can be palpated when the child is under anesthesia, this may influence the siting of the incision. The incision is aligned with the skin creases in a slightly oblique direction.

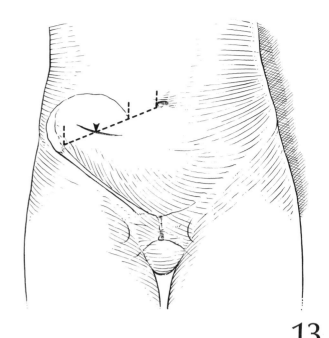

13

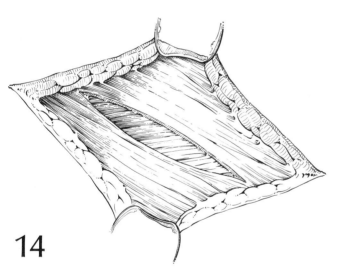

14

14 The subcutaneous tissues are divided with diathermy and swept aside with a swab to expose clearly the external oblique aponeurosis; this facilitates subsequent closure. The external oblique muscle is incised and then divided along the line of its fibers and separated from the underlying muscle.

15 The internal oblique muscle is opened by passing blunt scissors or artery forceps into the muscle and spreading it at right angles to the direction of the fibers. Two Langenbeck retractors are inserted into the space and used to separate the fibers widely. The underlying transversus abdominis muscle and the fatty layer covering the peritoneum are opened in a similar fashion.

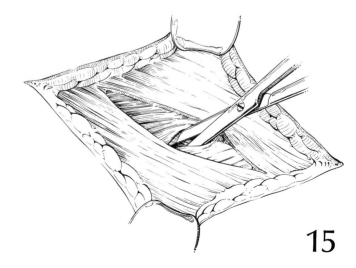

15

16 The peritoneum is grasped with two pairs of artery forceps, taking care to avoid the underlying bowel. The forceps are lifted and the peritoneum is incised transversely with a scalpel; the opening is enlarged using scissors.

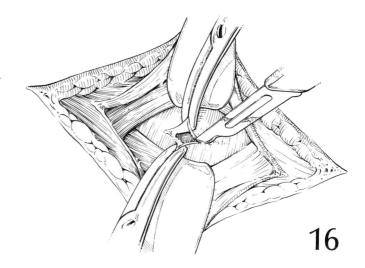

16

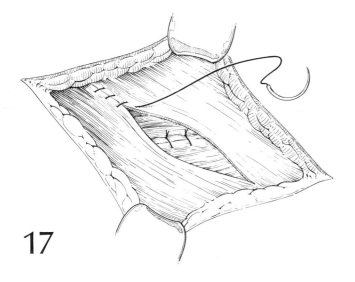

17

Wound closure

17 The edges of the peritoneum are grasped with artery forceps and closed with a continuous absorbable suture.

The fibers of the transversus and internal oblique muscles are closed as a single layer, using two or three interrupted sutures which are loosely tied to avoid muscle ischemia. The external oblique muscle is closed with a continuous absorbable suture. The subcutaneous fat seldom requires sutures.

For skin closure, if adhesive strips alone are not adequate, a subcuticular suture of 5/0 absorbable material is used. In children the skin is always closed after appendectomy, regardless of the degree of contamination; appropriate prophylactic antibiotic cover must be given.

Extending the incision

Circumstances may require the incision to be extended laterally; this is done by dividing the abdominal muscles in layers using the diathermy, as shown in *Illustration 5*.

18 To extend the incision medially, the incision in the external oblique muscle is carried onto the anterior rectus sheath. The rectus muscle is retracted medially. The internal oblique and transversus muscles are divided medially and this incision is extended to open the posterior rectus sheath and peritoneum. If necessary, the rectus muscle is also divided. The incision is closed in layers, as for a transverse abdominal incision.

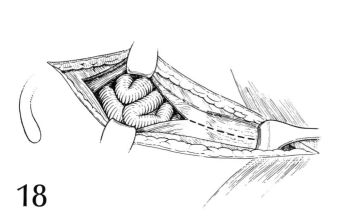

18

OBLIQUE MUSCLE CUTTING (LANZ) INCISION

In the left iliac fossa this incision is used for colostomy formation. It may be extended medially as the 'hockey stick' incision to provide access to the pelvis.

19 The skin is incised in an oblique direction at the midpoint of a line from the umbilicus to the anterior superior iliac spine. The external oblique muscle is incised along the line of its fibers, as for a grid-iron incision. The internal oblique and transverse muscles are cut obliquely in the same direction as the external oblique muscle, using the diathermy.

For the 'hockey stick' extension the incision is continued medially, parallel to the skin creases. The rectus muscles and peritoneum are cut transversely.

Wound closure

The incision is closed in layers, as for a transverse abdominal incision.

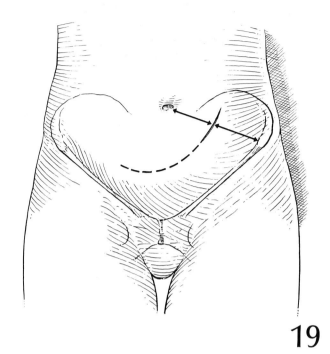

19

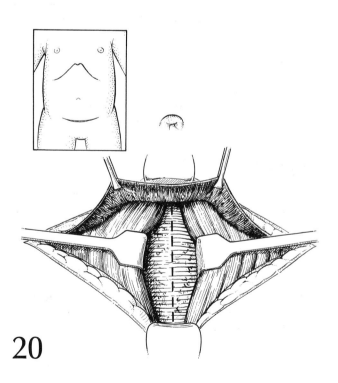

20

PFANNENSTIEL INCISION

This lower abdominal incision provides access to the pelvic organs, in particular the bladder, uterus and ovaries, without dividing the rectus muscles.

20 The skin and subcutaneous tissues are incised transversely between the lateral borders of the two rectus muscles. The incision is slightly curved to follow the skin creases, and is centered about 2 cm above the pubic symphysis. The anterior rectus sheaths are divided transversely and dissected off the rectus muscles by blunt and sharp dissection, extending cranially well up to the umbilicus and caudally to the pubic symphysis. The rectus muscles are separated vertically in the midline and retracted laterally. The transversalis fascia and peritoneum are then opened vertically, taking care to avoid the bladder.

Wound closure

The incision is closed in layers, as for a transverse upper abdominal incision. The rectus muscles are approximated in the midline with interrupted sutures.

Illustrations by Marks Creative Illustrations

Gastroesophageal reflux: Nissen fundoplication

Lewis Spitz PhD, FRCS, FRCS(Ed), FAAP(Hon)
Nuffield Professor of Paediatric Surgery, Institute of Child Health, University of London, and Consultant Paediatric Surgeon, Great Ormond Street Hospital for Children, London, UK

Gastroesophageal reflux is more common in infancy and childhood than is generally recognized. Although in the majority of cases (>90%) the reflux resolves spontaneously within the first year of life as the lower esophageal sphincter matures, a small but significant proportion of cases develop complications requiring prolonged medical or surgical treatment.

Principles and justification

Clinical presentation

Early infancy

The child presents with recurrent vomiting which may be regurgitant or projectile. The vomitus may contain altered blood (the 'coffee-grounds' appearance). The infant fails to thrive and may be constipated.

Older child

Vomiting is a major feature. In addition, the child complains of heartburn and dysphagia and may occasionally present with iron-deficient anaemia secondary to chronic blood loss.

Mental retardation

A significant proportion of severely retarded children suffer from repeated vomiting which is often due to gastroesophageal reflux. It is notable that there is a high failure rate of medical treatment in this group.

Anatomic anomaly

Gastroesophageal reflux is more common in infants with esophageal atresia, diaphragmatic hernia, anterior abdominal wall defects and malrotation.

Aspiration syndromes

There is a small but definite association of aspiration symptoms (asthma, pneumonitis, cyanosis, apneic episodes) and gastroesophageal reflux.

Other presentations

Other presentations include rumination, Sandifer's syndrome (torsion spasms of the neck), protein-losing enteropathy, irritability, hyperactivity.

Pathologic anatomy

Reflux may, or may not, be accompanied by an associated hiatus hernia. Two types of hiatus hernia are recognized.

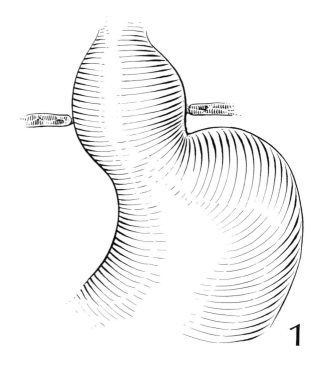

1 Sliding hiatus hernia, characterized by ascent of the cardia into the mediastinum.

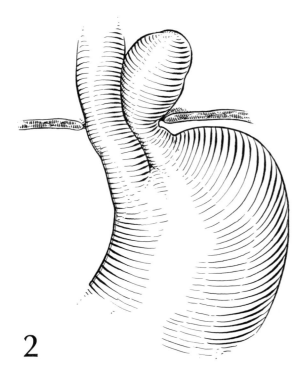

2 Paraesophageal or rolling hernia, in which the gastroesophageal junction remains in the abdomen while part of the gastric fundus prolapses through the esophageal hiatus into the mediastinum.

The sliding hernia is frequently associated with reflux, while gastric stasis in the paraesophageal hernia predisposes to peptic ulceration, perforation or hemorrhage.

Normal mechanisms preventing reflux

Physiologic control of reflux depends on the following factors:

1. Anatomic
   (a) length and pressure of the lower esophageal sphincter;
   (b) the intra-abdominal segment of the esophagus;
   (c) the gastroesophageal angle (angle of His);
   (d) the lower esophageal mucosal rosette;
   (e) the phrenoesophageal membrane;
   (f) the diaphragmatic hiatal pinchcock effect.
2. Physiologic
   (a) coordinated effective peristaltic clearance of the distal esophagus;
   (b) normal gastric emptying.

Pathophysiology of reflux

The squamous epithelium of the esophagus is unable to resist the irritant effect of gastric juices. The acid pepsin causes a chemical inflammation with erythema of the mucosa. With continued reflux, the mucosa becomes friable and bleeds easily on contact. Later, frank ulceration develops which, with repeated attempts at repair and relapse, eventually leads to stricture formation. This process is summarized in *Figure 1*.

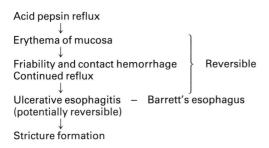

Figure 1   Pathophysiology of reflux

Indications for antireflux surgery

Antireflux surgery should be undertaken in the presence of an established esophageal stricture or if conservative measures of treatment have failed. Surgery may also be considered at an early stage (1) in the presence of an anatomic anomaly, e.g. esophageal atresia, malrotation, exomphalos; (2) in the presence of associated neurologic damage, where the response to conservative measures is notoriously poor. Surgery may also be necessary if the patient is suffering from apneic episodes and repeated respiratory infections due to aspiration of refluxed material, or if the infant fails to thrive despite adequate therapy.

Preoperative

Investigations

A number of preoperative investigations should be performed.

Barium esophagogram, with particular attention to the anatomy of the esophagus (presence of strictures, ulcerative esophagitis, abnormal narrowing or displacement); presence of a hiatus hernia; peristaltic activity of the esophagus and rate of clearance of contrast material; the degree of gastroesophageal reflux (grade I: distal esophagus; grade II: proximal/thoracic esophagus; grade III: cervical esophagus; grade IV: continuous reflux; grade V: aspiration into tracheobronchial tree); and evidence of gastric outlet obstruction.

Esophageal pH monitoring. Continuous 24-h monitoring of the pH in the distal esophagus is the most accurate method of documenting reflux. A pH of less than 4 is regarded as significant. During the 24-h recording the following parameters should be examined: (1) the number of episodes where the pH falls below 4; (2) the duration of each reflux episode; (3) the number of episodes lasting more than 5 min; and (4) the total duration of reflux, expressed as a percentage of recording time.

Esophageal manometry. Pressure recordings are made with continuously perfused open-tipped catheters or solid-state pressure transducers. A high-pressure zone is normally present in the distal esophagus. Individual pressure values are unreliable diagnostic indicators of reflux but may be useful in predicting cases which will eventually require surgical treatment.

Endoscopy and biopsy. Endoscopy will determine the degree of esophagitis; histology of the biopsy will provide pathologic grading of inflammatory cell infiltration. Four grades of esophagitis are recognized at endoscopy: grade I – erythema of mucosa; grade II – friability of mucosa; grade III – ulcerative esophagitis; grade IV – stricture.

Scintiscanning. Technetium (^{99}Tc) sulphur colloid scans may be useful in documenting pulmonary aspiration.

Medical management

Small, frequent, thickened feeds should be given. A 30° head-elevated, prone position is the most suitable posture for young infants. Antacids-alkalis with or without alginic acid (Gaviscon) should be administered. Histamine receptor antagonists (cimetidine, ranitidine) will suppress acid secretion and allow severe esophagitis to heal. Omiprasol is even more efficient. Metoclopramide, cisapride and bethanechol increase lower esophageal pressure and stimulate gastric emptying.

Anesthesia

General endotracheal anesthesia is administered, with the patient supine. A single dose of prophylactic broad-spectrum antibiotics should be given after induction of anesthesia.

Operation

Some surgeons insist on inserting a large-calibre bougie in the esophagus during the construction of the fundoplication to ensure that the wrap is not too tight. The author prefers a regular size nasogastric tube and constructs a very loose wrap.

Incision

3 In the majority of cases the ideal approach is via a midline upper abdominal incision extending from the xiphisternum to the umbilicus. This incision may be extended caudally to one side of the umbilicus.

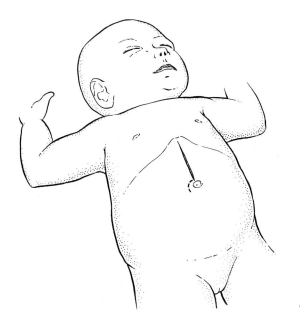

3

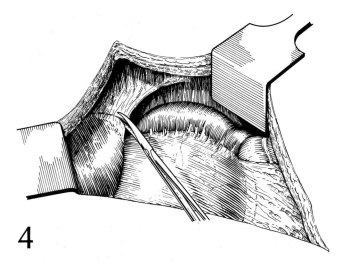

4

Exposure

4 Adequate exposure of the gastroesophageal junction will usually be obtained by retracting the left lobe of the liver anterosuperiorly. Additional exposure may be attained, if necessary, by dividing the left triangular ligament in the avascular plane and then retracting the left lobe of the liver to the right.

Mobilization of the fundus of the stomach

5a, b The proximal one-third to one-half of the greater curvature of the stomach is liberated from its attachment to the spleen by ligating and dividing the short gastric vessels in the gastrosplenic ligament. This is accomplished most safely by passing a right-angled clamp around each vessel in turn and ligating the vessel on the gastric and splenic side before dividing it.

When the vessels in the gastrosplenic ligament have been divided the spleen should be allowed to fall back into the posterior peritoneum, thereby avoiding inadvertent trauma. Splenectomy should rarely be necessary in this procedure. The fundus is now sufficiently free to allow for a loose ('floppy') fundoplication.

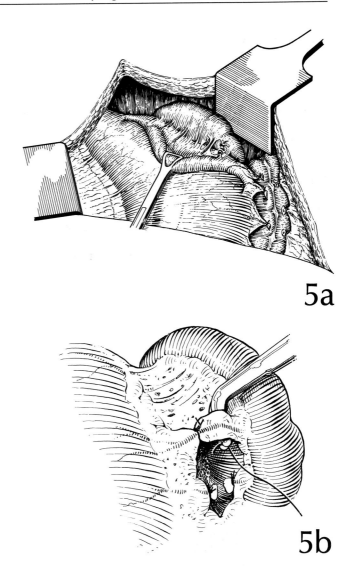

5a

5b

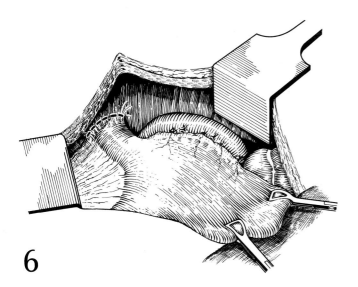

6

Exposure of the esophageal hiatus

6 The phrenoesophageal membrane is placed on stretch by downward traction on the stomach while the diaphragmatic muscle is retracted superiorly. The avascular membrane is incised with scissors and the musculature of the esophagus displayed. The anterior vagus nerve will be seen coursing on the surface of the esophagus. It should be carefully protected and preserved.

Mobilization of the distal esophagus

7 Using a combination of sharp and blunt dissection, the lower end of the esophagus is encircled, avoiding injury to the posterior vagus nerve. A rubber sling is placed around the esophagus incorporating the posterior vagus nerve which will be included in the fundoplication. The lower 2 or 3 cm of esophagus is now mobilized using blunt dissection with either a pledget or right-angled forceps. The esophageal hiatus is completely exposed by dividing the upper part of the gastrohepatic omentum above the left gastric vessels.

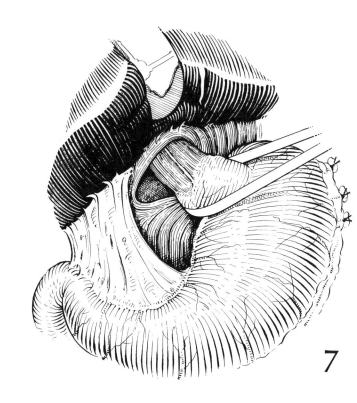

7

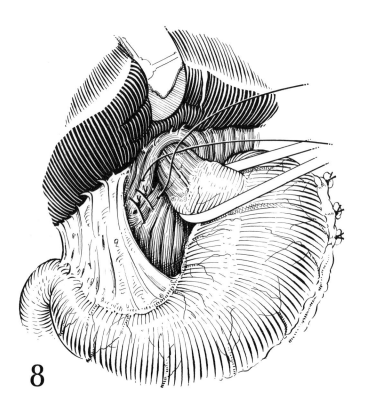

8

Narrowing of the hiatus

8 The esophageal hiatus is narrowed posterior to the esophagus by placing deep sutures through the crura of the diaphragm. The sutures are tied loosely to prevent them cutting through, but leaving sufficient space alongside the esophagus to allow the tip of a finger to pass. Two or three sutures may be required for this purpose.

Construction of the fundoplication

9a–c The mobilized fundus of the stomach is folded behind the esophagus so that the invaginated part of the stomach appears on the right side of the esophagus. It is important not to twist the stomach during this maneuver and to ensure that the stomach has been sufficiently mobilized to be able to fashion a loose wrap.

The length of the wrap varies from 1.0 cm in the infant to 2–2.5 cm in the older child. Commencing at the level of the gastroesophageal junction 3–4 sutures of non-absorbable material (3/0 or 4/0) are placed through the stomach and esophageal muscle. Each suture passes from left to right through the anterior wall of the stomach, through the esophageal muscle (taking care not to enter the lumen of the esophagus) and through the wall of the mobilized portion of the fundus of the stomach, which has been folded behind the esophagus. Traction on the first (untied) suture brings the rest of the operating field clearly into view and facilitates the insertion of the remaining two or three proximal parallel sutures through the anterior wall of the stomach, esophageal muscle and 'prolapsed' fundus. When all these sutures are in place, they are tied serially without tension on the wrap.

A second layer of non-absorbable sutures including the seromuscular surface of the stomach only may be placed superficial to the primary sutures to prevent disruption of the wrap.

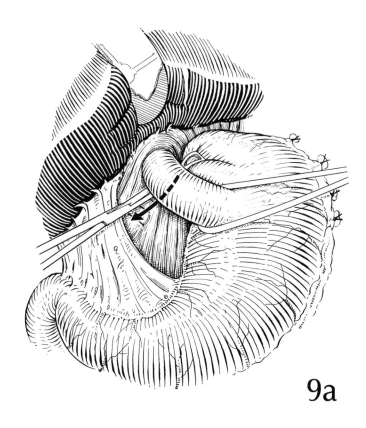

9a

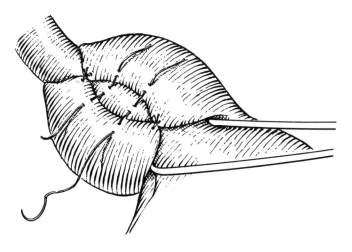

9b

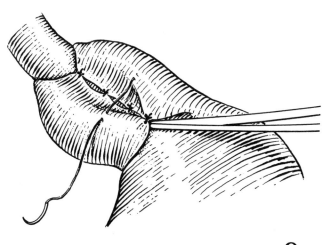

9c

10 The proximal suture of the second layer should be passed through the anterior wall of the esophageal hiatus in the diaphragm. An additional two or three sutures may be placed between the hiatus and the fundoplication to prevent the wrap migrating into the posterior mediastinum.

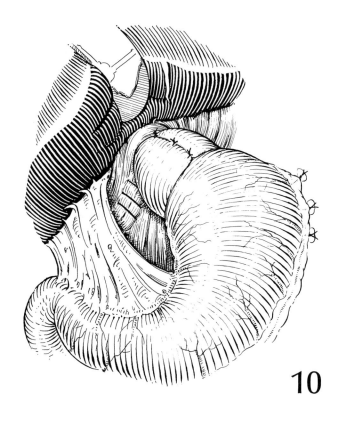

10

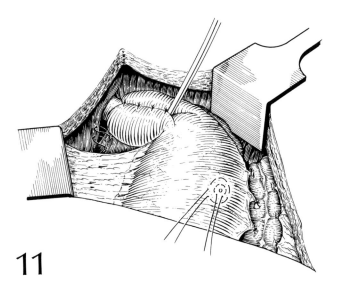

11

Gastrostomy

11 A feeding gastrostomy should be constructed in neurologically impaired children who are unable to eat normally. A suitable area on the anterior wall of the stomach is selected to permit the gastrostomy site to be anchored to the anterior abdominal wall without exerting traction on the fundoplication.

Two rows of circumferentially placed non-absorbable sutures are placed through the seromuscular layer of the stomach. A suitable size Malecot catheter is inserted through a centrally placed gastrotomy into the stomach and the sutures are tied, invaginating the gastrotomy site. The tube is brought out through a separate stab incision in the left hypochondrium and the stomach wall sutured to the anterior abdominal wall at the exit site to prevent leakage.

Closure

The wound is closed either in layers or with interrupted *en masse* sutures. A subcuticular suture approximates the skin edges.

Postoperative care

Nasogastric decompression and intravenous fluids are continued until postoperative ileus has resolved (usually 2–4 days).

Complications

Death following this procedure is extremely uncommon. In severely retarded children there is a small but not insignificant risk of mortality, related mainly to the underlying disease.

Wound infection and dehiscence occasionally occur.

Respiratory complications such as pneumonia or atelectasis particularly affect severely retarded patients and patients undergoing fundoplication for chronic respiratory complications secondary to aspiration.

Dysphagia may result from a wrap which is either too long or too tight.

The gastroesophageal reflux may recur either because of disruption of the fundoplication or herniation of the fundoplication into the posterior mediastinum.

Paraesophageal hernia occurs following inadequate approximation or disruption of the crural repair.

Gas bloat, hiccup, retching and dumping symptoms are usually transient.

Adhesion intestinal obstruction is particularly common if additional intra-abdominal procedures such as gastrostomy, incidental appendectomy, correction of malrotation are performed. N.B. It is important to alert the parents to the danger of intestinal obstruction as the inability to vomit may result in inordinate delay in establishing the diagnosis.

Further reading

Johnson DG. The Nissen fundoplication. In: Holder TM, Ashcraft KW, eds. *Pediatric Esophageal Surgery* Orlando: Grune and Stratton, 1986: 193–208.

Leape LL, Ramenofsky ML. Surgical treatment of gastro-esophageal reflux in children. Results of Nissen fundoplication in 100 children. *Am J Dis Child* 1980; 134: 935–8.

Randolph J. Experience with the Nissen fundoplication for correction of gastroesophageal reflux in infants. *Ann Surg* 1983; 198: 579–84.

Spitz L, Kirtane J. Results and complications of surgery for gastroesophageal reflux. *Arch Dis Child* 1985; 60: 743–7.

Spitz L, Roth K, Kiely EM, Brereton RJ, Drake DP, Milla PJ. Operation for gastro-oesophageal reflux associated with severe mental retardation. *Arch Dis Child* 1993; 68: 347–51.

Tunnel WP, Smith EI, Carson JA. Gastroesophageal reflux in childhood: the dilemma of surgical success. *Ann Surg* 1983; 197: 560–5.

Gastroesophageal reflux: Thal procedure

Keith W. Ashcraft MD

Professor of Surgery, University of Missouri – Kansas City School of Medicine, and Chief of Urology, Children's Mercy Hospital, Kansas City, Missouri, USA

The efficacy of the Thal anterior fundoplication is based upon the construction of a length of intra-abdominal esophagus and an acute angle of His to create a valve mechanism at the gastroesophageal junction. The fact that the fundoplication involves only half the circumference of the esophagus allows the patient to be able to vomit and belch; the inability to eructate and vomit is an undesirable aspect of Nissen's fundoplication. The Thal procedure is simple; it does not require division of the short gastric vessels thus reducing operating time and operative manipulation. The incidence of postoperative small bowel adhesive obstruction is much lower than after a Nissen fundoplication.

Operation

Incision

1 A transverse incision extending from nipple line to nipple line just below the costal margin is the preferred approach. It allows access to the upper abdominal contents. It is usually just above the transverse colon and, if the patient is relaxed, the transverse colon helps to prevent small bowel exposure and handling. A nasogastric tube is placed for purposes of identification and stabilization of the distal esophagus during the procedure.

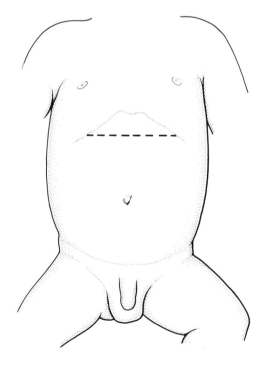

1

2 A transverse incision of the peritoneum over the gastroesophageal junction is made and the hiatus lifted so that the esophagus may be dissected anteriorly on either side. The left or anterior vagus nerve should be visible.

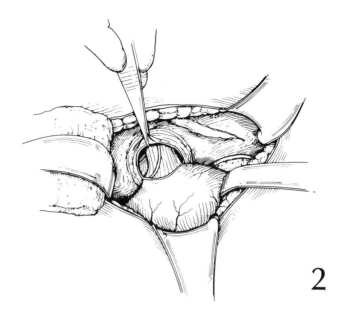

2

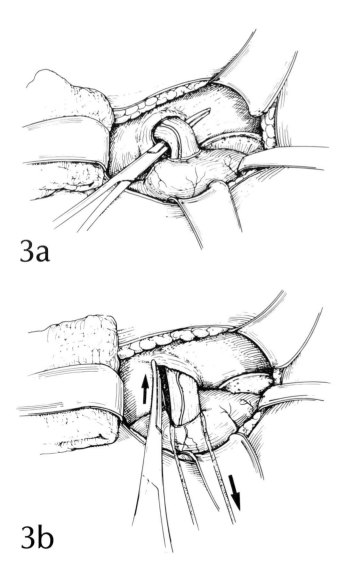

3a

3b

3a, b A blunt dissector is passed behind the esophagus from the right to the left of the patient and a polyester fiber tape (Dacron) is pulled back. Downward traction on the tape provides stability for the gastroesophageal junction as the hiatus on either side is pushed cephalad to expose an appropriate length of distal esophagus. The dissector is then passed behind the esophagus through the Dacron tape tract and the underside of the esophagus cleaned off by simply pushing the tissue cephalad. At this point it is important to ensure that the posterior vagus nerve is incorporated within the loop of the tape. If it is not, the tape is replaced.

4 The hiatus is narrowed posteriorly by a 'figure of eight' permanent suture using 2/0 or 3/0 silk on a cardiovascular needle. The hiatus is narrowed to an appropriate size for the age of the child, leaving a little more space in a child who is eating solid food than in one whose diet consists of liquids.

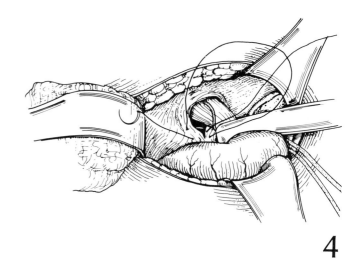

4

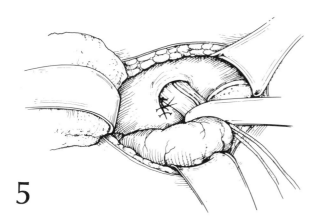

5

5 The figure of eight suture is tied to close the hiatus and the needle is used to fix the posterior aspect of the esophagus to the hiatus. Neither of these sutures is tied so tightly that muscle necrosis will result.

6 The arms of the tape are then separated and held in clamps. The anterior wall of the stomach is pulled up from beneath the tapes and prepared for application to the anterior half of the esophagus.

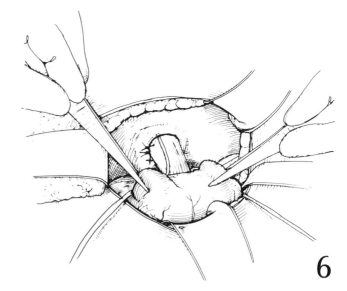

6

7 The fundoplication is accomplished by beginning a continuous suture at the greater curve gastroesophageal junction. A polytetrafluoroethylene (PTFE; Gore-Tex) suture of either 2/0 or 3/0 is preferred. Six knots are required to prevent the suture from slipping. The needle is passed through the seromuscular layer of the stomach about 1 cm down from the original stitch and then along the left lateral aspect of the esophagus coming from deep upward. These sutures are inserted without reloading the needle between stomach and esophagus to ensure that the point of the stomach fits easily and without tension against the point of esophagus selected.

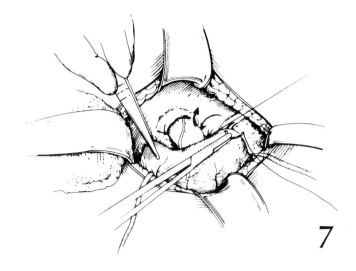

7

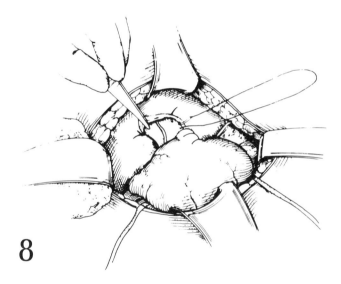

8

8 The continuous suture is carried up along the left side of the esophagus to the hiatus where the suture then incorporates stomach, esophagus and hiatus.

9 After the anterior portion of the suture line has been completed the suture line is turned downward toward the lesser curve gastroesophageal junction where it is tied. Thus a continuous inverted U-shaped suture line affixes the anterior free wall of the stomach to the exposed anterior half of the esophagus. The short gastric vessels are not divided for this procedure.

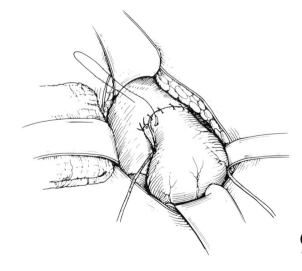

9

10 The completed fundoplication is shown with a nasogastric tube in place. The nasogastric tube is removed on the operating table, and the patient allowed to feed the following day and discharged usually within 48 h.

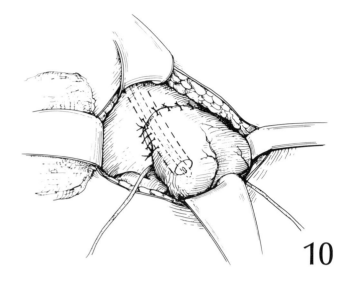

10

Postoperative follow-up

Follow-up consists of a wound check about 10 days after the operation, a barium study to confirm the integrity of the fundoplication at 4 months, and a repeat barium study at any time if a question of recurrent reflux arises. Repeat 24-h pH studies are done if the patient's symptoms are not relieved and to determine that the reflux has been successfully corrected.

Outcome

The author has performed 1400 of these procedures over a 20-year period; the reoperation rate has been 4% (58 patients). Recurrent gastroesophageal reflux has been due to either dehiscence of the fundoplication, recurrent herniation through the hiatus, or both.

Acknowledgments

Illustrations 2–10 are reproduced from *Pediatric Surgery*, 2nd edition, edited by K.W. Ashcraft and T. Holder (1993), published by W.B. Saunders Company, Philadelphia, with permission of the publishers.

Further reading

Ashcraft KW, Goodwin CD, Amoury RW, McGill CW, Holder TM. Thal fundoplication: a simple and safe operative treatment for gastroesophageal reflux. *J Pediatr Surg* 1978; 13: 643–7.

Ashcraft KW, Holder TM *et al*. The Thal fundoplication for gastroesophageal reflux. *J Pediatr Surg* 1984; 19: 480–3.

Thal AP. A unified approach to surgical problems of the esophagogastric junction. *Ann Surg* 1968; 163: 542–50.

Gastroesophageal reflux: Boix-Ochoa procedure

J. Boix-Ochoa
Professor of Pediatric Surgery, Autonomous University of Barcelona, and Chairman of the Department of Pediatric Surgery, Children's Hospital, Vall d'Hebron, Barcelona, Spain

J. M. Casasa
Head of Gastrointestinal Surgery, Department of Pediatric Surgery, Autonomous University of Barcelona, and Children's Hospital, Vall d'Hebron, Barcelona, Spain

Principles and justification

The aim of the Boix-Ochoa procedure is to restore the anatomic relationships and the physiologic characteristics of the lower esophageal sphincter mechanism. This may be achieved by: restoring the length of the intra-abdominal segment of the esophagus; repairing the widened esophageal hiatus in the diaphragm and anchoring the esophagus to its margins; and restoring the angle of His. The final step comprises the opening up or unfolding of the fundus of the stomach (as in opening an umbrella) by inserting suspending sutures between the fundus and the diaphragm.

The procedure has the effect of increasing the length of the intra-abdominal segment of esophagus, which restores the normal closing pressure mechanism. Reconstruction of the angle of His provides the mechanical mechanism for compressing and closing off the esophagus, while unfolding the fundus of the stomach buffers the effect of raised intragastric pressure and enhances the mechanical closing of the esophagus.

Operation

Position of patient and incision

1 A pillow is placed under the back of the patient at the level of the lower ribs to facilitate the approach to the distal esophagus. A nasogastric tube should be in place.

The distal esophagus is approached through a midline abdominal incision. Access is best achieved if this is a long incision from the left side of the xiphoid extending to 1 cm below the umbilicus, where the underlying umbilicus vessels are ligated to ease the handling of the liver.

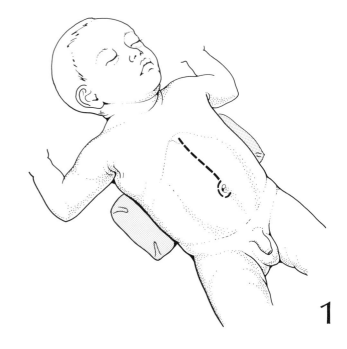

1

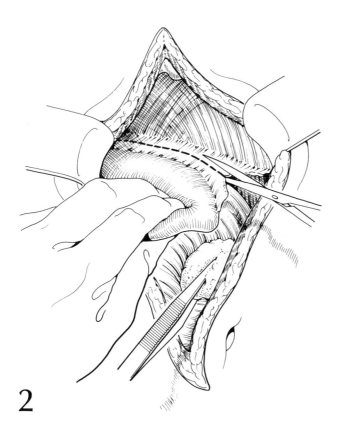

2

Mobilization of the left liver lobe

2 The left thoracic cage is elevated with a retractor by the second surgical assistant. The stomach is pulled caudally by the first assistant and the spleen is pushed aside. The liver is grasped with a sponge and retracted downwards to allow division of the left triangular ligament which attaches the left lobe to the undersurface of the diaphragm. Small vessels are cauterized, taking great care not to dissect beyond the right side of the hiatus in order to avoid injury to the suprahepatic veins.

Division of the esophagohepatic ligament

3 Once the left lobe of the liver is free, it is turned downwards protected by a sponge and retracted to the right by the second assistant who stands cranial to the surgeon. The first assistant retracts the stomach downwards, and separates the spleen and the splenic flexure of the colon away from the field. The fold of peritoneum extending from the esophagus and stomach to the liver is divided by sharp dissection, taking care not to injure the left gastric vessels.

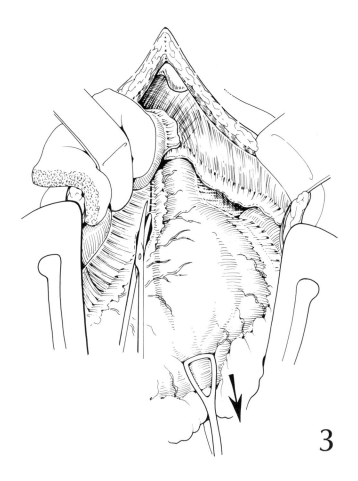

3

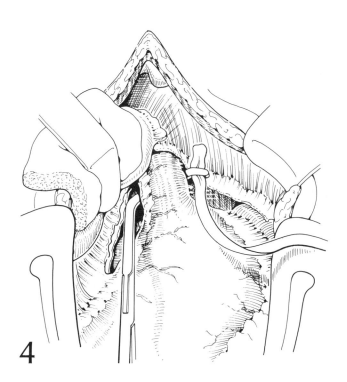

4

Mobilization of the distal esophagus

4 The distal esophagus is exposed by blunt dissection from surrounding tissues. A suitable instrument is then passed behind the esophagus so that an umbilical tape or rubber or plastic sling can be passed beneath the esophagus and used for downward traction.

Exposure of the distal esophagus

5   The distal 2–3 cm of the intrathoracic esophagus is exposed by blunt dissection and freed from the surrounding tissue. Care must be taken when mobilizing the intrathoracic distal esophagus to avoid injury to the pleura. The dissection should continue until 3–4 cm of distal esophagus has been exposed in small infants and 7–8 cm in older children. The pillars (right, left and anterior) of the hiatus are retracted by means of stay sutures. The hiatus should now be completely visible and the esophagus free and mobile.

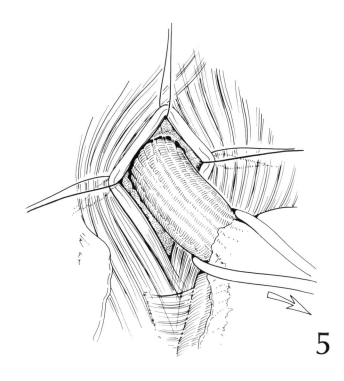

5

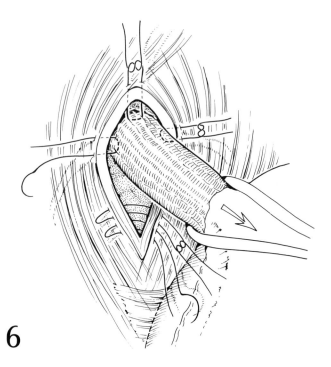

6

Anchoring the esophagus to the hiatal margins

6   To anchor the esophagus to the hiatal margins three U-sutures (pillar-esophagus-pillar) of 2/0 silk are inserted at the anterior, right and left pillar. The sutures are tied while pushing the diaphragm cranially and pulling on the esophageal tape. These anchoring sutures ensure as long an intra-abdominal esophagus as possible.

Closure of the posterior pillars

7 Once the esophagus is anchored to the hiatus, two or three snugly tied deep crural sutures are inserted to close the posterior pillars. The tip of the little finger should be able to be introduced into the hiatus alongside the esophagus. If the suture is left too loose it can lead to the development of a paraesophageal hernia, and if it is too tight it will result in dysphagia.

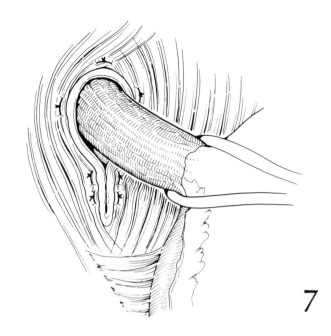

7

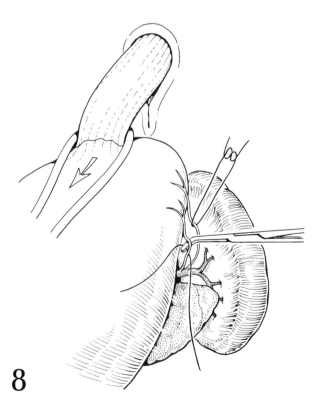

8

Restoration of the angle of His

8 The upper two short gastric vessels are dissected and ligated. Occasionally they are very short and require careful dissection to avoid a splenic injury. The greater curvature of the stomach has to be dissected and mobilized, so that the upper portion of the greater curvature can be placed without any tension over the right pillar of the hiatus, to restore and reinforce the angle of His.

Anchorage of greater curvature over right pillar and distal esophagus

9 Once the great curvature is mobilized, a suture of 0 silk is placed from the great curvature to the rim of the esophageal hiatus (right crus/pillar) in order to produce an exaggerated angle of His.

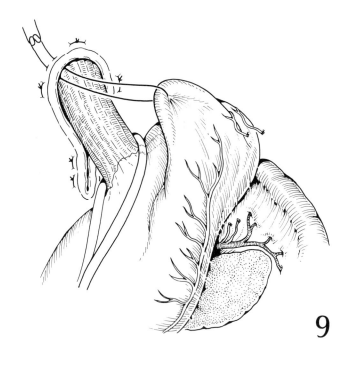

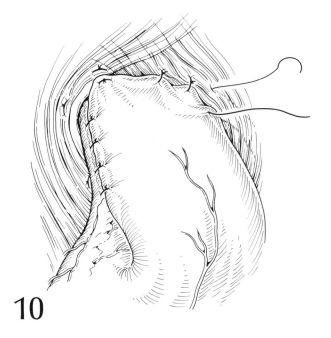

Reconstruction of angle of His

10 A further four or five silk sutures are inserted between the rim of the mobilized gastric fundus and the intra-abdominal segment of the esophagus. This consolidates the angle of His.

Fixation of the fundus to the diaphragm

To maintain an open fundus it must be unfolded upwards like an umbrella. To achieve this, three sutures are placed in a triangle between the fundus and the under surface of the left diaphragm. This maneuver allows any increase in intragastric pressure of the open fundus to be transmitted against the wall of the esophagus, thus closing it. It also reinforces the angle of His and diminishes tension in the sutures.

Optional anterior gastropexy

11 The anterior gastropexy (Boerema) is only recommended in severe cases, short esophagus, encephalopathies and Down's syndrome. Two or three sutures are placed from the lesser curvature to the anterior abdominal wall to facilitate healing free of tension by anchoring the intra-abdominal segment of the esophagus.

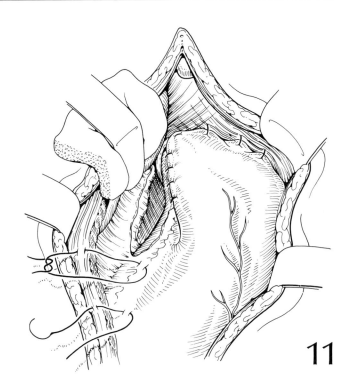

11

Postoperative care

Under normal circumstances the postoperative course should be smooth and uneventful. Routine intravenous fluids are administered. Prophylactic antibiotics will protect against wound infection. A nasogastric tube is left *in situ* for 5 days. Feeds are commenced via the nasogastric tube.

Three months after the operation radiological assessment for reflux is carried out and at 6 months a 24-h pH study is performed.

Outcome

Between 1966 and 1992 a total of 2566 patients were assessed for gastroesophageal reflux: 65 had major hiatal hernias. The total number undergoing antireflux surgery was 224 (8.7%). Follow-up studies on 180 patients 2–18 years after the operation revealed excellent radiological and clinical results in 168 (93.3%) cases. In 12 patients reflux could be demonstrated on radiological assessment but the children were asymptomatic. Two patients required reoperation. In this series the complications were: adhesion obstruction (3), postoperative pneumonia (5), mediastinitis secondary to perforation (1) and esophageal stenosis (2).

References

1. Boix-Ochoa J, Casasa JM. Surgical treatment of gastroesophageal reflux in children. *Surg Annu* 1989; 21: 97–118.

2. Gil-Vernet JM, Boix-Ochoa J. Valor clínico de la pHmetría intraesofágica en pediatría. Experiencia en 233 casos. *An Esp Pediatr* 1984; 21: 125–31.

3. Casasa JM, Boix-Ochoa J. Surgical or conservative treatment in hiatal hernias in children: a new decisive parameter. *Surgery* 1977; 82: 573–5.

4. Bettex M, Oesch I. The hiatus hernia saga: Ups and downs in gastroesophageal reflux: past, present and future perspectives. *J Pediatr Surg* 1983; 18: 670–80.

Illustrations by Patrick Elliott

Gastrostomy

Michael W. L. Gauderer MD
Professor of Pediatric Surgery and Pediatrics, Chief, Division of Pediatric Surgery, Case Western Reserve University, School of Medicine, Cleveland, Ohio, USA

History

Gastrostomy is one of the oldest abdominal operations in continuous use and its history is closely associated with the evolution of modern surgery[1].

Gastrostomies are important in the management of a wide variety of surgical and non-surgical conditions of childhood. Refinements in traditional procedures and the introduction of newer, and simpler endoscopically and laparoscopically aided gastrostomies have increased the safety and expanded the applicability of this operation[2–5]. The use of softer, minimally irritating materials in the manufacture of gastrostomy catheters and the development of skin-level gastrostomy devices have greatly facilitated long-term use of this type of enterostomy[1,6].

Principles and justification

Gastrostomy is performed in infants and children primarily for long-term feeding, decompression or a combination of both. Additional uses include gastric access for esophageal bougienage, gastroscopy and administration of medication[1,5].

Techniques

Three basic methods of constructing a gastrostomy are commonly used: (1) formation of a serosa-lined channel from the anterior gastric wall to the skin surface around a catheter; (2) formation of a tube from full-thickness gastric wall to the skin surface, a catheter being introduced intermittently for feeding; (3) percutaneous techniques, in which the introduced catheter holds the gastric and abdominal walls in apposition.

Formation around catheter

In the first group of techniques, the catheter may be placed parallel to (Witzel technique)[1] or perpendicular to (Stamm technique)[1] the stomach with a celiotomy (*see below*). The stomach is usually anchored to the abdominal wall with sutures. The essence of the Stamm-type gastrostomy is the use of concentric purse-string sutures around the gastrostomy tube, producing an invagination lined with serosa.

Gastrostomy brought to the surface

The gastric tube is constructed and then brought to the abdominal wall either as a direct conduit (Depage, Beck–Jianu, Hirsch and Janeway methods)[1] or interposing a valve or torsion of the tube to prevent reflux (Watsudjii, Spivack techniques)[1]. This conduit is secured to the layers of the abdominal wall and/or the skin. The main appeal of the Janeway-type stoma is that the patient does not need a catheter between feedings. The use of automatic stapling devices has greatly facilitated the construction of the tube from the anterior gastric wall.

Percutaneous techniques

In this third group the catheter is placed with endoscopic assistance without a celiotomy (Gauderer technique)[1,3,4]. Depending on the method of introduction of the catheter, this percutaneous endoscopic gastrostomy may be performed using a pull technique (Gauderer–Ponsky)[1,3,4] (*see below*), a push technique

(Sacks *et al.*)[1] in which a semi-rigid catheter guide is advanced over a Seldinger-type wire instead of being pulled into place by a string-like guide from inside the stomach to the skin level or the introducer technique (Russel *et al.*)[1] in which a Foley catheter is advanced through a removable sheath from the skin level into the stomach. This procedure was initially developed for children at high risk who were unable to swallow[3]. It was later adapted for use in adults[3].

Additionally, direct long-term access to the stomach may be gained with percutaneous non-endoscopic gastrostomy procedures using radiologic assistance[1].

Laparoscopically assisted gastrostomies may be performed using variations of the three basic modalities described above, either as single interventions or associated with other intracavitary procedures.

Indications

The type of gastrostomy, the preoperative work-up, the technique and the choice of gastrostomy device depend mainly on the indication for the procedure, the child's age and underlying disease, and the familiarity of the surgeon with the different operations.

Feeding and administration of medications

Placement of a gastrostomy for enteral feeding has two prerequisites: the upper gastrointestinal tract must be functional; and the need for enteral feedings must be long-term, at least 3–6 months. Children benefiting from gastrostomy fall into two broad categories: (1) those unable to swallow, and (2) those unable to consume adequate nutrients orally. The first group is the largest and composed primarily of patients with neurologic disturbances. The second group includes patients with a variety of conditions in which the central nervous system is intact: failure to thrive; complex bowel disorders (e.g. short gut syndrome, Crohn's disease, malabsorption); malignancy and other debilitating illnesses; and various congenital or acquired diseases interfering with growth.

In selected patients a gastrostomy is the most effective means of administering a non-palatable special diet (e.g. that used in chronic renal failure) or ensuring compliance with medication (e.g. administering cholestyramine in Alagille's syndrome).

All three basic gastrostomy types described above are suitable for this purpose (these are compared in *Table 1*). A comparison of devices used in all gastrostomy types (except gastric tube stomas) is given in *Table 2*.

Table 1 Comparison of the three most commonly used gastrostomies

	Serosa-lined channel (Stamm)	Gastric tube (Janeway)	Percutaneous endoscopic technique
Catheter/stoma device continuously *in situ*	Yes	No	Yes
Celiotomy	Yes	Yes	No
Laparoscopically feasible	Possible	Yes	Yes
Need for gastric endoscopy	No	No	Yes
Need for abdominal relaxation during operation	Yes	Yes	No
Procedure time	Short	Moderate	Very short
Postoperative ileus	Yes	Yes	No
Potential for bleeding	Yes	Yes	No
Potential for wound dehiscence/hernia	Yes	Yes	No
Potential for early dislodgement of catheter	Yes	No	No
Potential for gastric separation	Possible	Possible	Yes
Potential for infection	Yes	Yes	Yes
Potential for gastrocolic fistula	Possible	No	Yes
Incidence of external leakage	Moderate	Significant	Low
'Permanent'	No	Yes	No
Suitable for passage of dilators for esophageal stricture	Yes	No	No
Interferes with gastric reoperation (fundoplication)	No	Yes	No
Suitable for infants	Yes	No	Yes

Table 2   Comparison of commonly used gastrostomy devices

	de Pezzer, Malecot, T-tube	Foley (balloon type)	Skin-level (button type)
Suitable for initial insertion	Yes	Yes	Yes
Suitable for decompression	Yes	Yes	Yes*
Tendency for accidental dislodgement or external migration	Moderate[†]	Moderate	Very low
Tendency for internal (distal) migration	Moderate	High	Unlikely
Tendency for peristomal leakage (particularly large tubes)	Moderate	Moderate	Low
Reinsertion	Easy to moderately difficult	Easy	Easy to moderately difficult
Long-term (particularly ambulatory patient)	Adequate	Adequate	Best suited

*With special adaptor
[†]High with Malecot

Decompression with or without enteral feeding

When a gastrostomy is placed in conjunction with another intra-abdominal procedure (such as fundo-plication or repair of duodenal atresia), the tube is used initially for decompression and then for intragastric feedings. If prolonged gastric or duodenal dysmotility is anticipated a smaller, more flexible catheter is advanced into the lumen of the jejunum, exiting either along the gastrostomy tube or through a counter-incision[1].

A palliative decompressive gastrostomy can be of value in the management of patients with intestinal obstruction secondary to unresectable malignancy[1].

All gastrostomy types, except gastric tubes, are suitable for this purpose.

Contraindications

Contraindications to percutaneous endoscopic gastro-stomy are inability to perform upper tract endoscopy safely or to identify transabdominal illumination and see an anterior gastric wall indentation clearly. Anatomical abnormalities such as malrotation or marked scoliosis, ascites, coagulopathy, and intra-abdominal infection, if severe, may render the procedure inadvisable.

Preoperative

Gastrostomy for feeding

Gastroesophageal reflux, as a manifestation of foregut dysmotility, is a common problem in neurologically impaired children both before and after the placement of a gastrostomy[1]. Evaluation for reflux in these patients generally includes an upper gastrointestinal barium study, esophageal manometry and 24-h pH probe. In some children a gastric emptying study is also needed. Patients with severe reflux are best managed with an antireflux procedure and a Stamm gastrostomy. Children with mild or no reflux are candidates for gastrostomy only[5].

Gastrostomy as an adjunct in children with surgical lesions

The addition of a stoma to the surgical correction of a congenital or acquired lesion should be considered only if it will substantially facilitate perioperative or long-term care. Examples in neonatal surgery include complex esophageal atresias, certain duodenal obstructions, abdominal wall defects in which long-term ileus is anticipated, and short gut syndrome. Indications in older children include severe esophageal stricture, complex foregut trauma, intestinal pseudo-obstruction, malignancy and complex adhesive bowel obstruction.

Operations

STAMM GASTROSTOMY

This operation is performed using general endotracheal anesthesia. The child is positioned with a small roll behind the back to elevate the epigastrium, then prepared and draped. The author prefers to use a de Pezzer-type catheter ranging in size from 12 Fr (full-term neonates) to 20 Fr for adolescents, and a 10 Fr T-tube or Malecot catheter for preterm infants or neonates with very small stomachs. The procedure may be modified slightly to accommodate the initial placement of a skin-level device.

Incision

1 The stomach is approached through a short transverse supraumbilical incision. Fascial layers are incised transversely and the muscle retracted or transected. The catheter exit site is approximately at the junction of the lower two-thirds and the upper one-third of a line from the umbilicus to the mid-portion of the left rib cage, over the mid-rectus muscle. A vertical incision may be useful in children with a high-lying stomach or a narrow costal angle.

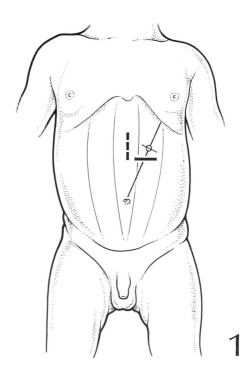

1

Production of gastrostomy site on anterior gastric wall

2 Traction guy sutures and a purse-string suture (synthetic, absorbable) are placed as shown. The opening should be away from the gastric pacemaker at the level of the splenic hilum; away from the greater curvature because that site may be needed for construction of a gastric tube for esophageal replacement; away from the fundus to allow for a possible fundoplication; and away from the antrum to prevent excessive leakage and pyloric obstruction by the catheter tip. If the catheter is to be placed cranially and close to the lesser curvature for a gastrostomy with antireflux properties care must be taken to avoid the vagus nerve.

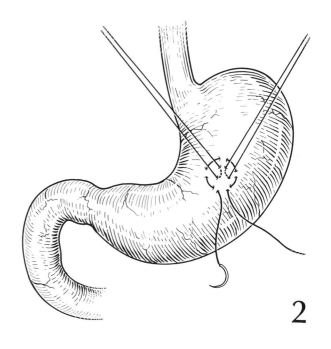

2

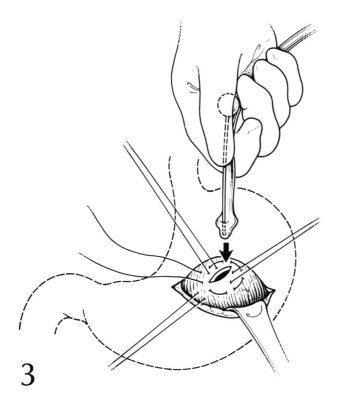

3

3 A lower guy suture pulls the stomach caudally, enhancing exposure and allowing better gastric access. The gastrotomy is performed with fine scissors or cautery while the upper guy sutures are lifted to prevent injuring the back wall. The de Pezzer catheter is introduced using a simple stylet while these sutures are elevated.

4 The purse-string suture is tied. A continuous synthetic absorbable monofilament suture (polydioxanone) is used to anchor the stomach to the anterior abdominal wall. A Kelly clamp is placed through the counter-incision and the abdominal wall layers pushed inwards. The posterior 180° of the anastomosis are completed, the peritoneum and fascia incised and the tip of the clamp pushed through. The catheter end is grasped and the tube brought out through the counter-incision.

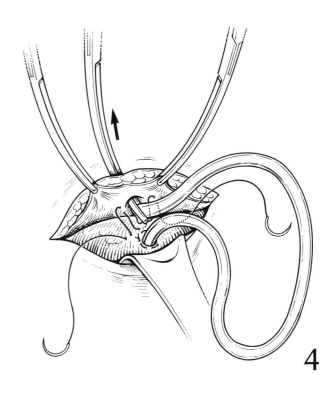

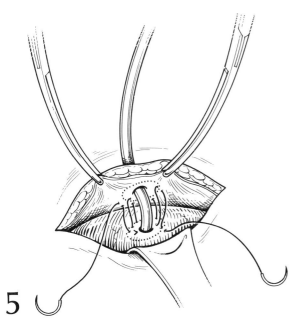

5 Placement of the continuous monofilament suture is now completed. When tied, this suture provides a 360° fixation with a watertight seal. In most cases this maneuver obviates the need for a second purse-string suture.

Wound closure

6 The abdominal wall layers are closed with synthetic absorbable sutures and the skin is approximated with subcuticular stitches and adhesive strips. The catheter is secured with synthetic monofilament sutures (polypropylene). These are removed 1–2 weeks after surgery and a small latex crossbar is placed to prevent distal catheter migration.

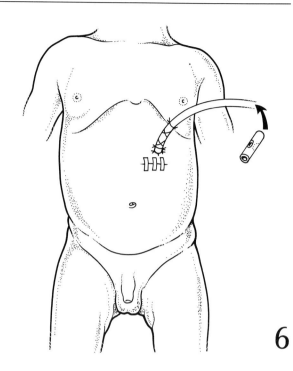

6

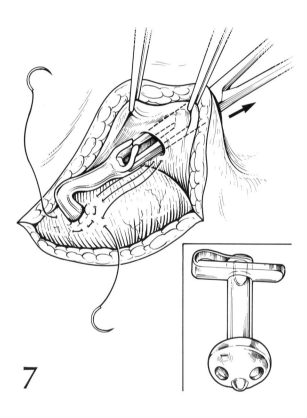

7

7 This standard procedure may be modified to allow insertion of a skin-level gastrostomy device. The gastrostomy 'button' (inset) is available in different shaft lengths and diameters[6]. The shaft length should encompass the invaginated gastric wall, the abdominal wall and an additional few millimeters of 'play' to allow for postoperative edema, ease of care and subsequent growth and weight gain.

8 The stomach is vented with a nasogastric tube or a special decompression device which, when inserted in the shaft, deactivates the one-way valve at the gastric end of the shaft.

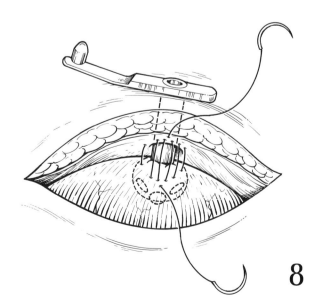

8

JANEWAY GASTROSTOMY

This procedure may be accomplished using either a conventional celiotomy and a GIA stapler or employing an Endostapler under endoscopic control.

9a, b The stapler is employed to tubularize the gastric wall. The gastric tube is brought out away from the incision if the open technique is used, or through one of the port sites if it is performed laparoscopically. The second row of sutures depicted here is optional.

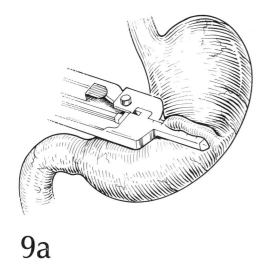

9a

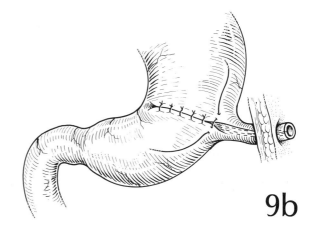

9b

PERCUTANEOUS ENDOSCOPIC GASTROSTOMY

The procedure is best performed in the operating room. Older children and those able to tolerate endoscopy without compromising the upper airway receive local anesthesia with sedation as needed. Younger children require general endotracheal anesthesia primarily because of anticipated difficulties with the airway management. A single dose of a broad-spectrum intravenous antibiotic is given shortly before the procedure. For the endoscopy, the smallest available pediatric gastroscope is used. The catheter and retaining crossbar or catheter head should be soft and collapsible enough to glide atraumatically through the oropharynx and esophagus. The 15-Fr silicone rubber catheter depicted in *Illustration 10* is well suited for children. Hybrid catheters leading to primary implantation of skin level devices are now also available.

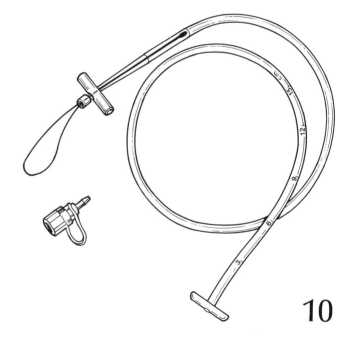

10 A pediatric catheter should be used, with a gastric retainer, markings on the shaft and dilating tapered end with steel wire loop. Also shown in this illustration are skin-level retainer (external crossbar), immobilizing ring and catheter adapter with Luer lock. The catheter is cut to an appropriate length after insertion.

10

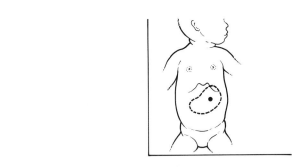

11 The gastroscope is inserted and the stomach insufflated. The stoma should be away from the rib cage to allow placement of an incision if a fundoplication becomes necessary in the future. Under-insufflation or overinsufflation should be avoided to minimize the possibility of accidentally piercing the transverse colon. Insufflation of the small intestine tends to push the transverse colon in front of the stomach and should also be avoided. Digital pressure is applied to the proposed gastrostomy site, which usually corresponds to the area where transillumination is brightest. Transillumination and clear visualization of an anterior gastric wall indentation are key points. Without these, an open or laparoscopic technique should be employed.

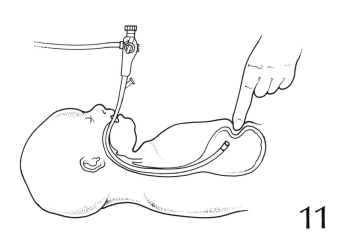

11

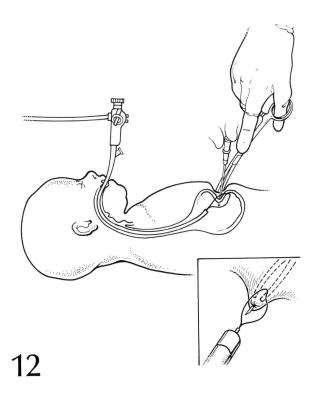

12

12 An incision of 8–10 mm is made in the skin and a Kelly-type hemostat applied to maintain the intragastric indentation. The endoscope is moved gently in small increments. The endoscopist then places the polypectomy snare around this 'mound'. The intravenous cannula is placed in the incision between the slightly spread prongs of the hemostat and then firmly thrust through the abdominal and gastric walls, exiting through the tip of the 'mound' into the loop of the polypectomy snare. The snare is partially closed, but not tightened around the cannula.

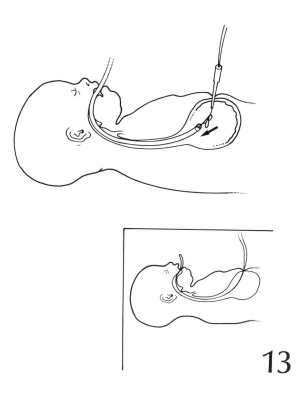

13 The needle is removed and the looped steel wire inserted through the cannula. The polypectomy snare is allowed to slide away from the cannula and is tightened around the wire. An alternative method is to retrieve the wire with alligator or biopsy forceps. The wire is then pulled back with the endoscope through the stomach and esophagus, exiting through the patient's mouth. A guiding tract is thus established.

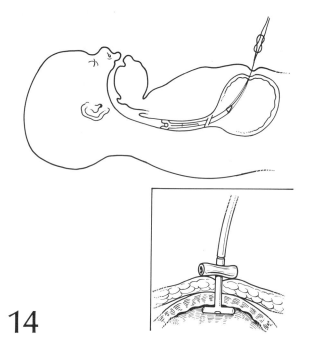

14 The catheter is attached to the guidewire by interlocking the two steel wire loops. Traction is applied to the abdominal end of the wire, guiding the catheter through esophagus, stomach and across gastric and abdominal walls. The collapsed wings of the gastric retainer minimize the risks of esophageal injury (for diagrammatic purposes a shortened catheter is shown). The tapered end of the catheter exits through the abdominal wall before the gastric retainer enters the patient's mouth, allowing complete control of the catheter during placement. Traction is continued until the gastric and abdominal walls are in loose contact. The external crossbar and immobilizing ring are slipped over the catheter and guided to the skin level, avoiding pressure from the retaining crossbar on the mucosa or skin. The catheter is cut to the desired length and the feeding adaptor attached. No sutures are used and the catheter is connected to a small clear plastic trap. A gauze pad and tape are applied.

Postoperative care

Enteral feedings begin following an open gastrostomy once the ileus has resolved, and on the day after surgery following percutaneous endoscopic gastrostomy. The dressing is removed after 1–2 days, the wound is examined and, in the case of a percutaneous endoscopic gastrostomy, the external crossbar and retaining ring loosened if necessary. Granulation tissue tends to form after a few weeks and is controlled with silver nitrate sticks. If a long catheter was used with the initial procedure, it can be changed to a skin-level device after 3 months.

Complications

Although generally considered a basic procedure, gastrostomy is associated with a long list of complications related to technique, care and catheter used[1]. Serious technique-related problems include separation of the stomach from the abdominal wall leading to peritonitis, wound separation, hemorrhage, infection, injury to the posterior gastric wall or other organs, and placement of the tube in an inadequate gastric position. Most complications may be avoided by careful choice of the procedure and stoma device, considering it a major intervention and using meticulous technique, approximating the stomach to the abdominal wall, exiting the catheter through a counter-incision and avoiding tubes in the midline.

One of the most serious long-term problems is severe leakage of the gastrostomy. Initially, this should be managed using conservative measures. If these fail, the stoma may be relocated using a simple non-endoscopic variation of the percutaneous endoscopic gastrostomy[1].

A new stoma site is selected and a small incision made. A large curved needle is placed through the leaking stoma, exiting through the new site. The suture is pulled through, establishing a tract. The catheter follows the tract, entering through the malfunctioning stoma and exiting through the new one. Once the catheter is in place, the leaking stoma is closed extraperitoneally.

Follow-up

All children with gastrostomies should be carefully followed to prevent long-term catheter-related complications and manifestations of foregut dysmotility, particularly gastroesophageal reflux.

References

1. Gauderer MWL, Stellato TA. Gastrostomies: evolution, techniques, indications and complications. *Curr Probl Surg* 1986; 23: 661–719.

2. Haws EB, Sieber WK, Kiesewetter WB. Complications of tube gastrostomy in infants and children: 15 year review of 240 cases. *Ann Surg* 1966; 164: 284–90.

3. Gauderer MWL, Ponsky JL, Izant RJ Jr. Gastrostomy without laparotomy: a percutaneous endoscopic technique. *J Pediatr Surg* 1980; 15: 872–5.

4. Gauderer MWL, Stellato TA. Percutaneous endoscopic gastrostomy in children: the technique in detail. *Pediatr Surg Int* 1991; 6: 82–7.

5. Gauderer MWL. Percutaneous endoscopic gastrostomy: a 10 year experience with 220 children. *J Pediatr Surg* 1991; 26: 288–94.

6. Gauderer MWL, Olsen MM, Stellato TA, Dokler ML. Feeding gastrostomy button: experience and recommendations. *J Pediatr Surg* 1988; 23: 24–8.

Esophagogastroduodenoscopy

Robert E. Cilley MD
Assistant Professor of Surgery and Pediatrics, Division of Pediatric Surgery, Department of Surgery,
Pennsylvania State University College of Medicine, The Milton S. Hershey Medical Center, Hershey,
Pennsylvania, USA

Peter W. Dillon MD
Associate Professor of Surgery and Pediatrics, Division of Pediatric Surgery, Department of Surgery,
Pennsylvania State University College of Medicine, The Milton S. Hershey Medical Center, Hershey,
Pennsylvania, USA

History

Endoscopists in the 19th century used open rigid tubes to visualize the upper gastrointestinal tract. The characteristics of rigid endoscopes were improved by the addition of conventional lenses that provided magnification and some increase in the viewing angle. When miniaturized for pediatric applications the narrow viewing angle and the poor light transmission inherent in these devices limited their usefulness. A major advance in small diameter endoscopes was the development of the rod-lens telescope first available in 1966, together with the development of bright distal light sources. Since the development of flexible fiberoptic endoscopes in 1958, technical improvements, combined with the development of a wide variety of specialized equipment, have expanded the diagnostic and therapeutic potential of this technique. Flexible endoscopes for upper gastrointestinal endoscopy are now available in small sizes ideally suited to pediatric applications[1].

Principles and justification

Indications

Endoscopy of the upper gastrointestinal tract is indicated from the history or the cardinal signs of bleeding, dysphagia or pain.

Upper gastrointestinal tract bleeding

Flexible fiberoptic esophagogastroduodenoscopy definitively diagnoses most upper gastrointestinal tract bleeding. Definitive or palliative treatment may be provided for certain lesions. Esophageal varices may be treated by endoscopic sclerotherapy or variceal banding. Ulcer bleeding may be controlled by injection of sclerosants or coagulation using electric current, heat or laser energy.

Esophageal obstruction

Endoscopy is crucial in the diagnosis and treatment of foreign bodies, tumors, strictures and achalasia. The diagnosis can be made by direct inspection or by obtaining biopsy material. Foreign bodies may be removed. Achalasia may be treated by balloon dilatation and esophageal strictures may be treated by a number of dilatation techniques. Dilatation may be made easier and safer using endoscopy to visualize and assist in the passage of guidewires, strings and dilators.

Caustic ingestion/esophageal injury

Upper gastrointestinal endoscopy is mandatory in the initial evaluation of ingestion of acid or caustic substances. Esophagitis may be diagnosed, graded and followed using endoscopy to assess the response to medical and surgical therapy.

Adjuncts to feeding

Endoscopic techniques may be used to place gastrostomy tubes (percutaneous endoscopic gastrostomy) and transpyloric feeding tubes.

Choice of endoscope

The choice of rigid or flexible endoscopes depends on the procedure planned and the experience and training of the surgeon. The safety and ease of flexible endoscopy makes it the procedure of choice for most pediatric upper gastrointestinal endoscopic procedures. The ability to insufflate air and thus distend the esophagus and allow complete visualization ahead of the advancing esophagoscope is the principal advantage of the fiberoptic endoscope. Removal of an impacted foreign body may be easier with the rigid esophagoscope. The endoscopist should be familiar with both techniques.

Rigid esophagoscopes

The Storz–Hopkins rod lens telescope is utilized almost exclusively in performing rigid esophagoscopy. Unlike a conventional telescope that uses small lenses with long intervening air spaces, this system uses long glass rods with their ends shaped in the form of a lens and small intervening air space. This lens system allows transmission of a brilliant magnified image through a small diameter tube. A wide variety of endoscopic instruments are available to perform such tasks as foreign body retrieval and sclerotherapy. General anesthesia with endotracheal intubation is required under most circumstances.

Flexible fiberoptic endoscopes

Adult endoscopes are typically 11.0–12.6 mm in diameter and, although they may be passed into the esophagus of children, they are too large for maneuvers such as intragastric retroflexion for fundic visualization or transduodenal passage. Large endoscopes with two channels may have some advantages in emergency sclerotherapy for bleeding since one channel can be used for suction and irrigation while the other is used to direct the sclerotherapy needle. Endoscopes of intermediate size, 9.0–10.0 mm, are versatile and may be used in both adults and older children. Smaller instruments with an outside diameter of 7.9 mm were designed specifically for infants and children. High resolution 5-mm instruments are now becoming available, allowing complete upper gastrointestinal endoscopy to be performed on the smallest of infants.

Image processing systems

Image processing systems that allow the endoscopic image to be projected onto a video monitor are invaluable for teaching and documentation (hard copy imaging). Also, by allowing everyone in the operating room or endoscopy suite to visualize the procedure, there is a greater sense of participation among all involved. It is worth emphasizing that live video turns a room full of disinterested assistants into a gallery of involved participants. Modern endoscopes that utilize a video image processor located at the working end of the endoscope and are not dependent upon optical fibers to carry the image over the length of the instrument offer incredibly sharp images.

Preoperative

Patients should be nil by mouth for an appropriate period of time before sedation or anesthesia (e.g. 4 h in infants and 6 h in toddlers and young children). The mouth should be examined for loose and potentially dislodgeable teeth. Explanations appropriate to the age of the child should be given

Anesthesia

Upper gastrointestinal endoscopy should be performed either in the operating room or in an appropriately equipped, dedicated endoscopy suite. Equipment should be immediately available to provide airway and breathing support, including suction devices, supplemental oxygen, airways, bag/mask devices, and equipment for endotracheal intubation. Adjuncts to circulatory support including intravenous therapy, fluids, intraosseous devices and available resuscitation medications are essential. The equipment and personnel to manage vomiting, seizures, anaphylaxis and cardiopulmonary arrest must be available. Cardiorespiratory monitoring and pulse oximetry should be performed. An assistant for patient monitoring is essential. This may be either an anesthetist, nurse anesthetist, or nurse

assigned to the patient. It is preferable that this person is not the endoscopy assistant whose attention is focused more on the procedure and equipment. Guidelines for monitoring and management of pediatric patients undergoing pharmacologic sedation for diagnostic and therapeutic procedures have recently been published[2].

General endotracheal anesthesia provides the most secure airway during endoscopic manipulations and is preferred by many surgeons. General anesthesia may be avoided using techniques of conscious sedation. Most commonly, a benzodiazepine is used in combination with a narcotic (*Table 1*). Alternatively, a barbiturate may be used.

Table 1

Medication	Dose	Administration
Midazolam	0.1–0.15 mg/kg	One or two doses separated by 5 min.
Meperidine	1.0 mg/kg	Given after midazolam. Two doses separated by 5 min. Additional dose during procedure if needed

Operation

The following endoscopic techniques are commonly used by pediatric surgeons.

Passage of the rigid esophagoscope

1   For this procedure the child is anesthetized and endotracheally intubated. Supporting towels are placed under the shoulders to maintain the head in full extension. The oropharynx is suctioned. Although the esophagoscope may be passed directly into the cervical esophagus by visualizing through the esophagoscope as it is passed, this maneuver is facilitated by lifting the tongue and epiglottis with a laryngoscope and directly visualizing the entry into the esophagus. It is critically important that the oroesophageal axis is straight ('sword-swallower's' position) during rigid esophagoscopy. The teeth, if present, are protected by a gauze pad or plastic guard.

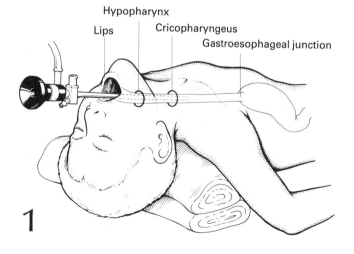

Lips   Hypopharynx   Cricopharyngeus   Gastroesophageal junction

1

2 The esophagoscope is grasped with the supporting hand much as one would grasp a pencil, while the remaining fingers of that hand rest against the maxilla or upper teeth.

The esophagoscope is then advanced – in the words of Chevalier Jackson[3]. '. . . the word insinuate is better than introduce, since it implies to introduce slowly, as through a winding and narrow passage. . . the esophagoscope is advanced. . .watching the folds as they unfold and recede.'

If any difficulty is encountered in negotiating the lumen of the esophagus, a small soft catheter may be used as a lumen finder. Again, Chevalier Jackson[3] advises: 'When no lumen is visible a search for a lumen is made by gentle palpation with the lumen finder. When the lumen is found the esophagoscope may be gently and safely advanced. The lumen finder is not, in any sense, a mandril for blind introduction. . .When it has found and entered deeply into the lumen, the esophagoscope is advanced.'

The narrowest points along the way are the cricopharyngeus and the gastroesophageal junction. Once the stomach has been entered, the esophagoscope is withdrawn. It is during the removal of the esophagoscope that the best view is obtained.

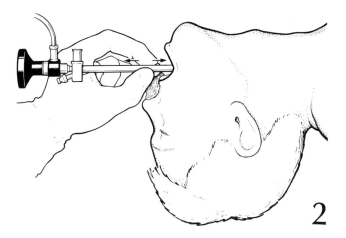

2

Passage of the flexible endoscope for esophagoscopy, gastroscopy or esophagogastroduodenoscopy[4]

In an awake child, conscious sedation is established. Topical anesthetic is applied to the mouth and the child is encouraged to swallow. The patient is positioned laterally with the left side down. Using a mouth guard to protect the endoscope, the instrument is introduced by directly visualizing the oropharynx and the entry into the esophagus through the cricopharyngeus. Entry can be facilitated by coordinating the advancement of the endoscope with spontaneous swallowing. The primary advantage of the flexible endoscope during advancement through the esophagus is the ability to insufflate air easily through the endoscope and with precise control in order to distend the esophageal lumen. Controlled air insufflation not only lessens the danger of esophageal injury during insertion of the endoscope, but also provides a valuable tool for examining the esophageal lumen since the degree of distensibility of the esophageal wall may be altered in pathologic conditions. It must be emphasized that the same dangers found in using rigid instruments are present during flexible esophagoscopy. The esophagoscope should never be forcibly or blindly advanced. The esophagus

may be injured just as easily during manipulations with flexible instruments.

The flexible endoscope may be just as easily passed in the supine, anesthetized, endotracheally intubated patient. Here the entry of the endoscope may be facilitated by digital manipulation in the hypopharynx or visualization of the cervical esophagus using the anesthetist's laryngoscope. Anterior traction on the larynx by an assistant grasping the neck 'opens up' the cricopharyngeus and may facilitate entry of the endoscope.

Air insufflation, although invaluable in visualizing the esophagus, must be controlled, especially in infants and small children. Gaseous distension of the abdomen can compromise ventilation. The lowest adjustment possible of the air insufflation rate is used, and the abdomen is left uncovered so that it may be continuously inspected. The child's temperature may need to be supported by elevating the room temperature, external warming lights and a warming mattress.

After the stomach is entered, insufflation is used to allow a panoramic view. Excessive fluid is suctioned to allow complete visualization of the mucosa. A gastrostomy, if present, must be occluded to allow the stomach to fill. Orientation and endoscopic maneuvers are similar in the lateral and supine positions. Once the stomach is filled with air, the endoscope is retroflexed through 180° and the gastroesophageal junction visualized. The endoscope is straightened and the remainder of the stomach is visualized. With the pylorus in view the endoscope is advanced. Entering the pylorus may be facilitated by rotation of the endoscope. Often it will 'pop' through the pylorus into the duodenal bulb. The best visualization of the pyloric channel may be obtained during the slow removal of the endoscope. In a patient with a pronounced angulation at the incisura (the 'J-shaped' stomach), a considerable length of the endoscope may need to be advanced before the tip will enter the pylorus. Changing the patient's position from supine to lateral or from lateral to supine may also be helpful. The endoscope is advanced to the third or fourth portion of the duodenum and slowly withdrawn. The ampulla of Vater is recognized by the drainage of bile. Cannulation of the ampulla for retrograde cholangiopancreatography is beyond the scope of this discussion. The duodenum, including the bulb and pylorus, is carefully inspected as the endoscope is slowly withdrawn. If the endoscope rapidly exits the duodenum ('falls out') before adequate visualization of these structures, it must be replaced in the duodenum and withdrawn again.

Biopsy techniques

Small cup biopsy forceps that are easily passed through the suction channel of the flexible endoscopes and alongside the telescope within the rigid endoscopy instruments allow precise biopsies to be performed.

Grading of esophagitis

Endoscopic grading of esophagitis is not uniform and is subject to both inter-user and intra-user variability. Nevertheless, description of the mucosal appearance should be part of the language of the endoscopist. The severity of esophagitis can be roughly graded on the basis of the visual appearance alone. Mild esophagitis is indicated by abnormal erythema and friability of the mucosa, moderate esophagitis describes linear erosions and superficial ulcers and severe esophagitis refers to confluent erosions, deep ulcers and diffusely hemorrhagic mucosa[5].

Grading of caustic injury

The severity of esophageal damage should be assessed by direct endoscopic visualization preferably within 24 h of injury. The following is a practical classification that parallels the grading of esophagitis. Mild injury is indicated by mucosal erythema and edema, moderate injury by superficial ulcerations with significant intact mucosa, and severe injury refers to circumferential ulceration, eschar formation, or very deep ulceration[6].

Esophageal sclerotherapy and banding for variceal bleeding

Esophageal variceal bleeding usually stops spontaneously in children with conservative treatment and correction of coagulopathy. Emergency endoscopy to control bleeding is rarely required. If, however, emergency treatment is needed, it is important to have available a large, adult-size two-channel endoscope to facilitate visualization of the site of bleeding.

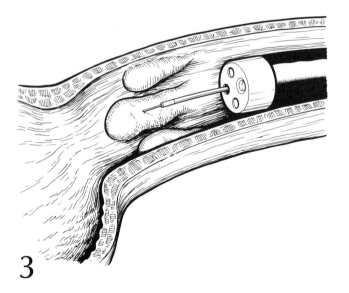

3 Under most circumstances varices are present circumferentially in the distal esophagus and extend a variable distance proximally. Each sclerotherapy session is limited to 0.5 ml of sclerosant per kg body weight. Sodium morrhuate, 50% dextrose and absolute alcohol have all been used for this purpose. The authors use a combination of perivariceal and intravariceal injection and preferentially obliterate an entire column of varices using injections at multiple levels rather than injecting circumferentially at one level. After injection of the varix, the endoscope is advanced and used to tamponade bleeding at the injection site.

3

4a, b

The newer technique of variceal banding requires an adaptor to release the band from the end of the endoscope after the varix is drawn into the end of the band applicator using suction[7]. The rubber band is released by traction on the tripwire. This technique avoids the pain and systemic reactions seen with the injection of sclerosant solutions.

Foreign body removal

Esophageal foreign bodies are encountered in infants (who will put any object into their mouths), children (who consciously put coins and toy parts into their mouths and accidentally swallow them), and patients with a functionally and anatomically abnormal esophagus (most commonly esophageal atresia). Although some advocate fluoroscopically guided balloon extraction as a safe and cost effective alternative to endoscopic foreign body removal, the authors have not adopted this technique. The controlled environment of the operating room is preferred, where adjunctive equipment is readily available to provide airway control. In addition, when the foreign body is removed endoscopically, the esophagus can be directly assessed for damage. The most important technical consideration in foreign body removal is the availability of the proper grasping forceps. A 'coin forceps' with small teeth at its distal end, allowing it firmly to grasp the edge of a coin or small solid object, is essential. Removal of an irregular object such as impacted food material may be facilitated by the passage of a balloon catheter beyond the material which is then withdrawn under direct vision while the airway is controlled by endotracheal intubation.

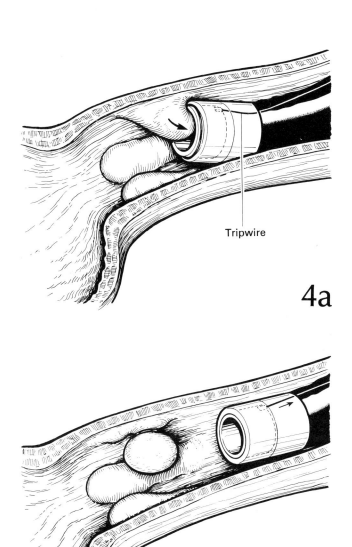

Tripwire

4a

4b

Percutaneous endoscopic gastrostomy

Percutaneous gastrostomy placement may be performed using either conscious sedation or general anesthesia in the endoscopy suite, intensive care unit or operating theater.

5 The gastroscope is passed and used to identify the anterior stomach in contact with the anterior abdominal wall. Orientation is provided endoscopically visualizing the deformation of the anterior wall of the stomach caused by indenting the proposed gastrostomy site with a probe or finger.

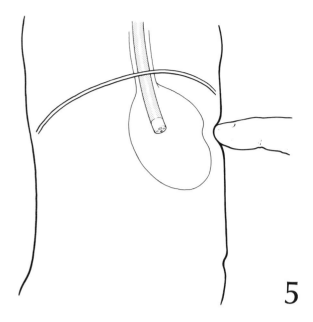

5

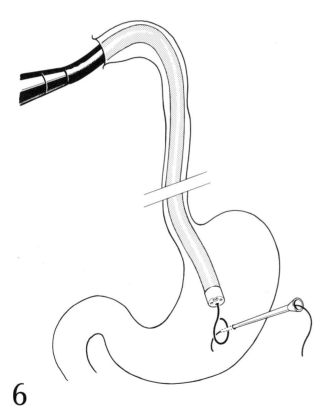

6 A needle is introduced through the gastrostomy site, full thickness of abdominal wall and into the stomach where its entry is visualized endoscopically. A suture passed through this needle is grasped with the endoscopic forceps or in a snare and withdrawn with the gastroscope out of the mouth.

6

7a, b

This suture (usually a plastic coated wire in commercially available kits) is used to guide a dilator on the end of which is a flanged feeding tube which will seat the stomach securely against the anterior abdominal wall when it is drawn out of the gastrostomy exit site. A small incision is made at the skin exit site to accommodate the gastrostomy tube.

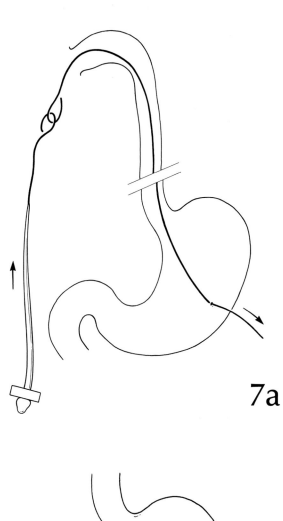

7a

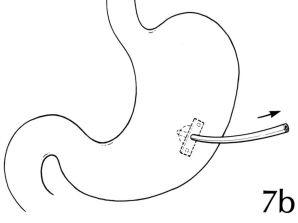

7b

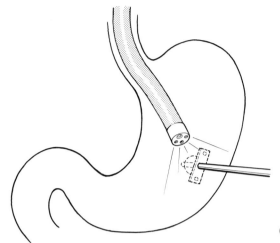

8 The gastroscope is again passed into the stomach and the proper positioning of the feeding tube is confirmed.

Dilatation of esophageal strictures

The flexible gastroscope may be used to facilitate the passage of a guidewire through an esophageal stricture, which may then be used for the passage of sequential over-the-wire dilators. Retrieval of the guidewire through a gastrostomy allows a string to be passed for string-guided dilators. The ease with which strictures can be traversed with a soft-tipped flexible guidewire using direct endoscopic visualization has nearly obviated the need to leave a permanent string through the stricture in all but the most difficult cases.

9 When balloon dilatation is performed for esophageal strictures, the flexible endoscope is essential to position the balloon properly. It is worth noting that, since the operating channel of pediatric gastroscopes is small and passage of the larger dilating balloons may be difficult, the balloon may be directly inserted into the esophagus alongside the gastroscope, and still be precisely positioned under direct vision. The dilating balloon is inflated to a preset pressure according to its diameter as recommended by the manufacturer, and held at that pressure for 2 minutes. The application of radial forces using a balloon results in much less shear force to the esophageal lining than an equivalent dilatation using prograde or retrograde techniques.

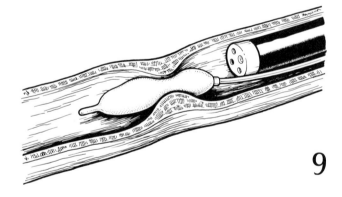

Postoperative care

The endoscopic procedure itself may be performed on an outpatient basis. Concurrent or underlying disease may necessitate hospitalization. A chest radiograph is obtained whenever significant manipulation of the esophagus has occurred such as during a dilatation procedure. The finding of mediastinal air or pneumothorax mandates esophagography with a water-soluble contrast medium to assess the degree of injury. Minor, self-contained perforations may be treated conservatively with antibiotics and hospitalization and possibly pleural drainage. Large perforations with significant pleural or mediastinal communication should be primarily repaired and drained.

Sclerotherapy may result in significant chest pain requiring narcotic analgesia. Esophageal ulceration and stricture may also result. Sucralfate is given by mouth for 1 week after sclerotherapy. Strictures following sclerotherapy usually respond to dilatation.

Percutaneously placed gastrostomy tubes may be used for feeding almost immediately, although the authors usually wait until the day after the procedure. Percutaneous gastrostomies require immediate operation for early tube dislodgement. Abdominal wall cellulitis will usually respond to antibiotic therapy. Failure to secure the gastric wall securely to the abdominal wall with resultant intraperitoneal leakage requires operative correction. Gastrocolic fistula may result from inclusion of a portion of the transverse colon in the path of the tube.

References

1. Gans SL. Principles of optics and illumination. In: Gans SL, ed. *Pediatric Endoscopy*. New York: Grune and Stratton, 1983: 1–8.

2. Committee on Drugs. Guidelines for monitoring and management of pediatric patients during and after sedation for diagnostic and therapeutic procedures. *Pediatrics* 1992; 89: 1110–15.

3. Jackson C. Difficulties and pitfalls in the insinuation of the esophagoscope. *Ann Otol Rhinol Largyngol* 1936; 45: 1109–13.

4. Cadranel S, Rodesch P. Fiberendoscopy of the upper gastrointestinal tract. In: Gans SL, ed. *Pediatric Endsocopy*. New York: Grune and Stratton, 1983; 67–86.

5. Schwesinger WH. Endoscopic diagnosis and treatment of mucosal lesions of the esopahgus. *Surg Clin North Am* 1989; 69: 1185–203.

6. Tunell WP. Corrosive strictures of the esophagus. In: Welch KJ, Randolph JG, Ravitch MM. O'Neill JA, Rowe MI, eds. *Pediatric Surgery*. Chicago: Year Book Medical Publishers, 1986; 698–703.

7. Pricolo VE. Gastrointestinal endoscopy. In: Wilmore DW, Brennan MF, Harken AH, Holcroft JW, Meakins JL, eds. *Care of the Surgical Patient*. New York: Scientific American, 1993: 1–25.

Laparoscopy in infants and children

Thom E. Lobe MD, FACS, FAAP
Chairman, Section of Pediatric Surgery, University of Tennessee and Le Bonheur Children's Medical Center, Memphis, Tennessee, USA

History

The use of laparoscopy in infants and children was introduced by Gans and Austin in the early 1970s. Since then other investigators have confirmed their early results and laparoscopy is now an established method of investigation and treatment in a wide variety of conditions in infants and children.

Principles and justification

Indications

Laparoscopy is indicated for *diagnosis* only when more simple studies are inadequate and when exploratory laparotomy would otherwise be considered. It is indicated for *therapy* only when such a procedure can be carried out safely without laparotomy and when the laparoscopic and open procedures are equally effective.

Laparoscopy is most commonly used to inspect the intraperitoneal contents, because all four quadrants of the abdominal cavity may be inspected through one tiny puncture. Investigative procedures carried out by this technique include exploration for occult pain, contralateral hernia, intra-abdominal testis, trauma, biliary atresia and for intersex. Laparoscopy is also used for operative procedures, which include appendectomy, cholecystectomy, Meckel's diverticulectomy, adhesiolysis for partial small bowel obstruction, fundoplication for gastroesophageal reflux, splenectomy, varicocelectomy, tumor staging and aspiration or excision of cysts.

Liver biopsy

Many patients have hepatobiliary conditions which, even after thorough study, may require a piece of liver tissue for accurate diagnosis. The simplest method of liver biopsy is using a percutaneous needle, but occasionally the results are unsatisfactory and open operation for liver biopsy is necessary. In the author's experience examination and biopsy using laparoscopy has distinct advantages over the open procedure:

1. The color, size, structure and feel of the liver can be evaluated and the presence of cysts, hemangiomas, nodules, tumors or diffuse hepatic processes noted before the biopsy needle or forceps is directed into the most promising areas. Focal or nodular lesions may be missed by blind needling and direct observation prevents penetration of vascular or other potentially harmful targets.
2. Any bleeding or leakage of bile persisting after biopsy is readily observed and controlled by suture or electrocoagulation.
3. A better view of the liver and even of the spleen is obtained.
4. The risks of adhesion formation and other surgical complications are reduced.
5. The operating time and stay in hospital are shorter and there is no abdominal scar.

Cholangiography

Percutaneous transhepatic cholangiography may be performed in well selected cases. It is not an easy maneuver but, when successful, it is definitive.

In a small number of older infants or children with jaundice, laparoscopy is considered after the usual investigations. The appearance of the liver and gallbladder is significant, and biopsy and percutaneous transhepatic cholangiography can be undertaken using this technique with acceptable safety, frequently avoiding open surgery. In some cases the findings on laparoscopy provide a definite indication for operation.

Ascites

Removal of the ascitic fluid, replacing it with carbon dioxide, followed by laparoscopy, may reveal the etiology of the condition.

Cysts and tumors

A clear view and biopsy of abdominal cysts and tumors sometimes surpass other procedures in providing necessary information for indications for surgery, or for the avoidance of open surgery when scattered metastases are seen. This is particularly true for tumors of the liver. In selected cases, second-look procedures may be appropriate.

Pelvic procedures

If the anatomic or hormonal status of the uterus, tubes and ovaries is in doubt, laparoscopy will find its greatest application in three different age ranges: (1) the newborn with ambiguous genitalia; (2) the child with pain or precocious puberty; (3) the postpubertal adolescent with pain.

Ovarian tumors may be biopsied, ovarian cysts aspirated and adhesions may be separated using electrocoagulation or the tine scissors.

Occult pain

Occult abdominal pain is categorized as recurrent, bizarre or chronic abdominal pain for which a satisfactory diagnosis cannot be established by the usual methods and for which laparotomy is now being considered. Non-surgical causes of such pain, for example regional enteritis and salpingitis, may be identified using laparoscopy and the appropriate medical therapy given. Laparoscopy is also helpful, if no pathology is found, in providing reassurance that the organs are normal and that no disease is present.

Ventriculoperitoneal shunt

Correction of malfunctions of ventriculoperitoneal shunts with the laparoscope is one of the most rewarding of its capabilities. Entrapment or encystation of the peritoneal catheter can be corrected by shifting its position to an appropriate site. Peritoneal fluid and tissue are easily obtained for culture. The entire peritoneal cavity is visualized and the region most suitable for repositioning of the shunt catheter is determined. Finally, the use of laparoscopy rather than laparotomy minimizes the formation of new adhesions within the abdominal cavity and may therefore reduce the risk of recurrent problems.

Trauma

Non-operative treatment for a ruptured spleen or liver is now preferred in abdominal trauma. When laparotomy is being considered, however (even when a considerable amount of blood is present in the peritoneal cavity), laparoscopy can be used to determine whether active bleeding is occurring, and which organ is bleeding. Furthermore, the infant or child with severe multiple organ system trauma, who is usually unconscious, requires rapid and accurate assessment, urgent respiratory and circulatory resuscitation and maintenance, and prompt therapeutic intervention. In a child who has sustained significant trauma to the head, chest, and extremities, the possibility of serious intra-abdominal injury must be ruled out before the priority of any particular regional or organ intervention is determined. Laparoscopy can be carried out quickly in the emergency room, intensive care unit, or in the operating room with portable equipment and will help provide the surgeons with information to make decisions.

Emergency laparoscopy

Indications for emergency laparoscopy are multiple organ system trauma, impaired sensorium, unexplained falling hemoglobin level, equivocal abdominal examination, or a stab wound with questionable abdominal wall penetration.

Contraindications

Laparoscopy is contraindicated in infants and children for whom general anesthesia is contraindicated, such as infants in shock. It is further contraindicated in conditions where a coagulopathy may lead to hemorrhage that is difficult to control. Pregnancy in adolescents, peritonitis, adhesions and intestinal obstruction warrant caution and possibly some modification in technique, but are no longer considered contraindications to laparascopy.

Preoperative

The stomach should be emptied if the upper organs are to be examined; the bladder and colon should be emptied if the lower organs or pelvis are to be examined. A Credé maneuver is usually sufficient to empty the bladder, except when pelvic exploration is to be undertaken, in which case an indwelling Foley catheter should be inserted.

Anesthesia

General anesthesia with endotracheal intubation is preferred because pneumoperitoneum significantly inhibits diaphragmatic movement.

Instruments

A wide variety of instruments are suitable for laparoscopy in infants and children. The Storz laparoscopic pediatric instruments are the standard for infants; all other instruments used should be compared with these.

A high-flow insufflating device is used to introduce carbon dioxide and to automatically control the flow and pressure of the gas. A xenon light source is also important.

The Veress needle with a spring-controlled stylet is used for closed access. A blunt trocar or Hasson cannula is used by many for open access.

Cannulas with trocars, instruments for grasping, retraction, biopsy, suction, electrocoagulation, palpation, cutting, and dissection complete the basic set. More advanced techniques require linear staplers, clip appliers, needle holders, and tissue extraction devices.

A video camera for projection onto multiple monitors is essential. Video recorders, printers, and slide makers are desirable accessories for documentation and for teaching.

Carbon dioxide insufflation

Position of patient

1 The patient is placed in the supine position on the operating table under endotracheal anesthesia and the operating team and equipment are appropriately positioned. The skin of the abdomen is prepared and draped.

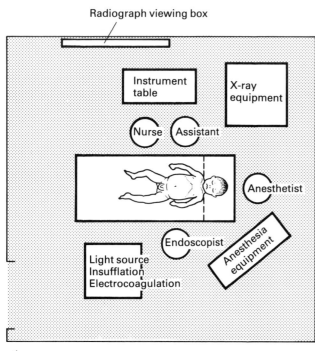

1

Incision

A stab wound is made in the skin with a pointed knife blade. This puncture is usually made in the rim of the umbilicus where the abdominal wall is thin; this central location permits examination of the entire peritoneal cavity and leaves an almost invisible scar. The tissues around the umbilicus may be too thin in the small or malnourished infant or in the infant with an umbilical hernia and air may leak out: in these patients the puncture should be made over the medial portion of one of the rectus muscles, above or below the level of the umbilicus, being careful to avoid damaging epigastric vessels.

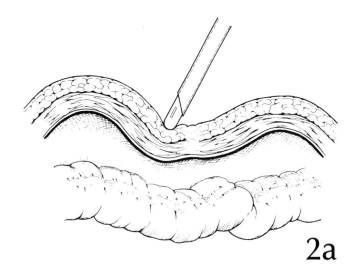

2a

2a–c The abdominal wall is tented upwards by the operator and assistant by grasping it above and below using a sponge between the fingers to maintain traction, and the Veress needle with the spring-controlled blunt stylet is introduced into the peritoneal cavity. As the needle pierces the peritoneum the blunt stylet springs out, thus protecting the abdominal contents from injury.

A 10 ml syringe is connected to the needle and aspiration is carried out to ensure that no bowel contents are present in the needle. Saline solution (5–10 ml) is then injected into the abdomen to demonstrate free flow. The meniscus of fluid in the hub of the Luer lock should descend when the abdominal wall is elevated.

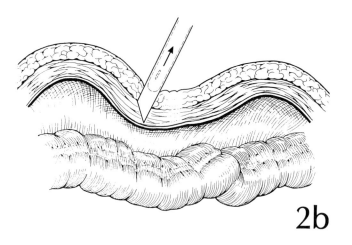

2b

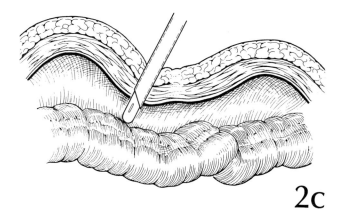

2c

3 Pneumoperitoneum is accomplished by connecting the needle to a carbon dioxide cylinder through the insufflating device so that flow and pressure can be controlled as desired or set automatically. Abdominal pressure should not exceed 8–10 mmHg in an infant, or 10–12 mmHg in the older child.

During insufflation the abdomen is gently percussed and palpated, and the needle is removed once the pneumoperitoneum is considered adequate. The skin puncture is enlarged by spreading it with a hemostat until it admits the trocar and cannula snugly.

Open access may be achieved using a blunt trocar/cannula system. After the umbilical incision is made the wound is spread and the midline fascia grasped with two hemostats, one on either side of the midline. Scissors are then used to incise the midline and the peritoneum is opened sufficiently to introduce the blunt trocar. A 2/0 suture is placed in the fascial edge to secure the cannula in place. The cannula is inserted under direct vision and the sutures are secured to the cleats on the cannula, as the tapered obturator fills the abdominal wall opening to prevent carbon dioxide from escaping.

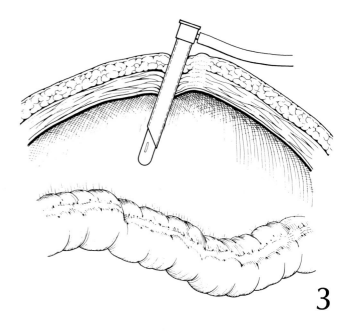

3

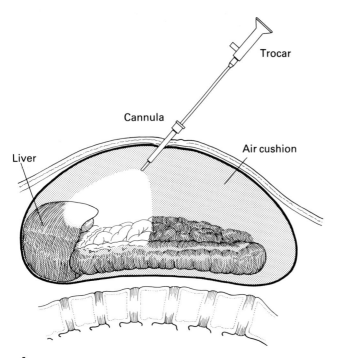

4

4 Once the pneumoperitoneum is established, the abdominal wall is again tented up by grasping it above and below the puncture, and the cannula with a pointed trocar is directed with a twisting motion through the abdominal wall and into the intra-abdominal air cushion. The trocar is then replaced by the appropriate telescope. The viscera underlying the puncture should be inspected before proceeding, to ensure that no injury has occurred.

Inspection of the peritoneal contents may then begin. Any fogging of the telescope may be cleared simply and easily by gently touching the bowel wall with the telescope end. Needles for biopsy or injection may be inserted directly through the abdominal wall under direct vision through the telescope.

5 For more involved manipulations, other appropriately sized cannulas are introduced separately through the abdominal wall, observing their introduction through the telescope. All the accessory instruments listed earlier may be introduced through these cannulas under direct vision.

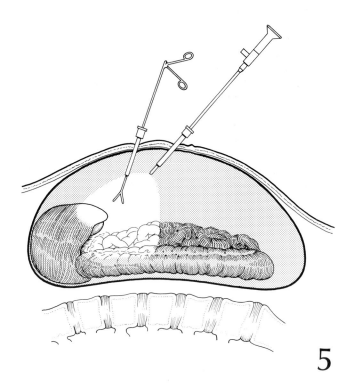

5

Operations

CHOLANGIOGRAPHY

6a, b A plastic needle with metal trocar is introduced through the abdominal wall and peritoneum (shown tented inward in *Illustration 6*), then through the liver and gallbladder bed into the gallbladder. The liver acts as a tamponade to prevent bile leakage. Under direct vision, radiopaque dye is injected and films are made under fluoroscopic guidance.

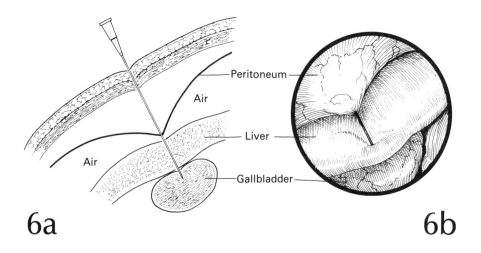

6a

6b

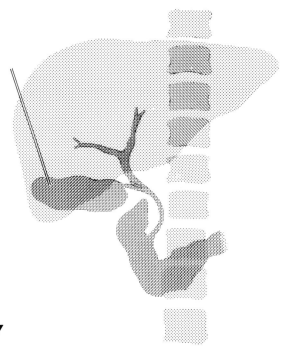

7

7 This method is useful in distinguishing neonatal hepatitis from biliary atresia and from bile duct hypoplasia. If the gallbladder is found to be absent on inspection, this is sufficient evidence to indicate exploration for biliary anomalies. If the gallbladder is present, cholangiography will demonstrate either a normal (as in *Illustration 6*) or an obstructed biliary duct system which could be an indication for open exploration.

CHOLECYSTECTOMY

Laparoscopic cholecystectomy has become the procedure of choice for cholecystitis and cholelithiasis. The procedure is particularly useful in children with sickle-cell disease because it is associated with fewer postoperative pulmonary complications.

8 Most surgeons use four cannulas: an umbilical cannula for the telescope; a subxiphoid cannula for instrumentation; and subcostal, mid-clavicular line and anterior axillary line cannulas for retraction.

9a–d The gallbladder is grasped using the two lateral cannulas for access and the cystic artery and duct are dissected free. Most surgeons believe that an operative cholangiogram should be performed to identify the ductal anatomy before dividing the cystic duct. The cystic duct and artery are divided between clips and the gallbladder is dissected free from the liver bed using electrocautery or laser.

Once hemostasis of the liver bed is assured the gallbladder is removed through the subxiphoid or umbilical cannula.

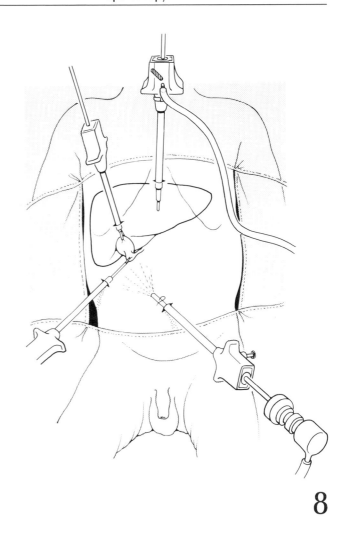

8

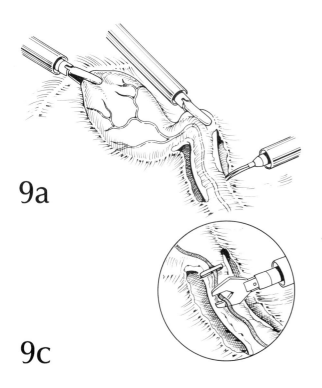

9a

9c

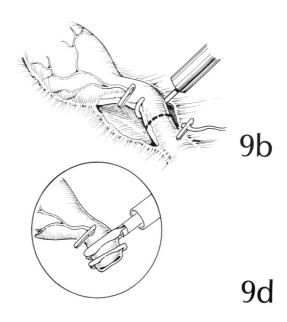

9b

9d

APPENDECTOMY

10 Three cannulas are sufficient for this procedure: an umbilical cannula is used for the telescope and right and left lower quadrant cannulas for instrumentation and removal of the inflamed appendix. Depending on the technique used, a cannula of 10 or 12 mm is inserted into one lower quadrant and one of 5 mm is inserted into the other.

If the appendix is to be removed using clips and endoscopic loops then the larger cannula should be inserted in the right lower quadrant. The appendix is grasped and the mesoappendix divided between clips to skeletonize the appendix. The appendix is freed to its junction with the cecum, pretied surgical loops are applied to base of the appendix and the appendix is divided and removed through the larger cannula.

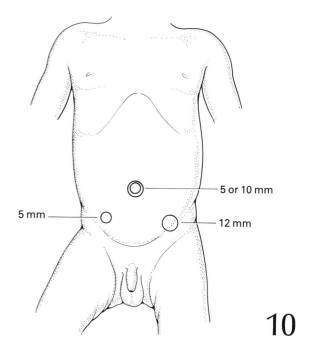

10

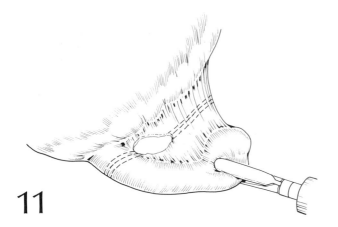

11

11 Alternatively, once the appendix has been grasped, a dissector may be used to create a window between the appendix and the mesoappendix at the junction of the appendix with the cecum. A linear stapler is then used to divide the appendix and the mesoappendix in turn. The appendix is then removed through the larger trocar, which is best placed in the left lower quadrant.

In the case of ruptured appendicitis, an irrigation/aspiration cannula is used to evacuate any pus, minimizing the risks of abscess formation.

FUNDOPLICATION

The indications for a laparoscopic fundoplication are the same as those for the open procedure.

12 The author uses a five-cannula technique: an umbilical cannula for the telescope of 5 or 10 mm; a cannula of 10 mm below the left costal margin in the midclavicular line for suturing; and two cannulas of 5 mm below the costal margin, either side of the suturing cannula. A fifth cannula may be placed below the right costal margin to elevate the liver from the esophageal hiatus.

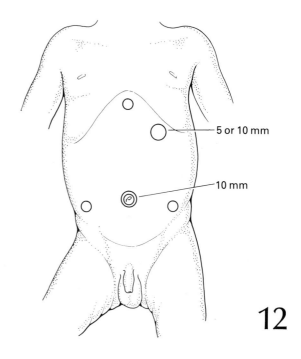

5 or 10 mm

10 mm

12

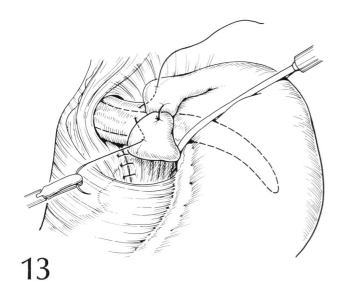

13

13 A bougie is inserted into the esophagus, the hiatus is exposed and the esophagus is mobilized and elevated with an encircling length of umbilical tape, thus exposing the diaphragmatic crura. These are then sutured closed and the fundus of the stomach is brought around the esophagus from behind. The wrap is then sutured into place in the same manner as at an open procedure.

Facility with endoscopic suturing is essential to the success of this procedure. A gastrostomy may be inserted if necessary under laparoscopic observation.

SPLENECTOMY

Laparoscopic splenectomy is useful for a small or moderately sized spleen, but may be difficult for the enlarged spleen. The procedure is most often carried out for hereditary spherocytosis, idiopathic thrombocytopenic purpura, or sickle-cell disease with life-threatening sequestration crises.

14 Five cannulas are used: a 5- or 10-mm umbilical cannula is inserted for use of the telescope; one of 12 mm is placed either in the midline below the xiphoid or to the left of the midline between the costal margin and the umbilicus for stapling the splenic hilum and for extracting the spleen; and two or three 5-mm cannulas are used for grasping forceps or retraction, one on either side of the 12-mm cannula in the upper abdomen and one in the lower left quadrant if necessary for retraction and manipulation of the spleen into the endoscopic bag.

The short gastric vessels are first divided between surgical clips. The patient must then be moved into a lateral decubitus position with the left side up. This allows the colon and other structures to fall out of the way to expose the spleen better.

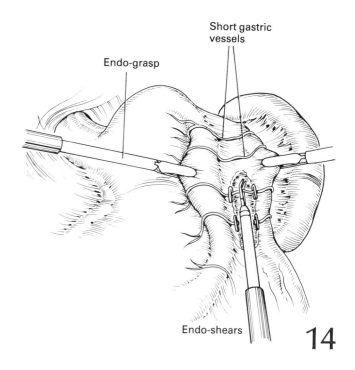

Endo-grasp

Short gastric vessels

Endo-shears

14

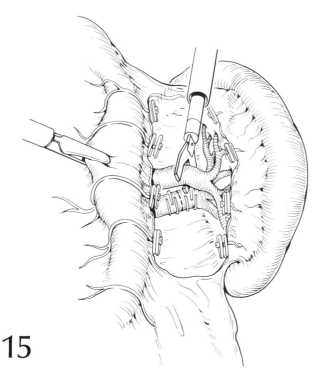

15

15 The splenic flexure of the colon is freed and displaced to expose the splenic hilum. The posterolateral attachments of the spleen are divided, as are remaining short gastric vessels. A linear stapler is then used to divide the splenic hilum – a quick and hemostatic process.

The patient is then returned to a supine position, an endoscopic bag is introduced into the peritoneal cavity and unfurled, and the spleen is placed into the bag. With the open neck of this bag exteriorized, the spleen may be extracted using ring forceps or a tissue morcellator.

Postoperative care

At the conclusion of laparoscopy, the carbon dioxide is allowed to escape from the peritoneal cavity through a cannula. Postoperative care consists of administration of appropriate analgesics and antinausea medications. The author uses oral metoclopramide and transcutaneous scopolamine patches in older children to ameliorate any nausea following laparoscopy.

Following fundoplication, patients are started on oral intake on the day of their procedure and are discharged from the hospital within 36 h. After splenectomy, the patient is started on oral intake the morning after surgery and is ready for discharge within 48 h.

Complications

Two serious complications occur rarely: (1) perforation of the bowel during blind puncture of the abdominal wall or in the use of manipulating instruments; and (2) uncontrollable bleeding from a biopsy site. Both of these complications are readily identified through the laparoscope at the time of occurrence, and appropriate treatment by laparotomy should be instituted immediately.

The incidence of these complications is not accurately known, but must be very low as they are absent from several large series. Considering that laparoscopy is performed only when laparotomy is the alternative, and that use of laparoscopy often avoids the need for laparotomy, the low risk of this procedure is acceptable provided that proper indications and precautions are followed.

Other complications include pneumothorax, gas embolism and thermal burns from laser or electrosurgical devices (recognition of this complication may be delayed). An understanding of the concepts of use of thermal energy in conjunction with intracavitary surgery helps to avoid such complications.

Further reading

Lobe TE, Schropp KP, eds. *Pediatric Laparoscopy and Thoracoscopy.* Philadelphia: WB Saunders, 1994.

Rodgers BM, Vries JK, Talbert JL. Laparoscopy in the diagnosis and treatment of malfunctioning ventriculoperitoneal shunts. In: Gans SL, ed. *Pediatric Endoscopy.* New York: Grune and Stratton, 1983: 179–87.

Stauffer UG. Laparoscopy in hepatology and hepatobiliary diseases. In: Gans SL, ed. *Pediatric Endoscopy.* New York: Grune and Stratton, 1983: 161–8.

Pyloromyotomy

Thom E. Lobe MD, FACS, FAAP
Chairman, Section of Pediatric Surgery, University of Tennessee and Le Bonheur Children's Medical Center, Memphis, Tennessee, USA

History

Sabricius Hildanus first described pyloric stenosis in 1646. Harald Hirschsprung elaborated on the clinical presentation and pathology of the condition in 1888. At this stage the preferred treatment was medical, using a combination of gastric lavage, antispasmodic drugs, dietary manipulation and the application of local heat, because the surgical mortality rate was almost 100%. In 1908 Fredet advocated longitudinal submucosal division of the thickened pyloric muscle, but recommended suturing the defect transversely. In 1912 Ramstedt simplified the Fredet procedure by omitting the transverse suturing, leaving the mucosa exposed in the longitudinal seromuscular defect: this operation was successful and its essential elements have remained virtually unmodified ever since. Surgery has now completely replaced medical measures for the treatment of pyloric stenosis.

Principles and justification

Incidence

The incidence of pyloric stenosis among white people is 2–3 per 1000 live births. Black people are less frequently affected. The male to female ratio is 4:1. The disorder often occurs in first-born boys, and there is a strong familial pattern of inheritance. Vomiting due to pyloric stenosis has been noted in twins whose symptoms began within hours of each other.

Diagnosis

Symptoms usually commence at 2–4 weeks of age, but can sometimes be seen in neonates or in infants closer to 2 months of age. Symptoms may consist of: projectile vomiting of non-bilious material, constipation, dehydration, lethargy or seizures, and failure to thrive. Hematemesis has been documented in a few cases.

Physical signs include variable degrees of dehydration, visible gastric peristalsis, and a palpable pyloric 'tumor'.

If one takes the time to perform a proper clinical examination the diagnosis can nearly always be made without further investigations but, more often, patients will be referred to the surgeon with diagnostic images suggestive of a pyloric tumor.

Special investigations

While diagnostic images may be helpful in difficult cases, none are necessary if clinical examination demonstrates a palpable 'tumor' or 'olive'. When physical examination fails to identify a pyloric mass, ultrasonographic images should be obtained. If ultrasonography is equivocal, then a barium swallow may be helpful. Endoscopy should not be necessary to make the diagnosis of pyloric stenosis, but may be useful in symptomatic patients with other causes for gastric outlet obstruction.

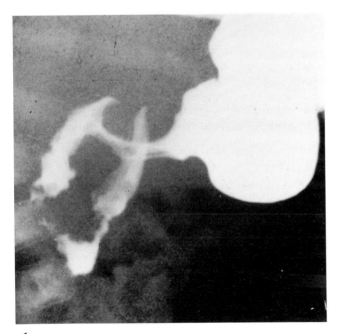

Barium swallow

1 The following features are diagnostic: 'string sign' of the narrow elongated pyloric canal; 'double track' in the pyloric canal owing to infolding mucosa; delayed gastric emptying; gastric hyperperistalsis; or the mushroom effect in the duodenal cap owing to indentation by the pyloric 'tumor'.

1

Ultrasonography

2 This typically shows a thickened pyloric musculature with a central sonolucent area representing the lumen of the pyloric canal. A cross-sectional image of the thickened muscle is easy to recognize as a donut or a bull's eye. Ultrasonographers also use the following measurement criteria to make the diagnosis: pyloric channel >17 mm in length and pyloric thickness >4 mm.

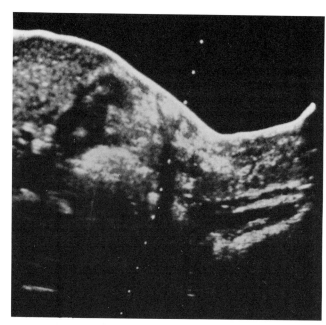

2

Preoperative

Preparation of patient

The operation of pyloromyotomy is *never* an emergency; correction of dehydration and acid–base imbalance take precedence. Parenteral correction of metabolic abnormalities is the safest way to prepare a patient for surgery. An intravenous infusion of isotonic saline or plasma (20 ml/kg) is administered over 60 min. Once urinary output has been established, potassium chloride (20–30 mmol/l) is added to the infusate of 5% glucose in 0.9% saline. The infusion is given at a rate of 150–180 ml/kg body weight per 24 h. It may take as long as 48–72 h for rehydration to be complete and for the infant to be ready for surgery. The goal is to correct the serum electrolytes to nearly normal. Accordingly, the serum potassium should be at least 3–4.5 mEq/l, the serum CO_2 should be <27–30 mEq/l and the serum sodium should be >130 mEq/l before surgery is considered. The serum chloride will usually correct itself to >100 mEq/l with the above measures.

Evacuation of retained contents in the stomach by gastric lavage with warm isotonic saline is also recommended. Preoperative nasogastric suction is not recommended because it will remove sodium, chloride and potassium, thereby depleting the patient of the very electrolytes that need replacement.

Anesthesia

Although local anesthesia has been used successfully, general endotracheal anesthesia is now preferred, particularly if laparoscopy is performed. The stomach should be emptied immediately before induction to avoid vomiting and aspiration. The bladder should be emptied using a Credé maneuver if laparoscopy is used. An intravenous infusion is set up for administration of perioperative fluids and for delivery of muscle relaxants. Some anesthetists may supplement the general anesthetic with a caudal block, particularly if an umbilical incision is used.

Operations

SURGICAL PYLOROMYOTOMY

Position of patient

The patient is placed supine on the operating table. A rolled towel under the mid-thoracic vertebra facilitates delivery of the pyloric tumor into the incision. The stomach should be emptied of any contents with a suction catheter before starting the operation.

Incision

3 A transverse incision 2–3 cm long is made in the right upper quadrant of the abdomen, one finger's breadth below the costal margin and starting immediately lateral to the lateral border of the rectus abdominis muscle. The incision is deepened through the subcutaneous tissues, and the underlying external oblique, internal oblique and transverse abdominis muscles are divided in the line of the incision, using electrocautery for hemostasis as needed. The peritoneum is opened transversely in the line of the incision.

An alternative approach is to enter the peritoneal cavity by splitting the muscles of the anterior abdominal wall in the direction of their fibers. This approach has the disadvantage of exposing unnecessarily wide tissue planes but is claimed to be associated with a lower incidence of dehiscence or later incisional herniation.

Some surgeons believe the transverse incision gives the best cosmetic result but others prefer a vertical, paramedian incision over the rectus muscle. In this case, the vertical incision is carried down through skin, subcutaneous tissues and peritoneum. Many surgeons combine a transverse skin incision with a vertical incision over the rectus fascia and muscle to combine good exposure and a good cosmetic appearance.

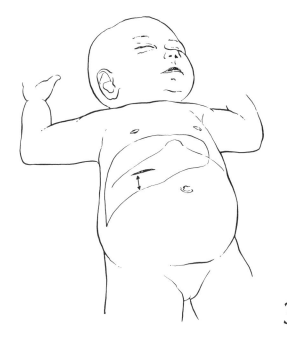

3

4 More recently, an umbilical incision has been used for a better cosmetic result. A curvilinear skin incision is made one-half to two-thirds around the superior circumference of the umbilicus in the umbilical fold. The subcutaneous tissues are spread with a hemostat to expose the midline fascia. The fascia is opened in the midline from the umbilical ring to as far cephalad as necessary to allow easy delivery of the pyloric mass.

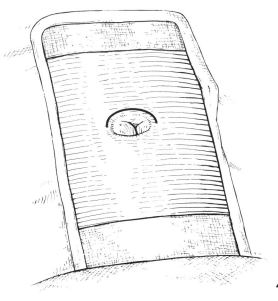

4

Identification of stomach

5 With the peritoneum opened, the liver covers the opening into the peritoneal cavity. The edge of the liver is gently retracted cranially using a malleable retractor protected by a moist gauze sponge.

No attempt should be made to grasp the pyloric tumor directly, as this only leads to serosal tears and hemorrhage. The greater curvature of the stomach is identified and grasped in a moist gauze sponge. If the stomach is not readily found, traction on the transverse colon will draw the greater curvature of the stomach into the wound.

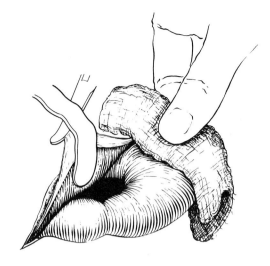

Delivery of pyloric tumor

6 With the greater curvature of the stomach firmly drawn across to the left and exerting traction on the antrum, the pyloric tumor is delivered out of the incision by applying a gentle to and fro rocking traction on the pylorus.

The distal extent of the tumor is marked by the pyloric vein of Mayo. Proximally the tumor is less obvious where it merges with the hypertrophied stomach musculature. The tumor has a glistening greyish appearance and is firm to palpation. There is a relatively avascular plane in the middle of the anterior surface where the vessels entering the pylorus superiorly and inferiorly merge.

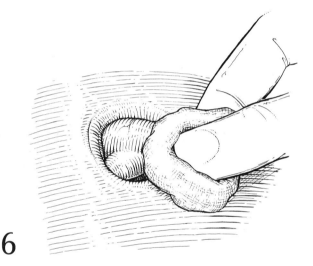

Incision of pylorus

7 A serosal incision is then made in the avascular area on the anterior surface of the tumor. It is carried distally as far as the pyloric vein of Mayo, which marks the pyloroduodenal junction, while proximally it extends well on to the anterior surface of the antrum of the stomach. The length of the incision is 2–3 cm. Protrusion of pyloric tumor into the lumen of the duodenum creates a critical zone of folded duodenal mucosa in a very superficial position at the distal end of the incision. It is in this area that perforation of the mucosa most often occurs.

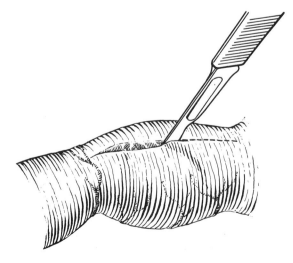

Splitting of pyloric musculature

8 Pressure with a blunt instrument (handle of a scalpel, MacDonald dissector) into the incision, with counter-pressure by a finger placed behind the tumor, allows splitting the hypertrophied muscle fibers down to the submucosa. This appears as a white glistening membrane in the depth of the incision of the pylorus. A twisting movement on the blunt instrument produces an extension of the split proximally and distally and widens the incision. Alternatively, the blunt instrument is gently 'rubbed' back and forth along the incision and over the muscle to split it.

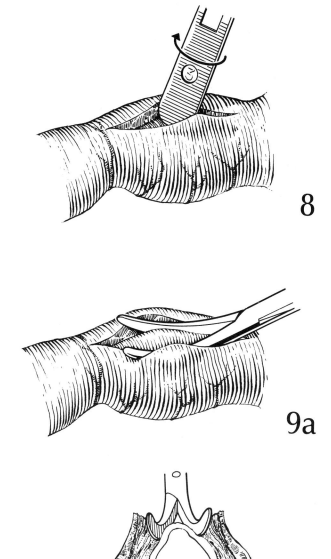

9a, b To ensure that all muscle fibers have been divided throughout the length of the incision, the edges of the split muscle are spread apart with either a pair of blunt forceps (ensuring that the points are held well away from the mucosa) or a pyloric spreader (Denis Browne or Benson and Lloyd) so that the submucosa bulges into the incision. Special care must be taken at the pyloroduodenal junction to avoid entering the lumen of the duodenum, which is particularly vulnerable because of the protrusion of the pyloric tumor into the duodenal lumen. The adequacy of the split is assured if the two halves of the muscle move independently of each other.

Testing for perforation

About 20–30 ml air is introduced into the stomach via the nasogastric tube and then gently milked through the pylorus into the duodenum and a gauze sponge is dabbed on the incision to detect any bile staining. Any perforation of the mucosa will become obvious at this juncture and should be closed by direct suture with 5/0 chromic catgut or polyglycolic acid.

Slight hemorrhage from the edges of the pylorotomy will cease once the tumor has been replaced into the peritoneal cavity and hence venous congestion relieved.

Wound closure

The wound is closed with a running suture of 4/0 polyglycolic acid. The subcutaneous fat layer is closed with continuous 4/0 polyglycolic acid suture and the skin edges are approximated with a 5/0 polyglycolic acid subcuticular suture. Incisions of the abdominal musculature should be closed in layers in the direction of the incision. The vertical fascial incision of the umbilical approach should be closed transversely as this gives a better cosmetic appearance to the wound.

LAPAROSCOPIC PYLOROMYOTOMY

A CO_2 pneumoperitoneum is first established. A 4- or 5-mm umbilical cannula is placed in the umbilicus for insertion of the laparoscope. Two 4-mm cannulae are placed in the left and right sides in the anterior axillary line, lateral to the rectus muscle, at or below the level of the umbilicus.

10 A 3/0 or 4/0 silk retraction suture is then passed through the abdominal wall, through the stomach proximal to the pyloric mass, and then back through the abdominal wall to hold this structure in place against the abdominal wall. A similar suture is placed in the duodenum just distal to the pyloric tumor.

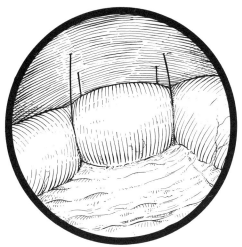

10

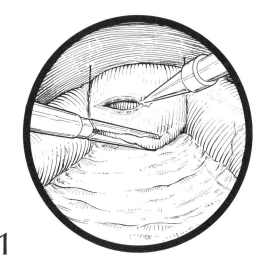

11

11 Using one pair of grasping forceps to secure the tissue, a serosa incision is then made along the pyloric muscle up onto the stomach. This can be made with a pylorotome or a thermal energy device such as a contact laser set at low power. Care should be taken not to extend the distal incision onto the duodenum. A dissector or spreader is then used to separate the edges of the hypertrophied muscle, taking care not to enter the mucosa.

12 It may be helpful during this maneuver to push and fix the pyloric muscle anteriorly against the abdominal wall with the grasping forceps to facilitate the spreading of the muscle. Alternatively, one grasper can be used from the patient's right to hold the pyloric tumor in place against the abdominal wall while the myotomy is made with an instrument inserted from the patient's left.

Unpublished data by Tan on 50 laparoscopic pyloromyotomies suggest that, with experience, the operation takes approximately 10 min to perform, and the patients are on full feed 7 h after surgery.

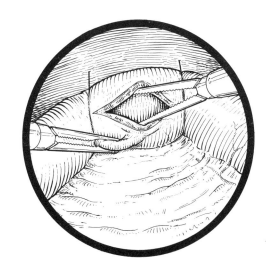

12

Postoperative care

The nasogastric tube is left *in situ* on gravity drainage until the infant is fully recovered from the anesthetic. In the event of a perforation the tube is left on suction for 24 h.

Many feeding regimens have been advocated, varying from commencing oral feeds within 2–4 h of surgery to delaying feeds for 24 h. It has been demonstrated that gastric peristalsis is abolished for 12–24 h after operation and that early introduction of feeds is associated with a high incidence of postoperative vomiting, which may delay discharge from hospital. Persistent vomiting is usually relieved after the stomach is emptied and lavaged with a mild bicarbonate solution; the feeds are then reinitiated. The regimen shown in *Table 1* has been found to be most acceptable.

Table 1 Feeding schedule after pyloromyotomy

Stage	Volume of feed	Type of feed	Interval
I	15 ml	Glucose-saline	3 hours
II	30 ml	Half-strength formula or breast	3 hours
III	60 ml	Half-strength formula or breast	3 hours
IV	90 ml	Full-strength formula or breast	4 hours

Complications

The operation is associated with few complications and operative mortality is extremely rare. Wound sepsis occurs in <5% of cases and is usually caused by *Staphylococcus*. Wound dehiscence occurs in <2% of cases. Recurrence is rare and is usually because of inadequate separation of muscle fibers (to allow submucosa to bulge to the surface) or failure to divide muscle far enough proximally onto the antrum of the stomach. In these cases, the pyloromyotomy should be redone 180° around the pylorus from the original procedure.

Further reading

Alain JL, Grousseau D, Terrier G. Extramucosal pylorotomy by laparoscopy. *J Pediatr Surg* 1991; 26: 1191–2.

Alain JL, Moulies D, Longis B, Grousseau D, Lansade A, Terrier G. Pyloric stenosis in infants. New surgical approaches. *Ann Pediatr (Paris)* 1991; 38: 630–2.

Benson CD. Infantile pyloric stenosis. Historical aspects and current surgical concepts. *Prog Paediatr Surg* 1970; 1: 63–88.

Schärli AF, Leditschke JF. Gastric motility after pyloromyotomy in infants. A reappraisal of postoperative feeding. *Surgery* 1968; 64: 1133–7.

Spicer RD. Infantile hypertrophic pyloric stenosis: a review. *Br J Surg* 1982; 69: 128–35.

Spitz L. Vomiting after pyloromyotomy for infantile hypertrophic pyloric stenosis. *Arch Dis Child* 1979; 54: 886–9.

Tan HL, Najmaldin A. Laparoscopic pyloromyotomy for infantile hypertrophic pyloric stenosis. *Pediatr Surg Int* 1993; 8: 376–8.

Duodenoduodenostomy

Robert E. Cilley MD
Assistant Professor of Surgery and Pediatrics, Division of Pediatric Surgery, Department of Surgery,
Pennsylvania State University College of Medicine, The Milton S. Hershey Medical Center, Hershey,
Pennsylvania, USA

Arnold G. Coran MD
Professor of Surgery and Head of the Section of Pediatric Surgery, University of Michigan Medical School, and
Surgeon-in-Chief, C.S. Mott Children's Hospital, Ann Arbor, Michigan, USA

History

Early in this century congenital duodenal obstruction was almost uniformly fatal. Its surgical correction was made difficult by a lack of appropriate suture material and the lack of understanding of the perioperative care needed by neonates. By the middle of the century enteroenterostomy, typically using a retrocolic side-to-side duodenojejunostomy, became the standard operation for this problem. Improved perioperative care of the sick neonate resulted in many more survivors. More recently, duodenoduodenostomy has been used to bypass congenital duodenal obstruction in an effort to hasten the return of intestinal function after surgery and to promote duodenal emptying[1-3]. Duodenoduodenostomy may be performed in either a standard side-to-side fashion or in an eccentric fashion commonly known as the diamond duodenoduodenostomy[4,5]. A more aggressive approach to the treatment of infants with trisomy 21, in whom duodenal atresia is relatively common, has also contributed to the increasing number of surviving infants who have undergone surgical correction to bypass congenital duodenal obstruction.

Principles and justification

The choice of surgical procedure for the treatment of duodenal obstruction is largely based upon the preference of the surgeon. There may be unusual anatomic variants that make one procedure obviously preferred at the time of surgery. Each surgeon should be familiar with all options. Although the evidence is not conclusive, there is reason to believe that the diamond duodenoduodenostomy is the procedure of choice in most circumstances[6]. Earlier postoperative feeding and shorter duration of hospitalization are purported advantages. This procedure is the choice of the authors and will be described below. The duodenoduodenostomy is applicable to almost all cases of duodenal obstruction, whether caused by stenosis or atresia, with or without annular pancreas. It may also represent the safest choice for the treatment of a duodenal web, since it does not risk damage to the pancreaticobiliary system which may occur with web excision. In the hands of those experienced with the technique, almost any atresia is readily handled using the mobility afforded by the dilated proximal duodenum in combination with mobilization of the distal duodenum beneath the superior mesenteric vessels. Both one-layer and two-layer anastomotic techniques have been used. It is unlikely that either has significant advantage. Although a decompressing gastrostomy was placed at the time of surgery in the past, this is no longer done routinely. Only in a child with multiple anomalies, in whom poor feeding is predictable, will a gastrostomy be added to the duodenoduodenostomy.

The only contraindications to surgery are the presence of multiple severe anomalies incompatible with life. The presence of other correctable anomalies or trisomy 21 no longer precludes surgery.

Preoperative

Neonates with congenital duodenal obstruction most often present with obvious symptoms on the first day of life. Feeding intolerance and vomiting that is usually bilious are noted from the outset. Dehydration and electrolyte depletion rapidly ensue if the condition is not recognized and intravenous therapy begun. Secondary complications such as aspiration and respiratory failure may also be present. The presence of a 'double bubble' on a plain abdominal radiograph is essentially pathognomonic of duodenal atresia. Contrast radiography is confirmatory and may be especially helpful in confirming the pathology when stenosis (incomplete obstruction) or aberrant pancreaticobiliary anatomy (pre- and post-atresia double ampulla) allows air into the distal intestinal tract. Differentiating intrinsic duodenal obstruction from malrotation with volvulus may be difficult and contrast radiography may also be helpful. Duodenal obstruction is treated less urgently than malrotation by some surgeons and thus differentiating between the two entities is critical. Many pediatric surgeons will operate as an emergency on every duodenal obstruction.

Trisomy 21, occurring in one-third of infants, and congenital heart disease must be suspected in all children with duodenal atresia. Concurrent malrotation, esophageal atresia and second intestinal atresias (most commonly in the duodenum itself) are gastrointestinal abnormalities that occur with increased frequency in patients with duodenal atresia[7,8].

Anesthesia

General anesthesia with rapid sequence endotracheal intubation is required. Epidural anesthetic supplementation is now used by many pediatric anesthetists for the operation as well as for postoperative analgesia. Prevention of hypothermia is accomplished by heating the operating room, warming the anesthetic gases, the use of external warming lights while the baby is uncovered, warming the intravenous fluids and the use of adhesive plastic drapes for surgical draping.

Operation

Incision and initial evaluation

1 A small transverse right upper quadrant incision provides adequate exposure. The type and location of the atresia as well as any pancreatic abnormality or the presence of a rare preduodenal portal vein are noted and carefully documented. The patient is checked for any abnormality of intestinal rotation. If present, a Ladd's procedure is carried out.

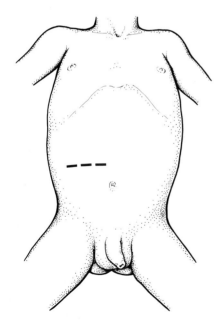

1

Mobilization and retraction

2a, b The hepatic flexure of the colon is mobilized sufficiently to expose the duodenum and the proximal obstructed duodenum is freed from its retroperitoneal attachments (Kocher maneuver). The requirements for distal mobilization vary according to the location of the atresia. If necessary, the entire distal duodenum may be mobilized from beneath the superior mesenteric artery. Rightward traction on the exposed distal duodenum allows these retroperitoneal attachments to be divided. A transpyloric tube is passed to determine if a 'windsock' abnormality is present. Injection of air or saline into the distal segment is conveniently performed at this stage to rule out a second atresia. Either hand-held or fixed, table-mounted retractors may be used.

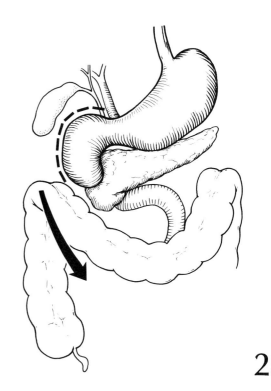

2a

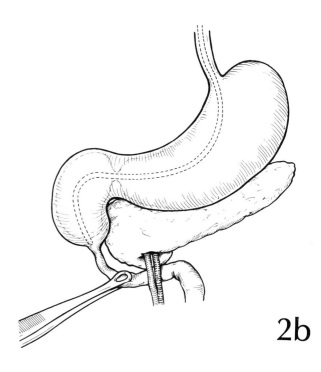

2b

Duodenoduodenostomy

3a–c A transverse duodenotomy is performed in the proximal segment. It is important that this incision be made 1 cm above the atresia to avoid any possibility of injuring the pancreaticobiliary system which may enter anywhere in the vicinity of the duodenal web, stenosis or atresia. A longitudinal duodenotomy of the same length is created in the distal segment. A single layer of interrupted sutures with posterior knots tied inside and anterior knots tied outside ensures symmetry. The orientation of the sutures in the 'diamond' anastomosis is shown in *Illustration 3b*. The completed anastomosis is shown in *Illustration 3c*.

A gastrostomy may be performed if the need is anticipated, and an appendectomy (excisional or inversion) may also be performed.

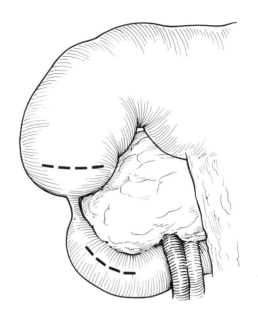

3a

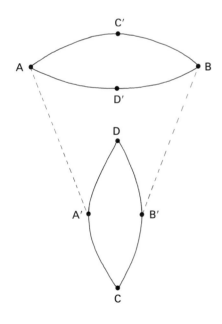

3b

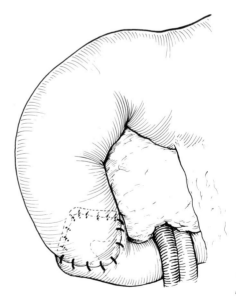

3c

Postoperative care

Postoperative care consists primarily of supportive measures to provide nutrition while awaiting the return of intestinal function. Immediate enteral feeding can be started if a transanastomotic tube is placed at the time of the initial operation. The disadvantages of tube dislodgement and anastomotic injury seem to outweigh the benefits. Parenteral nutrition is used to provide nutritional support postoperatively. To minimize the risks of parenteral nutrition (especially hepatotoxicity), total calories, protein and fat intake should be kept at the lowest levels possible to allow growth. Parenteral nutrition may be provided either peripherally or centrally. Placement of a central venous catheter at the time of surgery is often convenient. Unless the child was septic before surgery, only a prophylactic course of antibiotics is indicated. Ventilatory support is provided as needed. Nasogastric or gastrostomy drainage is maintained until gastric emptying begins as heralded by a change in the quality of the gastric drainage from bilious green to clear or yellow and a decrease in gastric residuals.

Feeding is instituted slowly and may require a period of several weeks before full enteral nutrition is tolerated. Standard infant formulas or breast milk are satisfactory and expensive partially digested formulas are usually unnecessary. If a gastrostomy was placed at the time of initial surgery, it may be removed before discharge from hospital if oral intake is adequate.

Outcome

The outcome depends almost entirely on the presence of other anomalies. Anastomotic leak, intra-abdominal sepsis and wound complications occur rarely. Missed second atresias have been reported. Duodenal atony or paresis with a functional duodenal obstruction in the face of an anatomically patent anastomosis is a rare but frustrating problem. Plication of the duodenum or an alternative method of duodenal bypass are surgical options if conservative observation is unsuccessful. Long-term complications are uncommon. Symptoms such as pain, vomiting and feelings of fullness may be present in up to one-third of patients when studied as adults[9]. Symptoms correlate poorly with objective findings on upper gastrointestinal radiographic studies and endoscopy.

References

1. Fonkalsrud EW, deLorimier AA, Hays DM. Congenital atresia and stenosis of the duodenum. *Pediatrics* 1969; 43: 79–83.

2. Weitzman JJ, Brennan LP. An improved technique for the correction of congenital duodenal obstruction in the neonate. *J Pediatr Surg* 1974; 9: 385–8.

3. Girvan DP, Stephens CA. Congenital intrinsic duodenal obstruction: a twenty-year review of its surgical management and consequences. *J Pediatr Surg* 1974; 6: 833–9.

4. Kimura K, Tsugawa C, Ogawa K, Matsumoto Y, Yamamoto T, Asada S. Diamond-shaped anastomosis for congenital duodenal obstruction. *Arch Surg* 1977; 112: 1262–3.

5. Kimura K, Mukohara N, Nishijima E, Muraji T, Tsugawa C, Matsumoto Y. Diamond-shaped anastomosis for duodenal atresia: an experience with 44 patients over 15 years. *J Pediatr Surg* 1990; 25: 977–9.

6. Weber TR, Lewis JE, Mooney D, Connors R. Duodenal atresia: a comparison of techniques of repair. *J Pediatr Surg* 1986; 21: 1133–6.

7. Nixon HH. Duodenal atresia. *Br J Hosp Med* 1989; 41: 134–40.

8. Stringer MD, Brereton RJ, Drake DP, Wright VM. Double duodenal atresia/stenosis: a report of four cases. *J Pediatr Surg* 1992; 27: 576–80.

9. Kokkonen M-L, Kalima T, Jääskeläinen J, Louhimo I. Duodenal atresia: late follow-up. *J Pediatr Surg* 1988; 23: 216–20.

Achalasia

Lewis Spitz PhD, FRCS, FRCS(Ed), FAAP(Hon)
Nuffield Professor of Paediatric Surgery, Institute of Child Health, University of London, and Consultant
Paediatric Surgeon, Great Ormond Street Hospital for Children, London, UK

History

Achalasia was first described by Willis in 1672. He treated the patient by fashioning a rod of a whale bone with a sponge on the end with which the patient was able to force food into his stomach. In 1877 Zenker and von Ziemssen, and in 1884 Mackenzie, suggested that achalasia was due to diminished contractile power of the esophageal musculature. In 1888 Meltzer and Mikulicz independently postulated that spasmodic contraction of the cardiac sphincter was the etiologic factor. In the same year Einhorn proposed that the condition was due to failure of relaxation of the cardia on swallowing.

Principles and justification

Achalasia is a motility disorder of the esophagus characterized by an absence of peristalsis and a failure of relaxation of the lower esophageal sphincter. The cardinal symptoms in childhood are vomiting, dysphagia, chest pains and recurrent respiratory infections, and weight loss. The child learns to eat very slowly and to drink large quantities of fluid to encourage food to enter the stomach. At first there is only regurgitation of food, but later vomiting of undigested food eaten days earlier occurs. The child with achalasia is often first referred to a psychiatrist for treatment of food aversion or anorexia.

Histopathology

Strips of muscle from the distal esophagus reveal varying pathologies from complete absence of ganglion cells to chronic inflammatory changes through to normal ganglia. Histochemistry reveals a significant reduction in all neuropeptides, particularly vasoactive intestinal polypeptide, galanin and neuropeptide Y.

Treatment

Medical treatment

Transient relief of symptoms can be achieved with nifedipine, a calcium antagonist that reduces the pressure at the lower esophageal sphincter.

Forceful dilatation

The aim of this treatment is to physically disrupt the muscle fibres of the lower esophageal sphincter by means of pneumatic dilatation. A fluid-filled (Plummer) or air-filled (Browne–McHardy, Rider–Möller, angioplasty catheter) bag of fixed diameter is radiologically positioned in the distal esophagus and gently inflated. Relief of symptoms in children is at best temporary but may occasionally last for prolonged periods.

Surgical treatment

The basis of all surgical procedures is the cardiomyotomy described in 1914 by Heller. Controversies concern the length of the myotomy, the extent to which the myotomy extends onto the stomach and the necessity for an antireflux procedure.

The principle of the procedure is to perform a myotomy over the distal 4–6 cm of esophagus, extending the incision for 1 cm onto the anterior wall of the stomach. The myotomy is covered by a short floppy Nissen fundoplication to protect against subsequent gastroesophageal reflux.

Preoperative

Diagnosis

Radiologic features

1 A plain chest radiograph may show a dilated food-filled esophagus with an air–fluid level. There may be radiologic signs of recurrent aspiration pneumonitis.

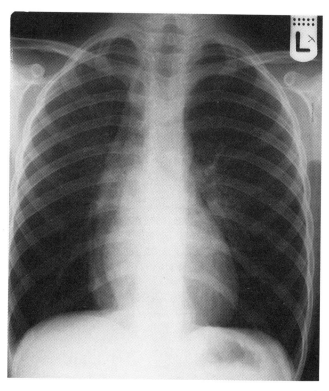

1

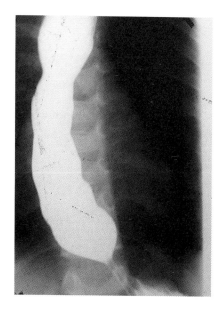

2

2 The diagnostic features of achalasia on barium swallow are a dilated esophagus, absence of stripping waves, incoordinated contraction and obstruction at the gastroesophageal junction with prolonged retention of barium in the esophagus. Failure of relaxation of the lower esophageal sphincter gives rise to the classical 'rat-tail' deformity of funneling and narrowing of the distal esophagus.

Endoscopy

The main value of esophagoscopy is to exclude an organic cause for the obstruction.

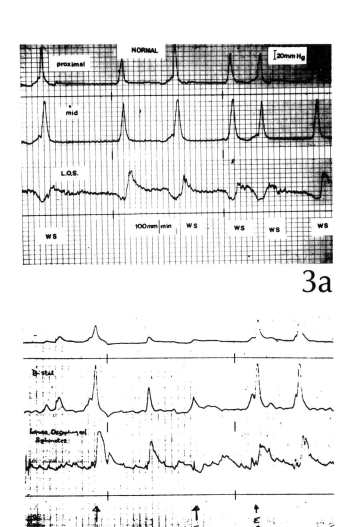

3a

3b

Esophageal manometry

3a, b The criteria for diagnosis include: (1) a high-pressure (>30 mmHg) lower esophageal sphincter zone; (2) failure of the lower esophagus to relax in response to swallowing; (3) absence of propulsive peristalsis; and (4) incoordinated tertiary contractions in the body of the esophagus.

Anesthesia

General endotracheal anesthesia is administered, with the patient supine on the operating table. Measures must be taken to avoid aspiration of esophageal contents during the induction of anesthesia. Preoperative esophagoscopy is recommended to ensure complete evacuation of retained food and secretions from the esophagus. A medium-caliber nasogastric tube is passed into the stomach.

Operation

Incision

4 The approach is via an upper abdominal midline incision extending from the xiphisternum to the umbilicus.

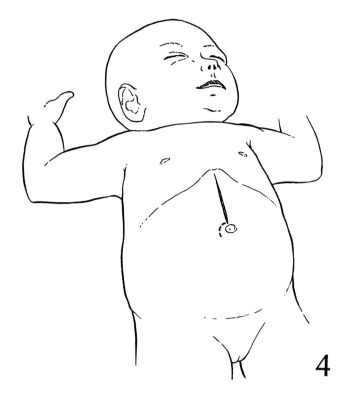

Exposure

5 In most cases adequate exposure of the abdominal esophagus can be obtained by retracting the left lobe of the liver anterosuperiorly with a wide retractor. If necessary, additional exposure may be attained by dividing the left triangular ligament in the avascular plane and retracting the left lobe of the liver towards the midline.

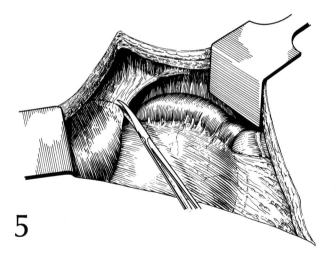

Mobilization of fundus of stomach

6a, b As a Nissen fundoplication will be performed in addition to the extended gastroesophageal myotomy, the operative procedure for fundoplication should be followed at an early stage.

The proximal one-third of the greater curvature of the stomach is liberated from its attachment to the spleen by ligating and dividing the short gastric vessels in the gastrosplenic ligament. This is accomplished most safely using a right-angled forceps passed around each vessel in turn and ligating the vessel on both the gastric and splenic sides before dividing it. When all the vessels in the gastrosplenic ligament have been divided, the spleen should be allowed to fall back into the posterior peritoneum, thereby avoiding inadvertent trauma. Splenectomy should never be necessary in this procedure. The fundus is now sufficiently free to allow for a loose ('floppy') fundoplication.

Exposure of esophageal hiatus

The phrenoesophageal membrane is placed on stretch by downward traction on the stomach while the diaphragmatic muscles are retracted superiorly. The avascular membrane is incised with scissors and the musculature of the esophagus displayed. The anterior vagal nerve will be seen coursing on the surface of the esophagus. It should be carefully protected and preserved.

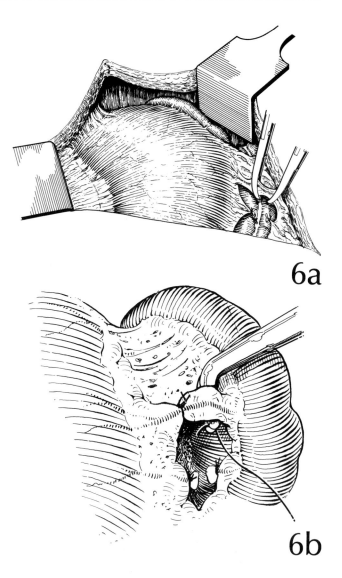

6a

6b

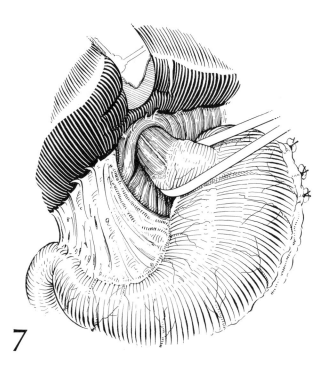

7

Mobilization of the distal esophagus

7 Using a combination of sharp and blunt dissection, the lower end of esophagus is encircled, taking care not to injure the posterior vagal nerve. A rubber sling is placed around the esophagus. The lower 5–8 cm of esophagus is now exposed through the esophageal hiatus into the posterior mediastinum by blunt dissection with either a moist pledget or right-angled forceps.

The esophageal hiatus is completely exposed by dividing the upper part of the gastrohepatic omentum above the left gastric vessels.

Gastroesophageal myotomy

8a–c The myotomy is performed on the anterior wall of the esophagus, extending for 1 cm onto the fundus of the stomach. A superficial incision (1–2 mm in depth) is made in the musculature of the distal 4–6 cm of the esophagus. The divided muscle is gently parted with a blunt hemostat until the underlying mucosa of the esophagus is encountered. The thickness of the muscle of the lower esophagus varies from a few millimeters to 0.5 cm or more. Great care must be taken to avoid opening into the lumen of the esophagus.

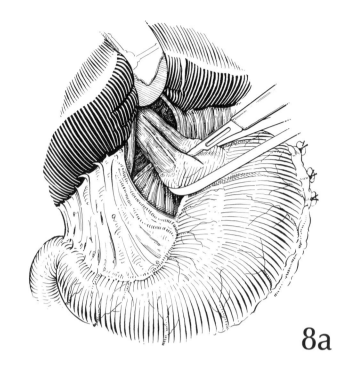

8a

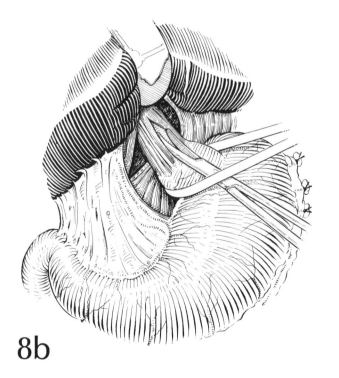

8b

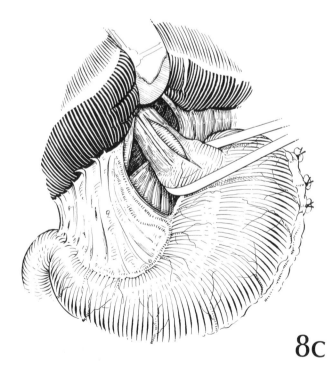

8c

9a, b

The divided muscle is now separated from the underlying mucosa by blunt pledget dissection in the submucosal plane. The dissection is continued until at least 50% of the circumference of the esophagus is free of the constricting muscle.

The myotomy is extended through the gastro-esophageal junction for 1 cm onto the fundus of the stomach and the musculature is similarly elevated from the underlying mucosa.

Testing for esophageal perforation

The stomach and esophagus are distended with air introduced through the nasogastric tube, and the exposed muscosa carefully inspected for perforation. A mucosal defect should be carefully closed with fine polyglycolic acid sutures.

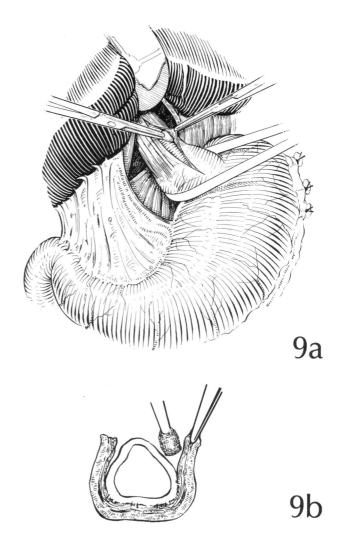

9a

9b

Narrowing of hiatus

10 The esophageal hiatus is narrowed posteriorly to the esophagus by placing deep sutures through the crura of the diaphragm. The sutures are tied loosely to prevent them from cutting through, leaving sufficient space alongside the esophagus to allow passage of the tip of a finger. Two or three sutures may be required for this purpose.

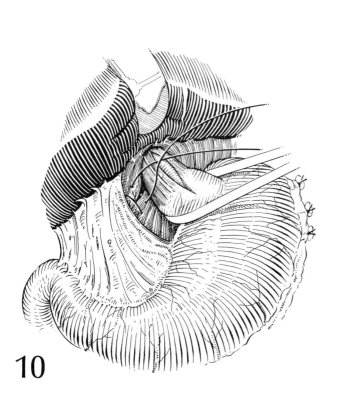

10

Fundoplication

11 A loose ('floppy') Nissen fundoplication is now constructed over the distal 1–1.5 cm of the esophagus. The esophageal sutures are only placed through one side of the divided esophageal muscle in order to prevent reapproximation of the edges of the myotomy (*see* chapter on pp. 265–273).

Wound closure

The wound is closed either in layers or with interrupted mass sutures of 3/0 polyglycolic acid. A subcuticular suture approximates the skin edges.

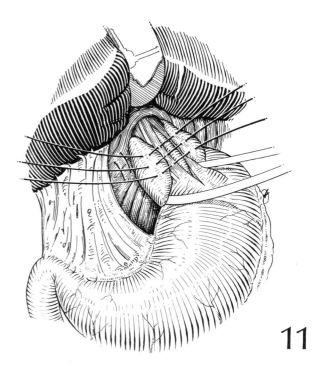

11

Postoperative care

Nasogastric decompression and intravenous fluids are continued until the postoperative ileus has resolved (mean of 3–4 days).

Complications

These can include mediastinitis due to failure to detect a mucosal perforation and recurrence of symptoms if the muscle is not separated from the underlying mucosa for at least half the circumference of the esophagus. Gastroesophageal reflux is due to an inadequate fundoplication, and dysphagia for solids is due to too tight a fundoplication.

Outcome

After myotomy alone, the long-term incidence of gastroesophageal reflux ranges from 15% to 50% depending on the length and extent of follow-up. Relief of the dysphagia and respiratory problems is usually complete, but residual or recurrent pain may occur in 25% of patients. The esophageal pain generally responds to pneumatic dilatation.

Further reading

Berquist WE, Byrne WJ, Ament ME, Fonkalsrud EW, Euler AR. Achalasia: diagnosis, management and clinical course in 16 children. *Pediatrics* 1983; 71: 798–805.

Buick RG, Spitz L. Achalasia of the cardia in children. *Br J Surg* 1985; 72: 341–3.

Donahue PE, Schlesinger PK, Bombeck CT, Samelson S, Nyhus LM. Achalasia of the esophagus: treatment, controversies and the method of choice. *Ann Surg* 1986; 203: 505–11.

Ellis FH, Gibb SP, Crozier RE. Esophagomyotomy for achalasia of the esophagus. *Ann Surg* 1980; 192: 157–61.

Emblem R, Stringer MD, Hall CM, Spitz L. Current results of surgery for achalasia of the cardia. *Arch Dis Child* 1993; 68: 749–51.

Vantrappen G, Janssens J. To dilate or to operate? This is the question. *Gut* 1983; 24: 1013–19.

Malrotation

Lewis Spitz PhD, FRCS, FRCS(Ed), FAAP(Hon)
Nuffield Professor of Paediatric Surgery, Institute of Child Health, University of London, and Consultant
Paediatric Surgeon, Great Ormond Street Hospital for Children, London, UK

The term 'malrotation' refers to a condition in which the midgut, that part of the intestine supplied by the superior mesenteric vessels extending from the duodenojejunal flexure to the mid-transverse colon, remains unfixed and suspended on a narrow-based mesentery.

History

The first description of intestinal development was written by Mall in 1898[1]. Frazer and Robins in 1915 expanded on the observations of Mall[2] and in 1923 Dott extended the embryological observations to the problems encountered clinically[3]. In 1936 William Ladd emphasized the importance of releasing the duodenum and placing the cecum in the left upper quadrant[4]. The principles of the modern procedure are almost unchanged from those of Ladd.

Principles and justification

Embryology

The alimentary canal initially develops as a straight tube extending down the midline of the embryo. As it lengthens, the intestine extends into the extra-embryonic celom of the umbilical cord but later returns to the abdominal cavity. The foregut – stomach and duodenum – is supplied by the celiac artery, the midgut – small intestine and proximal colon – by the superior mesenteric artery, and the hindgut – mid transverse colon to the rectum – by the inferior mesenteric artery. Three stages of development of the midgut are recognized[5].

Stage I

The first stage occurs during the fourth to 10th weeks of gestation. Owing to rapid growth, the celomic cavity is unable to contain the midgut within its confines. The midgut is forced out into the physiologic hernia within the umbilical cord.

Stage II

Stage II occurs at the 10th to 12th weeks of gestation, during which the midgut migrates back into the abdomen. The small intestine returns first and lies mainly on the left side of the abdomen. The cecocolic loop returns last, entering the abdomen in the left lower quadrant but rapidly rotating 270° counterclockwise to attain its final position in the right iliac fossa. The duodenojejunal loop simultaneously undergoes a 270° counterclockwise rotation, coming to rest behind and to the left of the superior mesenteric vessels. The cecocolic loop lies in front of and to the right of these vessels.

Stage III

During the 12th week of gestation various parts of the mesentery and the posterior parietal peritoneum fuse, notably the cecum and ascending colon which become fixed in the right paracolic gutter.

Consequences of errors of normal rotation

Errors may occur at any one of the three stages, with varying consequences.

Stage I

Failure of the intestine to return into the abdomen results in the formation of an exomphalos/omphalocele.

Stage II

During this stage a number of errors could occur:

1. Non-rotation – rotation may fail to occur following re-entry of the midgut into the abdomen.
2. Incomplete rotation – counterclockwise rotation is arrested at 180°. The cecum lies in a subhepatic position in the right hypochondrium. The duodeno-jejunal rotation is similarly arrested and the duodenojejunal flexure lies to the right of the midline and the superior mesenteric vessels. The base of the midgut mesentery is compressed and narrow and the entire midgut hangs suspended on the superior mesenteric vessels by a narrow stalk, which is prone to volvulus.
3. Reversed rotation – the final 180° rotation occurs in a clockwise direction, with the colon coming to lie posterior to the duodenum and superior mesenteric vessels.
4. Hyperrotation – rotation continues through 360° or more so that the cecum comes to rest in the region of the splenic flexure in the left hypochondrium.
5. Encapsulated small intestine – the avascular sac which forms the lining of the extraembryonic celom returns *en masse* into the abdomen with the intestine.

The most common error is incomplete rotation. Treatment of this condition forms the basis of the rest of the discussion.

Stage III

Rotation occurs normally but fixation is defective, resulting in a 'mobile cecum'. It is estimated that this situation is present in 10% of asymptomatic individuals but it may predispose to cecal volvulus.

Incidence

Malrotation may go undetected throughout life. Approximately 60% of cases are encountered in the first month of life and over 40% of these within the first week. Sporadic cases occur throughout life. It is generally accepted that once the diagnosis of malrotation has been established, surgical correction is mandatory to prevent the development of volvulus which occurs in 40–50% of cases not treated surgically. Malrotation forms an integral part of exomphalos/omphalocele, congenital diaphragmatic hernia and prune-belly syndrome. It has also been found in conjunction with intrinsic duodenal obstructions, esophageal atresia, Hirschsprung's disease, biliary atresia and urinary tract anomalies. Associated anomalies are present in 30–45% of patients.

Clinical presentation

Neonatal period

Malrotation in early infancy may present either with acute strangulating obstruction or with recurrent episodes of subacute intestinal obstruction.

Acute life-threatening strangulating intestinal obstruction occurs as a result of midgut volvulus. The infant presents in a shocked and collapsed state with bilious vomiting (which often contains altered blood), abdominal tenderness with or (commonly) without distension, and the passage of dark blood rectally. Edema and erythema of the abdominal wall develop as the volvulus becomes complicated by intestinal gangrene, perforation and peritonitis.

Recurrent episodes of subacute intestinal obstruction are usually a forewarning of volvulus. The first, and often the only, sign may be bile-stained vomiting, the investigation of which must be vigorously and intensively investigated.

Infants and children

A wide spectrum of clinical symptoms has been ascribed to malrotation. The most common symptom is intermittent or cyclic vomiting which is occasionally bile-tinged. Failure to thrive and malnutrition may be a result of intestinal malabsorption secondary to lymphatic compression in the narrow-based mesentery of the small intestine. Older children may present with features of anorexia nervosa. Early satiety or pain associated with intake of food results in a reluctance to eat or food aversion.

Preoperative

Radiologic investigations

Plain abdominal radiography

1 The features suggestive of a volvulus on the plain abdominal radiograph are air-fluid levels in the stomach and proximal duodenum (a 'double-bubble' appearance) and a paucity of gas in the rest of the intestine. In the infant presenting in shock with features of acute strangulating obstruction, further radiologic investigations only delay definitive treatment.

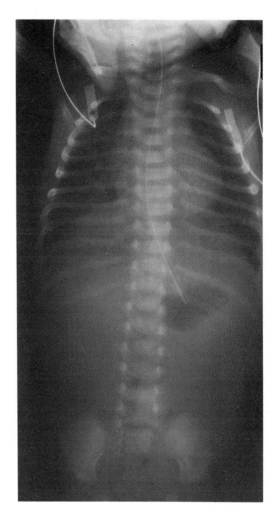

1

Contrast radiology

2 The investigation of choice is an upper gastro-intestinal contrast study. The features that should be elicited are an abnormal configuration of the duodenal C-loop, the identification of the duodeno-jejunal flexure to the right of the midline and small bowel loop on the right side of the abdomen. A 'twisted ribbon' and 'corkscrew' appearance of the duodenum and upper jejunum indicates a midgut volvulus.

Contrast enema gives information only about the position of the cecum, which may occasionally be normally placed even in the presence of a volvulus.

Preoperative resuscitation

Patients presenting with acute strangulating obstruction require rapid resuscitation before proceeding to surgery. This comprises rapid intravenous volume replacement (plasma 20 ml/kg body weight), naso-gastric decompression, correction of electrolyte and acid–base imbalance and administration of broad-spectrum antibiotics. Attempts should be made to correct hypothermia. The period of intensive resuscitation should not extend for more than 1–2 h before proceeding to surgery, as prolonging the time will expose the intestine to increased ischemia and may result in more extensive bowel necrosis.

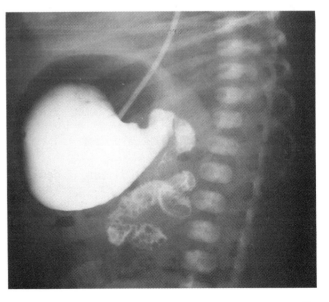

2

Operations

Surgical correction of the anomaly should always be regarded as an emergency even in patients presenting non-acutely. Volvulus may supervene at any stage and the operation should be scheduled as early as possible.

Incision

3 A laparotomy is performed via a generous upper abdominal transverse muscle-cutting incision, extending mainly to the right side. The obliterated umbilical vein in the free edge of the falciform ligament is ligated and divided. The entire bowel is delivered into the wound for careful examination. A small volume of yellowish free peritoneal fluid is usually present in any early intestinal obstruction, but blood-stained fluid is indicative of intestinal necrosis.

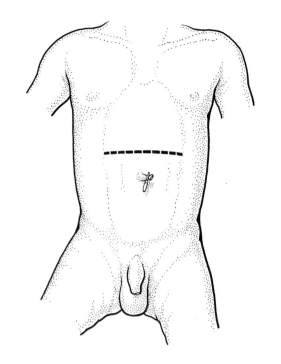

3

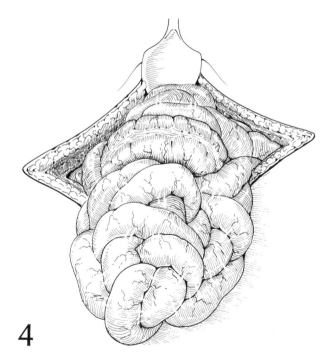

4

MIDGUT VOLVULUS

4 The volvulus occurs around the base of the narrow midgut mesentery. The twist usually occurs in a clockwise direction and is untwisted by as many 180° counterclockwise rotations as required.

5 Moderately ischemic bowel, which appears congested and dusty, rapidly resumes a normal pinkish color on reduction of the volvulus. Frankly necrotic bowel is extremely friable and may disintegrate on handling. Bowel of questionable viability should be covered, after untwisting, with warm moist swabs and left undisturbed for approximately 10 min before assessing the extent of ischemic damage. A Ladd's procedure for the malrotation is carried out (*see* below).

In patients with extensive intestinal gangrene, frankly necrotic bowel should be resected and the bowel ends either tied off or stomas fashioned with a view to performing a second-look laparotomy in 24–48 h when clearer lines of demarcation will be evident. At this stage an end-to-end anastomosis may be feasible. In the intervening period the patient is electively ventilated and resuscitative measures continued.

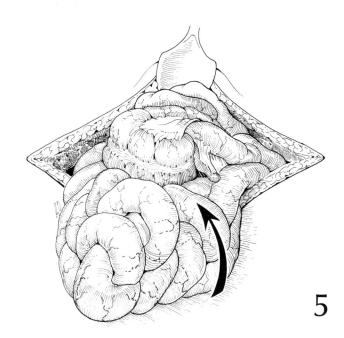

5

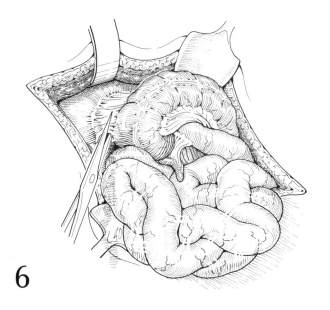

6

UNCOMPLICATED MALROTATION (LADD'S OPERATION)

The aim of this procedure is to restore intestinal anatomy to the non-rotated position with the duodenum and upper jejunum on the right side of the abdomen and the cecocolic loop in the left upper quadrant.

6 Folds of peritoneum extending from the cecum and ascending colon across the duodenum to the right paracolic gutter and to the liver and gallbladder are carefully divided. This maneuver leaves the cecocolic loop free laterally but dense adhesions in the base of the mesentery must be divided before the cecum and ascending colon can be fully separated from the duodenojejunal loop. Separation is achieved by opening the serosa of the mesentery between the duodenum and cecum and exposing the anterior surface of the superior mesenteric vessels coursing in the narrow-based mesentery to the midgut.

The mesentery in this part is often thickened and edematous, especially if an associated midgut volvulus needs to be untwisted. Care should be taken to avoid trauma to the main vessels and small branches may need to be ligated before being divided. Large fleshy lymph glands are often present in the base of the mesentery, and lymphatic channels that have been divided should be closed by ligation or electrocoagulation to avoid postoperative chylous leakage.

7 The mesentery is widened peripherally to allow the right colon to be mobilized. Centrally the dissection is continued into the base of the mesentery until the superior mesenteric artery and vein are freed of any fibrous compression.

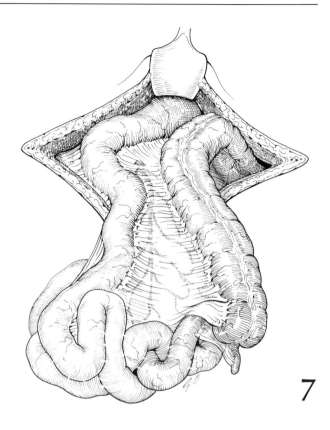

7

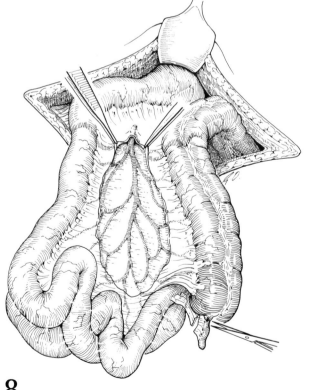

8

8 The duodenum is straightened by dividing the ligament of Treitz and should be carefully inspected for the presence of any intrinsic obstruction. If there is any doubt, a balloon catheter should be passed perorally through the duodenum into the proximal jejunum, inflated and carefully withdrawn into the stomach. Inability to pass the catheter through the duodenum or hold-up of the inflated balloon on withdrawal indicates an intrinsic obstruction.

An appendectomy should always be performed as the cecum will be placed in the left upper quadrant of the abdomen and the diagnosis of subsequent appendicitis could be extremely difficult to establish in the future.

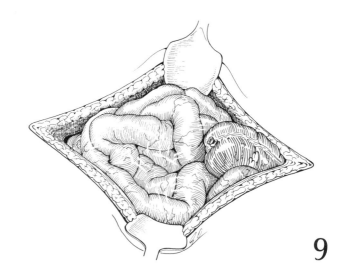

9 The intestine is replaced in the peritoneal cavity, commencing with the duodenum and proximal jejunum which lie on the *right* side and ending with the terminal ileum and cecum which are placed in the *left* hypochondrium. No attempt is made to fix the intestine in this position, although some authors[6] advocate stabilizing the position by suturing the duodenum to the right perinephric fascia and the cecum to the left paracolic gutter to prevent recurrent volvulus.

9

Closure

The abdomen is closed in layers or *en masse* with continuous or interrupted sutures. The skin is closed with a continuous subcuticular suture.

Postoperative care

Nasogastric aspiration and intravenous fluid and electrolyte support continue until bowel function returns. The period of ileus generally lasts 48–72 h, during which time intestinal fluid losses should be replaced with an equivalent volume of 0.45% sodium chloride in 5% dextrose solution containing 20 mEq/l potassium chloride.

Outcome

Recovery is generally prompt and uncomplicated. Infants who have suffered extensive bowel loss following midgut volvulus may experience problems of short bowel syndrome with prolonged parenteral nutrition. Recurrent volvulus is rare but adhesion intestinal obstruction is relatively common (3–5% of cases).

Acknowledgments

The illustrations in this chapter have been reproduced from *Operative Newborn Surgery* (ed. P. Puri) with permission from Butterworth-Heinemann.

References

1. Mall FP. Development of the human intestine and its position in the adult. *Bull Johns Hopkins Hosp* 1898; 9: 197.

2. Frazer JE, Robbins RH. On the factors concerned in causing rotation of the intestine in man. *J Anat Physiol* 1916; 50: 75–110.

3. Dott NM. Anomalies of intestinal rotation: their embryology and surgical aspects with report of 5 cases. *Br J Surg* 1923; 11: 251–86.

4. Ladd WE. Surgical diseases of the alimentary tract in infants. *N Engl J Med* 1936; 215: 705–8.

5. Skandalakis JE, Gray SW. *Embryology for Surgeons*. 2nd edn. Baltimore: Williams and Wilkins, 1994: 184–200.

6. Bill AH, Grauman D. Rationale and technic for stabilization of the mesentery in cases of nonrotation of the midgut. *J Pediatr Surg* 1966; 1: 127–36.

Further reading

Janik JS, Ein SH. Normal intestinal rotation with non-fixation: a cause of chronic abdominal pain. *J Pediatr Surg* 1979; 14: 670–4.

Powell DM, Othersen HB, Smith CD. Malrotation of the intestines in children. The effect of age on presentation and therapy. *J Pediatr Surg* 1989; 24: 777–80.

Simpson AJ, Leonidas JC, Krasna IH, Becker JM, Schneider KM. Roentgen diagnosis of midgut malrotation: value of upper gastrointestinal radiographic study. *J Pediatr Surg* 1972; 7: 243–52.

Yanez R, Spitz L. Intestinal malrotation presenting outside the neonatal period. *Arch Dis Child* 1986; 61: 682–5.

Congenital atresia and stenosis of the small intestine

S. Cywes MMed, FACS, FRCS, FRCS(Ed), FRCPS(Glas), FAAP
Professor of Paediatric Surgery, University of Cape Town and Chief Surgeon, Institute of Child Health, Red Cross War Memorial Children's Hospital, Rondebosch, South Africa

H. Rode MMed, FCS(SA), FRCS(Ed)
Associate Professor of Paediatric Surgery, University of Cape Town and Principal Surgeon, Institute of Child Health, Red Cross War Memorial Children's Hospital, Rondebosch, South Africa

History

In 1911 Fockens[1] of Rotterdam reported the first successfully treated case of small intestinal atresia. Up until 1952, however, the mortality rate of atresia of the small intestine remained prohibitive even at the best pediatric surgical centers in the world, e.g. 84% at the Children's Medical Center, Boston[2] and 88% at the Hospital for Sick Children, Great Ormond Street, London[3]. In a comprehensive review of the world literature up to 1950, Evans[4] could find reports of only 39 successfully treated cases of jejunoileal atresia.

1 In 1952 Louw[3] published the results of an investigation of 79 patients treated at Great Ormond Street, London, and suggested that jejunoileal atresia was probably due to a vascular accident rather than being the result of inadequate recanalization, as had previously been the commonly accepted hypothesis. At his instigation, Barnard perfected an experimental model in pregnant mongrel bitches[5]. This not only confirmed the hypothesis and supported changes in the surgical procedure, but also paved the way for further fetal experiments.

Since then there has been a steady improvement in the results of treatment of atresia and stenoses of the small intestine[6–10]. More recently, Tibboel *et al.*[11] showed in chick embryo studies that intrauterine perforation of the small intestine may also produce atresia.

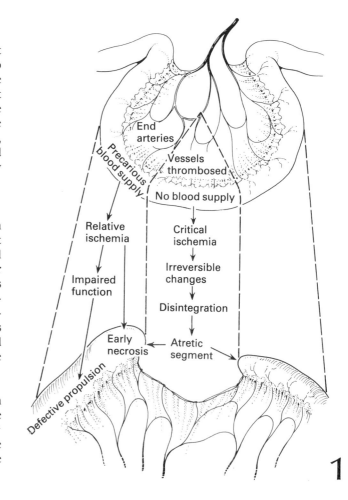

1

Principles and justification

Indications

Many cases of intestinal atresia are now being diagnosed prenatally by ultrasonographic investigation of the fetus, showing dilated and obstructed fetal intestine, particularly in pregnancies complicated by third trimester polyhydramnios. Postnatally, atresia or severe stenosis of the small intestine presents as neonatal intestinal obstruction with persistent bilious (green) vomiting dating from the first or second day of life, varying degrees of abdominal distension, and perhaps some abnormality in evacuating meconium. Erect and supine abdominal radiographs will reveal distended small intestinal loops and air–fluid levels. An inverted radiograph is useful to distinguish between low small intestinal and colonic obstruction.

In some cases the first abdominal radiograph reveals a completely opaque abdomen due to a fluid-filled obstructed bowel. Emptying of the stomach by means of a Replogle nasogastric tube and the injection of a bolus of air will demonstrate the level of the obstruction. When intestinal stenosis is present, an abnormal differentiation in caliber of the proximal obstructed intestine and the distal tract will be evident. The diagnosis may be difficult and delayed. When the radiograph suggests a complete low obstruction, a contrast enema is given to rule out associated colonic atresia or functional obstruction, e.g. total colonic aganglionosis or meconium ileus, which may be confused with atresia of the distal ileum. When an incomplete small intestinal obstruction is diagnosed, an upper gastrointestinal contrast study is indicated to demonstrate the site and nature of the obstruction. Differentiation between atresia, intrinsic and extrinsic intestinal obstruction due to midgut volvulus or internal hernia is the most important urgent consideration.

Appearance of atretic segment

This depends on the type of occlusion, but in all cases the maximal dilatation and enlargement of the proximal intestine occurs at the point of obstruction, and this segment is often aperistaltic and of questionable viability.

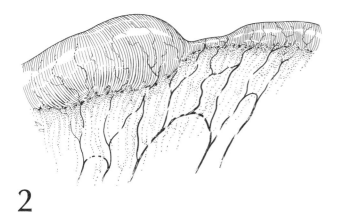

2

Stenosis

2 The proximal dilated intestine and distal intestine are in continuity with an intact mesentery, but at the junction there is a short, narrow, somewhat rigid segment with a minute lumen which may simulate atresia type I. The small intestine is of normal length.

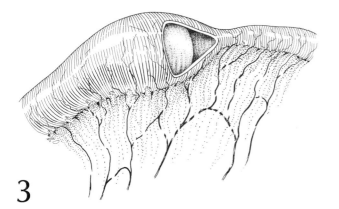

3

Atresia type I (membrane)

3 The dilated proximal and collapsed distal intestine are in continuity and the mesentery is intact. The pressure in the proximal intestine tends to bulge the membrane into the distal intestine, so that the transition from distended to collapsed intestine is conical in appearance: the 'wind-sock' effect. The distal intestine is completely collapsed. The small intestine is of normal length.

Atresia type II (blind ends joined by a fibrous cord)

4 The proximal intestine terminates in a bulbous blind end which is grossly distended and hypertrophied for several centimeters. This blind end is often aperistaltic and cyanosed, and may be necrotic with a perforation. The intestine proximal to this is usually considerably distended and hypertrophied for a further 5–10 cm, but more proximally assumes a normal appearance. The distal, completely collapsed intestine commences as a blind end which is occasionally bulbous, owing to the remains of a fetal intussusception. The two blind ends are joined by a thin, fibrous band. The corresponding intestinal mesentery is usually normal but may occasionally be absent, leaving a small V-shaped gap. The small intestinal length is usually normal.

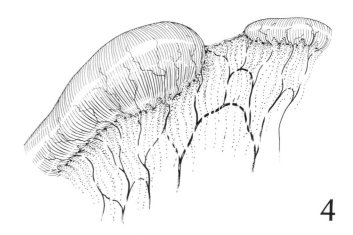

4

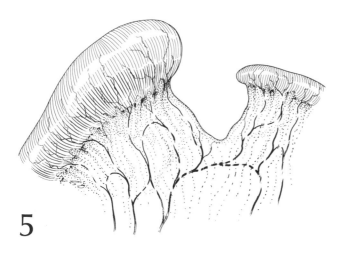

5

Atresia type IIIa (disconnected blind ends)

5 The appearance is similar to that in type II, but the blind ends are completely separate. There is always a mesenteric defect of varying size and the proximal intestine may, as a secondary event, undergo torsion or become overdistended with necrosis and perforation. The total length of intestine is reduced to a varying extent.

Atresia type IIIb ('apple peel' atresia)

6 As in type IIIa the blind ends are unconnected but the mesenteric defect is large. The atresia is in the proximal jejunum near the ligament of Treitz, with absence of the superior mesenteric artery beyond the origin of the middle colic branch and absence of the dorsal mesentery. The distal intestine assumes a helical configuration around an attenuated single perfusing vessel arising from the ileocolic or right colic arcades. Occasionally atresia type I or II is found in the distal intestine. Vascularity of the distal intestine may be impaired.

There is always a significant reduction in intestinal length.

Atresia type IV (multiple atresia)

Multiple atresias can be combinations of types I–III. The intestinal length is always reduced.

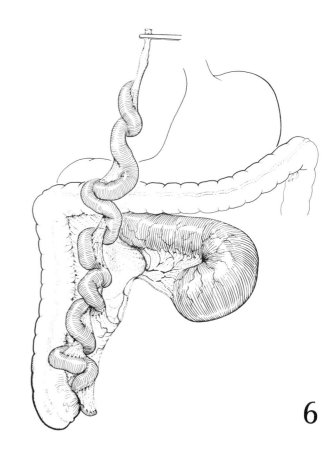

6

Preoperative

Preparation

The principles of successful perioperative management are early diagnosis, appropriate investigations, comprehensive perioperative care and performing the correct surgical procedure. The neonate tolerates operative intervention better after a few hours of preoperative preparation, particularly if diagnosis has been delayed. The preparation should pay particular attention to hypothermia, hypoxia, hypovolemia, hypoglycemia and hypoprothrombinemia.

The patient is nursed in a warmed, well-humidified incubator. A Replogle nasogastric tube is passed to decompress the stomach and prevent aspiration of vomitus. The aspirate is cultured. Blood gas levels are monitored and the fractioned inspired oxygen level is adjusted as required. An intravenous infusion is set up by means of a 'push in' into the vein of the scalp or dorsum of the hand or foot, to re-establish fluid and electrolyte balances, to correct any acid–base abnormality and to facilitate blood transfusion during operation. One unit of fresh blood is cross-matched. In a shocked patient, colloid solution, 10–20 ml/kg, is infused over 30 min. Maintenance fluid consisting of 0.25% saline in 10% dextrose with added potassium, at a volume of 30–120 ml/kg/day, depending on the number of days after birth, is administered. Additional fluid may be required to maintain an adequate blood pressure (mean 45–50 mmHg) and urine flow (1 ml/kg/h). Hyperbilirubinemia when present is treated by phototherapy, but if severe requires preoperative exchange transfusion. Blood glucose levels are closely monitored.

The neonate is washed with chlorhexidine, and vitamin K_1 is given to counteract prothrombin deficiency. The lungs are kept clear by nasopharyngeal aspiration. When respiration is impeded by severe abdominal distention and/or pulmonary infection, ventilation is often life-saving. Prophylactic broad-spectrum antibiotics are given immediately before operation, if not already administered for an associated complication.

Temperature regulation

Heat is conserved by having the theater comfortably warm (24°C), and by placing the patient supine on a thermostatically controlled, warm-water blanket through which water at 40°C is circulated. Further heating can be achieved by an infrared lamp. The baby is well covered with warm cotton wool blankets until anesthetized and connected to all the monitoring devices, e.g. rectal thermometer, electrocardiograph, esophageal stethoscope, pulse oximeter and non-invasive blood pressure device.

Anesthesia

Endotracheal anesthesia with warm humidified air, oxygen and halothane and assisted ventilation is used and is supplemented with a non-depolarizing relaxant (atracurium besylate or pancuronium bromide). Complementary epidural anesthesia avoids the need for intraoperative and postoperative opiate analgesics. Fentanyl citrate may be given to those patients requiring postoperative ventilation. Local infiltration of the wound with 0.25% bupivacaine hydrochloride, 2 mg/kg, supplements analgesia.

Sterilization of skin and draping

The umbilical cord is cleansed with 70% alcohol and is transected flush with the abdominal wall. The abdominal skin is prepared by cleansing with prewarmed 2% povidone-iodine in 70% isopropyl alcohol. Sterile, warm, cotton wool rolls are placed alongside the patient, who is then draped with towels, and a large sterile, transparent adhesive drape is applied over the operative field.

Perioperative supportive care

During the operative procedure the patient is given a balanced electrolyte solution containing 10% dextrose, by slow intravenous infusion, to provide 10% of blood volume during the first 30 min of surgery and 5% of blood volume/h thereafter. Blood lost during the operation is carefully measured colorimetrically and, when exceeding 10% of blood volume, is replaced to maintain a hematocrit between 36% and 42%. After the first 30 min, third space losses are replaced with a colloid solution at a volume of 5–10% of the baby's blood volume.

Operation

Incision

An adequate incision is required. Exposure is obtained by a supraumbilical transverse incision transecting the rectus muscles 2–3 cm above the umbilicus.

Exploration

7 In uncomplicated cases the intestine can easily be delivered into the wound by gentle exertion of pressure on the wound edges. If free gas escapes on opening the peritoneum, or if there is contamination of the peritoneal cavity, the perforation should be sought immediately and closed before further exploration. The intestine proximal to the obstruction is distended while the intestine distal to the obstruction is collapsed, tiny and worm-like. All the intestine is exteriorized to determine the site and type of obstruction and to exclude other areas of atresia or stenosis as well as associated lesions, e.g. incomplete intestinal rotation or meconium ileus.

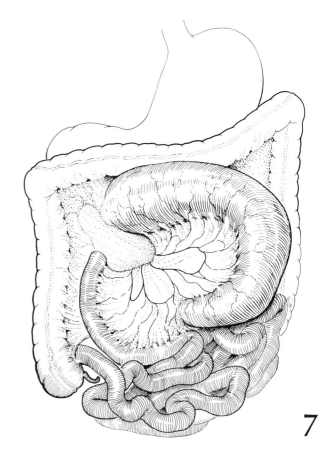

7

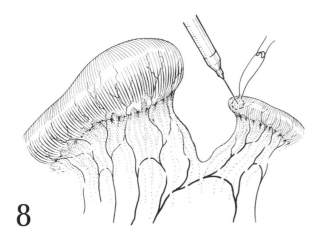

8

Detection of other atretic areas

8 After the location and type of lesion have been identified, the distal intestine is carefully examined to untwist any volvulus present and to exclude other atretic segments, which occur in 6–21% of cases. Intraluminal membranes are best detected and localized by injecting 0.5 N saline into the lumen of the collapsed intestine and milking it down to the caecum.

The total length of small intestine is measured. The normal length at birth is approximately 250 cm and in the preterm infant 160–240 cm.

Distension of distal end

9 After complete patency of the distal small intestine has been established, the next task is to splice the disproportionate proximal and distal blind ends. This is facilitated by applying an atraumatic bowel clamp about 6–8 cm from the distal blind end and distending the intervening segment with 0.5 N saline, taking care not to split the serosa. The needle puncture is closed with an encircling 5/0 polypropylene (Prolene) or polydioxan-one (PDS) suture to prevent leakage.

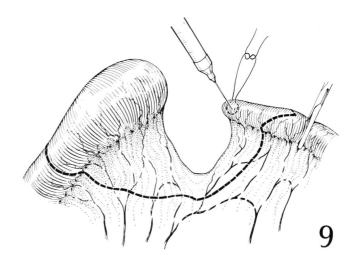

Resection

The atretic area and adjacent distended and collapsed loops of intestine are isolated by replacing the rest of the intestine and walling off the rest of the abdominal cavity with moist packs. To ensure adequate postoperative function the proximal distended and hypertrophied intestine must be liberally resected, even if it appears viable; usually 10–15 cm are removed.

10 After milking the intestinal contents into the proximal bulbous end, or in high jejunal atresia into the stomach, from where it is aspirated, an atraumatic bowel clamp is applied across the bowel a few centimeters proximal to the site selected for transection. The mesentery adjoining the portion to be resected is clamped, divided and ligated up to the proposed lines of section of proximal and distal intestine. The proximal intestine is transected. The blood supply at this point should be excellent, and therefore the intestine is divided at right angles, leaving an opening about 1.5 cm in width. Some 4–5 cm of the distal intestine is then removed using a slightly oblique line of transection and continuing the incision along the antimesenteric border to create a 'fish-mouth' that renders the opening about equal to that of the proximal intestine.

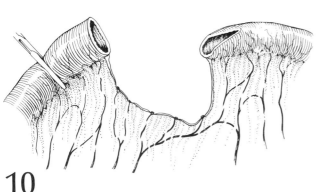

Uniting the mesenteric borders

11 A 5/0 or 6/0 polypropylene or polydioxanone inverting mattress suture unites the mesenteric borders of the divided ends, and temporary stay sutures are inserted at the antimesenteric angles to facilitate accurate approximation.

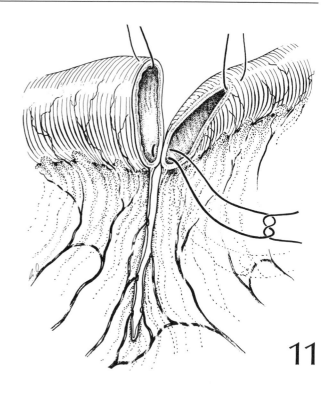

11

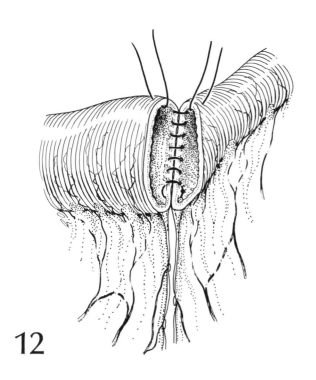

12

'Posterior' sutures

12 The 'posterior' edges of the loops are united with interrupted through-and-through or inverting Connell stitches, tied on the mucosal aspect.

'Anterior' sutures

13 The 'anterior' edges are joined by similar through-and-through sutures tied on the serosal surface. Alternatively Connell, Gambee or Lembert stitches may be used.

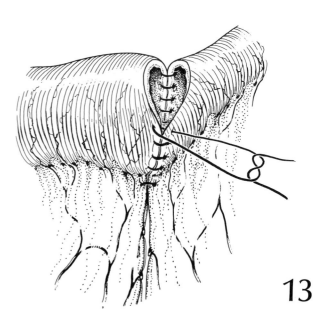

13

Completion of anastomosis and closure of mesenteric gap

14 The completed anastomosis is not strictly end-to-end but a modification of Denis Browne's 'end-to-back' method. The suture line is tested for leakage, and reinforcing sutures are inserted as required. The defect in the mesentery is repaired by approximating (and overlapping if necessary) the divided edges with interrupted sutures, taking great care not to kink the anastomosis. It is pertinent to measure the length of the residual intestine. Thereafter the intestines, well moistened with warm saline, are returned to the peritoneal cavity.

A similar technique is used for stenosis and intraluminal membranes. Procedures such as simple enteroplasties, excision of membranes, and bypassing techniques are not recommended because they fail to remove the abnormal segment of intestine. Side-to-side anastomosis is avoided because of the increased risk of creating blind loops.

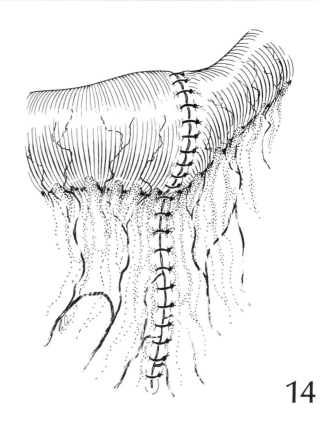

14

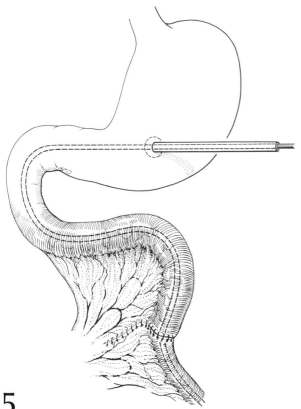

15

Gastrointestinal decompression

15 A complementary Stamm gastrostomy performed on the lesser curvature in neonates with high jejunal atresia serves as an avenue for gastric decompression and as a conduit for a transanastomotic soft Silastic tube, which is placed with its tip 10 cm beyond the intestinal anastomosis, allowing early intraluminal feeding. The Silastic tube is stabilized at the anastomotic site by a single tethering stitch which prevents retrograde displacement. In addition, a Replogle tube decompresses the stomach until prograde intestinal function has been established. Alternatively, gastric decompression alone with a transnasal Replogle tube placed on continuous low-pressure negative suctioning will decompress the foregut adequately, and is the preferred current method.

Closure of abdominal wound

Before closure, the whole peritoneal cavity is irrigated with saline and all blood clots and particulate matter are removed.

The abdominal wound is closed in a single layer using continuous 3/0 or 4/0 polydioxanone sutures to include all layers of the abdominal wall excluding Scarpa's fascia and skin. The fascial and adipose layers are approximated with absorbable sutures. The skin is sutured with a continuous subcuticular 5/0 polydioxanone or polyglycolic acid suture or approximated with adhesive strips and then covered with a thin, sterile, skin dressing. No drains are used.

Special surgical considerations

Bowel-saving procedures

If the measured intestinal length is less than 80 cm, two alternative surgical procedures should be contemplated.

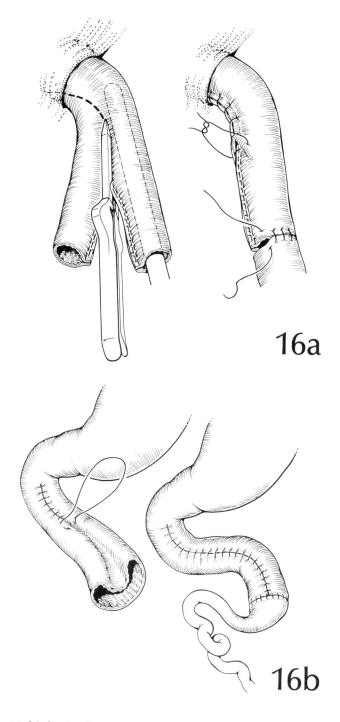

16a

16a, b A tapering jejunoduodenoplasty is accomplished by resection of the antimesenteric segment of the dilated proximal intestine over a 22–24-Fr catheter to ensure adequate luminal size. An intestinal autostapling instrument may greatly facilitate this procedure. The linear anastomosis is reinforced with absorbable 5/0 or 6/0 Lembert sutures. Tapering can safely be done over an extended 10–20 cm length.

Antimesenteric intestinal plication involves infolding more than half of the intestinal circumference into the lumen over an extended length. The infolding is accomplished with non-absorbable sutures.

16b

Exteriorization

Exteriorization of proximal and distal intestine may be required with established peritonitis or questionable vascularity of the remaining intestine. The authors do not favor the fashioning of stomas.

Intestinal atresia and gastroschisis

Primary anastomosis may be difficult and hazardous and the favored option is reduction of the eviscerated intestine with the atresia left intact, closure of the abdominal wall defect and delayed resection and primary anastomosis of the atresia at 14–21 days.

Multiple atresias

Multiple atresias are often localized to a 15–50-cm segment of intestine, and resection with one anastomosis is preferred if sufficient intestinal length remains.

Bowel lengthening

Bowel-lengthening procedures have no place at the initial operation.

Postoperative care

On completion of the operative procedure the patient is transferred to an intensive care unit. Supportive respiratory care is an integral component of the postoperative phase and additional oxygen or mechanical ventilation may be required. Vital signs, weight, temperature, hemodynamic status, blood gases, packed cell volume, electrolytes, blood glucose and bilirubin levels are regularly monitored. The position of the patient is changed regularly and pharyngeal secretions cleared. Nasogastric drainage is facilitated by placing the Replogle tube on negative pressure (-3 to -4 kPa) and the gastrostomy tube on free drainage, the aim being to prevent gastric distention, vomiting and inhalation. Urine output is carefully monitored, aiming at 1 ml/kg/h.

A balanced electrolyte maintenance solution in 10% dextrose is administered at 80–120 ml/kg/day. Gastric losses are measured at 4-h intervals and replaced volume for volume with 0.5 N saline in 5% dextrose. Stabilized human serum in bolus doses (10 ml/kg) or continuous infusion (1–2 ml/kg/day) may be required for continuing third space losses. Low serum albumin levels are corrected with daily albumin infusions (1 g/kg/day). Acidosis is corrected with 4.2% sodium bicarbonate after correction of any fluid deficits.

Therapeutic antibiotics are continued for 5–7 days or longer and an oral antifungal agent is given prophylactically. Bilirubin levels are closely monitored and phototherapy continued or exchange transfusion performed when necessary.

Nasogastric decompression is usually required for 4–6 days after the operation (longer for high jejunal atresias). Oral intake is commenced when the patient is alert, sucks well and with evidence of prograde gastrointestinal function, that is, a clear gastric effluent of low volume, a soft flat abdomen, propulsive peristaltic activity and clinical evidence that flatus or feces have been passed.

If a gastrostomy was performed the tube is elevated as a chimney and, if no excessive nasogastric drainage or vomiting occurs, oral intake can commence.

If at any time there is suspicion of a leak at the anastomosis (suggested by sudden collapse, abdominal distention and vomiting), a plain erect radiograph of the abdomen should be taken. If this reveals free air in the abdomen more than 24 h after operation laparotomy should be performed immediately and the leaking site sutured.

In neonates with less than 75 cm of small intestine remaining, diarrhea and excessive water loss may be problematic. In these and in every case in which normal enteral feeding is not expected to be established within 5 days after operation, parenteral feeding is indicated. Intravenous carbohydrate, amino acid and fat-containing solutions are introduced in a graduated manner over a period of 3 days. Peripheral venous push-in lines are used in preference to central, surgically placed venous catheters in the short term. The aim is to have the patient on the complete parenteral feeding regimen by the fifth day after operation. Small-volume feeding through a transanastomotic tube may be very beneficial for intestinal nourishment, thereby shortening the period of adaption. Once intestinal function has been re-established, the neonate is gradually weaned from parenteral to enteral feeding. Careful tailoring of the diet is required, as each patient has different tolerance thresholds.

Predictions of the degree of intestinal hypofunction are based on the known residual length of small intestine. When gross intestinal insufficiency is expected, isotonic liquid feeding is introduced in accurately titrated volumes. Regular monitoring for clinical signs and/or biochemical evidence of intestinal overload is required. Disaccharide intolerance and the rare monosaccharide intolerance, indications of gross brushborder malfunction of the intestine, should be detected by regular biochemical assessment of samples of stool fluid before severe clinical signs become manifest.

A falling pH and an associated increasing level of reducing substances denote unsatisfactory carbohydrate assimilation. The patient's oral intake is gradually increased in volume and in energy content, while the small intestine is allowed time to adapt, until maximum intake tolerance is reached. This can take up to 1 month or more. Pharmacologic control of intestinal peristaltic activity has been achieved more effectively since the introduction of loperamide hydrochloride. Vitamin B_{12} should be given if the terminal ileum has been resected.

In predicting the ultimate functional outcome the following factors must be taken into consideration: (1) early introduction of intraluminal feeding facilitates and shortens the period of intestinal adaption; (2) the ileum adapts to a greater degree than the jejunum – the neonatal small intestine still has a period of maturation and growth ahead of it and the actual residual small intestinal length is difficult to determine accurately; (3) the proximal obstructed intestinal segment is dilated and its length may be overestimated, while the distal, unused, collapsed intestine should have its measured length at least doubled when calculating the residual small intestine.

Outcome

Before 1952 the mortality rate for congenital atresias of the small intestine in Cape Town was 90%. Between 1952 and 1955, 28% of the neonates survived. At that stage most were treated by primary anastomosis without resection. With liberal resection of the blind ends and end-to-end anastomosis the survival rate increased to 78% during the period 1955–1958. During the 34-year period 1959–1992, 211 patients with jejunoileal atresia and stenosis were admitted to the pediatric surgical service at the Red Cross War Memorial Children's Hospital, of whom 26 have died, giving an overall mortality rate of 12.3% (*see Figure 1*). Five neonates were moribund on admission with infarction of the proximal intestine due to volvulus of the bulbous end and established peritonitis (type I, II, IIIa and two type IIIb). Five infants died from infection related to pneumonia and septicemia. Further management was withheld from two patients with less than 10 cm of residual small intestinal length. One infant died from bleeding due to vitamin K deficiency and 13 died from the short gut syndrome (nine early and four late deaths).

The survival in relation to birth weight and associated anomalies is shown in *Table 1* and the mortality rate in relation to type is outlined in *Table 2*.

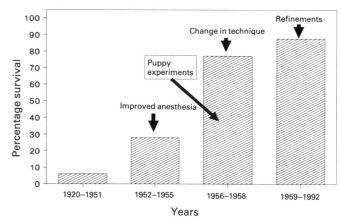

Figure 1   Results in congenital atresia and stenosis of the small intestine in 211 cases

Table 1   Survival in relation to weight and associated anomalies in 211 cases

	No. of patients	Survivors	
		No.	Percentage
Weight			
> 2300 g	110	105	95.5
1800–2200 g	67	55	82.0
< 1800 g	34	25	73.5
Associated anomalies			
Insignificant or nil	140	132	94.3
Moderate	37	30	81.1
Severe	34	23	67.6
Total	211	185	87.6

Table 2   Mortality rate related to type in 211 patients, 1959–1992

Type	No. of patients	Mortality rate		
		No.	Percentage	Overall (%)
Stenosis	24	0	0	0
Type I	44	4	9.1	1.9
Type II	20	3	15.0	1.4
Type IIIa	35	6	17.1	2.8
Type IIIb	40	9	22.5	4.3
Type IV	48	4	8.3	1.9
Total	211	26	—	12.3

References

1. Fockens P. Ein operativ geheilter Fall von kongenitaler Dünndarmatresie. *Zentralbl Chir* 1911; 38: 532–5.

2. Ladd WE, Gross RE. *Abdominal Surgery of Infancy and Childhood*. Philadelphia: WB Saunders, 1941.

3. Louw JH. Congenital intestinal atresia and severe stenosis in the newborn: report on 79 consecutive cases. *S Afr J Clin Sci* 1952; 3: 109–29.

4. Evans CH. Atresias of the gastrointestinal tract. *Int Abstr Surg* 1951; 92: 1–8.

5. Louw JH, Barnard CN. Congenital intestinal atresia: observations on its origin. *Lancet* 1955; ii: 1065–7.

6. Nixon HH. An experimental study of propulsion in isolated small intestine, and applications to surgery in the newborn. *Ann R Coll Surg Engl* 1960; 27: 105–24.

7. Benson CD, Lloyd JR, Smith JD. Resection and primary anastomosis in the management of stenosis and atresia of the jejunum and ileum. *Pediatrics* 1960; 26: 265–72.

8. Cywes S, Davies MRQ, Rode H. Congenital jejuno-ileal atresia and stenosis. *S Afr Med J* 1980; 57: 630–9.

9. Grosfeld JL. Jejunoileal atresia and stenosis. Section 3. The small intestine. In: Randolph JG, Ravitch MM, O'Neil JA, Rowe MI, eds. *Pediatric Surgery*, 4th edn. Chicago: Year Book Medical Publishers, 1986: 838–48.

10. Smith GHH, Glasson M. Intestinal atresia. Factors affecting survival. *Aust N Z J Surg* 1989; 59: 151–6.

11. Tibboel D, Molenaar JC, Nie CJ. New perspectives in fetal surgery: the chicken embryo. *J Pediatr Surg* 1979; 14: 438–40.

Illustrations by Sharon Teal and Peter Cox

Meconium ileus

Frederick J. Rescorla MD
Associate Professor, Section of Pediatric Surgery, James Whitcomb Riley Hospital for Children, and Indiana University School of Medicine, Indianapolis, Indiana, USA

Jay L. Grosfeld MD
Professor and Chairman, Department of Surgery, Indiana University School of Medicine, and Surgeon-in-Chief, James Whitcomb Riley Hospital for Children, Indianapolis, Indiana, USA

Etiology and classification

Cystic fibrosis is the most common serious inherited defect affecting the Caucasian population. Cystic fibrosis is transmitted as an autosomal recessive condition with a 5% carrier rate and an incidence of approximately 1:2500 live births. The cystic fibrosis transmembrane conductance regulator gene is located on the long arm of chromosome 7 and the delta F508 mutation at this locus is responsible for 70% of the abnormal genes[1]. Neonatal intestinal obstruction due to inspissated meconium has been identified since the early reports concerning cystic fibrosis and is referred to as meconium ileus. This presentation is observed in 10–15% of infants born with cystic fibrosis. The etiology of this abnormal meconium (mucoviscidosis) is due to deficient pancreatic and intestinal secretions as well as an abnormal concentration of the meconium within the duodenum and proximal jejunum. Instances of meconium ileus can be classified into uncomplicated and complicated cases.

Uncomplicated meconium ileus

Clinical presentation

1 In this condition the abnormal thickened meconium causes a simple obturator obstruction of the terminal ileum. The distal 15–30 cm of terminal ileum is filled with inspissated meconium pellets which are adherent to the bowel wall. The ileum just proximal to the obstruction fills with thick putty-like meconium and dilates to 3–4 cm in diameter. The colon is unused and small (microcolon) since meconium has not yet entered this segment of bowel.

The typical neonate with meconium ileus may appear relatively normal for the first 12–18 h of life and some tolerate several feeds. As the proximal bowel fills with swallowed air, however, abdominal distension and emesis (initially clear, later bilious) and failure to pass meconium are noted, heralding the presence of intestinal obstruction at 24–36 h of age.

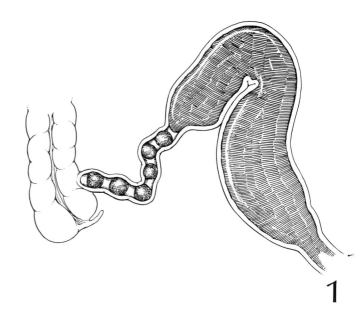

1

Initial management

The neonate with suspected bowel obstruction should be treated with oral gastric tube decompression of the stomach and intravenous fluids to replace pre-existing fluid deficits and ongoing losses. Antibiotics are administered as the infant is at increased risk of aspiration.

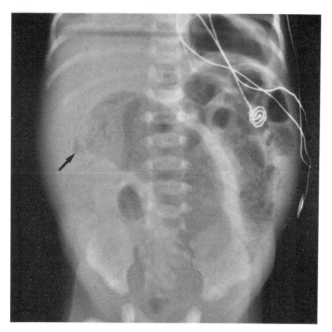

2

Radiographic evaluation

2 Plain abdominal radiographs and decubitus views usually demonstrate similar sized dilated loops of intestine without air-fluid levels. A 'soap bubble' appearance is often noted in the right lower quadrant (arrow), a result of air mixing with the thick meconium.

Diagnostic enema

3 The initial diagnostic test is a contrast enema. If the diagnosis of meconium ileus is not apparent from the plain radiographs, a barium enema is the diagnostic procedure of choice. This will demonstrate microcolon and may also document the presence of meconium pellets in the proximal ascending colon and terminal ileum.

This study will also exclude cases of colon atresia, small left colon syndrome and meconium plug syndrome, and document the location of the cecum to rule out anomalies of rotation and fixation. Neonates with distal ileal atresia and total colonic aganglionosis may have a similar appearance on a contrast enema examination, but they usually have air-fluid levels in the dilated proximal small bowel and absence of pellets in the distal ileum and proximal colon. If the neonate is stable and there is no evidence of complicated meconium ileus (peritoneal calcifications, giant cystic structure, etc.) non-operative treatment with a hypertonic contrast enema is recommended.

Therapeutic enema

The management of neonates with uncomplicated meconium ileus was significantly altered with the introduction of the diatrizoate meglumine (Gastrografin) enema by Noblett in 1969[2]. The efficacy of this procedure is related to the hyperosmolar nature of Gastrografin (1100–1900 mOsm/l), which contains a wetting agent (Tween 80) and draws large volumes of fluid into the bowel lumen, thus washing out the obstructing meconium. Although initial reports used full strength Gastrografin, most pediatric radiologists dilute the contrast material to approximately 3:1, and the Gastrografin currently used does not contain a wetting

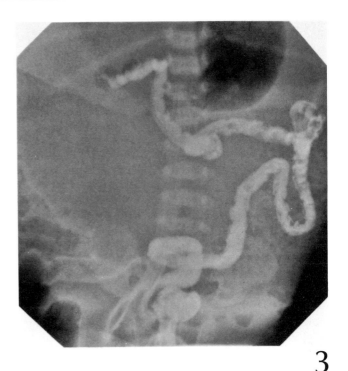

3

agent. Complications reported following Gastrografin enema include: perforation, necrotizing enterocolitis, shock and the occasional death. Most of these events are probably related to the hyperosmolar nature of the contrast material, causing fluid depletion, which results in decreased intestinal blood flow and perfusion. Some radiologists prefer using other agents such as diatrizoate sodium (Hypaque) or iothalamate meglumine (Conray), alone or in combination with N-acetylcysteine, but the authors prefer to use dilute Gastrografin.

4 The enema is gently administered under fluoroscopic control and the contrast material flushed around the obstructing meconium pellets in the terminal ileum.

Before the enema, an intravenous route is established and lactated Ringer's solution is administered at 20 ml/kg over 0.5 h. Intravenous fluids are infused at a rate of 1.5 times maintenance after the procedure. The infant's pulse rate and urine output are carefully monitored in anticipation of fluid shifts into the bowel lumen. Meconium pellets, followed by loose meconium, generally pass through the rectum over the next 4–8 h. If evidence of bowel obstruction persists and the infant remains clinically and hemodynamically stable, a second or third enema may be administered. N-acetylcysteine (2.5–5%, 5 ml in 6 h) may be administered by oral gastric tube to aid in clearing the thickened meconium. The Gastrografin enema is successful in resolving the obstruction in approximately 55% of cases. If these non-operative efforts fail, surgical exploration is required.

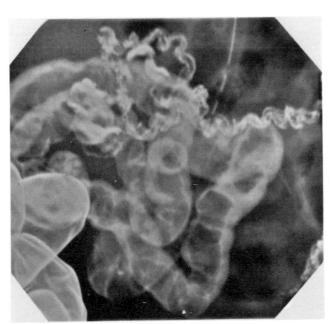

4

Complicated meconium ileus

Clinical presentation and initial management

5a—c Complicated cases include instances of volvulus, bowel perforation, intestinal atresia and giant cystic meconium peritonitis. Volvulus usually occurs when the distended segment of ileum twists at the level of the narrow pellet-filled distal small intestine (*Illustration 5a*). In some cases volvulus can result in bowel perforation, leading to meconium peritonitis (*Illustration 5b*) and, in others, the bowel may become necrotic and liquefy, resulting in a pseudocyst. This latter condition is referred to as a giant cystic meconium peritonitis. Bowel atresias are thought to arise when the base of the volvulus becomes ischemic (*Illustration 5c*).

Neonates with complicated meconium ileus usually present with abdominal distension at the time of, or shortly after, delivery. In addition, bile-stained fluid is usually noted in the stomach. On physical examination an abdominal mass may be noted. Neonates with meconium peritonitis occasionally have meconium in the scrotal sac or vagina as a result of passage of this material through a patent processus vaginalis or the fimbriated ends of the fallopian tubes, respectively. In addition, in one unusual report a meconium pseudocyst appeared as a buttock mass. The early management of these neonates includes intravenous hydration, antibiotics and oral gastric tube decompression of the stomach.

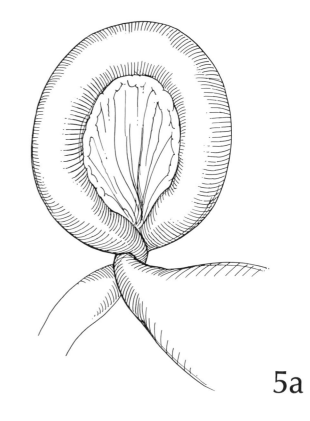

5a

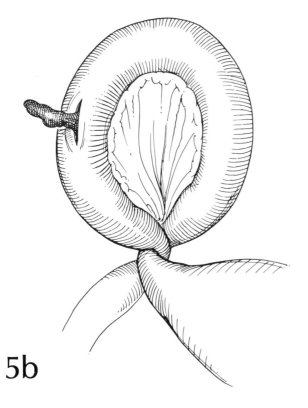

5b

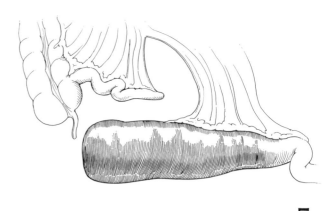

5c

Diagnosis

6 In contrast to neonates with uncomplicated meconium ileus, flat and erect or decubitus radiographs
of the abdomen in complicated cases may demonstrate
distended loops of small bowel of different size with
air-fluid levels. Intraperitoneal calcifications from the
extravasated meconium, characteristic of meconium
peritonitis, may be noted. A mass effect or ascites may
also be observed.

Neonates who can be identified as complicated cases
by plain abdominal radiographs are taken to the
operating room for prompt exploration. In uncertain
cases, a barium enema may be useful to exclude other
causes of distal obstruction.

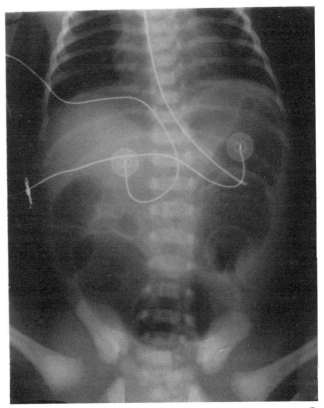

6

Operations

UNCOMPLICATED MECONIUM ILEUS

Mikulicz procedure

Meconium ileus was often considered a fatal condition until 1948 when Hiatt and Wilson reported a number of survivors after enterotomy and irrigation[3]. This technique was not widely utilized and, in 1953, Gross reported successful outcomes in infants with meconium ileus following bowel resection and use of a Mikulicz enterostomy[4].

7 The dilated bowel loop filled with thickened meconium is brought out of the abdomen and the small bowel proximal and distal to this segment is sutured together in a side-to-side fashion by interrupted seromuscular sutures. Following closure of the abdomen the exteriorized dilated bowel is resected, thus avoiding the risk of peritoneal contamination. This results in an enterostomy through which the distal bowel can be irrigated in the postoperative period to wash out the obstructing meconium pellets. A Mikulicz spur crushing clamp is applied, resulting in a common lumen, and the ostomy is then closed at a later date.

The disadvantages of this procedure are the loss of fluids from the mid–small bowel ostomy, the need for a subsequent procedure to close the stoma, and some reduction of bowel length due to the initial resection.

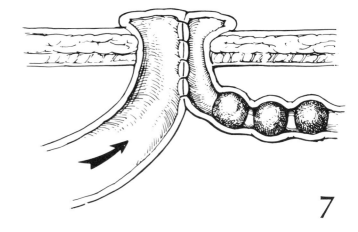

7

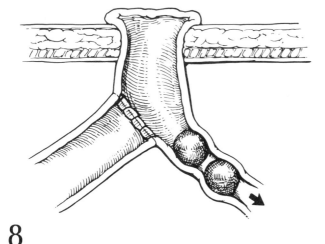

8

Bishop–Koop procedure

8 In 1957 Bishop and Koop reported resection of the large dilated loop followed by an anastomosis between the end of the proximal segment and the side of the distal segment[5]. The end of the distal bowel is then brought out as an end ileostomy. A catheter is passed into the distal segment to allow postoperative irrigation. As the distal obstruction is relieved the intestinal contents preferentially pass into the distal ileum and colon, thus decreasing loss of fluid and electrolytes from the stoma. The ostomy can be closed at a later date and, in some cases where it is trimmed beneath the skin, may close spontaneously.

The disadvantages of this technique include loss of bowel length at the time of the initial procedure, the need for an intraperitoneal anastomosis and the need for a second operative procedure.

Santulli–Blanc enterostomy

9 This modification of the Bishop–Koop procedure concept was reported in 1961[6]. The operation involves resection of the distal dilated bowel segment followed by a side-to-end anastomosis with proximal enterostomy.

Disadvantages are similar to those noted for the Bishop–Koop procedure.

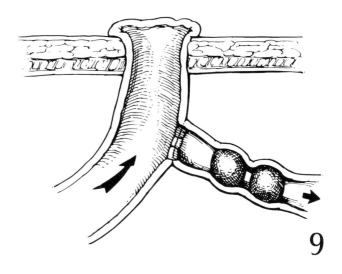

9

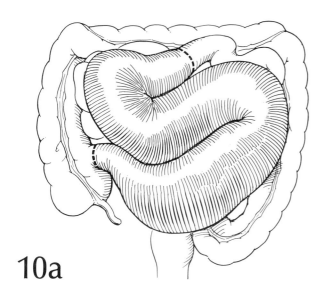

10a

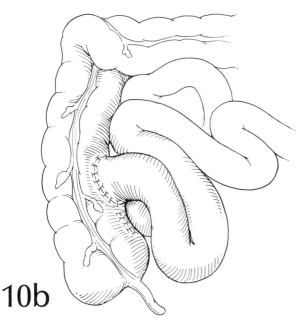

10b

Primary resection and anastomosis

The use of resection with primary anastomosis in the management of meconium ileus was first reported by Swenson in 1962[7].

10a, b After resection of the obstructed bowel segment the remaining pellets in the distal bowel are irrigated clear and an ileocolonic anastomosis is performed.

The disadvantage associated with this procedure is resection of additional bowel as the terminal ileum containing meconium pellets was usually resected along with the dilated segment of ileum. This, as well as concerns about an unvented intraperitoneal anastomosis, prevented wide acceptance of this procedure.

Tube enterostomy

11 In 1970 O'Neill and colleagues reported success with a simple procedure involving tube enterostomy with postoperative irrigation[8]. Their initial report of five neonates was followed by a report by Harberg *et al.* concerning nine of 11 neonates who had successful meconium washout using this technique[9].

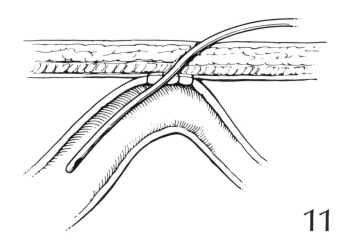

11

Enterotomy and irrigation

The technique of enterotomy with irrigation has been the procedure of choice at our institution since 1981. As previously noted, this procedure was originally described by Hiatt and Wilson in 1948[3]. Scattered reports by several other authors appeared in the literature between 1970 and 1990.

The infant is taken to the operating room and an endotracheal tube is placed before anesthesia to avoid aspiration.

12 After induction of general anesthesia, the procedure is carried out through a right-sided supraumbilical transverse abdominal incision. The right rectus abdominis muscle, as well as a portion of the right external and internal oblique and transversus abdominis muscles, is divided using electrocautery. The peritoneal cavity is entered and explored. The distended meconium-filled loops and pellet-filled distal small bowel are identified and delivered into the wound.

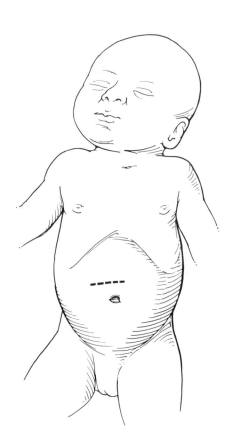

12

13 A purse-string suture of 4/0 silk is placed on the antimesenteric border of the dilated bowel 6–8 cm proximal to the narrow region containing the obstructing pellets. An 8–10-Fr red rubber catheter is placed through a small enterotomy, the purse-string suture is snugged, and the bowel lumen is irrigated by gently instilling saline through a syringe attached to an adapter and three-way stop cock. Fluid is irrigated into the proximal thick meconium and around the distal pellets.

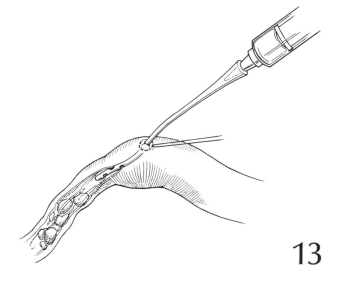

13

With irrigation, the thick meconium from the distended loop can be removed through the enterotomy, with gentle manual manipulation some of the distal obstructing pellets are 'milked' proximally out of the enterotomy. The remaining pellets are irrigated and washed out distally through the colon.

Occasionally the enterotomy may need to be extended to a 1.5–2.0-cm opening to allow removal of the thick meconium and pellets. Numerous irrigations are usually required. Dilute Gastrografin or 2.5–5% N-acetylcysteine solution may also be used for irrigation. There have been occasional reports documenting hypernatremia with some forms of N-acetylcysteine. When the pellets are cleared, saline is irrigated through the distal ileum and into the colon to exclude the possibility of atresia and also to flush some of the distal pellet fragments into the colon. The enterotomy is then closed in two layers, using an inner full-thickness layer of absorbable 4/0 or 5/0 polyglactin (running or interrupted) and an outer seromuscular layer with interrupted 5/0 silk suture. Irrigation of the bowel through the base of the appendix has also been described.

COMPLICATED MECONIUM ILEUS

The anesthetic management is similar to that described for uncomplicated cases. The abdomen is entered through a transverse supraumbilical incision. The operative findings and ease of procedure may vary significantly, from volvulus and bowel atresia to meconium peritonitis or giant cystic meconium peritonitis. These conditions will, therefore, be discussed separately.

Volvulus and atresia

In instances of meconium ileus associated with bowel volvulus or atresia, the pathology is usually easily identified at laparotomy, and a primary anastomosis is nearly always possible.

14a–c
In cases of volvulus, the involved loop is resected and an end-to-oblique anastomosis constructed between the dilated proximal bowel and smaller distal bowel. The proximal bowel is divided at a 90° angle with respect to the mesentery and the distal bowel at a 45° angle. The distal meconium pellets should be removed through the open bowel, and the distal segment should also be irrigated to facilitate return of bowel function and to avoid a postoperative obturator obstruction distal to the anastomosis. The anastomosis is constructed with one or two layers of interrupted 5/0 silk sutures.

In cases of atresia, if adequate bowel length is present, the proximal dilated segment (usually 10–15 cm) is resected, since it is frequently atonic, and an end-to-oblique anastomosis is fashioned.

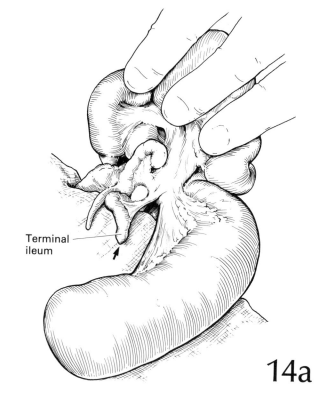

Terminal
ileum

14a

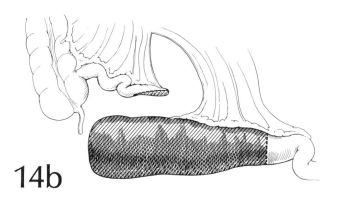

14b

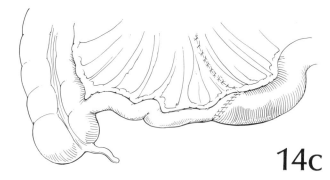

14c

Meconium peritonitis and giant cystic meconium peritonitis

Neonates with these two disorders generally have numerous adhesions throughout the abdomen and may have significant blood and fluid losses during the operation. The abdomen is explored and the small bowel and colon carefully identified and dissected free from the numerous adhesions.

The necrotic dilated segment is resected and, if possible, an end-to-end or end-to-oblique anastomosis is constructed. In some cases this is not possible and a temporary enterostomy is required. The bowel opening may be found within the pseudocyst. Most of the pseudocyst wall should be resected, if possible. This may result in some blood loss requiring transfusion. The proximal end may be brought out as a temporary stoma through the corner of the wound or through a separate incision. The distal bowel can either be closed with sutures or staples and left in the abdomen, or brought out as a separate mucous fistula to allow irrigation as well as refeeding of the effluent from the proximal ostomy into the distal bowel.

Postoperative care

Uncomplicated meconium ileus

In the early postoperative period an oral gastric tube is left in place until bowel function returns. Use of N-acetylcysteine (2.5–5%, 5–10 ml in 6 h) through an oral gastric tube may further aid passage of inspissated meconium. When bowel function returns, the tube is removed and enteral feedings are initiated along with pancreatic enzyme supplementation. The diagnosis of cystic fibrosis is confirmed by obtaining an elevated sweat chloride level on testing and the actual chromosomal defect is identified to assist in genetic counseling. The management of these patients requires a multidisciplinary team, including the pediatric respiratory physician, in order to optimize the pulmonary status which is the major cause of morbidity and mortality. Parents are carefully instructed regarding methods of chest percussion and postural drainage.

Long-term complications include the development of meconium ileus equivalent or the distal intestinal obstruction syndrome. This obturator obstruction often occurs after an intercurrent illness in which the child has a decreased oral intake and frequently stops taking the pancreatic enzyme supplement. This may require treatment with Gastrografin enemas or administration of a balanced intestinal lavage solution orally or though an oral gastric tube. Other complications can be related to pulmonary infections, hemoptysis, gallstones and cirrhosis of the liver. Recent advances in gene therapy and lung transplantation may serve further to prolong survival of these children.

Complicated meconium ileus

Neonates with complicated meconium ileus are managed in a similar manner to uncomplicated cases, although return of bowel function may be somewhat slower, particularly in cases of perforation. Some infants may require total parenteral nutrition if bowel function is slow to return, or if a proximal enterostomy does not provide an adequate absorptive surface to support the infant with enteral nutrition alone. Infants with both a proximal and distal stoma can often be managed with oral feeds combined with refeeding of the proximal ostomy effluent into the distal stoma. Enterostomy closure is generally performed 5–6 weeks after the initial procedure.

Outcome

The results of medical and surgical management of 62 neonates with meconium ileus treated between 1972 and 1993 at the James Whitcomb Riley Hospital for Children have been reviewed recently[10]. The study included 21 girls and 41 boys. A family history of cystic fibrosis was present in six neonates.

Twenty-six neonates had uncomplicated meconium ileus due to intraluminal obstruction of the terminal ileum with concretions of abnormal meconium. The treatment of these patients can be divided into two time periods, 1972–1980 and 1981–1993. Ten infants presented during the first time period, and only two of them were successfully cleared with a diatrizoate meglumine (Gastrografin) enema. The eight remaining infants underwent resection of the dilated segment of bowel filled with putty-like meconium, operative irrigation and enterostomy formation. A Bishop–Koop stoma was constructed in two infants, and six had a double-barrel (side-by-side) enterostomy. Of the 16 neonates treated during the later time period eight (50%) were successfully cleared with a Gastrografin enema. The remaining eight infants required laparotomy: seven were treated with enterotomy and intraoperative irrigation with saline or dilute contrast agent (Hypaque or Gastrografin) and one with irrigation and double barrel enterostomy.

Thirty-six neonates presented with 59 complications of meconium ileus, including volvulus (23), atresia (20), perforation (7) and giant cystic meconium peritonitis (8). Clinical presentation in these neonates included abdominal distension, bilious vomiting, and failure to pass meconium; these symptom were usually noted earlier than in uncomplicated cases. Neonates with perforation and giant cystic meconium peritonitis often had abdominal distension at the time of delivery. Neonates with atresia and volvulus also presented with signs and symptoms of obstruction earlier than neonates with uncomplicated meconium ileus, but occasionally tolerated several feeds.

In cases of meconium ileus complicated by atresia or volvulus, abdominal radiographs demonstrated marked dilation of the distal small bowel with air–fluid levels. In cases with perforation and giant cystic meconium peritonitis, radiographs frequently showed peritoneal calcification with a mass effect. In three recent cases prenatal ultrasonography documented the presence of intestinal obstruction and an associated mass. Two of these neonates were found to have giant cystic meconium peritonitis and the third a volvulus with peritonitis. Many of the children with atresia or volvulus underwent contrast barium enema examination if the plain films did not demonstrate definite evidence of complicated meconium ileus. Operative management of patients with atresia, volvulus and perforation included resection and anastomosis in 16 and enterostomy in 12. The eight patients with giant cystic meconium peritonitis underwent excision of the pseudocyst and enterostomy.

The diagnosis of cystic fibrosis was confirmed in all cases by a sweat chloride test. Pancreatic enzyme therapy was instituted along with a routine formula feed. Enterostomy closure was usually accomplished between 4 weeks and 3 months of age. All patients have been followed by the Indiana University Cystic Fibrosis Clinic at the James Whitcomb Riley Hospital for Children. Survival at 1 year was 92% (24/26) in patients with uncomplicated meconium ileus and 89% (32/36) in complicated cases. The mortality in the uncomplicated cases was due to pulmonary problems, and both occurred during the early time period. Deaths in the complicated cases were the result of sepsis (two), renal failure (one) and severe cholestatic jaundice progressing to liver failure (one).

Acknowledgments

Illustrations 1, 5a, 5b, 5c, 6, 7, 8, 9, 10a, 10b, 11, 12, 13, 15a and *15b* are reproduced with permission of the copyright holders, Indiana University School of Medicine.

References

1. Kerem BS, Rommens JM, Buchanan JA, *et al*. Identification of the cystic fibrosis gene: genetic analysis. *Science* 1989; 245: 1073–80.

2. Noblett HR. Treatment of uncomplicated meconium ileus by Gastrografin enema: a preliminary report. *J Pediatr Surg* 1969; 4: 190–7.

3. Hiatt RB, Wilson PE. Celiac syndrome: therapy of meconium ileus: report of eight cases with a review of the literature. *Surg Gynecol Obstet* 1948; 87: 317–27.

4. Gross RE. *The Surgery of Infancy and Childhood: its Principles and Techniques*. Philadelphia: Saunders, 1953: 175–91.

5. Bishop HC, Koop CE. Management of meconium ileus: resection, Roux-en-Y anastomosis and ileostomy irrigation with pancreatic enzymes. *Ann Surg* 1957; 145: 410–14.

6. Santulli TV, Blanc WA. Congenital atresia of the intestine: pathogenesis and treatment. *Ann Surg* 1961; 154: 939–48.

7. Swenson O. *Pediatric Surgery*, Vol 1, 3rd edn. New York: Appleton-Century Crofts, 1969: 672.

8. O'Neill JA, Grosfeld JL, Boles ET, Clatworthy HW, Jr. Surgical treatment of meconium ileus. *Am J Surg* 1970; 119: 99–105.

9. Harberg FJ, Senekjian EK, Pokorny WJ. Treatment of uncomplicated meconium ileus via T-tube ileostomy. *J Pediatr Surg* 1981; 16: 61–3.

10. Rescorla FJ, Grosfeld JL. Contemporary management of meconium ileus. *World J Surg* 1993; 17: 318–25.

Vitellointestinal (omphalomesenteric) duct anomalies

Spencer W. Beasley MS, FRACS
Senior Lecturer, Department of Paediatrics, University of Melbourne, Consultant Surgeon, Royal Children's Hospital, Melbourne, and Chairman, Division of Paediatrics, PANCH, Preston, Victoria, Australia

The vitellointestinal (omphalomesenteric) duct is an embryonic communication between the yolk sac and the midgut. This communication normally disappears at about the sixth week of fetal life. Persistence of the duct between the intestinal tract and the umbilicus, or persistence of its embryonic blood supply, results in a variety of lesions which usually present in early infancy, but occasionally appear later in life.

Types of anomalies

A Meckel's diverticulum represents persistence and patency of the inner or intestinal component of the vitellointestinal tract (*see Illustration 1*). In a small proportion of patients there will be a fibrous band extending from the apex of the Meckel's diverticulum to the undersurface of the umbilicus (*see Illustration 2*), but more often there is a band representing the remnants of the vitelline vessels joining the Meckel's diverticulum to the mesentery of the small bowel (*see Illustration 3*). Meckel's diverticulum has diverse clinical presentations (*Table 1*), but frequently remains quiescent throughout life. The chances of an asymptomatic Meckel's diverticulum causing symptoms later in life are such that *en passant* removal of the structure when it is observed during operation for some other reason is arguably justified in children, but is probably not justified in adults when the chances of it becoming symptomatic are remote.

Table 1 Presentation of Meckel's diverticulum

Melena and anemia	Ectopic gastric mucosa in the Meckel's diverticulum releases hydrochloric acid which causes ulceration of adjacent ileum, producing major gastrointestinal bleeding
Abdominal pain (Meckel's diverticulitis)	Inflammation of a Meckel's diverticulum, particularly if long and with a narrow lumen, causes clinical features similar to those of acute suppurative appendicitis. Perforation of an adjacent ileal ulcer may also cause an inflammatory mass, pneumoperitoneum and peritonitis
Intussusception	A Meckel's diverticulum may invert and act as a lead point for an intussusception. This is responsible for about 2% of intussusceptions
Meckel's band obstruction	A band extending from a Meckel's diverticulum to the root of the small bowel mesentery or to the umbilicus may cause a loop of bowel to become entangled around it, producing a bowel obstruction
Incidental finding	During laparotomy for other conditions, e.g. appendicitis, a Meckel's diverticulum may be found

1 The typical appearance of a Meckel's diverticulum is shown in cross section. Parts of the inner surface may contain ectopic pancreatic or gastric mucosa. Ectopic gastric mucosa produces hydrochloric acid which can ulcerate adjacent non-gastric mucosa, either in the diverticulum itself or in adjacent ileum, and cause bleeding.

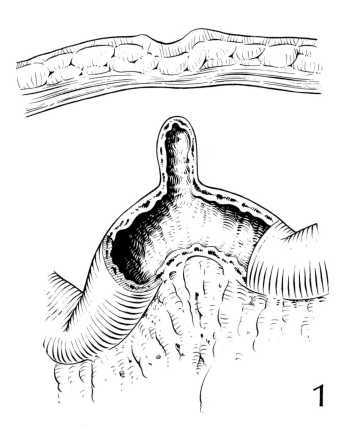

1

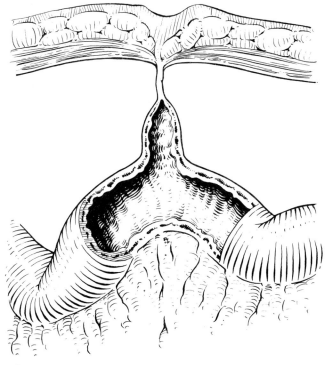

2

2 The vitellointestinal band (Meckel's band) is the remnant of the duct in which the lumen has been obliterated, but a fibrous cord or band persists. This runs from the deep surface of the umbilicus to the ileum or to a Meckel's diverticulum. There is always a risk that a loop of bowel may become entangled around it, producing intestinal obstruction, often with a closed loop.

3 The Meckel's diverticulum is often bound down by remnants of the vitelline vessels from its apex and is adherent to the mesentery of the ileum. (Division of the vessels at the apex and of the peritoneal fold reveals its typical antimesenteric origin.)

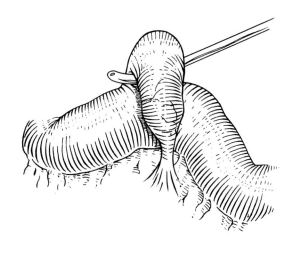

3

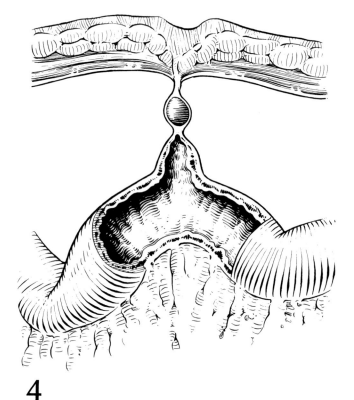

4

4 This form of Meckel's diverticulum has a cord containing a cystic remnant which may slowly increase in size. A cyst is the result of partial obliteration of the duct. It may become infected and form an abscess; if it has a sinus, pus may discharge from the umbilicus.

Bleeding Meckel's diverticulum

Principles and justification

This is the most common clinical presentation of a Meckel's diverticulum, and results from the presence of ectopic gastric mucosa in the lining of the diverticulum. Hydrochloric acid produced by the gastric mucosa causes ulceration of the adjacent small bowel mucosa and, less commonly, of the diverticulum itself. This may result in rapid hemorrhage which usually presents as painless but profuse 'brick-red' rectal bleeding. The resultant anemia may necessitate blood transfusion, but the bleeding usually stops spontaneously without the need for emergency surgery. The definitive investigation is surgery, but a technetium scan may confirm the presence of ectopic gastric mucosa.

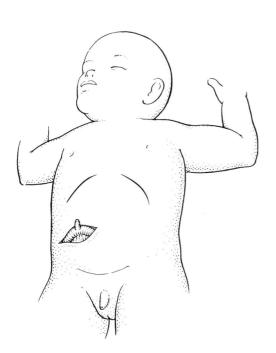

5

Indications

Surgery is indicated where the clinical presentation of major and painless intestinal hemorrhage is consistent with a bleeding Meckel's diverticulum, irrespective of the results of the technetium scan.

Preoperative

Anesthesia

The procedure is performed under general anesthesia and muscle paralysis, using the same technique as for any acute abdominal procedure. Blood transfusion is required very occasionally in the perioperative period for major blood loss from the ileum, although the operative procedure itself is relatively bloodless. Electrolytes and fluid balance must be monitored. Perioperative antibiotics are administered.

Operation

Incision

5 The surgical approach is through a right transverse infraumbilical, muscle-splitting or muscle-cutting incision. This can be extended medially by retracting the rectus towards the midline or even dividing the muscle, if necessary. A Meckel's diverticulum can be excised easily through the standard incision used for an appendectomy. Alternatively, laparoscopic-assisted Meckel's diverticulectomy through an umbilical incision has also been described.

Identification of lesion

At laparotomy for bleeding the Meckel's diverticulum will not usually be inflamed. A blue discoloration will be seen in the ileum and colon distal to the diverticulum if recent bleeding has occurred. The diverticulum causing bleeding is delivered through the wound.

Control of ileum and its contents

6 Compression of the ileum with fingers or a non-crushing bowel clamp (fingers are preferred because they are less traumatic to the bowel) reduces the amount of bleeding and soiling that occurs when the ileum is opened and the diverticulum is excised. Packs are placed on either side of the loop of ileum containing the Meckel's diverticulum. Suction is kept nearby to reduce accidental spillage of liquid ileal contents when the ileum is opened. Stay sutures (3/0) are placed on the ileum on either side of the diverticulum.

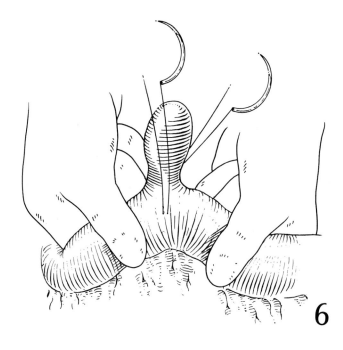

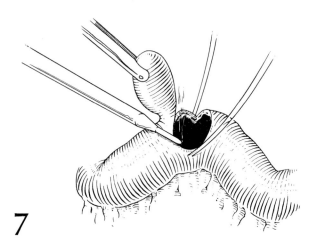

Excision of diverticulum

7 A longitudinal or oblique elliptical incision is made in the ileum near the base of the diverticulum using scissors or diathermy. It is *essential* that the entire diverticulum is removed because a remnant of acid-secreting mucosa left at the base of the diverticulum could continue to cause ulceration and bleeding of adjacent ileum.

8 The stay sutures are then held apart to transform the longitudinal or oblique elliptical incision into a transverse one. This allows closure of the wound without narrowing the lumen of the ileum.

Closure of ileum

A 4/0 polyglycolic acid continuous or interrupted all-layers suture is used to close the bowel. A second seromuscular continuous layer can be employed.

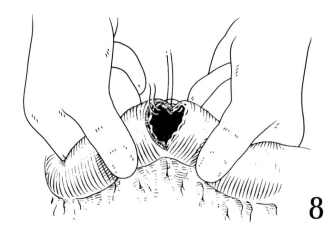

Alternative method for narrow-necked diverticulum

9 A curved artery forceps or crushing clamp is placed across the base of the diverticulum at 45° or more to the long axis of the ileum. This avoids the narrowing which might be caused by an incision closed longitudinally. Mattress sutures of 3/0 polyglycolic acid are inserted under the clamp and tied. The diverticulum is cut away at the distal border of the clamp.

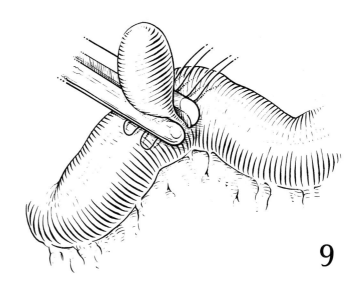

9

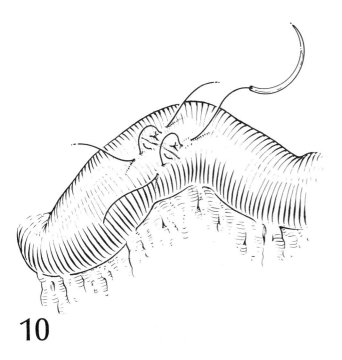

10

10 The clamp is removed and the line of section buried by a second layer of sutures.

Wound closure

The peritoneal cavity is irrigated with antibiotic saline before closure. The wound is closed in layers with 2/0 or 3/0 absorbable polyglycolic acid sutures.

Postoperative care

Oral fluids can be commenced on about the second day after operation when the abdomen is becoming soft to palpation and there is no nausea, i.e. no clinical evidence of ileus. Most children can be discharged on the third or fourth day after operation.

Meckel's diverticulitis

Principles and justification

Meckel's diverticulitis is an extremely unusual presentation in children. When it does occur, the child is assessed clinically as having acute suppurative appendicitis, but at laparotomy the appendix is found to be normal and there is an inflammatory process involving a Meckel's diverticulum. In all operations for suspected appendicitis in which the appendix is found at laparotomy to be normal, the distal 100 cm of ileum should be inspected to exclude inflammation of a Meckel's diverticulum as being responsible for the symptoms. The inflamed Meckel's diverticulum is often palpable in the abdomen on opening the peritoneum. An inflammatory mass around a Meckel's diverticulum may result from perforation of an ulcer in ileum adjacent to the base of the diverticulum. Perforation may also cause pneumoperitoneum and peritonitis.

Indications

The indication for surgery for Meckel's diverticulitis is when the appendix is found to be normal at the time of laparotomy for suspected appendicitis and an adjacent inflammatory mass (inflamed diverticulum) is identified.

Preoperative

Anesthesia

The procedure is performed under general anesthesia and muscle paralysis using the same technique as for acute appendicitis. Perioperative antibiotics are administered.

Operation

Incision and exposure

When the diagnosis is known or suspected before operation, a small transverse right infraumbilical incision can be used. If the diagnosis is made during operation at the time of exploration for suspected appendicitis, the inflamed Meckel's diverticulum and adjacent ileum can be delivered easily through the appendectomy wound and the diverticulum excised outside the abdomen.

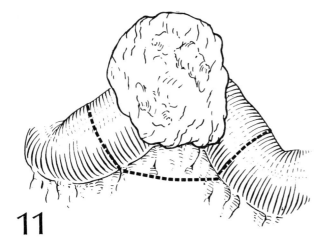

11

Extensive inflammatory mass

11 If there is severe or long-standing inflammation of the diverticulum causing edema and involving the surrounding ileum or if the base of the Meckel's diverticulum is very broad, it is appropriate to excise it with a small sleeve of ileum and perform an end-to-end small bowel anastomosis along conventional lines. Otherwise, the inflamed Meckel's diverticulum is excised in the same way as for a bleeding Meckel's diverticulum.

Meckel's band obstruction

Indications

These children present with a distal small bowel obstruction, the exact cause of which cannot usually be determined clinically. Laparotomy is performed for obstruction. Closed loop obstruction is common.

Operation

12 A right supraumbilical or subumbilical incision is standard where the pathology is not certain before operation. The band running from the Meckel's diverticulum is identified and divided, releasing the entrapped loops of bowel. Most commonly, the band runs to the root of the small bowel mesentery (*see Illustration 2*), but may be attached to the undersurface of the umbilicus (*see Illustration 3*).

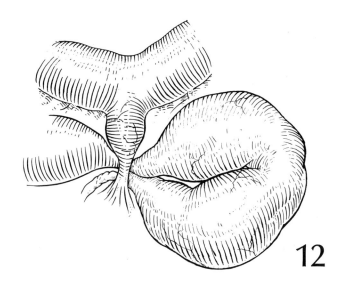

Intussusception of Meckel's diverticulum

Meckel's diverticulum is the most common cause of intussusception in which a pathologic lesion at the lead point is identified. It may occur at any age during childhood, but is most common in the first 2 years of life.

Indications

Peritonitis or other clinical evidence of the presence of ischemic bowel is an absolute indication for surgery in patients with intussusception. Otherwise, the child is treated initially by gas (or barium) enema. Where the intussusception is due to a Meckel's diverticulum, however, enema reduction is unlikely to be successful and surgery is indicated because the enema has failed to reduce the intussusception.

Operation

Incision

A right transverse supraumbilical incision is deepened as a muscle-cutting incision through the rectus abdominis.

Technique

13 The intussusception is located and an attempt made to reduce it manually by gentle compression of the colon in a proximal direction at the level of the lead point. Much of the intussusception can be reduced, but when there is a Meckel's diverticulum at the lead point the final portion often cannot be reduced and must be resected in continuity with the diverticulum.

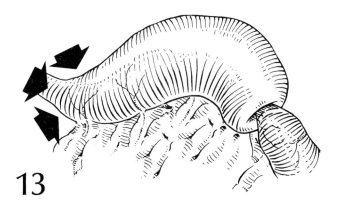

Complete persistence of the vitellointestinal duct (fistula)

Principles and justification

14 When the entire vitellointestinal (omphalomesenteric) duct persists and remains patent there is an open communication between the ileum and the umbilicus. This allows intermittent discharge of the contents of the ileum (gas and ileal fluid) and causes periumbilical excoriation. The tract may be of sufficient caliber to allow prolapse of ileum as a 'pair of horns'.

Diagnosis

Escape of air and feces through an opening in the umbilicus is pathognomonic of a patent vitellointestinal tract. When there is doubt about the nature of the discharge from the umbilicus (often because of its intermittency) a sinogram will usually demonstrate direct communication with the ileum.

Indications

Surgery is indicated in all cases where a patent vitellointestinal tract has been demonstrated.

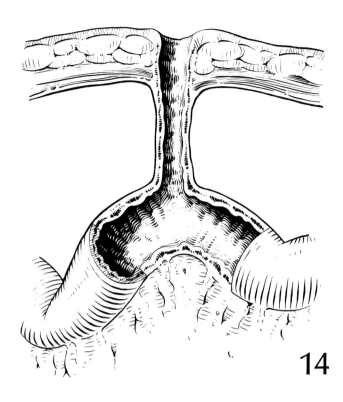

14

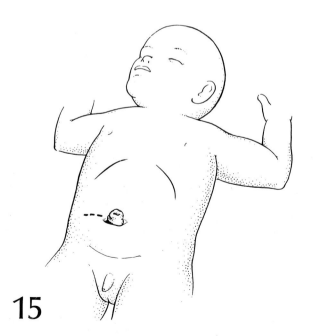

15

Operation

Incision

15 A right transverse incision immediately lateral to the umbilicus through the rectus muscles allows adequate exposure of the vitellointestinal tract from within, avoiding the need to circumcise the umbilicus. After dissection of the tract, the defect in the umbilicus can be repaired from its deep surface.

16 Alternatively, an incision in the umbilicus, circumcising the external opening of the patent vitellointestinal tract, can be made. The tract is mobilized by separating it from the tough fascia of the linea alba surrounding it, and the peritoneum is opened. To improve exposure, the incision usually needs to be extended lateral to the umbilicus by dividing the medial 1–2 cm of rectus abdominis, including the anterior rectus sheath, medial fibers of the rectus abdominis muscle and the posterior rectus sheath.

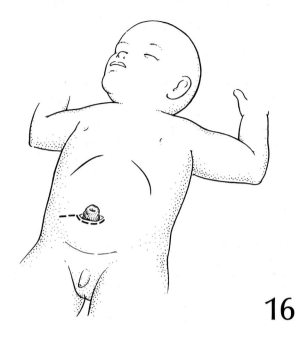

16

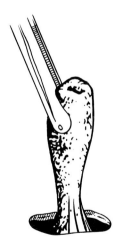

17

Dissection of tract

17 Dissection of the vitellointestinal tract is continued into the peritoneal cavity where its communication with the ileum is readily seen.

Division at junction with ileum

Two stay sutures are placed on the ileum and the vitellointestinal tract is divided at this point. The communication with the ileum may be narrow, resembling a fibrous cord, or broad as in many patients with a Meckel's diverticulum. The ileum is closed in one or two layers with absorbable 3/0 or 4/0 polyglycolic acid sutures.

Reconstruction of umbilicus

The defect in the umbilical ring is repaired in the same way as for an umbilical hernia. When the incision has been extended to the right, the posterior and anterior rectus sheath should be closed with 3/0 polyglycolic acid sutures.

Prolapse of patent vitellointestinal tract

Principles and justification

18 When the channel is a short and broad vitellointestinal tract, the ileum may intussuscept through it onto the surface of the umbilicus, producing a double-horned or 'Y-shaped' segment of bowel, inside out, with a lumen evident on each horn.

Operation

As long as the bowel is not necrotic (which is rare) it should be reduced manually, after which the vitellointestinal tract can be excised as a semielective procedure. In extremely rare situations there is a single-horned prolapse of the vitellointestinal tract. This is occasionally seen in the neonatal period and suggests that there is an atresia of one horn which will necessitate excision of the vitellointestinal tract and end-to-end ileoileostomy to reconstitute gastrointestinal continuity. This is usually an isolated lesion, not associated with other abnormalities.

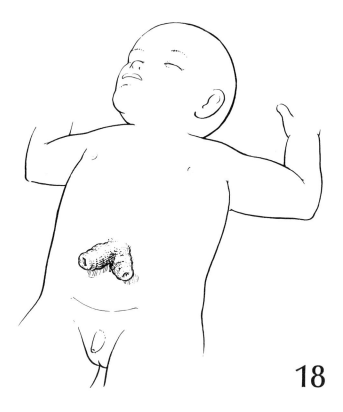

18

Ectopic mucosa

Principles and justification

Discharge of mucus from the umbilicus may be caused by a small sequestrated nodule of ectopic alimentary mucosa (representing persistence of the external part of the vitellointestinal tract). It appears as a shiny, spherical, deep red nodule in the depths of the umbilical cicatrix, but may be pedunculated. Crusts may form on the cicatrix and on the surrounding skin. It should be distinguished clinically from the more common umbilical granuloma which presents as a small mass of heaped pink or greyish granulations accompanied by a chronic seropurulent discharge: the granuloma can be treated with topical application of silver nitrate.

Contraindications

If a sinus opening is evident, it is likely that all or part of the vitellointestinal tract is present and patent. Likewise, discharge of air or fecal fluid suggests complete patency of the vitellointestinal tract (vitellointestinal fistula). In this situation, surgical excision of the whole tract will be required.

Operation

19 Pedunculated ectopic mucosa can be ligated within the umbilical ring; alternatively, a wider based lesion may be excised by diathermy dissection across its base. Suture is required only occasionally.

Further reading

Campbell J, Beasley SW, McMullin N, Hutson JM. Clinical diagnosis of umbilical swellings and discharges in children. *Med J Aust* 1986; 145: 450–3.

Oldham KT. Meckel's diverticulum and related disorders. In: Greenfield LJ, Mulholland MW, Oldham KT, Zelenock GB, eds. *Surgery: Scientific Principles and Practice*. Philadelphia: JP Lippincott, 1993: 1872–3.

Williams RS. Management of Meckel's diverticulum. *Br J Surg* 1981; 68: 477–81.

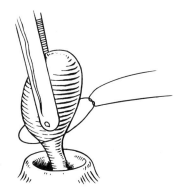

19

Illustrations by Paul Richardson

Duplications of the alimentary tract

Mark D. Stringer BSc, MRCP, MS, FRCS
Consultant Paediatric Surgeon, United Leeds Teaching Hospitals Trust and St James's University Hospital Trust, Leeds, UK

Principles and justification

Alimentary tract duplications are rare congenital malformations that may be found anywhere from mouth to anus[1] and include various other pathologic entities such as enterogenous and neurenteric cysts. Duplications are mostly single, more often cystic than tubular and vary widely in size. Duplications are typically located on the mesenteric aspect of the intestine but may occur at remote sites. They are lined by alimentary tract mucosa and usually share a common smooth muscle wall and blood supply with the adjacent gut, with which they may communicate. Heterotopic gastric mucosa may be found in any duplication but is more often seen in tubular lesions. Most duplications cause symptoms in infancy or early childhood but some present as an incidental finding in patients with other conditions.

There is no satisfactory single explanation for the development of duplications. The pathogenesis of those with associated vertebral anomalies is best explained by an abnormal adherence of the endodermal roof of the embryonic gut to the developing notochord (the 'split notochord' theory). Some hindgut duplications may arise from caudal twinning and some intestinal lesions may result from an intrauterine mesenteric vascular accident.

Distribution and variety

1   The distribution and variety of duplications is reflected by their diverse presentations[2], which include obstruction (respiratory, esophageal, intestinal), hemorrhage, infection/inflammation, perforation, intussusception or an asymptomatic mass. The distribution of 500 alimentary tract duplications[2] is shown in the illustration.

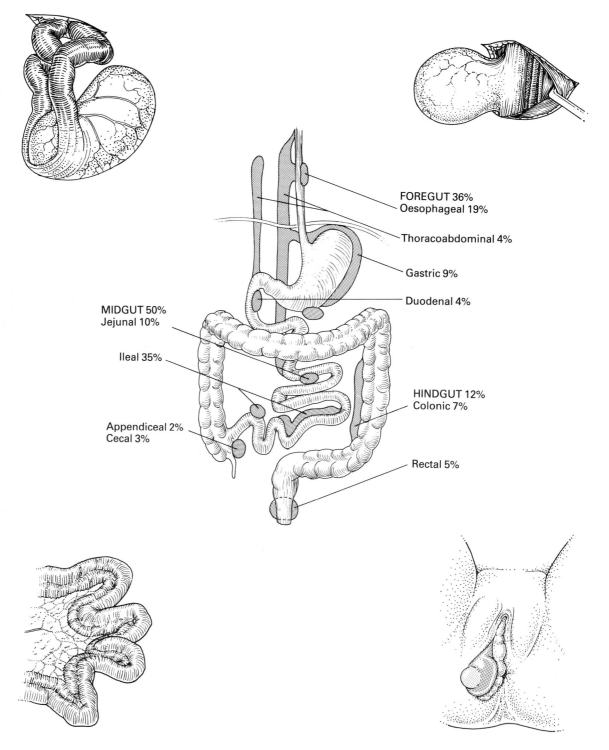

FOREGUT 36%
Oesophageal 19%

Thoracoabdominal 4%

Gastric 9%

Duodenal 4%

MIDGUT 50%
Jejunal 10%

Ileal 35%

Appendiceal 2%
Cecal 3%

HINDGUT 12%
Colonic 7%

Rectal 5%

1

Treatment of duplications

Alimentary tract duplications should be treated by early complete excision. Rarely, complete resection is too hazardous and alternative techniques such as mucosal stripping or fenestration are necessary. Asymptomatic appendiceal duplications found in association with cloacal or bladder exstrophy may be retained for use in reconstructive surgery later. With the possible exception of rectal duplications, the risk of late malignant degeneration is rare and overzealous surgery is not recommended.

Preparation of patient

Patients with intestinal obstruction should be fully resuscitated before surgery. In elective cases mechanical bowel preparation is advisable before operating on an intestinal duplication: oral intake is limited to clear fluids for 24 h before surgery and, for non-obstructing lesions of the large intestine, stimulant laxatives or whole gut irrigation may be combined with rectal washout.

Anesthesia

All patients should receive prophylactic parenteral broad-spectrum antibiotics at induction of anesthesia. Anesthesia should be tailored to the age of the patient and to the location and size of the lesion. Requirements for postoperative analgesia and possible respiratory support should be considered with the anesthetist before surgery. Cross-matched blood must be available and central access is useful during major operations.

Preoperative

Diagnosis

2 Vertebral anomalies are important diagnostic pointers and may also indicate the presence of related intraspinal pathology, particularly with foregut duplications. Other congenital malformations are found in 50% of patients. For example, intestinal malrotation or atresia may occur with midgut duplications and genitourinary duplication and bladder exstrophy with hindgut lesions.

Isolated duplications of the small intestine require few preoperative investigations; plain radiography, abdominal sonography and occasionally a radionuclide scan to detect heterotopic gastric mucosa. In contrast, thoracoabdominal lesions demand detailed radiologic imaging of mediastinal, abdominal and spinal components (including the cervical spine). Computerized tomographic (CT) scanning or magnetic resonance imaging (MRI) facilitate assessment of the cranial and caudal extent of the cyst. Supplementary investigations such as upper gastrointestinal contrast studies, endoscopy and myelography may be necessary. In older children, endoscopic retrograde cholangiopancreatography is helpful in evaluating some duodenal lesions and mesenteric angiography is useful for huge retroperitoneal cysts. Pelvic duplications are best imaged by CT or MRI in conjunction with contrast enema, fistulogram, and urinary tract sonography.

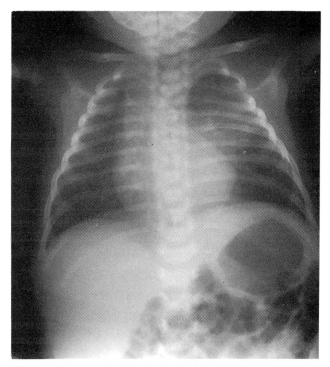

Chest radiograph of infant with foregut duplication cyst, showing thoracic vertebral anomalies and left mid-zone consolidation

2

Operation

The goal of each procedure should be complete excision of the duplication, but the surgeon must be familiar with a variety of alternative techniques that may be needed on rare occasions.

Small intestine

3a–c Cystic lesions of the ileum or jejunum, the most common duplications, may usually be excised without difficulty, but the continuous muscular coats of the normal and duplicated bowel make excision of the cyst alone difficult and impractical, and the duplication should be resected with the adjacent intestine after serial ligation and division of mesenteric vessels.

If the intestine is obstructed, atraumatic clamps placed across the intestine (but not the mesentery) will help prevent spillage. Before dividing the bowel with cutting needle diathermy or scissors the surgical field should be protected using gauze swabs soaked in warm dilute aqueous povidone-iodine. End-to-end anastomosis is performed using a single layer of interrupted extramucosal sutures such as 4/0 or 5/0 polyglactin (Vicryl) or polydioxanone (PDS), depending on the size of the intestine.

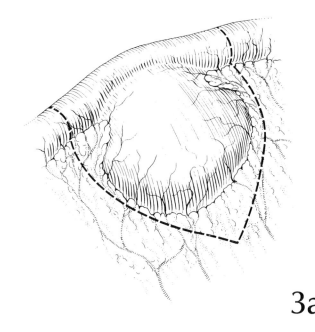

3a

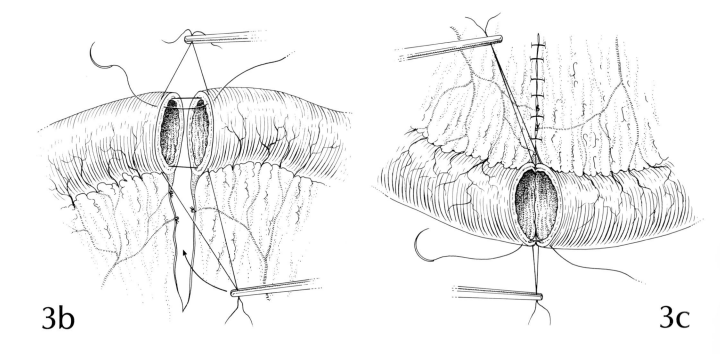

3b

3c

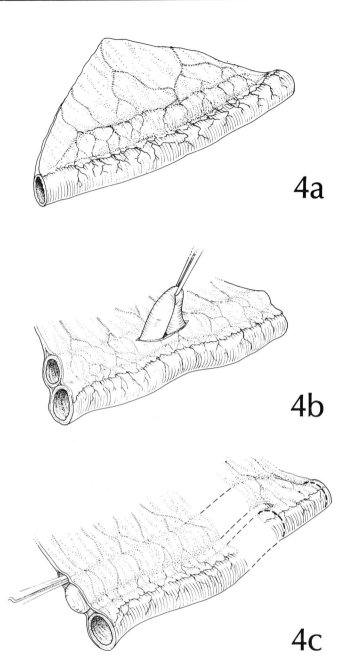

4a–c

Short tubular duplications may also be excised in continuity with adjacent intestine, but care should be taken to obtain complete excision at the proximal and distal margins of the lesion where the distinction between normal and duplicated bowel may be difficult.

Very extensive tubular duplications, where remaining intestinal length is an important issue, pose more of a problem. Alternative treatment for these unusual cases is submucosal resection[3]. The mucosal lining is stripped out using a series of longitudinal seromuscular incisions in the duplication. The submucosal injection of saline may help to define this plane. The residual seromuscular sleeve of the duplication may be safely left *in situ*. Bleeding within this sleeve almost always stops spontaneously.

For duplications that are within the mesentery yet are separate from the intestine, careful separation of the two leaves of the mesentery and division of vessels on one side only may enable enucleation of the duplication without jeopardizing the blood supply of the adjacent bowel[4].

Whichever technique is used, it is essential to resect the junction of duplicated and normal bowel because heterotopic gastric mucosa is frequently present in tubular small bowel duplications and also to check the viability of the remaining intestine carefully.

Associated intestinal malrotation requires a Ladd's procedure.

Esophagus

5a–c Duplications of the esophagus are usually intramural non-communicating cystic lesions, more often related to the right side of the esophagus, and are approached via a posterolateral transpleural thoracotomy. Cervical esophageal duplications may be removed via a supraclavicular approach.

The cyst is most easily excised by transecting the base of the lesion close to the esophagus and removing the residual mucosa, leaving a small circumferential muscle cuff. The proximity of the vagus and phrenic nerves and the thoracic duct should be noted. Any communication with the esophagus should be closed and the muscular defect repaired using the fringe of duplication muscle. Occasionally, an adjacent esophageal stricture or ulcer will require a segmental esophageal resection. The chest is closed and pleural drainage is not usually necessary.

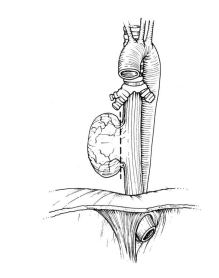

5a

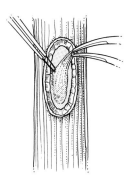

5b

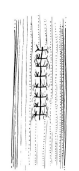

5c

Thoracoabdominal duplications

6 A thoracoabdominal duplication usually lies to the right of, but separate from, the esophagus in the posterior mediastinum and communicates through the diaphragm with the stomach, duodenum, jejunum or ileum. These lesions are best resected by separate thoracic (posterolateral thoracotomy) and abdominal incisions. On rare occasions laminectomy may also be necessary to deal with an intraspinal component. A staged approach, excising each component sequentially, should be avoided if possible as complications may occur in the interval; it is least hazardous when an asymptomatic abdominal component is temporarily left *in situ* but an undrained thoracic segment may be dangerous. Complete excision of the duplication involves dissecting its often thin upper extremity free from any bony vertebral attachment, which may require use of a gouge or chisel. The duplication is traced distally, where it usually passes behind the diaphragm and may become very tenuous; however, it rarely terminates at this level. The lesion should be pulled up into the chest and divided between ligatures and the chest closed with pleural drainage. The abdominal portion most often appears as a tubular lesion communicating with the jejunum but may end blindly along the greater curve of the stomach. It is usually excised without difficulty. Some thoracoabdominal duplications present with hemoptysis due to erosion into the lung from peptic ulceration; successful excision requires oversewing the fistula or, rarely, lobectomy.

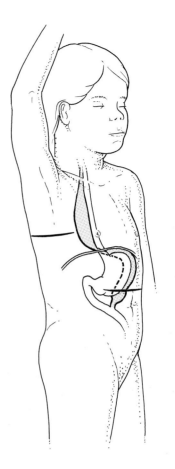

6

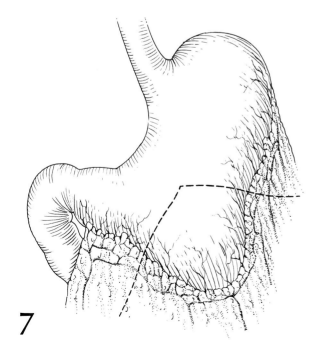

7

Stomach

7 Many duplications of the greater curve or pylorus may be completely excised by dissecting the cyst from the gastric submucosa and repairing the residual seromuscular defect with interrupted inverting absorbable sutures. After a difficult dissection, the stomach can be inflated with air to detect an unsuspected perforation before beginning the repair. Cystic gastric duplications rarely communicate with the stomach lumen. Small lesions may be more simply excised by wedge resection of the cyst and a margin of stomach followed by two-layer gastric closure.

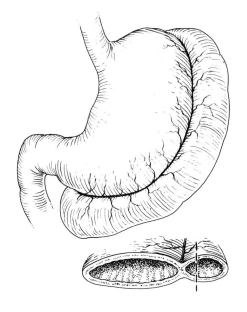

8a, b Extensive duplications of the greater curve can be treated by partial resection, stripping the residual mucosal lining and repairing the defect. Alternatively, the septum separating the duplication from the gastric lumen can be divided with linear staplers introduced via proximal and distal gastrotomies. The septum should be divided completely but this procedure must be regarded as second best because it does not remove the mucosal lining of the duplication.

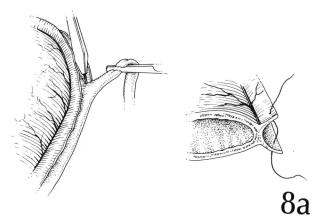

8a

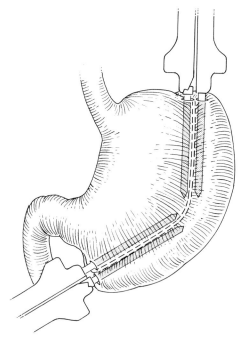

8b

Duodenum

9 Although some duodenal duplications are simple cystic lesions and are easily excised, those related to the second part of the duodenum in particular may be extremely complex and may communicate with the pancreatic and/or biliary ducts. Previous pancreatitis or peptic ulceration from heterotopic gastric mucosa may add to the surgical difficulties. Facilities for intraoperative cholangiopancreatography should be available and the child placed on a radiolucent operating table.

Alternative approaches are dictated by the anatomy and include complete excision of the cyst with ligation and division of any ductal communication, partial excision and mucosectomy, and fenestration into the duodenal lumen (when the duplication is adjacent to the ampulla of Vater). If this last technique is performed, the presence of gastric mucosa should be excluded by intraoperative biopsies and the window must be of sufficient size to allow good dependent drainage. The edges of the window should be cautiously oversewn with fine absorbable sutures to achieve hemostasis.

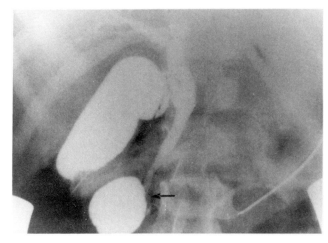

Intraoperative cholangiogram showing a duplication cyst (arrowed) communicating with the distal common bile duct

9

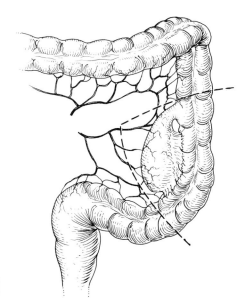

10

Colon and appendix

10 All cystic, and most tubular, duplications may be excised directly with an adjacent segment of colon. The bowel is repaired with an end-to-end, single layer, extramucosal anastomosis.

11 The rare total colonic duplication tends to lie lateral or medial to the normal colon rather than in the mesentery and commonly has a proximal connection[5]. Heterotopic gastric mucosa is very rarely present and if resection would necessitate total colectomy, distal fenestration may be undertaken by introducing a linear stapler through an enterotomy near the distal margin of the duplication. The distal end of the septum must be completely divided to avoid leaving a spur. If both colons reach the perineum a preliminary double defunctioning colostomy is recommended. The duplicated bowel may subsequently be divided at the rectal level and anastomosed to the normal rectum; the mucosa of the redundant distal segment is then excised.

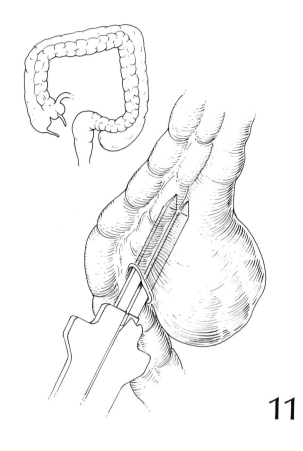

11

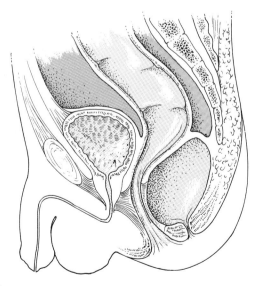

12

Rectum

12 Rectal duplications often present as a neonatal perianal mucosal swelling and/or perianal fistula. They may be excised by one of several approaches[6].

13 Small submucosal rectal lesions can be excised through an endorectal route. The anus is dilated and retracted causing the cyst to bulge forward. The rectal mucosa over the cyst is incised and, keeping in the submucosal plane of the rectum, the cyst is gradually dissected free. The cyst should not be aspirated until near the end of the dissection. The rectal incision is repaired with interrupted absorbable sutures.

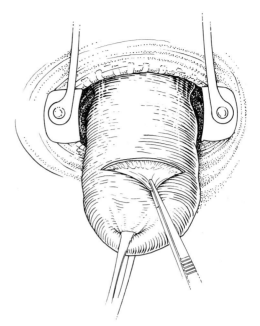

13

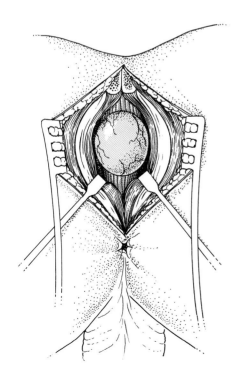

14

14 For larger or more complex duplications which may have a diverticulum, the posterior sagittal approach provides excellent exposure of the retrorectal space. Occasionally, a limited perineal excision is all that is required for a localized small mucosal duplication. With attention to bowel preparation and antibiotic prophylaxis, a defunctioning colostomy is rarely required.

Infected rectal duplication cysts should intially be treated by drainage and resected after the acute inflammation has settled.

Other sites

Retroperitoneal duplication cysts may be very large and frequently adhere to the pancreas. Some are undoubtedly unusual varieties of gastric duplication cysts and great care is required during surgery to avoid injuring mesenteric vessels and nearby viscera. Duplication cysts in the tongue tend to be small and may be removed by an intraoral sublingual approach. Intradural or extradural spinal duplications should be investigated and treated by pediatric surgeons with neurosurgical expertise.

Postoperative care

The postoperative course is dictated by the anatomy of the duplication and the complexity of the procedure. Surgical complications are related to size, location, communication with the gastrointestinal tract, presence of heterotopic gastric mucosa and involvement of mesenteric vessels[2]. Incomplete excision is a particular risk with thoracoabdominal duplications and potential consequences include meningitis, gastrointestinal bleeding and perforation and respiratory problems.

Outcome

An analysis of 72 children (41 boys, 31 girls) with alimentary tract duplications referred to the Hospital for Sick Children, London between 1973 and 1992 has been carried out, and the results are shown in *Table 1*. Vertebral anomalies were present in 21% of patients and heterotopic gastric mucosa in almost 30% of duplications. Twelve patients had incidental, asymptomatic duplications associated with other major congenital anomalies but the duplication was the principal pathology in 60 patients, with a median age of 3 months. In this group, foregut lesions were responsible for much of the overall morbidity and mortality: five patients died from postoperative complications.

A wide appreciation of the spectrum of these lesions, careful preoperative assessment and appropriate surgery are the essential steps to a successful outcome.

Table 1   Distribution and characteristics of 77 alimentary tract duplications in 72 children

Site of duplication	Number of duplications	Spherical/tubular	Heterotopic gastric mucosa*	Vertebral anomalies
Foregut	39	29/10	11	7
Oropharyngeal	2	2/0	0	0
Esophageal	15	12/3	3	2(C)
Thoracoabdominal	6	0/6	6	5(3C, 2D)
Gastric	10	9/1	—	0
body	4			
antrum and pylorus	6			
Duodenal	3	3/0	1	0
Retroperitoneal†	3	3/0	1	0
Midgut	30	16/14	7	5
Jejunal	5	3/2	3	1(D)
Ileal	13	8/5	4	1(D)
Ileocecal	3	3/0	0	0
Appendix	3	0/3	0	2(1D, 2S)
Cecum	3	2/1	0	0
Colonic	3	0/3	0	1 (1D+S)
Hindgut	7	4/3	0	3
Colonic	1	1/0	0	0
Rectal	6	3/3	0	3 (1D, 1D+S, 1S)
Spinal	1	1/0	0	0
Total	77	50/27	18	15

*The epithelial lining had been destroyed in five duplications
†Exact origin of cyst unknown
C = Cervical; D = dorsal thoracic; S = sacral vertebrae
In four patients more than one duplication was present, yielding an additional two gastric and three jejunal duplications

References

1. Ladd WE, Gross RE. Surgical treatment of duplications of the alimentary tract: enterogenous cysts, enteric cysts, or ileum duplex. *Surg Gynecol Obstet* 1940; 70: 295–307.

2. Stringer MD, Spitz L, Abel R *et al*. The management of alimentary tract duplication in children. *Br J Surg* 1994 (in press).

3. Wrenn EL Jr. Tubular duplication of the small intestine. *Surgery* 1962; 52: 494–8.

4. Norris RW, Brereton RJ, Wright VM, Cudmore RE. A new surgical approach to duplications of the intestine. *J Pediatr Surg* 1986; 21: 167–70.

5. Ravitch MM. Hindgut duplication: doubling of the colon and genital urinary tracts. *Ann Surg* 1953; 137: 588–601.

6. LaQuaglia MP, Feins N, Eraklis A, Hendren WH. Rectal duplications. *J Pediatr Surg* 1990; 25: 980–4.

Intussusception

Vanessa M. Wright FRCS, FRACS
Consultant Paediatric Surgeon, Queen Elizabeth Hospital for Children and University College London Hospitals, London, UK

Principles and justification

An intussusception is an invagination of proximal bowel (intussusceptum) into the lumen of the distal bowel (intussuscipiens). The leading point or apex of the intussusception is typically a Peyer's patch in the terminal ileum, the ileocecal valve itself, or a part of the cecal wall, but very rarely an intussusception has a pathologic lead point. The apex commonly reaches the transverse colon but can proceed so far distally as to be palpable on rectal examination, and on rare occasions may present at the anal margin, mimicking a rectal prolapse. The incidence is highest in infants between 4 and 10 months of age, but earlier and later presentations (up to 15 years) are not unusual.

Etiology

Very often the patient has a history of upper respiratory tract infection, gastroenteritis or a significant change in diet (i.e. weaning). Adenovirus infection has been implicated in intussusception. The finding at laparotomy of an edematous Peyer's patch as the leading point and of enlarged mesenteric lymph nodes suggests 'irritation' of the intestinal lymphoid tissue. No single etiologic factor predominates and the term 'idiopathic' is appropriate. Between 2% and 12% of patients have a pathologic lead point[1], the most common of which is a Meckel's diverticulum but polyps, duplication cysts and solid tumors may all initiate an intussusception. A pathological lead point should always be suspected if a child outside the usual age range presents. Almost all large series report the overall incidence of intussusception to be higher in boys, but the sex incidence is more equal if the condition has a pathologic lead point[1].

Clinical presentation

Sudden onset of spasmodic abdominal pain is characteristic, the episodes of pain occurring with remarkable regularity. Initially the child may behave normally between the spasms but after some hours lethargy and pallor occur. Vomiting is common but is rarely bile-stained in the first few hours. Overt rectal bleeding is not a consistent finding; in many cases blood in the rectum is apparent only on rectal examination. A palpable abdominal mass, most easily felt in the transverse colon, is the cardinal sign of an intussusception and may be present in the absence of all the typical symptoms. There may be an associated feeling of emptiness in the right iliac fossa. Tenderness and guarding over the mass may make palpation difficult and is sufficient to justify further investigation if the symptoms suggest an intussusception.

The characteristic radiologic features of a low small intestine obstruction usually occur late. Often the intestinal gas pattern is not particularly abnormal; a paucity of gas is often a feature in an early intussusception. The soft tissue mass of the intussusception may be visible as an opacity. Other radiologic features such as crescent and target signs may be recognized[2]. If there is doubt as to the diagnosis a contrast study or an abdominal ultrasound examination will confirm or exclude intussusception.

Non-operative reduction

Between 55% and 95% of intussusceptions are reducible by hydrostatic or pneumatic methods under fluoroscopic or ultrasonographic control[3, 4]. Individual radiologists will have their own exclusion criteria, but non-operative reduction is generally considered inappropriate in the seriously ill child requiring intensive resuscitation or in children with clinical or radiologic evidence of peritonitis or perforation. Attempts to identify factors that will predict the likelihood of success of enema reduction have all concluded that there is no single predictive factor. A combination of a history longer than 24 h, radiographic evidence of obstruction of the small intestine and extremes of age (under 3 months or over 2 years of age) significantly reduce the likelihood of successful reduction by enema[5].

Technique

Few centers use routine sedation. Ideally an intravenous infusion and a nasogastric tube should be inserted before starting the procedure, but this is not essential in early cases if the child is well.

Barium or a water-soluble contrast solution are instilled thorugh a well secured wide-bore tube from a reservoir 90–100 cm above the patient and its progress monitored on the fluoroscope. Air or oxygen is delivered at 80–150 mmHg; delivery is also monitored fluoroscopically. Initial reduction of the intussusception is often rapid and may be complete with filling of several loops of ileum. Quite often the intussusception lodges in the cecum, and if it does not move with pressure sustained for 3–4 min, the pressure should be reduced and reapplied after a short rest of 1–2 min. Reduction and reapplication of pressure should continue until it is obvious that progress has ceased. Pressure may gradually be increased, but this increases the risks of perforation[3]. If the colon is very irritable and the patient has difficulty in retaining the contrast, hyoscine or glucagon may help to reduce colonic peristalsis.

Occasionally there is doubt as to whether a persistent filling defect in the cecum is an unreduced terminal ileum or an edematous ileocecal valve. In these circumstances it is reasonable to return the child to the ward to see whether there is clinical improvement, in particular the absence of the previous colic. A plain radiograph taken an hour or so later may demonstrate reflux of contrast into the terminal ileum or a persisting intussusception.

The benchmark of successful reduction is reflux of contrast or air into several loops of ileum. Radiologic evidence of persistence of the intussusception, or the obvious continuation of symptoms during a short period of observation after the enema, necessitates laparotomy. The incidence of perforation during reduction is very low, and is usually immediately apparent. Perforation with air enemas seems to result in much less peritoneal contamination than occurs with fluid enemas. The effects of barium in the peritoneal cavity has prompted many radiologists to use a water-soluble contrast material in patients with increased risk of perforation.

After a successful non-operative reduction, the child should be encouraged to eat as soon as he or she is interested. Observation in hospital is probably advisable for 24–48 h to ensure that the symptoms have resolved completely, and to diagnose an early recurrence promptly.

ULTRASOUND-GUIDED HYDROSTATIC REDUCTION

The use of ultrasound to diagnose and treat intussusceptions is gradually gaining ground as experience with the technique increases[4]. Using color Doppler it is possible to identify an ischemic intussusceptum, and sonographic features suggesting peritonitis are being evaluated[6].

Technique

The intussusception is identified as a doughnut- or target-shaped configuration on transverse images and a pseudokidney appearance on the longitudinal image[4]. Saline solution or water are used in the reservoir instead of barium. Ultrasonography identifies the apex of the intussusception surrounded by fluid and follows its progress retrogradely along the length of the colon; reduction is confirmed when the mass disappears and loops of terminal ileum are obviously filled with fluid.

Surgical reduction and resection

The success of non-operative reduction means that children with a diagnosis of probable intussusception must be treated in a center offering the full range of diagnostic and treatment options.

Preoperative

Many children will require little preoperative resuscitation. Those with a long history, in whom peritonitis, gangrenous bowel and septicemia are likely, will benefit from a regime of intravenous fluids (including colloid or blood), antibiotics and gastric decompression with a nasogastric tube. Optimal resuscitation can be achieved within 2–4 h; delaying surgery beyond this time will not benefit the patient because this is a strangulating obstruction.

Antibiotics should be administered preoperatively, because appendectomy and bowel resection may be necessary and mucosal damage is almost inevitable, increasing the likelihood of bacteria or toxins entering the circulation.

Anesthesia

General anesthesia with endotracheal intubation and relaxation is essential.

Operation

Incision

1 A right transverse skin incision is made above the umbilicus. The lateral abdominal muscles, anterior rectus sheath and rectus muscle are divided, the extent of division being dictated by the exposure required to reach the apex of the intussusception.

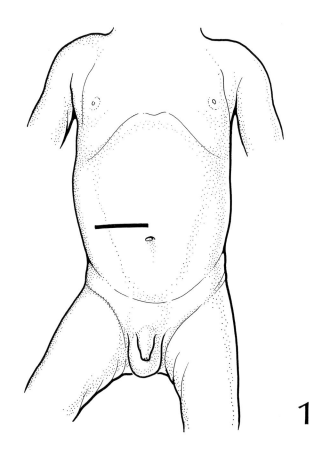

1

2

Reduction of intussusception

2 Delivery of the bowel involved in the intussusception, particularly the right colon, facilitates reduction and reduces manipulation of the remainder of the proximal bowel. To achieve this the bands between the right colon and paracolic gutter are divided by a combination of sharp dissection and sweeping with a pledget.

3 Once the affected section of bowel has been delivered, packs are positioned to absorb any fluid which escapes from the space between intussusceptum and intussuscipiens during the reduction. Reduction is achieved by squeezing the bowel distal to the apex as though squeezing a tube of toothpaste. Placing a layer of gauze between the bowel and fingers may facilitate manipulation. Traction on the intussuscepted bowel should be avoided but a gentle pull may establish the direction in which to apply the reducing push.

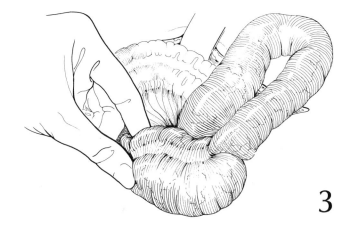

3

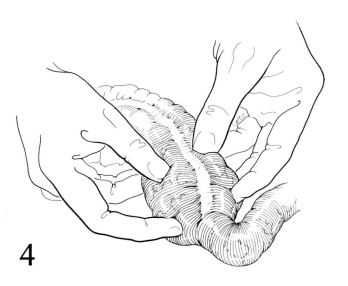

4

4 Reduction of ileum through the ileocecal valve requires patience. Using both thumbs to push on the apex while using the fingers to pull back the cecal wall is usually effective.

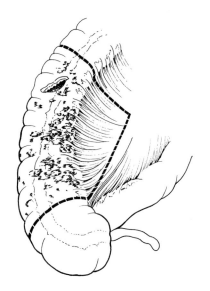

5a

Resection

5a–c Resection is necessary if the intussusception cannot be reduced, or if after reduction there is necrotic bowel or a pathologic lead point (e.g. a Meckel's diverticulum or a duplication cyst). It is occasionally necessary if reduction has caused serious trauma and perforation of the ascending colon or cecal wall which has already been stretched by the contained intussusception. Provided that the adjacent wall is sound, an acceptable alternative for a small perforation is to excise the edges and suture the perforation. Even if resection is necessary the intussusception should be reduced as far as possible and only the minimum of bowel compatible with a good blood supply to the two ends should be removed. Formal right hemicolectomy is rarely required. An edematous ileocecal valve or Peyer's patch can mimic an intraluminal mass – careful palpation and a knowledge of the likely etiology of this condition, particularly in the young infant, should prevent unnecessary resection. Appendectomy is not contraindicated if the adjacent cecal wall is normal.

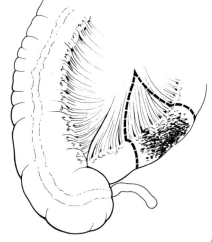

5b

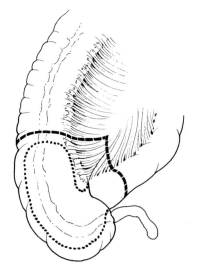

5c

Anastomosis

6 Care should be taken when using bowel clamps on the intestine of young infants because of the risk of trauma. If the contents of the proximal bowel are sucked out, the need for a clamp may be avoided. A single-layer anastomosis using interrupted sutures is used, the choice of suture material depending on individual preference. Any mesenteric defect must be closed. In seriously ill infants requiring resection it may be wiser to bring the ends of the bowel out through the wound as ostomies. Closure is then postponed until the child's general condition has improved and the proximal ileostomy is working – usually after 36–48 h.

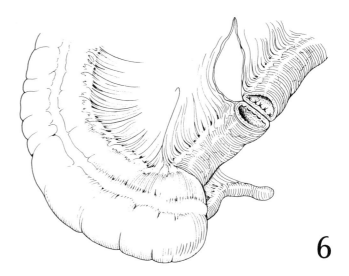

6

Postoperative care

Appropriate intravenous fluids are continued until oral feeds are tolerated. A nasogastric tube decompresses the stomach, and is left on free drainage and regular aspiration initially. Return of satisfactory bowel function is indicated by the absence of abdominal distension, minimal nasogastric aspirate and the passage of stools. Antibiotics may be continued if necessary for a maximum of 48 h after operation. A high temperature is common in the first 24–48 h and usually subsides without specific measures.

Outcome

Recurrence rates up to 10% have been reported, often occurring during the initial hospital admission[7]. More than one recurrence can occur, and may indicate the presence of a pathologic lead point. Although non-operative reduction is not contraindicated in these cases, if an intussusception recurs it is essential to look for radiologic/ultrasonographic evidence of a mass lesion, particularly in an older child.

Death following intussusception is rare unless there has been a significant delay in diagnosis.

If an extensive length of ileum has been resected, the child will require long-term follow-up to monitor vitamin B_{12} absorption. Loss of the ileocecal valve may also affect absorption and transit time.

References

1. Ong N-T, Beasley SW. The leadpoint in intussusception. *J Pediatr Surg* 1990; 25: 640–3.

2. Ratcliffe JF, Fong S, Cheong J, O'Connell P. The plain abdominal film in intussusception: the accuracy and incidence of radiographic signs. *Pediatr Radiol* 1992; 22: 110–11..

3. Stein M, Alton DJ, Daneman A. Pneumatic reduction of intussusception: 5 year experience. *Radiology* 1992; 183: 681–4.

4. Woo SK, Kim JS, Suh SJ, Paik RW, Choi SO. Childhood intussusception: US-guided hydrostatic reduction. *Radiology* 1992; 182: 77–80.

5. Beasley SW, Glover J. Intussusception: prediction of outcome of gas enema. *J Pediatr Surg* 1992; 27: 474–5.

6. Lam AH, Firman K. Value of sonography including color Doppler in the diagnosis and management of long standing intussusception. *Pediatr Radiol* 1992; 22: 112–14.

7. Palder SB, Ein SH, Stringer DA, Alton D. Intussusception: barium or air? *J Pediatr Surg* 1991; 26: 271–5.

Appendectomy: open and laparoscopic approaches

Christopher R. Moir MD, BSc, FRCS(C), FACS
Consultant in Pediatric Surgery, Mayo Foundation, Rochester, Minnesota, USA

History

The almost pedantic modern state of appendectomy belies a past history of tragedy, confusion and spirited debate. The recent introduction of operative laparoscopy promises to provide more controversy in the saga of this common childhood disease. Recognition and surgical treatment of appendicitis was popularized in the late 1800s, but Claudius Amyand, in 1735, was credited with the first successful appendectomy. He operated on an 11-year-old boy whose appendix was not inflamed and not in the right lower quadrant, but trapped in a scrotal hernia and perforated by a pin.

The appendix was first drawn by DaVinci in 1492, described and published by Vesalius in 1545, and recognized to take part in disease in 1554. Sadly, this and many other cases to follow were all described at post-mortem examination. A 7-year-old French girl who died with abdominal pain and diarrhea was found to have a free perforation in the region of the cecum. Throughout the next three centuries the cause of this tragic right lower quadrant affliction ('iliac passion') remained unrecognized and not specifically treated.

Progress was made in the early 19th century, when surgeons cautiously recommended drainage of those abscesses clearly localized to the right lower quadrant. Encouraged by early success, they expanded the indications for operation by the mid 1800s to include the diagnosis of spreading peritonitis. Finally, in 1886 Fitz clearly identified the appendix as the cause and recommended appendectomy within 48 h of symptom onset[1]. The appendicitis debate was thus clarified in the USA but each country has its own story. In London Treves instantly popularized appendectomy by curing King Edward VII in 1902. In Canada a country doctor named Abraham Groves is said to have diagnosed and successfully removed the inflamed appendix of a 12-year-old boy while on rounds of his farming area. This event apparently took place in 1883, three years before the Fitz[1] landmark presentation.

In reviewing the history of appendicitis, it is clear that even a century ago advances in surgical care were brought about by bold innovation and honest communication with colleagues, a principle that has served our pediatric patients well. The tragedy of appendicitis has been transformed to the satisfaction of a well planned operation and excellent outcome.

Principles and justification

Indications

Despite historical controversy, appendectomy has been recommended for appendicitis and other conditions of the appendix for over 100 years. The recent availability of a reliable laparoscopic approach should not change the basic indication for appendectomy. Laparoscopy is an invasive surgical procedure performed under general anesthesia in most children. With this in mind, candidates for laparoscopic appendectomy should undergo the same careful preoperative diagnostic evaluation as those children who will have an open procedure. Prompt operation by either approach is the most effective way of preventing the inexorable progression of acute appendicitis to gangrene and perforation. Most surgeons believe these sequelae will occur within 48 h of the onset of symptoms, and early perforation can be expected in young children or when there is complete obstruction of the lumen, such as by a fecolith. Once perforated, operative drainage and appendectomy are not problematic, but vital for survival in most circumstances. Occasionally, a child with a well contained perforation will benefit from percutaneous drainage, intravenous antibiotics and delayed appendectomy 6 weeks to 2 months later. In these otherwise stable patients, appendectomy performed acutely has not been as successful. The delayed or 'interval' appendectomy, if performed at all, can be approached by laparoscopic or open methods.

Appendectomy is also recommended for small (<2 cm) carcinoid tumors at the tip of the appendix, other benign conditions of the appendix, and is part of Ladd's procedure for midgut malrotation. Incidental removal of a normal appendix is often a part of other gastrointestinal operations, such as pull-through procedures for Hirschsprung's disease in small children. The removal of a normal appendix in an older child not undergoing a gastrointestinal procedure is open to debate.

Contraindications

Most children with perforated appendicitis can and should undergo immediate operation for control of intra-abdominal sepsis and prevention of recurrence. However, stable patients with a well contained abscess will benefit from the non-operative approach detailed above. A laparoscopic appendectomy cannot be justified for patients with perforation and sepsis, or a large appendiceal mass. In addition to the difficulty of laparoscopic dissection under these circumstances, the benefits of laparoscopy such as early hospital dismissal are negated by the need for inpatient treatment that includes intravenous antibiotics, pain control and intravenous fluids for resolving peritonitis. It is usually too difficult to assemble these therapies on an outpatient basis. For these reasons, it is essential to continue the time-honored practice of abdominal examination under general anesthesia before appendectomy. If a mass has been palpated, a laparoscopic approach should probably be abandoned in favor of an open procedure or conservative therapy.

Incidental appendectomy is relatively contraindicated as part of an abdominal procedure when the intestine will not otherwise be opened. A normal appendix should also not be removed if vascular or other prosthetic materials are used.

Preoperative

Appendicitis remains one of the most critical but elusive intra-abdominal diagnoses. Although appendicitis is the most common abdominal emergency of childhood, misdiagnosis is not only tolerated but encouraged. Timely operation despite a paucity of corroborating evidence is still the best treatment since delaying until diagnosis is obvious usually means waiting for perforation. Mortality from perforation has been greatly reduced by antibiotics and fluid support, but morbidity remains high, and long-term complications of perforation are still seen. For this reason, a 15% 'negative' laparotomy (or laparoscopy) rate is the accepted norm[2].

The approach to the diagnosis of acute appendicitis in this era of sophisticated preoperative imaging still relies on the history of a visceral prodrome that progresses to localized somatic symptoms in the right lower quadrant. The delight of dealing with children means the history is not always classical, but the physical examination will reveal the diagnosis. In most instances no further testing is required. When the diagnosis is questionable, ultrasonography has been very helpful not only to visualize an inflamed appendix, but more importantly to exclude other abdominal or pelvic conditions, especially in teenage girls. Radiographic evaluation is non-specific except to identify a fecolith, and barium studies are usually contraindicated. Computed tomographic scanning is rarely needed.

Children with appendicitis must also be evaluated for degree of sepsis and dehydration. Most will have vomited or not eaten for over 24 h. For this reason alone, intravenous isotonic fluid resuscitation before operation is mandatory for all patients with appendicitis. Superimposed sepsis will indicate more aggressive fluid support before operation. Infectious complications are best prevented and treated in all patients by using perioperative antibiotics. The typical 'triple antibiotic' regime is designed to control the aerobes and anaerobes of the lower gastrointestinal tract. In the author's experience, the approach of universal antibiotic coverage for all patients with appendicitis has resulted in a wound infection rate and an intra-abdominal abscess incidence of 1.7% of patients with perforated or gangrenous appendicitis[3].

The most efficient way to control preoperative pain is immediate appendectomy, but in the rare instances of unavoidable delay, a small dose of intravenous narcotics is acceptable.

Patients undergoing a laparoscopic procedure must have nasogastric and bladder catheter decompression. Once again the abdomen must be palpated before insufflation to rule out the presence of a large intra-abdominal mass.

Finally, psychological preparation of the child and the parents is essential for a successful procedure. For many patients this is their first introduction to hospital and surgery. The family must be informed of what to expect, including the location of the incision, the possibility of drains and the remote possibilities of complications and stomas. Many children want to know when they will be able to leave the hospital but usually brighten up when told that their parents may stay with them.

Anesthesia

Premedication is generally unnecessary. A general anesthetic with muscle relaxation, hypnosis, analgesia and amnesia provides the best exposure for the surgeon and is kindest to the child. Local or regional anesthetic blocks are not helpful, especially in infected or septic cases.

Operation

OPEN APPENDECTOMY

Incision

1 With the child supine on the operating table and positioned closer to the surgeon's side when using an adult table, the abdomen is again palpated for the presence of a mass. If detected, the incision should be placed in close proximity to the mass, allowing for local topography and possible extension as needed. The principles of skin incision for appendicitis should include a transverse right lower quadrant skin crease approach, allowance for extension medially or laterally, and avoidance of the large periumbilical fat pad of the plump child. The thin child who has exquisite point tenderness will probably have an anterior appendix that will be easy to remove, tempting the surgeon to make a very low, short skin crease incision that can be extended medially if required. This approach is risky and best avoided by placing the incision just at or above and slightly medial to the anterior superior iliac spine. The incision then courses medially just through or below McBurney's point. Placement just above the anterior superior iliac spine allows lateral extension to the flank and medial enlargement across the rectus sheath. As a general rule, a higher and longer incision will provide more room for exploration, a satisfactory and faster dissection, and a more prolonged and painful hospital stay.

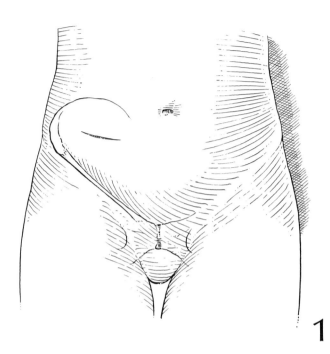

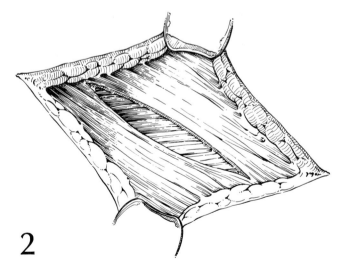

2 Following sharp dissection, the external oblique muscle is split along the direction of the fibers, out to and including the muscular belly. A liberal split of the external oblique muscle will provide adequate operative exposure.

3 The internal oblique and transverse muscles are split in the direction of their fibers using blunt-tipped scissors. Generally, both muscle bellies are split in tandem as the transverse muscle is nearly parallel with the internal oblique muscle. The aponeurosis of the transverse muscle occurs more laterally, and the fibers may run more obliquely from lower right to upper left than those of the internal oblique. Once split over a short distance, small retractors are then placed to continue the muscle division in the direction of the fibers.

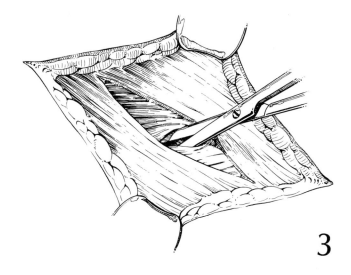

3

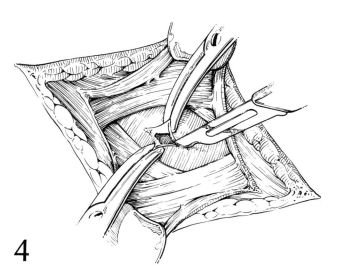

4

4 The peritoneum is grasped after blunt dissection of the transversalis fascia and lateral preperitoneal fat. Edema from appendiceal inflammation may obscure the peritoneum laterally; it is best identified medially. On opening the peritoneum with a scalpel, free fluid is suctioned and sent for culture. The peritoneal opening is enlarged with scissors.

5 The key to successful exposure of the appendix is delivery of the cecum into the wound. The anterior tenea coli is grasped and the cecum delivered using an up-and-down rocking motion, first pulling down then up. If the cecum cannot be delivered easily, lateral peritoneal attachments may require dissection under direct vision using cautery. This division should never be performed blindly or medially to the appendix. An appendiceal mass is almost always bound down laterally and inferiorly. Medial attachments are usually to the terminal ileum and its mesentery. These should be dealt with once the mass has been safely delivered through the wound.

A difficult dissection becomes easier with wound extension. The muscle-splitting incision can be extended medially across the anterior and posterior rectus sheaths using cautery. The rectus muscle is retracted and the inferior epigastric vessels divided between hemostatic ties. Lateral incision enlargement is also helpful if the wound has been placed too medial or further dissection is required in the flank.

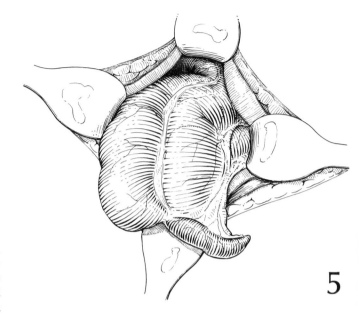

5

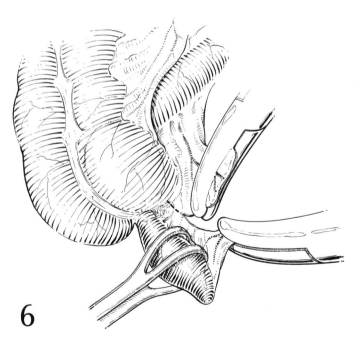

6

6 The inflamed appendix and any overlying omentum should not be allowed to touch the wound once delivered. Attached omentum is divided between hemostatic ties, and the mesoappendix is gently grasped with large Babcock forceps encircling, but not touching, the appendix. With traction on the Babcock forceps, the appendix is easily controlled and any further lateral attachments divided with cautery. The mesoappendix is then serially divided between hemostats and tied in sequence. The inflamed mesentery does not hold ties well. Excessive upper traction during tying may lead to delayed knot slippage and hematoma. The mesenteric division should continue to Treves' fold and end with careful evaluation of a small group of veins on the inferior cecal wall. These veins usually do not require division, but excessive traction on the appendix may tear them.

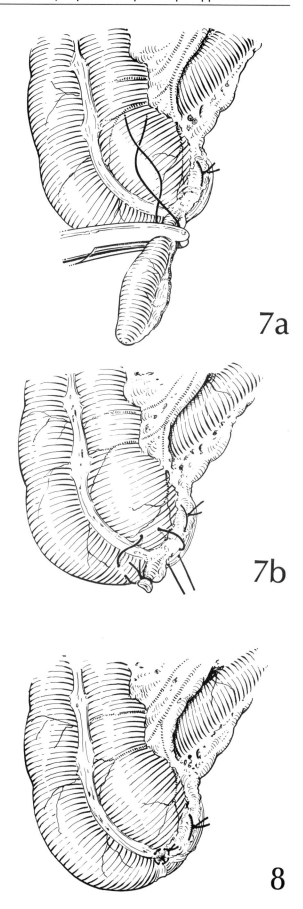

7a, b The base of the appendix is crushed 5 mm above its origin and the clamp drawn distally a few more millimeters. The area crushed is then tied with an absorbable suture and the appendix removed by sharp division just proximal to the clamp. The mucosa of the remaining stump is cleansed with antiseptic solution and may be cauterized. Stump inversion is not necessary[4] but, if performed, a purse-string absorbable suture is placed through the seromuscular base of the cecum, taking care to avoid the inferior cecal veins. The stump is inverted with the help of a hemostat, which is then removed from the operating field. Rarely the appendix is pedicled on a very broad and inflamed base that cannot be safely ligated with a free tie. In this case, a double row of inverted Lembert sutures will satisfactorily avoid a blown stump.

8 Before replacing the cecum, the operative field and mesoappendix ties are inspected for hemostasis. The distended cecum may prove difficult to return to the abdomen. Gentle alternating finger compression avoids tearing by forceps or stump blow-out from excessive pressure.

The pelvis and right paracolic spaces are suctioned and irrigated with saline if pus is found. Large well developed abscesses may be drained using closed wound suction through a separate stab wound. This is rare in children since most fibrinopurulent debris can be removed atraumatically and the areas irrigated clear. When there has been free perforation, the surrounding bowel loops and omentum should be checked for abscesses. Intra-abdominal antibiotics are not helpful when perioperative antibiotics have been used.

The wound is closed in layers with absorbable sutures after irrigation of each consecutive layer. The peritoneum is run and the internal oblique and transverse muscles are closed in one by apposition of the internal oblique epimesium using interrupted absorbable sutures. The external oblique aponeurosis is closed with a running suture, followed by Scarpa's fascia and skin. Even when there has been perforation and gross contamination, the skin is usually closed with an absorbable running subcuticular suture.

LAPAROSCOPIC APPENDECTOMY

Incision

9a–d A 10–11-mm vertical infraumbilical incision provides the most cosmetic approach for the laparoscopic port. In smaller children, a curvilinear incision is necessary. It may also be wise to open the umbilicus in the small child rather than attempt percutaneous placement of these ports. If an open technique is used, a horizontal mattress suture around the port provides satisfactory air seal without the necessity of using a more complex cannula. The abdomen is insufflated in a standard fashion and the laparoscope inserted for diagnosis and assessment of operative feasibility.

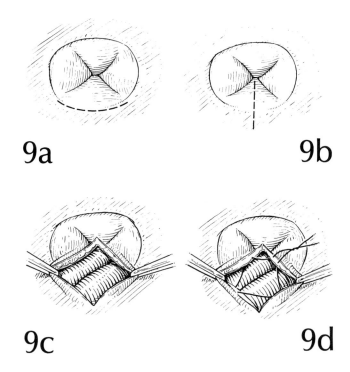

9a   9b

9c   9d

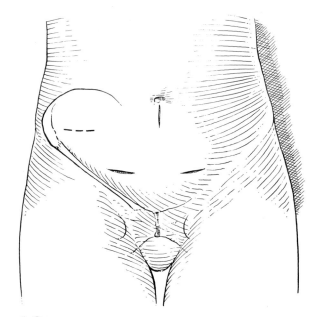

10

10 Two separate 5-mm infraumbilical incisions are placed on either side of the midline under direct laparoscopic control to avoid the inferior epigastric vessels. An optional third 5-mm incision is placed in the right lower quadrant for control of the appendix during lateral dissection. A trial of laparoscopic dissection should precede the use of this incision.

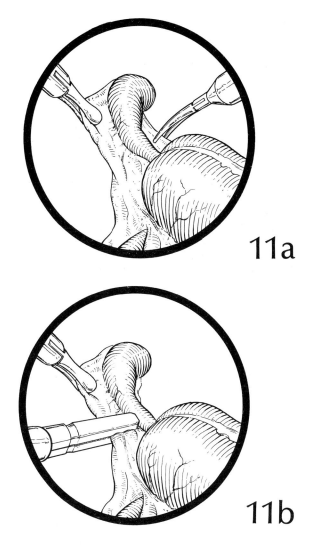

11a, b The appendix is grasped by the free edge of the mesentery or with a preformed loop when the lateral incision is used. A laparoscopic Babcock forceps through the right lower quadrant lateral wound may also be very helpful when necessary. With traction of the appendix, the lateral peritoneal attachments are divided to free the appendix and its mesentery. The dissection does not require extension onto the cecum since it will not have to be elevated through the wound. The lateral mobilization of the cecum is only desirable if the appendix is to be pulled through the 10-mm umbilical port for extra-corporeal appendectomy.

The mesoappendix is divided using cautery, clips or a vascular/gastrointestinal stapler. The larger stapling instruments may be inserted through the umbilical 10-mm port to avoid enlarging the infraumbilical or lateral incisions. The stapler is placed under direct vision with a 5-mm camera placed through one of the other ports.

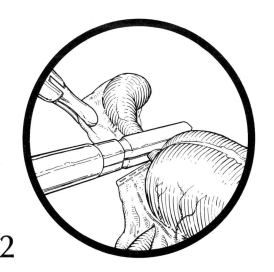

12 Once pedicled on the cecum, the appendiceal stump is ligated with two preformed loops or the gastrointestinal stapler. These sutures must be reinforced by two or three more free ties that may be tied intracorporeally or extracorporeally and pushed down with a knot pusher. Care must be taken with the stapler to ensure that only the base is ligated, avoiding the cecal wall.

The appendix is then removed through the sheath of the largest trocar so that the infected appendix does not touch the anterior abdominal wall. If the appendix is large, it is placed in a sterile bag and removed through the largest wound following trocar removal. After a final check for hemostasis, the abdomen is suctioned and irrigated as necessary. The laparoscopes and trocars are removed, the abdomen desufflated and the umbilicus closed with fascial sutures. The 5-mm incisions require subcutaneous skin closure only.

Postoperative care

If the appendix was not perforated, a nasogastric tube is not required and patients begin oral diet within 24 h. Antibiotics are discontinued after two postoperative doses. Intravenous narcotics are given on demand or by patient controlled analgesia pump for older children during the first day. Pain control transitions to oral medication as needed on the second postoperative day. Most children are up and active the day after surgery and are discharged home that day or early the next.

The amount of peritoneal contamination and visceral inflammation will determine the need for nasogastric tube decompression and nil-by-mouth status in patients with perforated appendices. Intravenous fluid resuscitation is vital for the first 24 h after operation to compensate for ongoing third space losses from peritoneal inflammation. Antibiotics are continued until the temperature is normal (37°C) and the white blood cell count <9000 with absence of left shift (<80% neutrophils). Occasional bladder catheter decompression is necessary. Patients are encouraged to ambulate, deep breathe and cough. Intravenous narcotics may be continued for two to three days.

Complications

Infections

The harbinger of wound infection or intra-abdominal abscesses is persistence of fever, white blood cell count elevation and pain. It is rare that patients with entirely normal vital signs and white blood cell count will return with an abscess, but recrudescence of these symptoms will signal the complication. Wound infections may be drained locally, but intra-abdominal abcesses will require antibiotics and probable drainage. Intra-abdominal abscesses usually occur in the right pelvis. Percutaneous drainage, under radiologic control, and antibiotics have been very successful. Large phlegmonous infections are not amenable to drainage but require several weeks to subside on intravenous antibiotics. These patients often do not eat well and may require total parenteral nutrition.

Hemorrhage

Significant postoperative hemorrhage requires reoperation to control bleeding and prevent infection.

Stump leak

A blown appendiceal stump can present with diffuse feculent peritonitis and sepsis and requires immediate reoperation. Occasionally stump leaks have been discovered only after continued leakage of feculent material from the wound or a percutaneous drain. These patients may be managed non-operatively with the hope that the tract will eventually seal. If not, reoperation weeks to months later to excise and close the tract will effect a cure. Persistent drainage may also indicate retained foreign material such as a fecolith that escaped detection at initial operation.

Outcome

A prospective study of a specific protocol for treatment of appendicitis in 420 children evaluated the use of perioperative intravenous antibiotics for all patients, peritoneal lavage and skin closure without deep or superficial drains[3]. The overall infection rate was 1.7% for the wound and 1.7% for intra-abdominal abscess formation. Hospital stay was 2.1 days for acute appendicitis and 6.9 days (range 3–40) for gangrenous or perforated appendicitis. These results indicate the efficacy of perioperative intravenous antibiotics and careful peritoneal and wound cleansing to decrease infection rates in children.

References

1. Fitz RH. Perforating inflammation of the vermiform appendix; with special reference to its early diagnosis and treatment. *Trans Assoc Am Phys* 1886; 1: 107–44.

2. Berry J Jr, Malt RA. Appendicitis near its centenary. *Ann Surg* 1984; 200: 567–75.

3. Neilson IR, Laberge JM, Nguyen LT *et al*. Appendicitis in children: current therapeutic recommendations. *J Pediatr Surg* 1990; 25: 1113–16.

4. Engstrom L, Fenyo G. Appendicectomy: assessment of stump invagination versus simple ligation: a prospective, randomized trial. *Br J Surg* 1985; 72: 971–2.

Necrotizing enterocolitis

William J. Pokorny MD
Professor of Surgery and Pediatrics, Baylor College of Medicine, Houston, Texas, USA

Principles and justification

Necrotizing enterocolitis represents a disease or diseases with a wide spectrum of intestinal involvement and systemic manifestations. It is widely accepted as a complication of prematurity in which there is intestinal hypoxia, usually due to a low perfusion state which results in mucosal injury and allows translocation of bacteria into the intestinal wall and portal venous system. There is probably an inverse relationship between the bacterial content within the intestinal lumen and the degree of mucosal injury required for clinical invasion of the intestinal wall by bacteria and the development of necrotizing enterocolitis. The process typically occurs after commencing feeding which provides a medium on which bacteria flourish in the distal ileum. Prematurity may also lead to decreased or abnormal peristalsis with intraluminal stasis contributing to the relative bacterial overgrowth. Factors associated with decreased gut perfusion include: (1) low flow states as seen in sepsis, asphyxia, patent ductus arteriosus and hypotension; (2) hypovolemia associated with hyperosmolar formulas and diarrhea; (3) selective mesenteric constriction associated with hypoxia and hypothermia; and (4) mesenteric artery occlusion due to a spasm or emboli associated with vascular catheters[1,2]. Although none of these etiologic factors has been clearly shown to cause necrotizing enterocolitis in controlled studies, they are common to a population of very sick, small and vulnerable infants.

Many authors will accept only infants with radiographic pneumatosis intestinalis as having acute necrotizing enterocolitis; others consider all preterm infants with acute segmental intestinal necrosis and perforation to have this syndrome, once other etiologies have been excluded. The radiographic findings of pneumatosis intestinalis may be fleeting and may be missed if radiographs are not taken during the initial 12–24 h of the illness; after this time the radiographs are more typical of ileus associated with ischemic intestine. Infants with acute ileal perforation following indomethacin therapy and infants with localized ileal meconium plugs with proximal dilatation leading to perforation are difficult to differentiate from those with necrotizing enterocolitis and are therefore grouped with them. The last two situations result in an isolated injury and perforation which can usually be closed primarily. The prognosis for these infants is much better than that for those with a more extensive process.

Most infants who develop necrotizing enterocolitis are preterm and weigh less than 1500 g; less than 10% of infants who develop the condition are full-term, and as many as 8% of preterm infants with birth weights of 750–1500 g develop the condition. Two-thirds of patients respond to medical management; only about one-third require surgical intervention[3].

Symptoms

The onset of symptoms is inversely related to the infants' weight and gestational age. Full-term neonates typically show signs within the first few days of life but a preterm neonate of 800 g usually does not manifest the syndrome for 2–3 weeks after birth. The age at which the infant develops necrotizing enterocolitis appears to be related to the onset of feeding, which is delayed in the small preterm infant.

Most sufferers have had a stressful event such as respiratory distress syndrome, congenital heart disease (usually with a left to right shunt), hypoxia or arrhythmia, hypoglycemia or sepsis. Initial symptoms may be subtle and include increased gastric residual volume ileus, abdominal distension and blood-streaked stools, or symptoms may be fulminant with signs of shock and frankly bloody stools.

The physical condition of infants with necrotizing enterocolitis varies with the extent and severity of the disease and with the development of intestinal perforation. Early findings include abdominal distension and tenderness. As the intra-abdominal inflammatory process progresses the abdominal wall may become erythematous and inflamed loops of intestine may become matted together to form a mass, most commonly in the right lower quadrant. A tender mass with platelet count persistently below 40 000 may indicate areas of intestinal necrosis that have been walled off by other intestinal loops, but by itself is not an indication for immediate surgical intervention. If the intestine perforates into the free peritoneum there are usually signs of generalized peritonitis which include generalized tenderness, diffuse abdominal wall erythema followed by cellulitis and rapidly increasing abdominal girth. Free air may be seen about the right lobe of the liver on the left lateral decubitus radiograph of the abdomen. Occasionally an otherwise healthy preterm infant develops a distended, bluish colored abdomen or will have free intraperitoneal air on radiograph; these patients typically have an isolated perforation or necrotic segment and have a good prognosis.

Radiographic findings

Radiographic findings of necrotizing enterocolitis vary with the duration and extent of the disease. The radiographic finding of pneumatosis intestinalis and portal vein gas are pathognomonic but are rarely present after 48 h. Portal vein gas is not by itself an indication for operative intervention but it has been found to indicate more extensive disease and an increased likelihood that operative care will be required. Other radiographic findings suggestive of the diagnosis include dilated loops of intestine, ascites and edema of the intestinal wall[4] (these findings are also seen in infants with sepsis and shock syndromes). By the third or fourth day the intraluminal gas has been absorbed and the radiograph shows a gasless abdomen with ascites and fluid-filled loops of intestine.

Differential diagnosis

Midgut volvulus

This diagnosis should be considered in any neonate with bloody stools and dilated edematous intestine without pneumatosis intestinalis or a localizing inflammatory process. Volvulus associated with malrotation is diagnosed by a limited gastrointestinal contrast study demonstrating the abnormal location of the duodenum.

Sepsis with ileus

The neonate with sepsis may develop an ileus and present with abdominal distension and vomiting. If the sepsis is not reversed shock will develop, primarily of the intestine. Intestinal ischemia and edema may progress to frank intestinal necrosis. Ascites commonly develops. In many of these sick neonates it is not clear whether the sepsis and shock syndrome result in the intestinal changes or if the intestinal process precedes the sepsis and shock syndrome. If the intestinal changes result from the sepsis and shock syndrome and are extensive, surgical intervention is of little value, but if the shock syndrome is secondary to intraperitoneal sepsis associated with necrotizing enterocolitis and segmental intestinal necrosis, surgical resection of the segment of intestine involved may be life saving.

Infectious enterocolitis

Neonates with infectious enterocolitis commonly have bloody stools but rarely have abdominal tenderness or abdominal wall erythema.

Non-operative treatment

This condition is treated non-operatively as follows. The patient is placed on bowel rest for 10–14 days, is allowed nothing by mouth and undergoes naso/orogastric tube decompression. While on bowel rest, parenteral nutrition is administered and intravenous antibiotics are given to cover both aerobic and anaerobic intestinal flora. Fluid, acid–base and ventilatory support are necessary and all vital signs, hemoglobin, platelet count, electrolyte levels, blood gases and urine output must be monitored closely in a neonatal intensive care unit. Abdominal radiographs, including left lateral decubitus radiographs, should be obtained every 6–8 h during the first 48 h and if any sudden change in abdominal girth or appearance occurs.

Operative treatment

Surgery may be necessary to treat complications of necrotizing enterocolitis. These complications include, first, free perforation into the peritoneum (as indicated by free air on radiograph or fecal material and bacteria on paracentesis); and, second, contained perforation, in which there is evidence of intestinal perforation or necrosis but no contamination of the general peritoneum and which is not responding to non-operative therapy. Infants with a contained perforation usually present with an inflammatory mass on physical examination and a mass effect with displacement of loops of intestine visible on radiograph. Although many of these patients will recover without operative intervention, others continue to have signs of sepsis with poor perfusion, an inflammatory abdominal mass and platelet consumption and require surgical removal of the source of sepsis. Intestinal obstruction is a third complication of the condition.

The indications for operative intervention in neonates with necrotizing enterocolitis (other than free perforation of the intestine with air and feces in the peritoneum) are quite complex, and the surgeon must consider multiple variables, including white cell and platelet consumption, partial or complete intestinal obstruction, changing ventilatory and acid–base requirements and change in abdominal findings (mass, erythema, abdominal wall edema, ascites). For this reason, algorithms for surgical intervention are difficult to develop as each neonate presents a unique challenge.

Early operative intervention may be harmful if areas of ischemia are walled off by adjacent loops of intestine, preventing free intraperitoneal perforation when transmural necrosis occurs. If the protecting loops are freed from the necrotic segment of intestine during surgical exploration, free perforation results. Although an argument can be made for early excision of the necrotic segment, these segments usually heal, albeit commonly with a stricture. The survival rate associated with resection of necrotizing enterocolitis strictures and primary anastomosis is much better than that for laparotomy for acute necrotizing enterocolitis with resection, enterostomy and subsequent closure. In addition, the surgeon who operates too early during acute necrotizing enterocolitis will find no clear demarcation of viable–ischemic–necrotic–perforated intestine and risks removing too much (or, worse, too little) intestine.

Operations

All areas of the intestine may be affected but the terminal ileum and right colon followed by the left and sigmoid colon are the most commonly involved sites. The entire intestine should be examined before a decision regarding operative repair or resection is made. The surgeon should aim to help the infant to survive with a functional gastrointestinal tract. As much of the intestine as possible should be saved but infants with as little as 20% of their small intestine do well with relatively normal intestinal function. Likewise, retention of even a relatively short segment of sigmoid colon and rectum will have a great impact on fluid and electrolyte absorption.

Incision

A standard transverse supraumbilical incision is used. Care must be taken not to injure the thin fascia and musculature of the extremely preterm infant. Electrocautery should be used sparingly and only for point hemostasis.

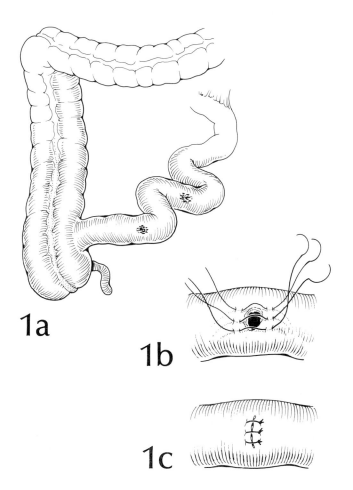

1a

1b

1c

CLOSURE OF ISOLATED, SIMPLE PERFORATIONS

1a–c Isolated perforations usually occur on the antimesenteric border of the terminal ileum but are seen throughout the small intestine and colon. The surrounding tissue typically appears viable and may even appear quite healthy. If possible the perforation should be closed primarily with oiled 5/0 silk Lembert sutures placed transversely to the intestine so as to narrow the lumen as little as possible. Manipulation and debridement should be limited. This technique may also be used to imbricate small foci of necrotic bowel on the antimesenteric border.

RESECTION WITH PRIMARY ANASTOMOSIS

This procedure is used to treat patients with isolated, necrotic and perforated segments with no involvement of the remaining bowel and whose condition is stable.

In order to be considered for primary anastomosis the necrotic and/or perforated segment must be entirely resected with no involvement of the remaining intestine. The anastomotic ends should appear normal and bleed briskly when cut. The patient should be stable with good general perfusion and acid–base balance.

In deciding whether to perform a primary anastomosis or enterostomy, the length of the segment is not as important as the appearance of the remaining intestine and the condition of the patient. Resection and anastomosis may be undertaken for short, 2–3-cm segments, or for long segments such as the terminal ileum and right colon, provided that the remaining intestine appears healthy with no involvement at the anastomotic line and that the infant's general condition is stable with good general tissue perfusion. The patient's weight does not affect the decision whether to perform an anastomosis or stoma, unless it is below 600 g.

In infants weighing less than 600 g the intestine is very fragile and the sutures easily pull through. If the sutures cannot be tied without pulling through the intestinal wall during the anastomosis, the procedure should be abandoned in favor of a stoma. The surgeon should remember that stomas in these small patients are also fraught with complications such as stenosis and perforation.

In patients with a necrotic and perforated segment with involvement of the remaining bowel or in unstable patients the necrotic segment should be resected, provided that it does not include more than 80% of the small intestine. The proximal end is brought out through a separate incision well away from the primary abdominal incision. If the functioning stoma is too close to the abdominal incision, wound complications, including wound separation, will be high. Primary anastomosis should not be attempted if the infant is unstable with poor perfusion of the intestine or if other areas of bowel show signs of ischemia or pneumatosis.

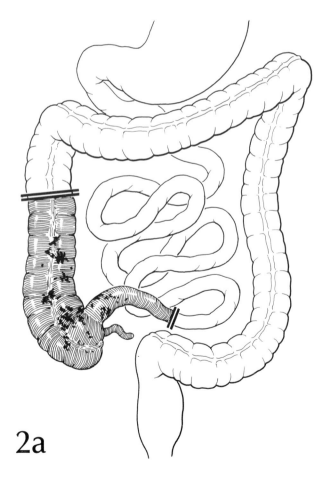

2a

2a–i The anastomosis is performed using an open technique. Sterile rubber bands may be brought through the mesentery to encircle the intestine several centimeters from the intestinal ends; this will prevent persistent spillage of feces into the field without compromising the perfusion of the anastomosis. The intestine is cut at an angle of 30–45° to increase the anastomotic circumference. A one-layer anastomosis with oiled 5/0 silk is used. The first stitch is placed at the mesenteric border and the second at the antimesenteric border, with the knots in the lumen. The back row of simple full-thickness sutures is completed, placing the knots on the inside of the lumen; this inverts the anastomotic edges. The anastomosis is completed with an anterior row of seromuscular inverting Lembert sutures.

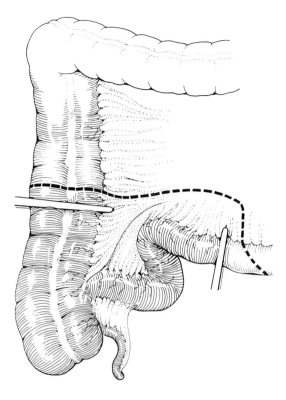

2b

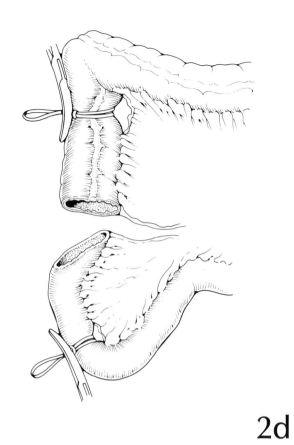

2d

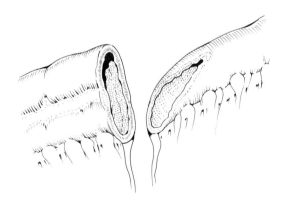

2c

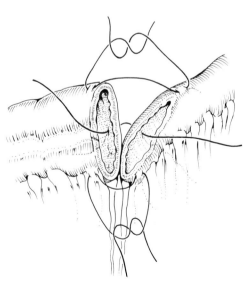

2e

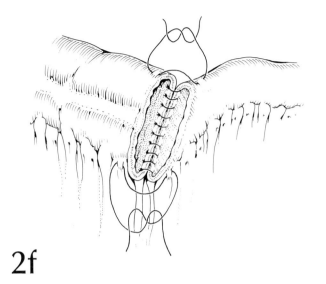

2f

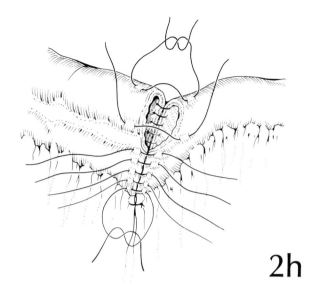

2h

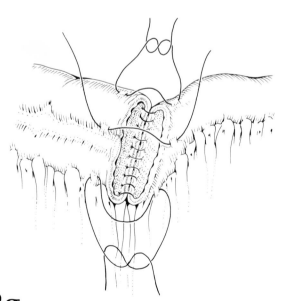

2g

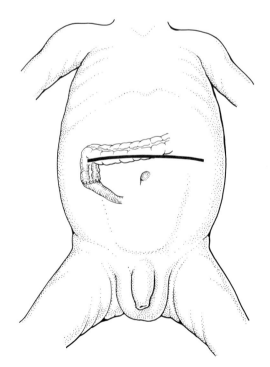

2i

CREATION OF A PROXIMAL STOMA

3a–j In full-term and large preterm infants proximal stomas are brought out through a separate lower quadrant incision. The bowel is sutured to the peritoneum and fascia and matured as a Brooke ileostomy.

In very small preterm infants the intestine does not tolerate excessive manipulation, traction and suturing and must be handled with great care. As in larger neonates, the functioning stoma should be placed away from the incision, usually in the lower quadrant. Care must be taken to ensure an adequate length to allow the end of the stoma to pass through the abdominal wall and approximately 1 cm beyond. As the submucosa tends to separate from the muscular layers, a ligature should be placed about the end of the intestine so that it can be pulled *en masse* gently through the abdominal wall. A limited number of sutures (three or four) should be used to secure the intestine to the abdominal wall. No attempt should be made to mature the stoma because the sutures may further compromise it; perfusion of the stoma will rapidly mature itself. Stenosis is a common problem for stomas of the small preterm infant, regardless of whether or not they are matured. Dilatations must be done with great care to avoid perforation.

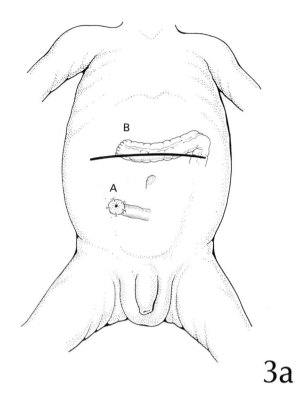

3a

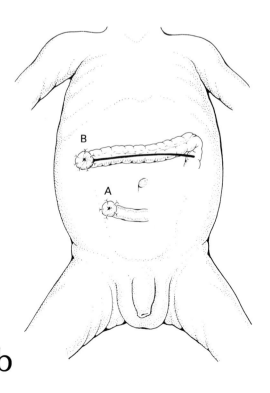

3b

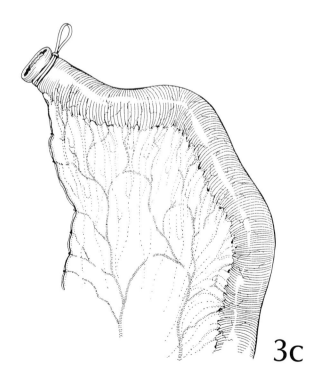

3c

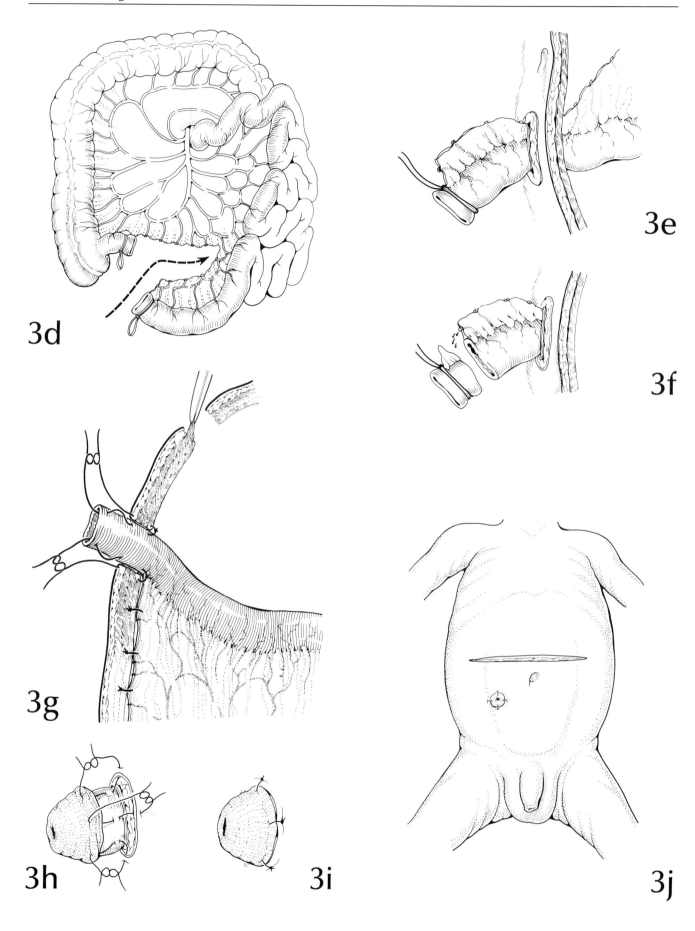

3d

3e

3f

3g

3h

3i

3j

CREATION OF A DISTAL STOMA

The end of the distal segment of intestine can be brought out through the end of the wound or simply closed. The decision to close the distal segment depends on the extent of involvement. If the distal bowel is involved so that stricture formation is a concern, a mucous fistula should be established to allow decompression of that segment proximal to the stricture. If there is no distal involvement, the distal intestine may be closed and expected to vent through the anus.

Involvement of non-adjacent segments of the intestine

4a, b In infants with necrotizing enterocolitis affecting the right and left colon with sparing of the transverse colon, the frankly necrotic segments are resected to conserve as much intestine as possible. The terminal ileum is brought out as an end ileostomy. The proximal end of the right transverse colon is closed and the distal end of the transverse colon brought out as a stoma. The sigmoid colon is closed off and dropped back into the peritoneal cavity.

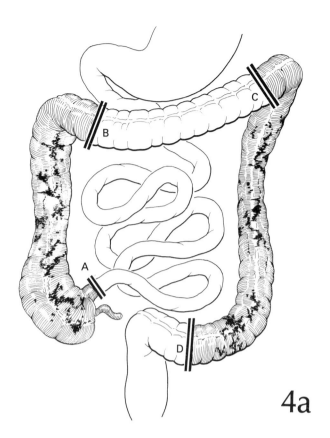

4a

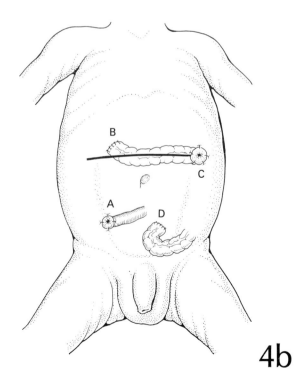

4b

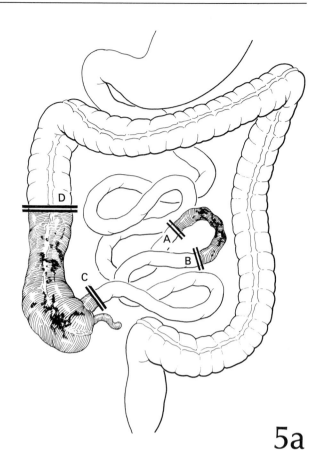

5a

5a, b Following resection of the frankly necrotic segments in patients with necrotizing enterocolitis affecting the mid ileum and cecal region, an end proximal ileostomy is performed through a separate opening in the right lower abdomen. The terminal ileum is brought out at the right end of the abdominal incision and the colon is closed off as a Hartmann's procedure.

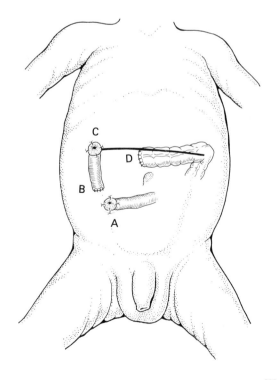

5b

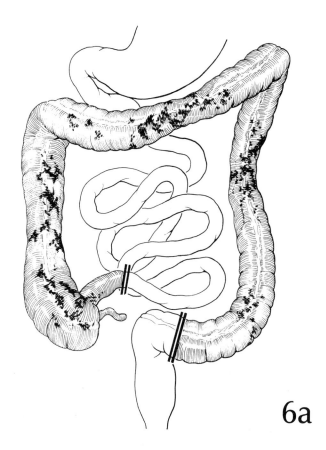

6a

Total colonic necrotizing enterocolitis

6a, b All frankly necrotic colon including a short section of terminal ileum is resected. The distal ileum is brought out through a separate opening in the right iliac fossa as an end ileostomy and the end of the sigmoid colon is closed off as a Hartmann's procedure.

Wound closure

Closure is performed in two fascial layers when possible, using a running absorbable suture. Unfortunately, in the extremely preterm infant weighing less than 600 g the fascia tears easily and is difficult to define so that a single layer closure, including both fascial layers and the rectus muscle, is usually performed, leaving the subcutaneous tissue and skin open. These wounds typically heal with very little scarring.

PERITONEAL DRAINAGE

Peritoneal drainage under local anesthesia is a valuable adjunct in the resuscitation of the very unstable small preterm infant[5]. A complete recovery without further surgery has been reported in up to 40% of infants who were treated only by drainage. This has led some surgeons to recommend drainage only for all preterm patients weighing less than 1500 g who require surgical intervention but this author continues to reserve peritoneal drainage under local anesthesia only for infants considered too hemodynamically unstable to undergo laparotomy.

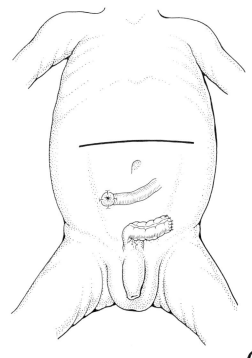

6b

Postoperative care

Intestinal stricture

Stricture formation is a late sequela of necrotizing enterocolitis, typically following an extensive, usually circumferential, intestinal injury. The incidence of stricture formation following medical intervention is about 10%[6].

Stricture formation distal to a diverting enterostomy is quite common[7]. For this reason, a contrast study of the distal bowel is mandatory before closing the enterostomy. If this is not performed or if it incompletely defines the distal intestine, the intestine should be examined carefully for narrowing at the time of laparotomy by passing a 14-Fr catheter and distending the distal segment with air and saline under direct vision. Multiple strictures may be present, separated by segments of normal bowel.

Strictures that develop following non-surgical management of necrotizing enterocolitis usually become clinically apparent only after oral feeding begins. They typically present as feeding intolerance as the diet is increased. After feedings are resumed and the infant begins to defecate, blood streaking may be seen in the feces as a result of bleeding from the granulation tissue lining the stricture where mucosal loss has occurred. Nearly 40% of strictures occur in the small intestine[7] and, for this reason, a series of radiographs of the small intestine should be obtained as well as a barium enema. The partial obstruction associated with the acute inflammatory process may resolve and, if possible, the infant should be supported nutritionally until 3–4 weeks after the acute process before operating for a stricture.

Enterostomy closure

If the infant thrives, the enterostomy may be closed safely when the infant reaches 5 kg and is in good nutritional balance. Distal stricture formation is quite common, occurring in approximately 30% of patients. Before closing the enterostomy a contrast study of the intestine distal to the enterostomy should be obtained. The enterostomy is closed using the same techniques described for resection and anastomosis for acute necrotizing enterocolitis.

Outcome

Early experience with 78 neonates with necrotizing enterocolitis who required laparotomy was reported in 1986[3]. At that time 38 patients underwent resection and primary anastomosis with a 92% survival rate; 29 neonates underwent resection of the necrotic segment and an enterostomy with a 62% survival rate; 11 were opened and closed or only drained (no survivors). Although the overall survival of the neonates treated surgically was 68%, if only those patients who had a resection of the involved segment with primary anastomosis or enterostomy as the initial procedure are included, 44 of 52 survived 30 days (85%) and 40 survived to leave the hospital.

In a recent review in 1993 of over 200 patients undergoing laparotomy for acute necrotizing enterocolitis, nearly 50% of the author's patients continued to undergo enterorrhaphy for focal perforation or resection of a well demarcated and necrotic segment of intestine with a primary anastomosis. The 30-day survival was 95% and in-hospital survival 90%. An additional 35% underwent resection and enterostomy with a 71% survival. Unfortunately, 15% were treated only by drainage or laparotomy with a 29% survival.

The overall survival reported by other authors using different operative techniques is similar, including drainage only in infants less than 1500 g or routine enterostomy during the acute process, suggesting that the extent of disease and condition of the infant determines survival, not the operative technique.

References

1. Kliegman RM, Fanaroff AA. Necrotizing enterocolitis. *N Engl J Med* 1984; 310: 1093–103.

2. Kosloske AM. Pathogenesis and prevention of necrotizing enterocolitis: a hypothesis based on personal observation and a review of the literature. *Pediatrics* 1984; 74: 1086–92.

3. Pokorny WJ, Garcia-Prats JA, Barry YN. Necrotizing enterocolitis: incidence, operative care, and outcome. *J Pediatr Surg* 1986; 21: 1149–54.

4. Bell RS, Graham CB, Stevenson JK. Roentgenologic and clinical manifestations of neonatal necrotizing enterocolitis. *Am J Roentgenol Rad Ther Nucl Med* 1971; 112: 123–34.

5. Ein SH, Marshall DG, Girvan D. Peritoneal drainage under local anesthesia for perforations from necrotizing enterocolitis. *J Pediatr Surg* 1977; 12: 963–7.

6. Schwartz MZ, Hayden CK, Richardson CJ, Tyson KRT, Lobe TE. A prospective evaluation of intestinal stenosis following necrotizing enterocolitis. *J Pediatr Surg* 1982; 17: 764–70.

7. Pokorny WJ. Discussion. *J Pediatr Surg* 1994 (in press).

The death of Dr Pokorny was announced shortly before the book went to press.

Anorectal anomalies

Alberto Peña MD
Chief, Division of Pediatric Surgery, Schneider Children's Hospital and Professor of Surgery, Albert Einstein College of Medicine, New York, USA

History

Anorectal malformations have been known for centuries. Previously, most children with these malformations received an operation consisting of the creation of an orifice on the perineum. With this simple procedure many children survived, probably because the rectum was located very close to the skin. Many of them also died, however, probably because the rectum was located high in the pelvis. In 1835 Amussat reported for the first time suturing of the rectal wall to the skin edges. This could be considered the first description of an anoplasty.

For many years surgeons performed a perineal operation, without a colostomy, for the so-called low malformations. High imperforate anus, on the other hand, was usually treated with a colostomy performed during the neonatal period, followed by an abdominoperineal pull-through sometime later in life. The specific recommendation was often made to pull the intestine as close to the sacrum as possible to avoid trauma to the genitourinary tract. Stephens performed the first objec-

tive anatomic studies of human specimens with these defects, and in 1953 proposed an initial sacral approach to separate the rectum from the urinary tract and preserve the puborectalis sling (considered a key factor in maintaining fecal continence)[1]. He also suggested opening the abdomen, if necessary, after the sacral approach. Following Stephens' recommendations, several different surgical techniques were proposed. The common denominator in all these techniques is the protection and utilization of the puborectalis sling. In 1982 a new approach was described in the literature[2, 3] – posterior sagittal anorectoplasty, which allows direct exposure of this important anatomic area. With this approach it became possible to correlate the external appearance of the perineum with the operative findings, and subsequently with the clinical results. The approach has implications for understanding the anatomy of these defects, terminology, classification, and most importantly, treatment.

Principles and justification

Incidence

Anorectal malformations occur in one in 4000 neonates. They seem to occur slightly more commonly in boys than in girls. The most common defect in girls is a rectovestibular fistula[4]; this is followed by perineal fistula, and the third most common defect seems to be persistent cloaca[4]. As opposed to most publications, this author has found that girls with rectovaginal fistula represent a real exception; most of the 'rectovaginal fistulas' reported in the literature are probably cases of misdiagnosed cloacas or rectovestibular fistulas. Therefore, the third most common defect in girls is persistent cloaca[4]. The most common defect in boys is a rectourethral fistula[4], followed by perineal fistula. Rectum–bladder neck fistulas in boys represent 10% of the entire group of defects. Imperforate anus without fistula in both boys and girls is unusual and represents only 5% of the entire group of defects. The estimated risk for a couple having a second child with an anorectal malformation is approximately 1%[5].

Classification

The classification shown in *Table 1* is proposed because it is therapeutically oriented.

Table 1   Classification of anorectal anomalies

Boys	
Perineal (cutaneous) fistula	No colostomy required
Rectourethral fistula	
Bulbar	
Prostatic	
Rectovesical fistula	Colostomy required
Imperforate anus without fistula	
Rectal atresia	
Girls	
Perineal (cutaneous) fistula	No colostomy required
Vestibular fistula	
Persistent cloaca	
Imperforate anus without fistula	Colostomy required
Rectal atresia	

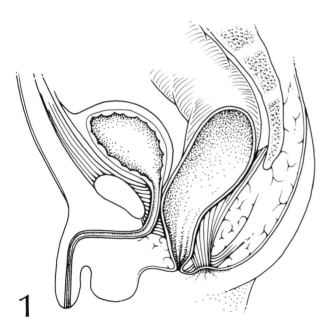

1

Boys

Perineal (cutaneous) fistula

1 This type of defect is also known as a low imperforate anus. The rectum is located within most of the sphincter mechanism. Only the lowest part of the rectum is anteriorly displaced.

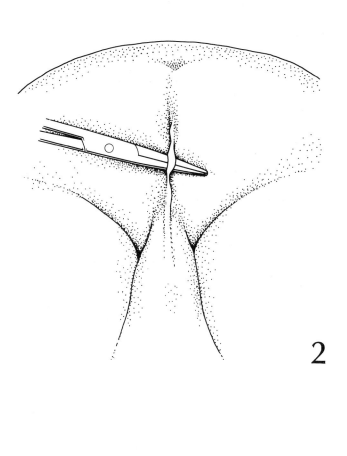

2

2, 3 Sometimes the fistula follows a subepithelial midline tract opening along the midline perineal raphe, scrotum or penis. The perineal findings in these kinds of defect include a prominent skin tag below which an instrument can be passed known as a 'bucket-handle' malformation (*Illustration 2*), a black ribbon-like midline structure that represents a subepithelial fistula filled with meconium, or a very well-formed anal dimple suggesting the presence of a very low defect (*Illustration 3*). All these perineal findings are highly suggestive of the presence of this kind of defect. The diagnosis is established by perineal inspection. No further investigations are required.

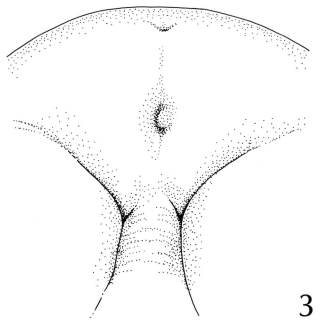

3

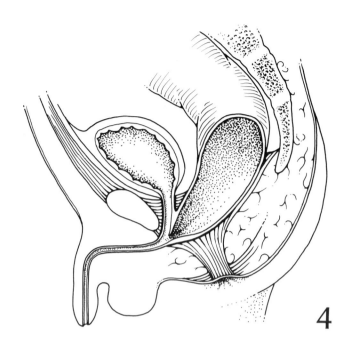

4

Rectourethral fistula
This is the most common defect in boys.

4, 5 The rectum may communicate with the lower part of the urethra (bulbar urethra) or with the upper urethra (prostatic urethra). Immediately above the fistula site the rectum and urethra share a common wall with no plane of dissection.

This anatomic fact has important technical and surgical implications. The rectum is surrounded laterally and posteriorly by the levator muscle mechanism. Between the end of the rectum and the perineal skin, there is a portion of striated voluntary muscle arbitrarily called the 'muscle complex'. The contraction of the levator muscle pushes the rectum forward. The contraction of the muscle complex mechanism elevates the skin of the anal dimple. At the level of the skin and located on both sides of the midline there is a group of voluntary muscle fibers called parasagittal fibers.

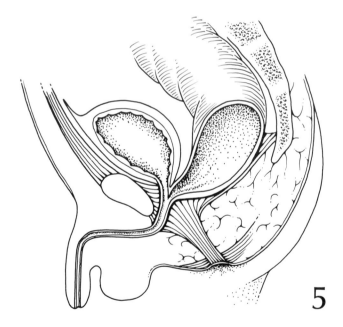

5

6 Patients with rectourethral bulbar fistulas usually have a 'good-looking perineum' consisting of a prominent midline groove and a normal sacrum.

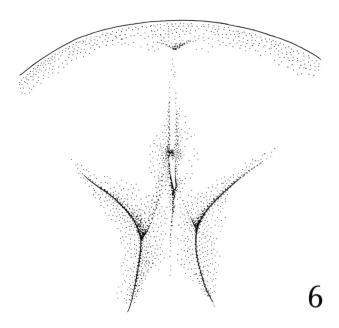

6

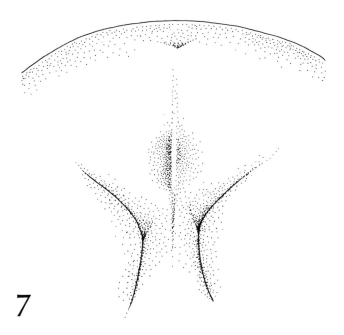

7

7 Patients with rectoprostatic fistulas tend to have a higher incidence of abnormal sacrum, under-developed sphincter mechanism and flat perineum. For some unknown reason, the external sphincter (anal dimple) is often located very close to the scrotum. Exceptions to these rules do exist, however. Neonates with rectourethral fistulas may pass meconium through the urethra, usually after 20 h of life, an unequivocal sign of rectourethral fistula.

Rectovesical fistula

8 In these malformations the rectum communicates with the urinary tract at the bladder neck. Levator muscle, muscle complex and parasagittal fibers are often poorly developed. The sacrum is often deformed or even absent. The entire pelvis seems to be under-developed, and its anteroposterior diameter seems to be foreshortened. The perineum is usually flat (*see Illustration 7*). For all these reasons, the prognosis for bowel function is usually poor.

Imperforate anus without fistula

In these cases the rectum is completely blind and is almost always found at the same level as in those cases with rectourethral bulbar fistula. The sacrum and sphincteric mechanism are usually normal, and therefore these patients have a good prognosis.

Rectal atresia

This is a very unusual defect, as it occurs in only 1% of the entire series. These are the only patients with imperforate anus who are born with a normal anal canal. Externally the anus looks normal, and the malformation is often discovered during an attempt to take a rectal temperature or after the onset of symptoms and signs of

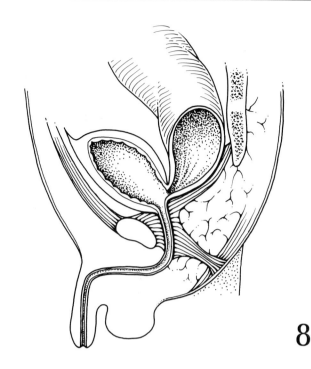

8

low intestinal obstruction. About 2 cm from the anal verge there is an atretic or stenotic area. The upper blind rectum is usually located very close to the anal canal. The sacrum is normal and the sphincteric mechanism is excellent, and therefore the prognosis is good.

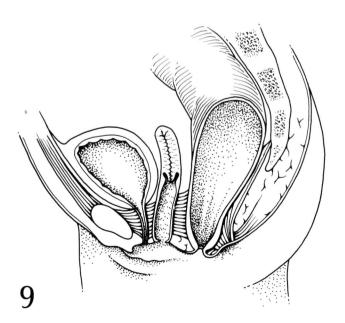

9

Girls

Perineal (cutaneous) fistula

9 This defect is equivalent to the perineal fistula described for boys. The rectum and vagina are well separated. The sphincteric mechanism is very good, and therefore the prognosis is also good.

Vestibular fistula

This is the most important and common defect seen in girls. The importance of this defect resides in the facts that it is the most common defect, it has an excellent functional prognosis and, paradoxically, in the author's experience, these patients are often referred from other institutions because of unsuccessful repairs.

10 The intestine opens in the vestibule of the female genitalia immediately posterior to the hymen. The most pertinent anatomic characteristic of this defect is that immediately above the fistula site the rectum and vagina share a very thin common wall. These patients usually have good muscles and a normal sacrum. The diagnosis is established by perineal inspection. These patients are commonly mislabeled as having rectovaginal fistula, which only reflects a careless inspection of the newborn genitalia.

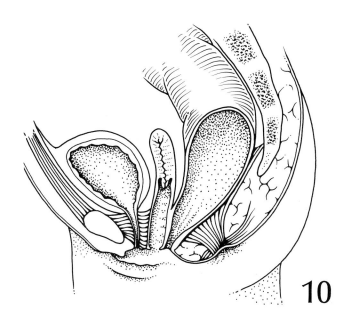

10

Persistent cloaca

11 This group of defects represents a separate spectrum of malformations. A cloaca is defined as a defect in which the rectum, vagina and urinary tract meet and fuse into a single common channel. The length of the common channel varies from 1 cm to 10 cm, which has important technical and prognostic implications. Patients with short common channels (shorter than 3 cm) usually have well-developed sacrums and good sphincters. A common channel longer than 3 cm usually suggests that the patient has a more complex defect and often has a poor sphincteric mechanism and poor sacrum. The rectum and vagina share a common wall as well as the vagina and urethra.

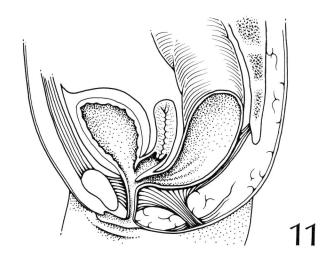

11

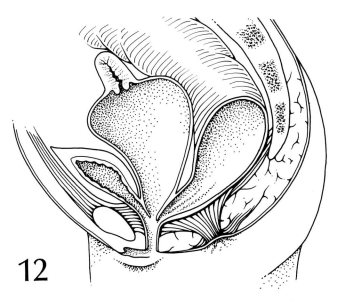

12

12 In more than 50% of these cases the vagina is abnormally distended and full of mucous secretions (hydrocolpos).

13 The vagina and uterus commonly show degrees of septation. A distended vagina (hydrocolpos) compresses the trigone and is often associated with megaureter. The sacrum and the sphincteric mechanism show different degrees of abnormalities.

Imperforate anus without fistula and rectal atresia
These two defects in girls have the same anatomic characteristics as those described in boys, and therefore similar prognostic implications.

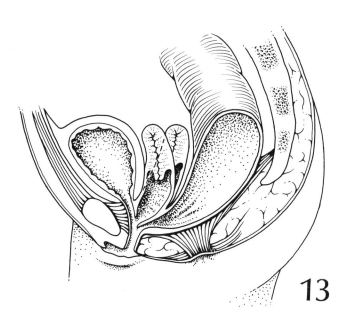

13

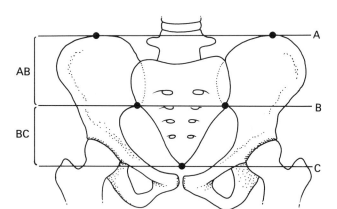

14a

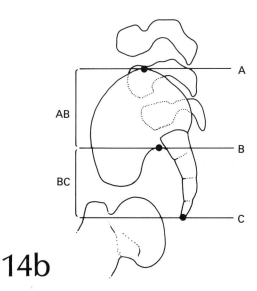

14b

Associated defects

Sacrum and spine
The sacrum is often abnormal in these types of malformations. There appears to be a very good correlation between the degree of sacral development and the final functional prognosis. Traditionally, the number of vertebrae has been the most useful criterion for evaluation of the sacrum. One missing vertebra does not have important diagnostic implications[4]. More than two absent vertebrae represent a poor prognostic sign.

14a, b In order to improve the prognostic accuracy based on sacral abnormalities, a new method of evaluation has been devised. This consists of comparing the size of the sacrum with pelvic and bony reference points to obtain a ratio that expresses the degree of sacral development. For this measurement, three lines are traced: line A extends across the uppermost portion of the iliac crests; line B joins the opposite inferior and posterior iliac spines; and line C runs parallel to lines A and B and passes through the lowest sacral point visible radiologically. In 100 normal children at the author's institution the ratio of the distances BC:AB was 0.7–0.8. Children with anorectal malformations suffer from different degrees of sacral hypodevelopment with the ratio varying between 0 and 0.8. In the author's experience a ratio of less than 0.4 usually signifies a poor functional prognosis.

15a, b

Two different examples of sacral abnormalities and poor ratios are shown.

Higher spinal abnormalities include hemivertebrae located in the lumbar or thoracic spine. The prognostic implications of these types of defects in terms of bowel and urinary control are not known.

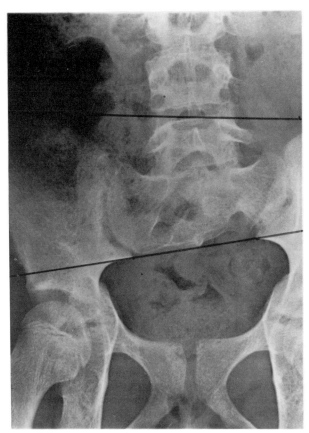

15a

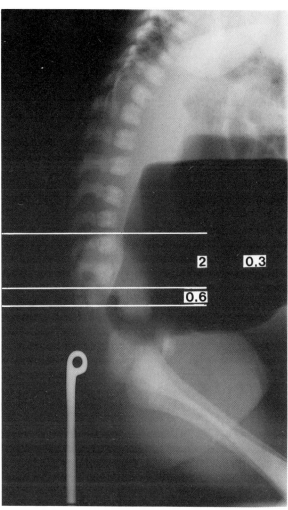

15b

Urogenital defects

The frequency of associated urogenital defects varies from 20% to 54%[6,7]. The reported variation may reflect the accuracy and thoroughness of the urologic investigations in different institutions. In the author's series, 48% of the patients (55% of girls; 44% of boys) had associated urologic anomalies[7]. Patients with persistent cloaca or rectovesical fistulas have a 90% chance of having an important associated urologic abnormality[7]. Children with minor defects (perineal fistula) have less than a 10% chance of suffering from an associated urologic defect. The most common urologic malformation associated with imperforate anus is absent kidney,

followed by vesicoureteric reflux. Hydronephrosis, urosepsis and metabolic acidosis from poor renal function represent the main source of mortality in neonates with anorectal malformations. Patients with anorectal malformations should have an ultrasonographic study of the abdomen during the first 24 h after birth. If this study shows some abnormalities, a thorough urologic evaluation is indicated.

Other defects

Other congenital malformations are commonly associated with this defect, including esophageal atresia, duodenal atresia and cardiovascular defects.

Management of anorectal malformations during the neonatal period

The most important decisions to be made during the neonatal period are whether the patient needs a colostomy or urinary or vaginal diversion to prevent sepsis or metabolic acidosis. The timing and establishment of priorities are the key to success.

Boys

The decision-making algorithm used by the author for the management of neonatal boys with anorectal malformations is shown in *Figure 1*. In more than 80% of boys, perineal inspection and urinalysis provide enough clinical evidence to make a decision regarding a diverting colostomy. All patients with perineal fistulas, 'bucket-handle' malformations or midline raphe subepithelial fistula are treated with a minimal posterior sagittal anorectoplasty.

The presence of a flat bottom and the demonstration of meconium in the urine is an indication for a diverting colostomy. Colostomy decompresses the intestine in the neonatal period, and will subsequently provide protection against infection during the healing process after the main repair.

It is important to wait 16–24 h before making a decision, for these patients do not show abdominal distension during the first few hours of life. Even if a perineal fistula is present, meconium is not usually seen in the perineum until 16–24 h after birth. A significant amount of intra-abdominal pressure is required for the meconium to force its way through a perineal or urinary

fistula. Moreover, this length of time is needed for the intraluminal rectal pressure to reach a level high enough to overcome the voluntary muscle tone that keeps the most distal part of the rectum compressed. Radiologic evaluations have often been thought inaccurate because of the presence of meconium in the blind pouch of the intestine, interfering with the migration of air into the pouch and giving a false image of a high defect. The author believes that the accuracy of these films depends mostly on the intraluminal intestinal pressure. It must be remembered that, in most cases of anorectal malformation, the most distal part of the rectum is surrounded by a striated muscle mechanism that keeps the rectum collapsed (*see Illustrations 1, 4, 5*). To distend that most distal part of the rectum it is necessary to exert significant intraluminal pressure. Radiologic evaluations performed during the first hours of life are, therefore, unreliable.

Shortly after birth an intravenous cannula must be established for the administration of fluids. A nasogastric tube is inserted to keep the stomach decompressed and thus avoid the risk of vomiting and aspiration. Antibiotics must be administered and an ultrasonographic study of the abdomen is indicated to rule out the presence of other anomalies (mainly urologic). A piece of gauze is placed on the tip of the penis, and the nurses are then instructed to check for particles of meconium filtered through this gauze.

If after 16–24 h of observation there is no clinical evidence indicating the need for a colostomy or a perineal operation, the patient must then have a radiologic evaluation (*Figure 1*). A cross-table lateral film with the patient in the prone position helps to determine the position of the rectal pouch and seems to

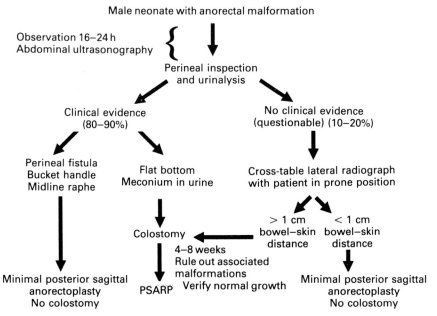

Figure 1   Decision-making algorithm for management of neonatal boys with anorectal malformations. PSARP = posterior sagittal anorectoplasty.

be equally as useful as the traditional invertogram[8]. At the author's institution the images obtained with this technique were comparable with those obtained from a traditional invertogram. It was much simpler, however, to do the study in the lateral position. The anal dimple is marked with radiopaque material. The presence of intestine located more than 1 cm from the skin represents an indication for a colostomy. If the image is questionable it is preferable to construct a diverting colostomy. When the intestine is located close to the skin (less than 1 cm), it is justifiable to approach these patients through a minimal anoplasty. The later situation is extremely unusual, however, for most of these cases have a tiny perineal fistula that has not been recognized.

After recovering from the colostomy the patient is discharged from the hospital. If the patient is growing well and has no other associated defects (cardiovascular or gastrointestinal) that require treatment, he is readmitted at 4–8 weeks of age for a posterior sagittal anorectoplasty. This early repair can be performed safely only if the surgeon has experience in dealing with the delicate anatomy of the infant.

Performing the definitive repair at 1 month of age has important advantages for the patient, including less time with an abdominal stoma, less size discrepancy between proximal and distal intestine at the time of colostomy closure, simpler anal dilatation, and no recognizable psychologic sequelae from painful perineal maneuvers. In addition, at least theoretically, placing the rectum in

the right location early in life may represent an advantage in terms of potentially acquired local sensation[9].

Some surgeons have proposed primary repair of all anorectal malformations during the neonatal period without a protective colostomy. There is no question that this can be done and that it has the potential of avoiding the morbidity related to the formation and closure of a colostomy. The disadvantages include the fact that the anatomy of the neonate is not as well defined as in older patients. Also the diagnostic tests used to determine the level of the defect are not accurate enough, and the surgeon is actually subjecting the patient to an exploration of the perineum. If the rectum is located high in the abdomen, the surgeon may damage other unexpected structures during the search for a very high rectum. Such structures include the posterior urethra, seminal vesicles, vas deferens and ectopic ureters. In addition, there is a risk of dehiscence and infection.

Girls

A decision-making algorithm for the initial management of girls is shown in *Figure 2*. Perineal inspection usually provides more information in girls than in boys. The principle of waiting 16–24 h before making a decision is valuable in this group of patients.

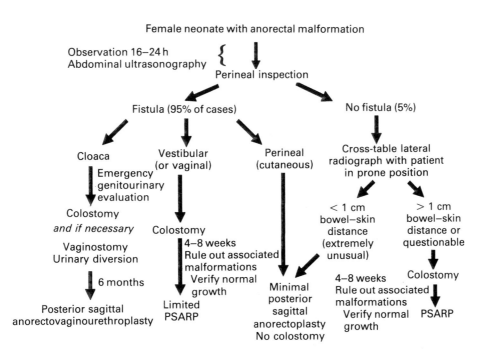

Figure 2   Decision-making algorithm for management of neonatal girls with anorectal malformations. PSARP = posterior sagittal anorectoplasty.

16 The presence of a single perineal orifice is pathognomonic of a cloaca. These patients also have rather small genitalia. Sometimes patients with cloacas have a palpable lower abdominal mass that represents a distended vagina (hydrocolpos). Many patients with cloacas are referred to the pediatric surgeon with the erroneous diagnosis of rectovaginal fistula. Failing to recognize the presence of a cloaca in a neonate may be dangerous, as more than 90% of these patients have important associated urologic defects.

Once the clinical diagnosis of a cloaca has been established, the next step is to perform an emergency urologic evaluation. Abdominal ultrasonography is the most important screening test. If this shows hydronephrosis or hydroureter, a urologic evaluation must be performed before a colostomy is constructed. The surgeon must be prepared to divert the urinary tract at the time of colostomy. The type of diversion depends on the specific urologic problem. In patients who have hydrocolpos it is important to drain the vagina. A distended vagina compresses the trigone of the bladder and interferes with drainage of the ureters. The most common error at this stage is to perform only a colostomy in a patient with severe obstructive uropathy. Once the patient has been subjected to a colostomy and urinary diversion (when indicated), the recovery is usually uneventful. The final repair of this defect is called posterior sagittal anorectovaginourethroplasty and is usually carried out after 6 months of age. Attempts to drain the urinary tract through the

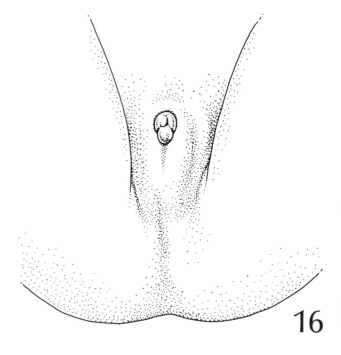

single perineal orifice (common channel) by way of intermittent catheterization or dilatations is not recommended, as it is unpredictable whether the catheter will enter the bladder or the vagina. This particularly applies in cases of long common channels. Blind dilatations of the single external orifice may also provoke local damage that can interfere with further management.

Perineal inspection may reveal the presence of a vestibular fistula, which is the most common condition in girls. The diagnosis of a rectovaginal fistula may only be established if meconium is seen coming from inside the vagina.

17 In cases with rectovestibular fistula, the rectal orifice is located within the vestibule and outside the hymen.

Most of these cases are referred after the diagnosis of rectovaginal fistula, which only reflects a careless inspection of the genitalia. It is the author's conviction that these patients need a protective colostomy; however, this procedure does not always need to be performed as an emergency. These fistulas are usually large enough to decompress the gastrointestinal tract. Occasionally, the fistula is too narrow and the patient will suffer from abdominal distension. In these patients the fistula may first be dilated in order to facilitate emptying the rectum. The colostomy then becomes an elective procedure. Delaying the fashioning of a colostomy for weeks or months, however, may result in severe megarectum, which may become irreversible; this has been identified as a cause of constipation. After the colostomy is opened, the patient is sent home for 4–8 weeks of observation to confirm that growth is proceeding normally. The defect is then repaired with a limited posterior sagittal operation.

Some surgeons prefer to perform a primary definitive operation on vestibular fistulas without a protective colostomy. Although this method is feasible, the author prefers to construct a protective colostomy before the main repair because patients with vestibular fistula are

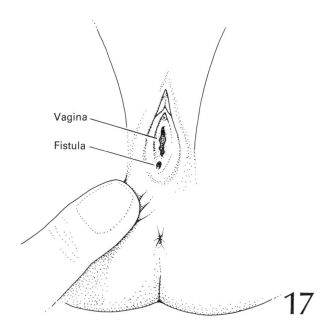

the ones most often referred after a failed attempt at primary repair without a colostomy. In addition, patients with this particular defect are usually continent after a successful operation. An infection and/or dehiscence must be considered an unacceptable complication because it is not only a wound infection but it also may damage the continence mechanism. The prognosis for fecal continence after a secondary procedure is not as good as after a primary repair[4].

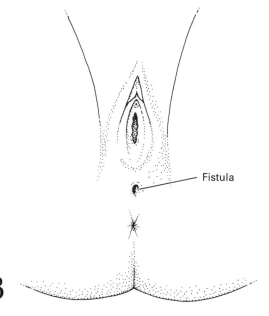

18 The presence of a perineal (cutaneous) fistula represents the simplest defect in the spectrum of female malformations. These patients can be treated with a minimal posterior sagittal anoplasty without a colostomy during the neonatal period.

Most girls with imperforate anus have a fistula (95%). Sometimes, after 16–24 h of observation, the neonate's abdomen may become distended and yet there is no evidence of meconium passing through the genitalia. The neonate is a candidate for radiologic evaluation; the same principles already discussed for male neonates are followed (*see Figures 1* and *2*).

Operations

COLOSTOMY

A descending colostomy with separated stomas best fulfils the requirements for the management of anorectal malformations. Transverse colostomies have several disadvantages: the mechanical preparation of the distal colon before the definitive repair is much more difficult and, in the case of a large rectourethral fistula or rectal–bladder neck fistula, the patient often passes urine into the colon, where it remains and is absorbed, leading to metabolic acidosis. A more distal colostomy allows urine to escape through the distal stoma without significant absorption. Loop colostomies often permit the passage of stool from the proximal stoma into the distal intestine, which can cause urinary tract infections and impaction of stool in the distal rectal pouch. Prolonged dilatation of the rectal pouch may provoke irreversible intestinal damage, which translates into severe constipation later in life.

Colostomy prolapse is more common with loop colostomies.

A colostomy created too distally in the area of the rectosigmoid colon may interfere with mobilization of the rectum during the pull-through procedure. The incidence of prolapse in descending colostomies is almost zero owing to the fact that the proximal stoma is opened immediately distal to the fixed descending colon.

During the opening of the colostomy, the distal intestine must be irrigated to remove all the meconium, preventing the formation of a megasigmoid.

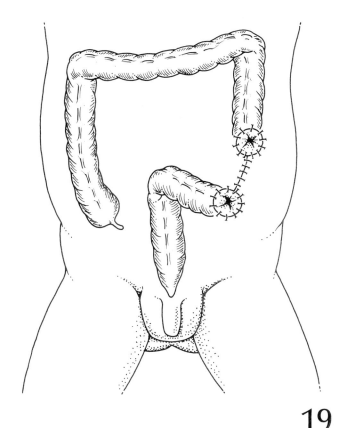

19

19 The colostomy is constructed through a left lower quadrant oblique incision. The proximal stoma is exteriorized through the upper and lateral part of the wound and the mucous fistula is placed in the medial or lower part of the wound. The mucous fistula is intentionally opened minimally to prevent prolapse. The stomas should be separated so as to allow the use of a stoma bag.

Distal colostography

Before the definitive repair, distal colostography is carried out. It is the most valuable and accurate diagnostic study for anorectal malformation. Water-soluble contrast medium is instilled into the distal stoma, filling the distal intestine in order to demonstrate the location of the blind rectum and the precise site of the rectourinary fistula. The rectum is surrounded by striated muscle which keeps it collapsed and prevents filling of the most distal part. This may give the erroneous impression of a very high defect and may prevent demonstration of the rectourinary fistula, which is always located at the most distal part of the rectum.

To avoid this problem, the contrast medium must be injected with considerable hydrostatic pressure under fluoroscopic control. The use of a Foley catheter is recommended; it is passed through the distal stoma, the balloon is inflated (2–5 ml) and it is pulled back as far as possible to occlude the stoma during the injection of the contrast medium. This maneuver permits exertion of enough hydrostatic pressure (syringe manual injection) to overcome the muscle tone of the striated muscle mechanism, fill the rectum, and demonstrate the urinary fistula when present[10].

In cases of rectourethral fistula (prostatic and bulbar) the surgeon knows precisely where to find the rectum. In cases of rectal–bladder neck fistulas the surgeon does not expect to find the rectum by using the posterior sagittal approach and so avoids dangerous, searching maneuvers. In this latter case the surgeon can prepare the patient for an additional laparotomy to mobilize a very high rectum.

DEFINITIVE REPAIR

Incision

All anorectal malformations can be correcte.' by the posterior sagittal approach. The size of the incision changes depending on the specific defect. The patient is placed in the prone position with the pelvis elevated. The use of an electric stimulator is strongly recommended to elicit muscle contraction during the operation as a guide to remain exactly in the midline. A long incision that starts in the middle portion of the sacrum and extends all the way to the single perineal orifice is necessary in cases of persistent cloacas. Smaller incisions (limited posterior sagittal anorectoplasty) are adequate for defects such as vestibular fistula. Perineal fistulas require a very small posterior sagittal incision (minimal posterior sagittal anoplasty).

The anatomic relationship of the rectum to all genitourinary structures is complex. The separation of the rectum from these structures represents the most risky part of the procedure.

About 90% of male defects can be repaired via the posterior sagittal approach without opening the abdomen. In cases of persistent cloacas the abdomen has to be opened in approximately 40% of cases.

Perineal (cutaneous) fistulas

The repair of these defects consists of a small anoplasty with minimal mobilization of the intestine, sufficient for it to be transposed and placed within the limits of the external sphincter. This is a meticulous operation and can be done during the neonatal period without a colostomy. These patients, both boys and girls, have an excellent prognosis, even without operation, except in cases where the intestine is dissected unnecessarily. If the surgeon has no experience with this type of procedure, a simple 'cut-back' may be enough to repair this defect with good functional results, although cosmetically the results are less than desirable.

Rectourethral fistula

A Foley catheter is inserted through the urethra. In about 25% of cases this catheter goes into the rectum rather than into the bladder. To avoid this, the catheter must be intentionally directed anteriorly to find its correct path by the use of a lacrimal probe inserted in the distal tip of the Foley catheter.

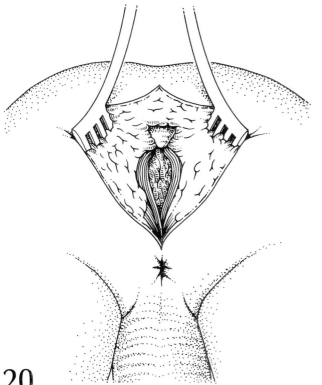

20 The skin is opened through a mid-sagittal incision, and the parasagittal fibers and muscle complex are divided exactly in the midline by use of a fine needle cautery. The fibers of the muscle complex run perpendicular and medial to the parasagittal fibers. The crossing of the muscle complex fibers with the parasagittal fibers creates the anterior and posterior limits of the new anus. These limits can be seen most clearly with the use of an electrical stimulator. The levator muscle, which lies deep in the incision, is then divided in the midline. The higher the malformation, the deeper the levator muscle is found. The levator muscle fibers run parallel to the skin incision. Levator muscle and muscle complex are in continuum.

20

21 When all muscle structures have been divided, the rectum can be seen. In cases of rectourethral bulbar fistulas, the intestine is prominent and it almost bulges into the wound. In cases of rectoprostatic fistulas, the rectum is located much higher and is not as prominent. In cases of rectal–bladder neck fistulas, the rectum is not visible through this approach, and searching for it is not recommended.

22 Two silk sutures are placed in the posterior rectal wall on both sides of the midline. The rectum is opened between the sutures and the incision is continued distally exactly in the midline, down to the fistula site. Temporary silk sutures are placed on the edges of the open posterior rectal wall for traction.

The anterior rectal wall immediately above the fistula is a thin structure. There is no plane of separation between rectum and urethra in that area. A plane of separation must be created in the common wall. Multiple 6/0 silk sutures are placed through the rectal mucosa immediately above the fistula in semicircumferential fashion. The rectum is then separated from the urethra, creating a submucosal plane for approximately 5–10 mm above the fistula site. During this delicate dissection, it is very helpful to dissect the rectum laterally, very close to the rectal wall, intermittently, until both dissections (lateral and medial) meet, separating the rectum completely from the urinary tract. Once the rectum is fully separated, a circumferential perirectal dissection is performed to gain enough rectal length to reach the perineum.

In cases of a fistula opening into the bulbar urethra, the dissection necessary to pull the rectum down to the perineum is rather minimal, whereas in cases of prostatic fistula the perirectal dissection is considerable. In both cases enough rectal length must be gained in order to perform a comfortable, tension-free anastomosis between the rectum and the skin. As traction is exerted on the mucosal stitches plus the stitches previously placed in the rectal edge during the opening of the rectum, some grooves can be seen in the rectal wall that demonstrate the tension lines that hold the rectum. These tension dents are nerves and vessels that must be divided. The implications of this denervation are unknown, though possibly it might provoke some degree of a pseudo-Hirschsprung's type of disorder. Thus, patients with higher malformations that require more dissection would be expected to suffer from more severe constipation. In the author's experience, however, patients with lower defects treated with this approach suffer more constipation than patients with higher defects.

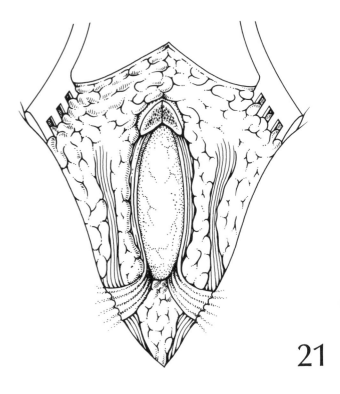

21

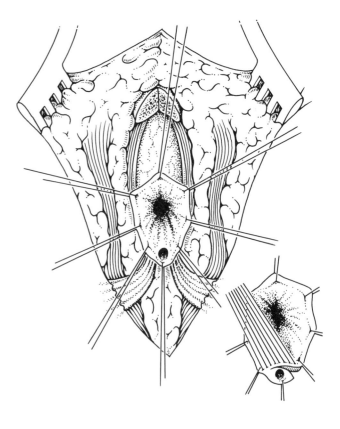

22

23 Once the rectum has been fully mobilized, a decision must be made concerning the need for tailoring the rectum. The size of the rectum can be evaluated and compared with the available space. If necessary, the rectum can be tapered by removing part of the posterior wall. The rectal wall is reconstructed with two layers of interrupted long-lasting absorbable sutures. The anterior rectal wall is often damaged to some degree as a consequence of the separation between rectum and urethra. To reinforce this wall, both smooth muscle layers can be sutured together with interrupted 5/0 long-lasting absorbable sutures. The urethral fistula is sutured with the same material.

The tapering of the rectum must always be done on the posterior rectal wall. The part of the intestine that will be adjacent to the closed end of the urethral fistula must be normal rectal wall to avoid a recurrent rectourethral fistula.

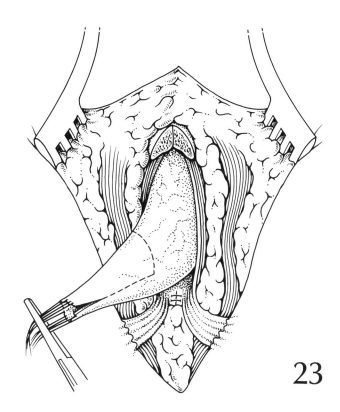

23

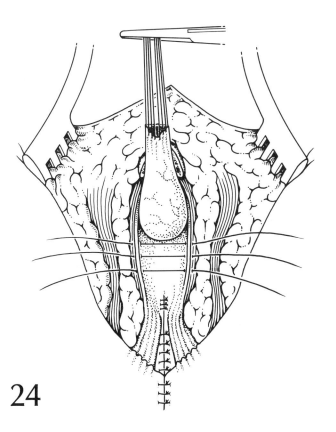

24

24 The rectum must be placed in front of the levator and within the limits of the muscle complex and external sphincter. The electrical stimulator is always helpful in identifying the limits of the muscle structures. Anterior and posterior limits of the external sphincter are temporarily marked with silk sutures. In cases where the incision is extended anteriorly beyond the limits of the sphincter, it is necessary to repair the anterior perineum with interrupted 5/0 long-term absorbable sutures to bring together both anterior limits of the external sphincter. Long-lasting 5/0 and 4/0 absorbable sutures are placed on the posterior edge of the levator muscle. The posterior limit of the muscle complex must also be reapproximated behind the rectum. These sutures must include part of the rectal wall in order to anchor it and to avoid rectal prolapse.

25 The anoplasty is performed with 16 interrupted long-lasting absorbable sutures. The wound is then closed, special care being taken in bringing together corresponding sphincteric structures in the midline.

The Foley catheter is left in place for 5 days. The patient receives broad-spectrum antibiotics for 3 days.

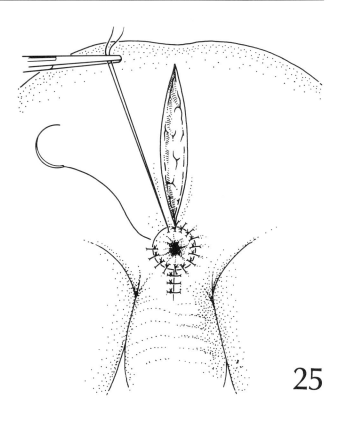

25

Rectovesical (bladder neck) fistula

26 For the repair of cases with rectal–bladder neck fistulas, the initial approach is the posterior sagittal one. All the muscle structures are divided in the midline. The urethra is exposed, and a rubber tube is placed in the presacral space in front of the levator muscle and within the limits of the muscle complex and external sphincter, where the rectum will subsequently be placed. The size of the tube should be chosen to represent the space available for the pull-through.

The patient is then turned into the supine position and a total body preparation is performed. The entire lower part of the patient's body is included in this sterile field, so that the surgeon can work simultaneously in the abdomen and the perineum. The abdomen is entered and the rectosigmoid colon is mobilized. In this very high defect, the rectal–bladder neck fistula is located approximately 2 cm below the peritoneal reflection of the rectum and communicates with the urinary tract in a T fashion, which means that there is no common wall between the distal part of the rectum and the urinary tract. This facilitates the dissection, which is minimal. The surgeon must be careful to avoid damage to the vas deferens which runs very close to the bowel.

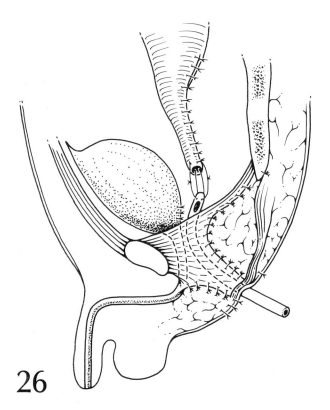

26

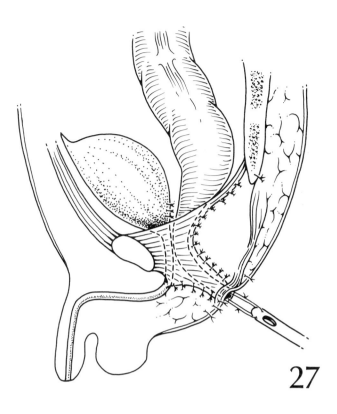

27 The rectum is separated from the bladder neck, and the bladder end of the fistula is sutured with interrupted absorbable sutures.

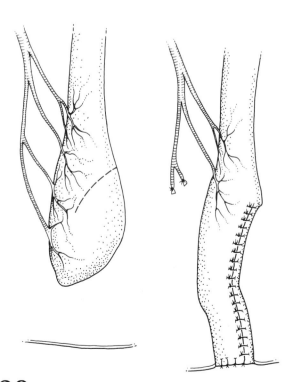

28 As this is a very high defect, mobilization of the rectum to reach the perineum requires special maneuvers. The first alternative is ligation of the inferior mesenteric vessels as high as possible, very close to their origin near the aorta. This maneuver may be sufficient to mobilize the rectum, but before ligating these vessels, a temporary clamp must be used to ensure that this maneuver does not compromise the blood supply of the rectum. Ligating these vessels sometimes causes ischemia in the distal rectum. Under these circumstances, another alternative consists of ligating the most distal branches of the inferior mesenteric vessels close to the rectum. If this is done, the more proximal branches of the inferior mesenteric vessels must be left intact to guarantee a good blood supply to the rectum. This last maneuver is possible only because the rectum has an excellent intramural blood supply.

The last maneuver to gain extra length consists of a plasty of the distal dilated portion of the rectum. A combination of these maneuvers usually allows the intestine to reach the perineum, provided the colostomy does not interfere with the pull-through of the rectum. This can be avoided by the use of colostography, which demonstates the precise length of intestine available from the colostomy to the end of the rectum. The rectum is tapered if necessary. The rectum is then anchored to the rubber tube and pulled down through the pelvis. The anoplasty is performed as previously described.

Imperforate anus without fistula

About 5% of the author's entire series consist of patients with imperforate anus but without a fistula. In both boys and girls the rectum lies about 2 cm from the perineal skin. Most of these patients have a very good sacrum and good muscles. The fact that these patients have no fistula does not necessarily mean that the repair is simpler. The rectum must be carefully separated from the urethra, because the two structures have a common wall. The rest of the repair must be performed as described for the rectourethral fistula type of defect.

Rectal atresia and stenosis

These defects are repaired through a posterior sagittal approach. All the sphincteric mechanisms are divided in the midline. The upper rectal pouch is opened as well as the small distal anal canal. An end-to-end anastomosis is performed under direct vision, followed by a meticulous reconstruction of the muscle mechanism posterior to the rectum. The wound is closed by following the same principles already described.

REPAIR IN GIRLS

Perineal (cutaneous) fistula

The treatment of a perineal (cutaneous) fistula in girls is the same as discussed for boys.

Vestibular fistula

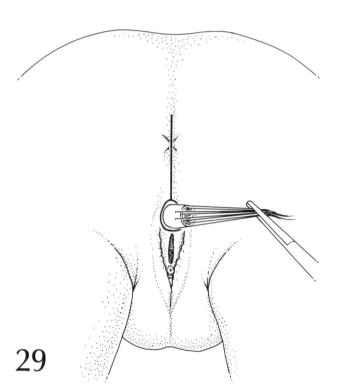

29

29 Most surgeons underestimate the complexity of this defect. Multiple 5/0 silk sutures are placed at the edge of the fistula in order to exert uniform traction on the rectum to facilitate its dissection. The incision used to repair this defect is shorter than the one used to repair rectourethral fistulas in boys. The incision continues around the fistula into the vestibule in a racket-like fashion. All the sphincteric mechanism is divided in the midline until the rectal wall is located. This helps to locate the plane of dissection during the entire mobilization of the rectum. Once the rectal wall has been identified, a lateral dissection is performed from the posterior midline, while placing traction on the fistula to make the plane of dissection more obvious.

Hemorrhoidal vessels are usually found on the lateral aspects of the rectum. The most delicate part of this dissection is that of the anterior rectal wall. The rectum and the vagina share a common wall, which is often very thin. This thin wall has no plane of separation and the surgeon has to make two walls out of one. This dissection is performed by using a very fine needle cautery and suction, which allows each one of the little vessels that are encountered during the dissection to be meticulously cauterized. This is continued up to the point where rectum and vagina separate and have full-thickness walls. The most common error in performing this operation is that vagina and rectum are not completely separated. This may create a tense anastomosis between the rectum and the skin, which may provoke dehiscence and recurrence of the fistula.

30 Once the dissection has been completed, the electrical stimulator is used to determine the limits of the sphincteric mechanism. The anterior limit of the external sphincter and the anterior edge of the muscle complex are reapproximated as previously described. The levator muscle is usually not exposed and therefore does not have to be reconstructed. The muscle complex must, however, be reconstructed posterior to the rectum. The anoplasty is performed as previously described.

Vaginal fistula

As previously mentioned, a vaginal fistula is a very unusual defect. Its repair requires a full posterior sagittal incision. Basically, the operation is the same as that described for a vestibular fistula, except that in these cases it is necessary to dissect much more of the rectum to gain enough length to pull it down to the perineum.

Persistent cloaca

Surgical management of a persistent cloaca represents the most complex technical challenge in pelvic pediatric surgery. The goal of the operation is to separate the rectum from the vagina and the vagina from the urinary tract, place the rectum within the sphincteric mechanism, open the vagina in its normal location and reconstruct the old common channel as a neourethra.

31 A long mid-sagittal incision is performed that extends from the middle portion of the sacrum through the external sphincter and down into the single perineal opening. All of the muscle structures are divided in the midline. The likely first visceral structure to be found is the rectum. This is opened in the midline as described in the surgical treatment of rectourethral fistula. The surgeon must be prepared to find bizarre anatomic arrangements of rectum, vagina and urethra. The incision in the posterior rectal wall is continued all the way down to the single perineal orifice, exposing the entire malformation.

At this stage, the surgeon has an objective idea of the complexity of the defect and can measure the length of the common channel. If it is longer than 3 cm, it usually means that the surgeon will have to open the abdomen to mobilize the vagina and a very high rectum. If the common channel is shorter than 3 cm that usually means that it will be possible to mobilize the entire vagina and rectum without opening the abdomen. The prognosis is also better in the latter group as compared with the former.

The rectum and vagina have a common wall, as described in cases of vestibular fistulas. The vagina and urinary tract also have a more extensive common wall.

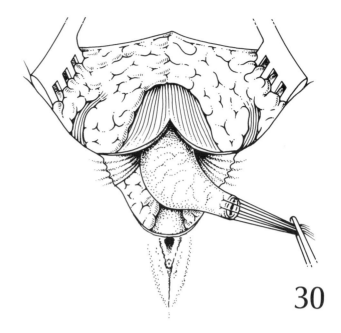

30

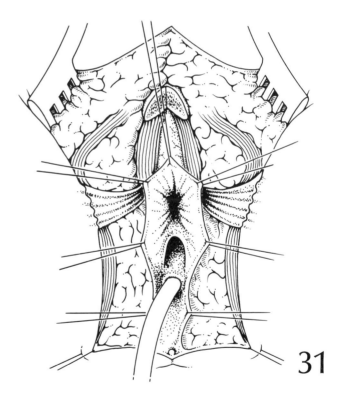

31

The separation of rectum and vagina is no more difficult than described in cases of rectovestibular fistula. On the other hand, separation of the vagina from the urinary tract represents the most difficult challenge of these procedures. The vagina and urinary tract are less elastic than the rectum and their common wall is thin. This common wall often extends into the trigone and, therefore, includes the opening of both ureters.

32 These structures are separated by following the same principles described above. Multiple 5/0 silk or 6/0 silk traction sutures are placed to include the rectal and vaginal mucosas in order to facilitate the dissections. The vagina surrounds the urethra and the bladder neck. Approximately 2–3 cm of dissection between vagina and urinary tract should be adequate to mobilize the vagina down to the perineum. If this is not enough to reach the perineum, as in cases with common channels longer than 3 cm, some form of vaginal elongation or replacement should be chosen. Over-zealous dissection of the structures may result in devascularization of the vagina or urethral injury.

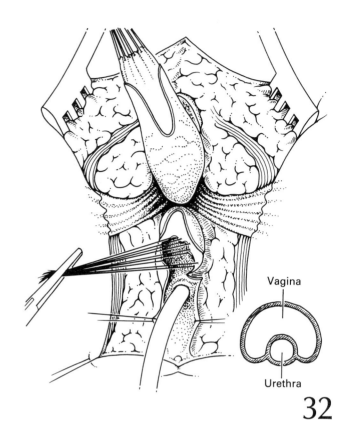

Vagina

Urethra

32

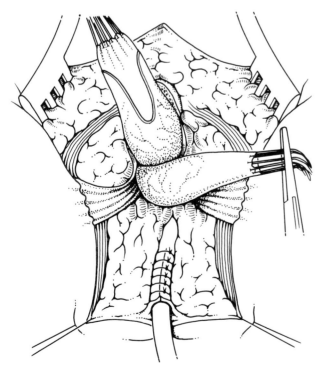

33

33 In cases of common channels of less than 3 cm the urethra is reconstructed using the whole common channel. This is performed over a Foley catheter with two layers of 5/0 long-term absorbable sutures.

The vagina is then sutured to the perineum with multiple long-term absorbable sutures in a circumferential manner creating a new introitus immediately behind the urethra.

The perineal body is reconstructed as previously described, the rectum is pulled down, and the sphincteric mechanism is reconstructed as in other defects.

In cases of long common channels the wound is packed with a gauze soaked in an antiseptic solution and the patient is prepared for an abdominal approach as described for cases of rectal–bladder neck fistula. The abdomen is opened, the bladder is opened in the midline and ureteric catheters are introduced into both ureters to facilitate identification of the ureters during the dissection between the vagina and the bladder. Heavy traction sutures are placed in the single uterus or in both hemiuteri. Traction sutures are also placed in the dome of the bladder. With the use of traction on both structures, dissection is initiated between the urinary tract and the vagina. This dissection is continued all the way down to meet the previous dissection initiated from below. In order to reconstruct a very high vagina, two maneuvers can be used.

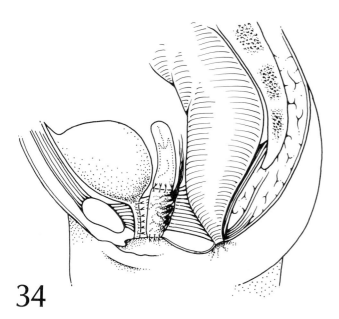

34

Vaginal replacement with a segment of small intestine

34 This procedure is suggested in cases of a very long gap or in cases of total vaginal replacement. A segment of small intestine is selected, preserving its mesentery. The continuity of the small intestine is re-established with an end-to-end anastomosis. Two more anastomoses are necessary: the upper between the segment of small intestine and the upper vagina, and the lower between the lower part of the intestine and the perineal skin[11].

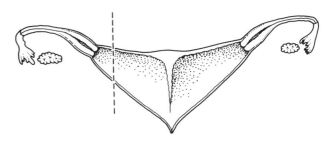

35a

Vaginal switch

35a, b These patients often have two hemi-vaginas divided by a midline septum. After separation of the vagina from the urinary tract has been completed, the vagina may be too short to fill the gap between vagina and perineum, and it is therefore impossible to move the vagina down. Despite this, the transverse diameter of both hemivaginas together may be such that it is possible to reach the perineum, provided one of the hemiuteri is sacrificed. Therefore, one of the hemiuteri is excised as well as the vaginal septum, the blood supply for the hemiuterus and the hemivagina is divided, and that same hemivagina is switched down to the perineum. This has proved to be a valuable maneuver in the reconstruction of this specific type of defect.

During separation of the vagina from the urinary tract, it must be remembered that the blood supply to both hemiuteri and hemivaginas reaches the hemiuterus laterally. That blood supply must be preserved until a decision is reached concerning the type of vaginal mobilization to be performed.

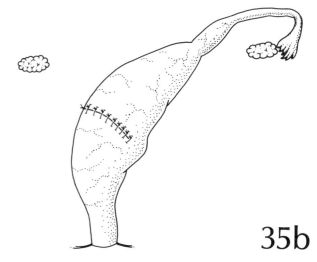

35b

Postoperative care

Patients generally have a smooth postoperative course. Pain is not a prominent symptom, except in those patients who have undergone a laparotomy. In cloacal repairs with short common channels (less than 3 cm) a Foley catheter is left in place for 5–7 days. In more complex cloacal defects a suprapubic cystostomy tube is placed. One month after the operation a suprapubic cystostogram is performed to verify the patency of the urethra and rule out the possibility of urethrovaginal fistulas. The tube is then removed.

In cases of rectourethral fistula in boys the urethral catheter is left in place for 5 days. If the urethral catheter is accidentally dislodged, the patient must be observed for spontaneous voiding. If voiding is not possible, as in cases of very abnormal sacrum, a percutaneous suprapubic cystostomy tube is inserted. Attempts to reintroduce a urethral catheter can be dangerous and must be avoided.

Intravenous antibiotics are administered for 72 h. An antibiotic ointment is applied locally for 8–10 days. The patient is discharged after 3–4 days in cases of a posterior approach without a laparotomy and after 5–7 days in cases of an abdominal approach.

Two weeks after the operations anal dilatations are started. On the first occasion, the dilator that fits snugly into the anus is used to instruct the parents. Dilatations must be carried out twice daily by the parents. Every week the size of the dilator is increased until the rectum reaches the desired size, which depends on the patient's age (*Table 2*). Once the desired size is reached, the colostomy may be closed. The frequency of dilatations may now be reduced once the parents state that the dilator passes easily without pain. The frequency of dilatations may be reduced according to the following schedule: at least once a day for 1 month; every third day for 1 month; twice a week for 1 month; once a week for 1 month; and every 2 weeks for 3 months.

After the colostomy is closed, patients often suffer from severe nappy rash as a consequence of multiple bowel movements. The number of bowel movements eventually decreases and patients develop their own bowel movement pattern. This pattern has a very significant prognostic value by 6 months after the closure of the colostomy. A baby who has one to three bowel movements each day, remains clean between bowel movements and pushes during each bowel movement — indicating that there is some feeling during the defecation process — has, in general, a good functional prognosis, and therefore is most likely to respond to toilet training. On the other hand, an infant who passes stool constantly, without any evidence of feeling or pushing, usually has a poor functional prognosis. In addition, on the basis of the results obtained in the author's series, it may be possible to predict the final functional result from the precise anatomic diagnosis and the status of the sacrum.

Functional disorders after repair of anorectal malformations

Most patients who have undergone a repair of anorectal malformations suffer from some degree of functional disorder due to congenital deficiencies that are not correctable.

Deficiencies in sensation

Except for patients with rectal atresia, most patients with these defects are born without an anal canal. This means that they do not have the exquisite sensation that normally resides in this anatomic area. Most patients, however, still preserve a vague sensation of proprioception generated from the distension of the rectum, and therefore stretching of the voluntary muscles around it. Liquid stools, which do not distend the rectum, are not felt by most of these patients.

Sphincteric mechanism

Anorectal malformations are represented by a spectrum of defects. Most of these patients have a sphincteric mechanism represented by parasagittal fibers of the external sphincter, muscle complex and levator muscle with different degress of development, which varies from almost non-existent muscle to almost normal sphincteric mechanism. Therefore, most of these patients have a limited capacity to hold stool inside the rectum.

Coordinated rectosigmoid motility

Most patients with anorectal malformations suffer from abnormal rectosigmoid motility. Patients who have undergone a surgical procedure in which the rectosigmoid colon is lost, as in endorectal procedures, do not have a normal fecal reservoir, but have a segment of sigmoid or descending colon pulled down to the perineum, and therefore they have a tendency to pass stool constantly, similar to a perineal colostomy.

Table 2   Size of dilator required in different age groups

Age group	Hegar dilator size
1–4 months	12
4–8 months	13
8–12 months	14
1–3 years	15
3–12 years	16
Over 12 years	17

On the other hand, patients who have undergone repair in which rectosigmoid colon was preserved (e.g. posterior sagittal anorectoplasty, sacroperineal pull-through or simple anoplasty) behave as if they had too large a fecal reservoir. Clinically this translates into different degrees of constipation. Mild cases of constipation can be treated very efficiently with laxatives, and the children usually live a normal life. Severe cases of constipation, particularly if they are not treated properly, may suffer from fecal impaction, constant soiling and, therefore, overflow pseudo-incontinence. This constipation seems to be more severe in patients with lower defects. Patients with vestibular fistula in particular are more prone to these problems. The author suspects that an ectatic distended colon (sometimes associated with a loop colostomy which allows fecal impaction in the distal blind pouch) eventually provokes severe constipation.

Complications

In the author's series of 740 patients, the following complications were encountered.

Wound infection

Five patients suffered wound infections. Three of them had a defective loop colostomy which allowed the passage of stool from proximal to distal stoma. The infection affected only the skin and subcutaneous tissue and had no repercussions on the function of the sphincteric mechanism.

Anal strictures

One patient suffered from an intractable anal stricture, which required a secondary operation; a very clear correlation was found in this case with intraoperative devascularization of the distal rectum.

The protocol of dilatations was not followed for several patients who disappeared from the clinic for several weeks. When they returned, the patients were suffering from anal stricture. This stricture was only a ring-like fibrous band at the mucocutaneous junction, however, which was easily treated. This was completely different from a long, narrow stricture secondary to ischemia.

It is important to emphasize that before the advent of the posterior sagittal approach, most surgeons would try to create a very big neoanus to avoid strictures and cumbersome anal dilatations. At that time, surgeons did not recognize the existence of a sphincteric mechanism. With new concepts based on objective knowledge of the sphincteric mechanism obtained via the posterior sagittal approach, the surgeon is obliged to create an anus no bigger than the size of the external sphincter and usually one that is smaller than a normal anus for that age. In addition, the new anus is surrounded by voluntary muscle that keeps the anus closed. If this is not dilated, it will heal closed and, therefore, anal dilatations are mandatory. Tapering of the rectum was not responsible for stricture formation in any of the patients. Those patients who underwent tapering of the rectum did not suffer more constipation.

Constipation

This was the most common functional disorder observed in this series.

Urethrovaginal fistula

This was the most common complication in cases of persistent cloaca, occurring in 8 of the first 80 cloacas evaluated. At the present time, the author feels that this complication can be avoided by always leaving a healthy vaginal wall in contact with the urethral suture line. The vagina can be rotated 90° to prevent this complication. A devascularized vagina with a perineal suture under tension must be avoided, and the abdomen should be opened without hesitation to effect some form of vaginal replacement as previously described.

Acquired vaginal atresia

Three patients suffered from complete vaginal fibrosis. This was secondary to an excessive dissection in a useless attempt to mobilize a very high vagina. In retrospect, one of the described vaginal replacement maneuvers should have been selected in these cases.

Transient femoral nerve pressure

This occurred in three adolescent patients owing to excessive pressure in the groin during a posterior sagittal operation. This problem can be avoided by adequate cushioning of the patient's groin area.

Recurrent rectourethral fistula

One patient developed this complication after a secondary operation. Fortunately, this fistula closed spontaneously. In retrospect, this patients had a severe inflammatory process in the pelvis, secondary to the presence of a foreign body left in place during the previous procedure.

Ureteric injury

Ectopic ureters were injured in two cases (in one boy with a very high defect during the search for the rectum). This patient required a laparotomy for the ureteric reimplantation during the same procedure. The second patient was a girl with a persistent cloaca and the injury occurred during the separation of the bladder from the vagina. This patient underwent a ureteric reimplantation via a posterior sagittal approach. A good distal colostogram in boys shows exactly where the rectum opens into the urinary tract and will allow the surgeon to identify those patients who have a rectal–bladder neck fistula in whom the rectum is too high to be mobilized from below.

Neurogenic bladder

Difficulty in voiding after a posterior sagittal approach has occurred only in patients with a very abnormal or absent sacrum or with a myelomeningocele, in whom the presence of a preoperative neurogenic bladder can be predicted.

Difficulty in voiding after the operation in patients with a normal sacrum has been observed only in cases of complex cloacas with hydrocolpos. These patients are born with a very large bladder that seems unable to contract well. Neurogenic bladder following a posterior sagittal approach in patients with favorable anatomy has not occurred. Such an occurrence could only be secondary to nerve damage due to a defective technique, where the surgeon does not follow the principles of this approach and veers off the midline. In addition, placing Weitlander's retractors deeper than is necessary may compress the nerves that come from the sacral area, causing a neurogenic bladder.

Medical management for fecal incontinence

As shown in *Table 3* there remains a significant number of patients who suffer from fecal incontinence, despite optimal surgical technique used for the repair of their malformations. For these patients a program of bowel management has been designed. This consists of training the parents and children to clear out the colon once a day with the use of suppositories, enemas or colonic irrigations and to avoid bowel movements between irrigations by the rational use of a specific diet and sometimes medication.

In addition to 740 patients followed up by the author, over 200 patients have been referred for management of fecal incontinence secondary to an operation for imperforate anus performed in another institution. All these patients are evaluated clinically and undergo a contrast enema study, voiding cystourethrography, radiologic evaluation of their sacrum, and magnetic resonance imaging. These evaluations allow the patients to be classified into the following groups.

Not trainable

These are patients who have a poor sacrum, poor muscles, very high defect, and a poor bowel movement pattern. The best treatment for these patients is a bowel management program. Because of the nature of their original defect and on the basis of statistics, these patients will always suffer from fecal incontinence. Therefore, time should not be wasted on biofeedback programs or behavior modifications, and perhaps more importantly, false expectations should not be created for the family. The bowel management program allows the patient to remain clean all day in order to be socially accepted.

This group is usually divided into two categories.

Constipated

These patients have undergone a procedure in which the rectum was preserved, as in anoplasties, via a sacroperineal approach or posterior sagittal approach. This group of patients tends to suffer from constipation. Management consists of the use of enemas or colonic irrigation, with volumes of fluids large enough to clean a large rectosigmoid colon. It is not usually necessary to use any kind of diet or medication because the

Table 3   Clinical results in the most common defects

	Type of fistula				
	Perineal	Vestibular	Bulbar	Prostatic	Bladder neck
Total number of cases	47	85	96	72	39
Number of cases evaluated	11	32	43	44	18
Voluntary bowel movement	11 (100%)	32 (100%)	30 (69.8%)	30 (68.2%)	3 (16.7%)
Soiling					
Minimal	0	4	10	8	0
Medium	0	4	4	6	1
Severe	0	0	3	2	1
No soiling	11 (100%)	24 (75%)	13 (30.2%)	14 (31.9%)	1 (5.6%)

constipation contributes to the patients remaining completely clean between enemas.

Patients with diarrhea

This group of patients has undergone a type of procedure in which their original rectosigmoid colon was resected, as in the Kiesewetter, Soave, or Rehbein types of operation. They have a natural tendency to suffer from the constant passing of liquid stools. A contrast enema shows that the colon runs straight from the splenic flexure down to the anus, and colonic haustrations are apparent all the way down to the perineum. They never suffer from constipation. This is the group that is most difficult to keep clean. Management consists of colonic irrigation followed by a very strict constipating diet and loperamide hydrochloride. Patients in whom colonic motility fails to slow down may be candidates for a permanent colostomy.

Trainable

These patients were born with a favorable type of defect (vestibular fistula, perineal fistula, rectourethrobulbar fistula), a good sacrum, and a good sphincteric mechanism and underwent an operation that placed the rectum in the correct position. In addition, these patients have a good bowel movement pattern. These patients undergo a behavior modification program to train them to have voluntary bowel movements, but they may need additional help with laxatives or suppositories to improve their quality of life.

Candidates for a reoperation

These patients were born with a favorable type of defect, good sacrum, and good sphincteric mechanism, and yet they underwent an operation that placed the rectum completely in the wrong place, as demonstrated clinically and confirmed by magnetic resonance imaging. Replacing the rectum within the limits of the sphincteric mechanism may significantly improve the functional result.

Candidates for a sigmoid resection

There is a subgroup of patients who have been born with a defect that had a good prognosis and who underwent a technically good operation but suffer from severe constipation and severe megasigmoid colon. They are incapable of emptying the rectosigmoid colon and suffer from chronic soiling and overflow pseudo-incontinence. A sigmoid resection, preserving the rectum and creating an anastomosis between the descending colon and the rectum above the peritoneal reflection, renders them continent. This operation is recommended only in patients with a good sacrum and a good sphincteric mechanism.

Outcome

Each type of defect has a different prognosis. Traditionally, defects have been classified as high, intermediate, or low. This type of classification represents an over-simplification that should be avoided. The so-called high defects often include individual malformations with very different prognoses for bowel function.

Patients should be evaluated without any medical treatment. Medical management, as described above, allows the author to keep most patients clean for 24 h and allows them to live a normal social life. This does not mean, however, that they have normal bowel function. Without medical help, many of these patients will suffer from fecal incontinence. Results presented in this chapter were obtained in patients without any medical management.

When medical management is given, all patients remain clean. *Table 3* shows the clinical results obtained in patients with the most common types of defects. When the sacrum is very abnormal, most patients remain fecally incontinent for life. All patients with low defects are continent. *Table 4* shows the clinical results obtained in a group of 54 cases with cloacas[12].

Table 4   Clinical results in cloacas[12]

	Voluntary bowel movement	Soiling	Diarrhea	Constipation	Urinary incontinence
Normal sacrum (19 cases)	18	14*	3†	2†	5
Abnormal sacrum (7 cases)	3	6‡	0	2†	5

*Six cases were grade 1, seven grade 2 and one grade 4.
†Grade 2.
‡Two cases were grade 1, two grade 2 and two grade 3.

References

1. Stephens FD. Imperforate rectum: a new surgical technique. *Med J Aust* 1953; 1: 202–6.

2. De Vries PA, Peña A. Posterior sagittal anorectoplasty. *J Pediatr Surg* 1982; 17: 638–43.

3. Peña A, De Vries PA. Posterior sagittal anorectoplasty. Important technical considerations and new applications. *J Pediatr Surg* 1982; 17: 796–811.

4. Peña A. Posterior sagittal anorectoplasty: results in the management of 332 cases of anorectal malformations. *Pediatr Surg Int* 1988; 3: 94–104.

5. Murken JD, Albert A. Genetic counselling in cases of anal and rectal atresia. *Progr Pediatr Surg* 1976; 9: 115–18.

6. Parrott TS. Urologic implications of anorectal malformations. *Urol Clin North Am* 1985; 12: 13–21.

7. Rich MA, Brock WA, Peña A. Spectrum of genitourinary malformations in patients with imperforate anus. *Pediatr Surg Int* 1988; 3: 110–13.

8. Goon HK. Repair of anorectal anomalies in the neonatal period. *Pediatr Surg Int* 1990; 5: 246–9.

9. Freeman NV, Burge DM, Soar JS, Sedgwick EM. Anal evoked potentials. *Z Kinderchir* 1980; 31: 22–30.

10. Gross GW, Wolfson PH, Peña A. Augmented-pressure colostogram in imperforate anus with fistula. *Pediatr Radiol* 1991; 21: 560–2.

11. Hendren WH. Repair of cloacal anomalies: current techniques. *J Pediatr Surg* 1986; 21: 1159–76.

12. Peña A. The surgical management of persistent cloaca: results in 54 patients treated with a posterior sagittal approach. *J Pediatr Surg* 1989; 24: 590–8.

Illustrations by Mark Iley

Surgery for anorectal anomalies: anterior perineal approach

P. Mollard
Professor and Head, Service de Chirurgie Pédiatrique, Hôpital Debrousse, Lyon, France

The anterior perineal approach was originally described for identification of the puborectalis sling and for accurate pull-through of the rectum within the sling without the need to divide it[1]. Attention has recently been directed to the preservation of various structures, which may improve the functional result[1]. These structures include the blind end of the rectum, the internal sphincter, the external sphincter and the perianal skin.

Preoperative

The preferred age for the pull-through procedure is 3–6 months. The theoretical advantage of an early operation is improved integration of the continence mechanism at the cortical level. Before surgery it is essential to obtain a radiograph of the distal end of the colon and a cystourethrogram to define the anatomy of the defect. The distal loop of the colostomy is washed out before operation.

Operation

Position of patient

The operation is performed with the infant in the lithotomy position. Access to the abdomen (if required) can be achieved by lowering the position of the left leg.

Incision

1 The anal site is identified by electrical stimulation and by palpating the ischial bones. A butterfly-shaped skin incision is outlined with the aid of a template. The anterior part of the incision borders on the scrotum, and the base of the flap will form the posterior limit of the neoanus. The flap must be wide enough to be sutured round a size 10–12 gauge Hegar dilator.

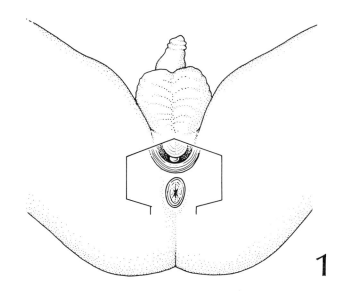

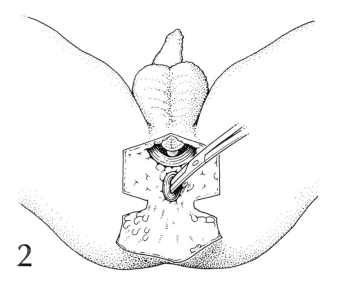

2 The flap is retracted downward and dissected off the fibers of the external sphincter which is developed to a greater or lesser extent and hence is more or less easy to identify.

In the best cases there is a well-developed ring, but sometimes this is only represented by a horseshoe with an anterior concavity. According to Peña the puborectalis sling and the external sphincter are 'mixed into a striated muscular complex'. The two components of this complex cannot be distinguished anatomically, but they are functionally independent. During the operation the external sphincter and the puborectalis sling appear to be separated by a mass of ischiorectal fat crossing the midline. The author has never found vertical striated fibers and it is his belief that these fibers exist only posteriorly. The external sphincter is always present and should be incorporated in the repair as much as possible.

3 The puborectalis sling is next identified. The bulbar urethra is easily identified as it has previously been catheterized with a sound. The membranous urethra is exposed immediately posterior to the bulbar urethra. The dissection then proceeds cranially, keeping in close contact with the urethra. All muscle fibers are gently retracted laterally and posteriorly. The puborectalis muscle can be seen and its upper limit is very easily identified. This step of the procedure is clear and easy. The anterior perineal approach allows an excellent definition of the puborectalis sling, which is left intact.

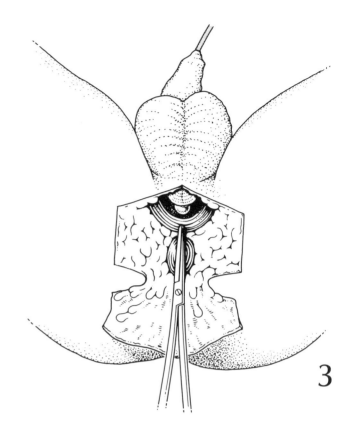

3

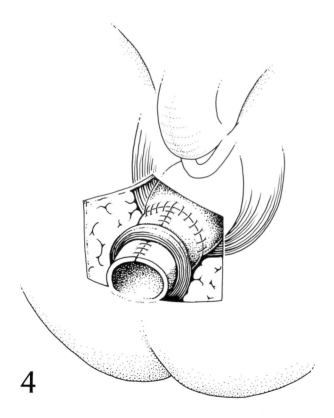

4

4 In infants with intermediate forms of imperforate anus, the cul-de-sac may be dissected entirely through the anterior perineal approach. This minimizes mobilization of the intestine, and the skin tube is long enough to reach up to it. The cul-de-sac is often near to the skin and the proportion of lesions operated on by the perineal approach is increasing in the author's series.

5a–c In infants with true high anorectal anomalies (supralevator) adding an abdominal approach is necessary. After lowering the left leg the surgeon stands on the left side of the abdomen which is opened through a lower left oblique incision. After division of one or two sigmoid arteries, and more occasionally the inferior mesenteric artery, the distal intestine is mobilized. The entire rectal cul-de-sac is preserved. It is certainly useful to obtain a reservoir compliant and sensitive to distention. Moreover, this avoids the propagation of sigmoid peristalsis to the anal margin. The dissection is kept in close contact with the wall of the cul-de-sac. In cases without fistula, dissection of the blind-ending pouch is relatively easy.

In infants with rectourethral (vaginal) fistula the procedure is much more difficult. It is necessary to dissect and suture the fistula flush with the urethra both in order to preserve the internal sphincter (see below) and to avoid fistula recurrence. The cul-de-sac is closely adherent to the urogenital structure, however, and the fistula is too high to approach from the perineal dissection and too low for an easy abdominal approach. Dissection and ligation of the rectourethral fistula is certainly more difficult than with Peña's technique[2]. In the author's series one fistula recurred. On the other hand, it is probably less dangerous for the pelvic nerves, and the author had no case of postoperative neurogenic bladder.

If dissection of the fistula appears too difficult or imprecise, it is possible to use a transvesical and transtrigonal approach (*Illustration 5c*).

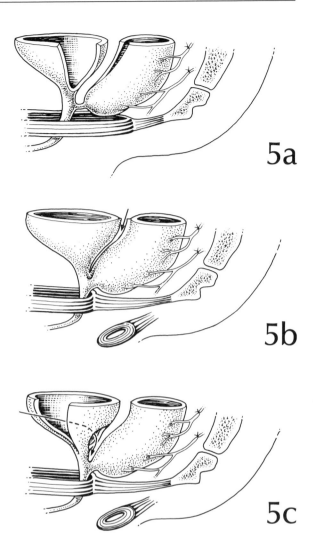

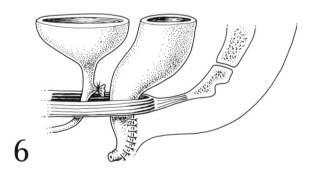

6 The distal cul-de-sac is often dilated and it may be impossible to pull it through the sling without causing compression of the intestine or excessive dilatation and disruption of the muscle fibers. In such cases the intestine should be tapered on a 35-gauge rubber tube. In order to preserve a compliant rectal reservoir the tapering must be as short as possible, and limited to the part of the cul-de-sac that will be pulled through the sling (3–4 cm). The tapering must leave the fistula intact in order to preserve the internal sphincter. The problem of the internal sphincter remains unsolved.

7a–c It is now increasingly acknowledged that the anlage of an internal sphincter can be expected to be found around the fistula or the most caudal part of the blind-ending rectum in patients without a fistula[3].

Even if it is hypoplastic and cannot be positively identified, its preservation around the anastomosis between the cul-de-sac and the skin is still desirable, Husberg *et al.*[4] reported good results using the fistula as a new anal canal. In the author's experience, although the fistula may appear to be very short after the division, it usually spontaneously widens sufficiently to permit it to be sutured to the newly constructed anal canal. When the fistula is long and narrow and in cases without a fistula, preservation of the hypothetical internal sphincter seems utopic. In fact, it is possible to use a progressive dilatation for 6–18h before the anastomoses are performed. For the present, however, this new development of the author's technique requires further study.

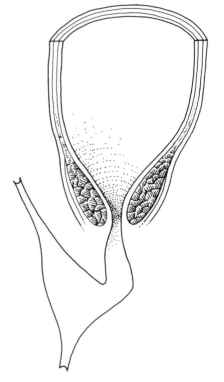

7a

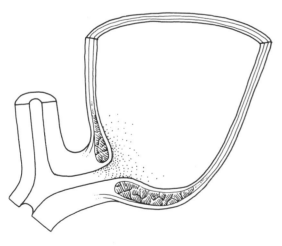

7b

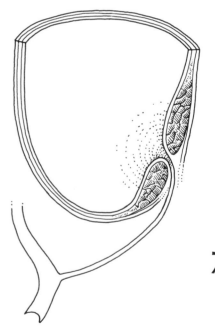

7c

8a–c The lateral edges of the skin flap are sutured together to form a tube. Whenever possible the tube is invaginated through the external sphincter and brought up to the intestinal edge, where it is sutured. If the abdomen has been opened the intestine is retracted upward from inside the abdominal cavity. Some of the sutures are passed through the intestine, the puborectalis, the external sphincter and subcutaneous tissue, in order to restore the continuity of the striated 'muscular complex' and its normal insertion onto the wall of the anorectum. The perineal wound is closed around the newly constructed anus.

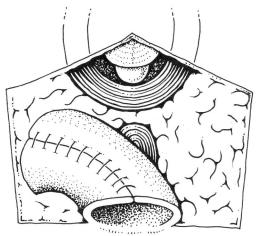

8a

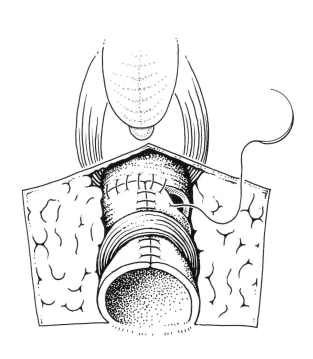

8b

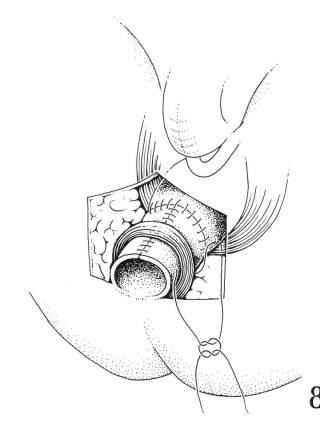

8c

Postoperative care

Anal dilatations with Hegar dilators are commenced on the 12th day after operation. When the anal orifice accepts a size 12 Hegar dilator, the colostomy may be closed. Dilatations are continued for 1 year.

In patients with a rectourethral fistula, the bladder is drained via a suprapubic catheter. A urethral catheter is strictly avoided.

Postoperative complications are rare. There has been no instance of necrosis of the terminal intestine and only one case of wound dehiscence and one recurrent fistula. None of the patients has developed a neuropathic bladder. The long-term anatomic result is excellent, with a well developed, skin-lined anal canal without mucosal prolapse. Functional results have been gratifying. This technique offers the patient the best chance of continence by overcoming many of the deficits associated with the anomaly.

References

1. Mollard P, Soucy P, Louis D, Meunier P. Preservation of infralevator structures in imperforate anus repair. *J Pediatr Surg* 1989; 24: 1023–6.

2. Peña A. Surgical management of anorectal malformations: a unified concept. *Pediatr Surg Int* 1988; 3: 82–93.

3. Lambrecht W, Lierse W. The internal sphincter in anorectal malformations. Morphologic investigations in neonatal pigs. *J Pediatr Surg* 1987; 22: 1160–8.

4. Husberg B, Lindahl H, Rintala R, Frenckner B. High and intermediate imperforate anus: results after surgical correction with special respect to internal sphincter function. *J Pediatr Surg* 1992; 27: 185–9.

Illustrations by Patrick Elliott

Malone procedure for antegrade continence enemas

Padraig S. J. Malone BSc, MCh, FRCS(I)
Consultant Paediatric Urologist, The Wessex Regional Centre for Paediatric Surgery, Southampton General Hospital, Southampton, UK

History

The Malone procedure for antegrade continence enemas was first performed in 1989 and a preliminary report of the first five cases was published in 1990[1]. Subsequently, larger series with intermediate-term follow-up have been published[2,3] and the procedure is now performed in many centres throughout Europe, but no long-term follow-up data are yet available. The procedure evolved to treat intractable fecal incontinence in neuropathic patients, particularly those with spina bifida, and more recently it has been used in patients with anorectal malformations, chronic idiopathic constipation and Hirschsprung's disease. Long-term studies are required to establish the precise role of the procedure in modern surgical practice.

Principles and justification

The main indication for the procedure is fecal incontinence secondary to neuropathy and anorectal malformations, which has not responded to conventional therapy. Although the procedure has been used in patients with chronic constipation and complicated Hirschsprung's disease, the results are variable and the author is reluctant to recommend its use under these circumstances. No patient should have a colostomy for fecal incontinence without having the opportunity of considering the Malone procedure as an alternative. The procedure can easily be reversed and does not preclude other surgical procedures.

1,2 The procedure combines the principles of the Mitrofanoff non-refluxing catheterizable channel and antegrade colonic washout to produce a continent, catheterizable colonic stoma through which washouts are delivered to produce complete colonic emptying and thus prevent soiling.

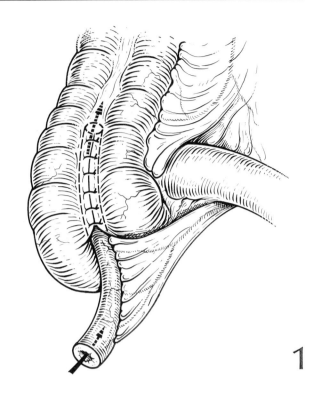

1

Preoperative

Assessment and preparation

Motivation of patients and carers is essential for a successful outcome. Intensive counseling is required and it must be stressed that the Malone procedure is not a 'magic' cure. A rigid, time-consuming regimen is required postoperatively and this is a lifelong commitment. A successfully working antegrade colonic enema takes approximately 45 min every day or on alternate days.

Most patients being considered for the Malone procedure will also have a neuropathic bladder, and it is vital that management of the bladder is assessed simultaneously. In many cases a combined lower urinary tract reconstruction and Malone procedure is appropriate. It is vital, therefore, to have a pediatric urologist involved in the assessment of these patients and in the planning of the operative procedure. Investigations may include ultrasonography, renography and urodynamics, but in the case of an isolated Malone procedure no special investigations are required.

A preoperative full blood count and cross-match are recommended and a full bowel preparation is important. The author favors a 48-h bowel preparation program using sodium picosulfate and rectal washouts, together with a 5-day course of broad-spectrum antibiotics including metronidazole. Preoperatively it is helpful to mark the site of the stoma at a convenient position for the patient.

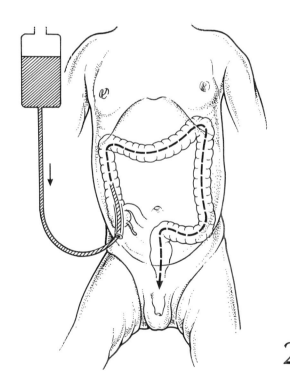

2

Anesthesia

This operation is performed under general anesthesia, but there are no special requirements.

Operation

Incision

3   When the Malone procedure is performed by itself a right lower quadrant muscle cutting incision is used, but a midline incision is better if a simultaneous bladder reconstruction is being carried out. A V-shaped skin incision is used for the stoma. For mobile patients the stoma is best sited in the right iliac fossa, but for wheelchair-bound patients a higher site is usually more suitable.

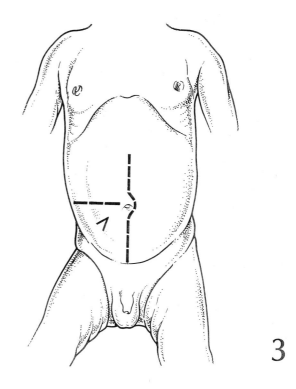

3

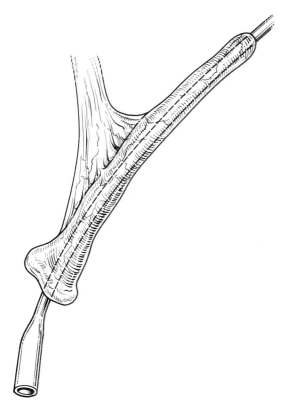

4

Amputation of the appendix

4   The cecum and ascending colon are mobilized and the appendix is amputated from the cecum (in a similar fashion to an appendectomy). The stump is crushed with an artery forceps and ligated with 4/0 chromic catgut and then buried using a 4/0 chromic catgut purse-string suture. If the appendix is short or the patient is obese, extra length may be obtained by excising a cuff of cecum with the appendix. The cecal defect is closed using a single layer of 4/0 or 5/0 interrupted extramucosal Maxon sutures. The tip of the appendix is amputated and its patency tested with a stiff 8-Fr catheter, and it is helpful to leave this catheter *in situ* to act as a retractor and thus avoid excessive handling. The appendix is mobilized by sharp dissection on its vascular pedicle until it is mobile enough to reimplant into the cecum.

Creation of cecal submucosal tunnel

5 The anterior tenia of the cecum is stretched using proximal, distal and two lateral stay sutures. The seromuscular layer of the tenia is incised with a scalpel down to the submucosa over a 5-cm length. The mucosa/submucosa is then freed from the overlying muscle using a combination of sharp and blunt dissection to leave an exposed strip of mucosa approximately 1 cm in width.

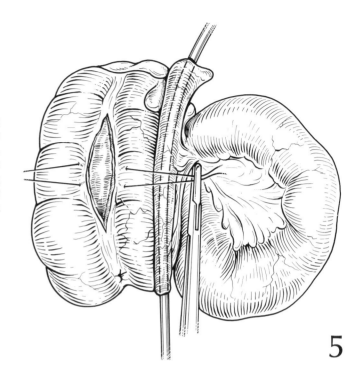

5

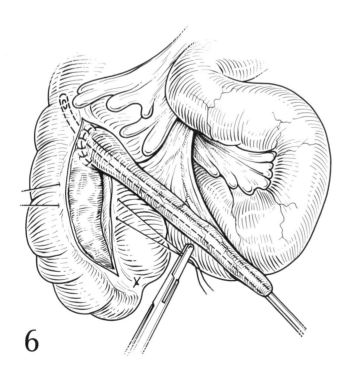

6

Appendiceal–mucosal anastomosis

6 A small hole is punched in the mucosa of the cecum using a pair of artery forceps. This is usually placed at the distal end of the mucosal tunnel but occasionally, if the stoma is to be placed on the upper abdominal wall, the hole may be proximal to facilitate a more direct track. The mucosa is anastomosed to the full-thickness appendix wall using interrupted 4/0 chromic catgut sutures over the appendiceal catheter. The appendix may be reimplanted in either a peristaltic or antiperistaltic fashion, whichever way the appendix lies best.

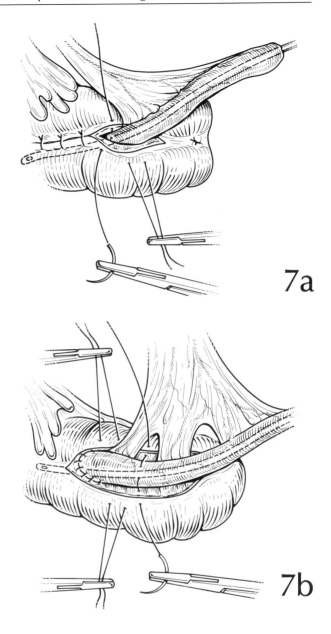

Closure of seromuscular tunnel

7a, b The seromuscular wall of the cecum is closed over the appendix using interrupted 5/0 Maxon sutures picking up a partial thickness of the appendix wall to prevent it slipping out of the tunnel.

At times the appendix has a broad mesentery that makes closure of the tunnel difficult. This can be helped by fenestrating the mesentery between the vessels and closing the seromuscular layer in bridges.

To avoid kinking and difficulties with catheterization, it is important that the length of appendix exiting from the cecum should only be sufficient to reach the abdominal skin flap, and where necessary it should be tailored to size.

Throughout the procedure it is important to ensure that catheterization is easy.

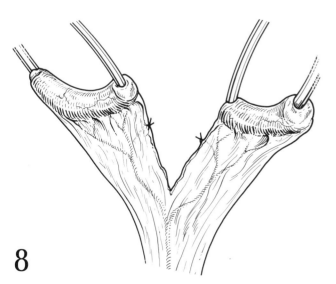

Simultaneous Mitrofanoff procedure/absent appendix

Split appendix

8 When both a Mitrofanoff and Malone procedure are required and the appendix is of sufficient length, it can be divided into two provided that the vascular anatomy is favorable.

Tubularized cecal flap

9a–c A flap of the anterior wall of the cecum, measuring approximately 4 cm × 1.5 cm, can be fashioned on the lateral vessels. This is then tubularized over an 8-Fr catheter using an interrupted extramucosal 5/0 Maxon suture. The tube should be snug on the catheter and the resulting cecal defect is closed as described above. This provides a tube of sufficient length to reach the skin flap and no special antireflux measure seems to be necessary.

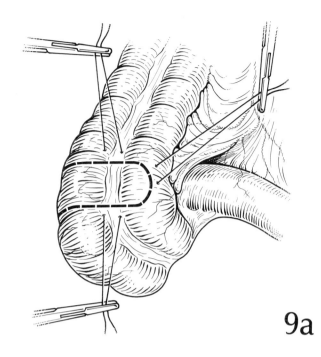

9a

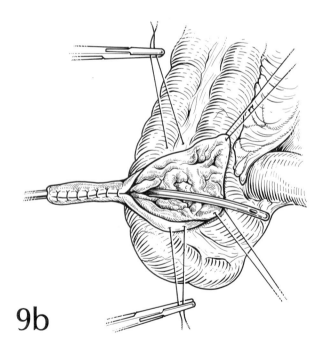

9b

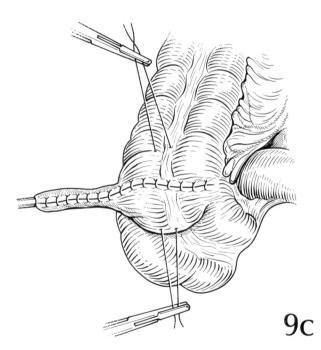

9c

Fashioning the stoma

$10a-f$ The V-shaped skin flap is mobilized and a hole is created in the abdominal wall, sufficiently wide to allow the appendix to pass freely. The cecum is sutured to the anterior abdominal wall to prevent tension on the stoma or volvulus of the cecum on the appendix.

The appendix or the cecal tube is fish-mouthed and the apex of the skin flap is sutured into the defect using 5/0 Maxon sutures with the knots outside the catheterizing channel. The skin flap is gradually sutured into the defect in the appendix until skin is anastomosed to its complete circumference. A short skin tube is then fashioned using only one skin–skin suture.

The skin defect is closed in layers using interrupted 4/0 Maxon and 4/0 polypropylene (Prolene). A 10-Fr Silastic Foley catheter is left *in situ* for 2 weeks after the operation.

In some centers the appendix is brought out directly to the skin without a skin flap and the results are reported to be very satisfactory. The author, however, believes that the skin flap offers several advantages: it provides a funnel that facilitates easy catheterization; and it separates the appendiceal mucosa from the air, which reduces mucous discharge and prevents irritation of the mucocutaneous anastomosis and thus reduces the risk of stomal stenosis.

Postoperative care

Following an isolated Malone procedure, intravenous fluids are required for 24–48 h but a nasogastric tube is seldom needed. A normal enteral diet can usually be established by 72–96 h and 24 h later the first antegrade continence enema is administered. Once the patient and carers are happy with the enema procedure they can be discharged with the indwelling Foley catheter, to return 2 weeks after operation for catheter removal and to learn the technique of stomal catheterization. This seldom takes longer than 48 h. The stomal sutures are also removed at this stage. The stoma should be catheterized twice daily, whether an enema is to be administered or not, as this seems to reduce the incidence of stomal stenosis. A standard 10-Fr Nelaton catheter is used, but for patients who experience difficult catheterization a Lofric catheter is worth trying. The patient should be given some 8-Fr catheters as well. If difficulty is experienced in passing the 10-Fr catheter the 8-Fr size should be used, and often the 10-Fr one will then pass without difficulty. If the patient cannot catheterize, a return to hospital is indicated for formal stomal dilatation under general anesthesia. Occasionally a stoma revision is required; uncommonly catheterization difficulties may be experienced because of kinking of the appendix itself and in these cases a complete revision of the procedure is indicated.

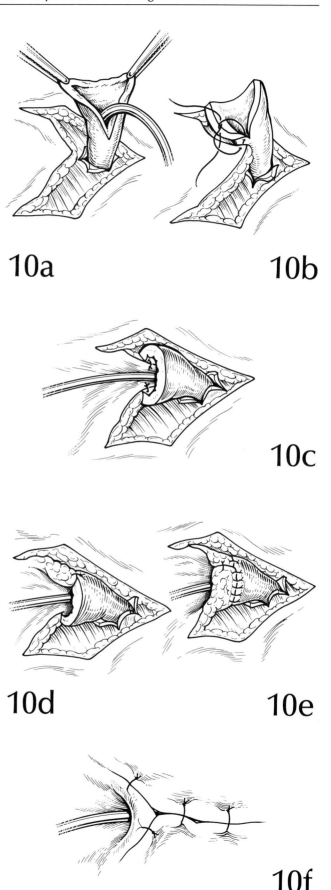

10a   10b

10c

10d   10e

10f

Stomal revision

11a–c The stenosis is usually caused by a fibrous bar at the level of the skin tube. It is corrected by fashioning a Y–V-plasty of peristomal skin. Full-thickness sutures using 4/0 Maxon are employed and a Silastic Foley catheter (10-Fr) is left *in situ* for 5–7 days. The author has successfully performed this revision on three occasions.

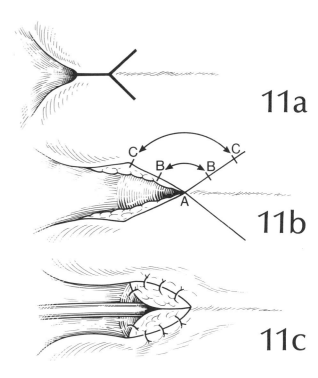

Enema regimens

There is no single correct enema regimen, and each patient develops an individual practice by trial and error. The author starts with 100 ml of a half-strength phosphate enema (Fletchers' phosphate): 50 ml phosphate plus 50 ml 1N saline. This is then followed by a variable volume of 1N saline (0–1000 ml). A daily enema is given for the first month and thereafter they continue daily, on alternate days or every third day in rare cases. The majority of patients continue to use an enema on a daily basis.

Initially some patients experience colicky abdominal pain, and this may be helped by reducing the concentration of the phosphate and the rate of saline infusion. If colic is persistent the administration of mebeverine hydrochloride 30 min before the enema can help.

If the enema does not produce a rapid result the concentration of phosphate can be increased in steps up to 100 ml of full strength enema, and in some patients this is used without saline lavage. Most patients, however, continue to use saline lavage, but if fecal leakage occurs between enemas the volume can be reduced or increased and this usually resolves the problem.

Complete failure of the antegrade colonic enema usually results from constipation with distal fecal impaction. This is best managed by the administration of arachis oil, 50 ml, via the stoma which is left *in situ* for at least 12 h before the next enema is given. Phosphate toxicity has been encountered in a few cases, particularly in younger patients, and it is of vital importance that if there is no response from the enema after 6 h the hospital is contacted and no further phosphate is given until a result has been obtained.

If the patient develops gastroenteritis, antegrade colonic enemas should be stopped until a complete recovery has been made.

Administering antegrade colonic enemas

12 Most patients use an infusion system. The bag is filled with the required phosphate and infused over a 10-min period. If a saline lavage is required the bag is refilled with saline and infused over the next 20–30 min. Evacuation usually starts within 15 min and is complete 30 min later.

Some patients prefer to use a large (50 ml) bladder washout syringe to administer the enema and find it very easy, but the majority favor the infusion system described above. As patients will spend a longer time sitting on the toilet than they ever did before, there is a risk of pressure sores in neuropathic patients. These can be avoided by using a padded toilet seat cover.

Complications

The common complications and their management have been discussed in the text. More uncommon complications include leakage of fecal fluid through the stoma, but the only occasion on which the author experienced this was when the appendix was not reimplanted into the cecum. Reimplantation is therefore recommended in each case. In a small number of patients the enema fails to pass through the rectum. It is worth attempting an anal dilatation or sphincterotomy in these circumstances, but if this does not work a colostomy may be considered. In the author's experience this failure seems to be caused by a functional obstruction in the rectosigmoid region.

Outcome

For patients with neuropathic incontinence the success rate for the antegrade colonic enema procedure is about 90%, and it is about 70% for those with anorectal malformations[3].

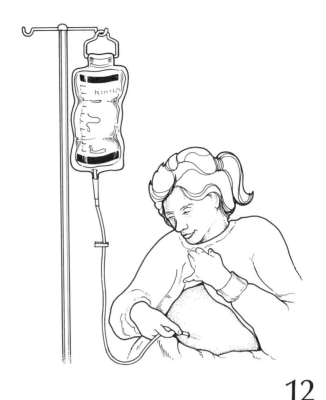

12

References

1. Malone PS, Ransley PG, Kiely EM. Preliminary report: the antegrade continence enema. *Lancet* 1990; 336: 1217–18.

2. Squire R, Kiely EM, Carr B, Ransley PG, Duffy PG. The clinical application of the Malone antegrade colonic enema. *J Pediatr Surg* 1993; 28: 1012–15.

3. Griffith DM, Malone PS. The Malone antegrade continence enema (MACE). *J Pediatr Surg* 1994 (in press)

Illustrations by Paul Richardson

Rectal suction biopsy

Mark Davenport FRCS
Senior Surgical Registrar, Department of Paediatric Surgery, Great Ormond Street Hospital for Children, London, UK

Lewis Spitz PhD, FRCS, FRCS(Ed), FAAP(Hon)
Nuffield Professor of Paediatric Surgery, Institute of Child Health, University of London and Consultant Paediatric Surgeon, Great Ormond Street Hospital for Children, London, UK

Hirschsprung's disease should be considered in neonates presenting with abdominal distension, delay in passing meconium and bile vomiting, and in the older child with intractable constipation. Although the diagnosis may be suggested by a contrast enema showing the 'transitional zone' or by anorectal manometry, it can only be established with certainty by histologic examination of the affected, aganglionic bowel wall. This can be achieved most easily by obtaining a biopsy of the mucosa and, most importantly, the submucosa of the rectum.

Principles and justification

Biopsy of the rectum using a suction biopsy tube is a common procedure in pediatric surgery and has generally superseded the former techniques of open rectal biopsy and punch biopsy with a sigmoidoscope or speculum. The technique needs to be carried out with meticulous attention to detail in order to obtain a suitable diagnostic specimen of rectal mucosa with sufficient submucosa attached on each occasion. The procedure may be performed in the ward or clinic without anesthesia, and is painless provided the biopsy is taken at least 2.5 cm above the anal verge in the neonate and 3.5 cm in the older child (i.e. above the sensitive zone of the anal canal).

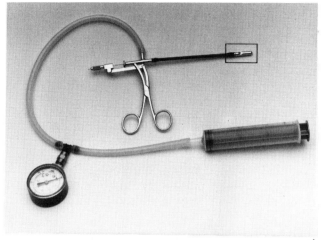

1

Instrumentation

1,2 The original suction biopsy instrument was devised by Noblett[1] and consists of a blunt-ended tube with a 3 mm side hole 1 cm from the tip attached to suction tubing. There are marks on the body of the instrument to indicate the level of biopsy. It has an inline manometer to measure the suction pressure. When inserted into the rectum and suction applied, a portion of the superficial rectal wall is drawn into the side hole. Triggering the concealed circular knife then completes the biopsy. Other similar biopsy instruments are available, all using the principle of the Noblett biopsy forceps.

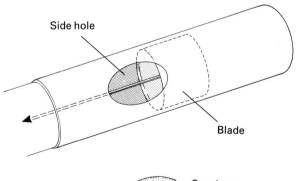

Side hole

Blade

Specimen

Submucosa

2

Operative technique

3 The neonate is usually held in the lithotomy position, although the left lateral knees-bent position is more comfortable to the older child. It is essential to confirm that vitamin K has been given to neonates. If the rectum is full a finger may be passed alongside the instrument, holding it firmly against the rectal wall. The lubricated instrument is inserted into the anus and the side hole positioned initially about 2 cm above the dentate line. This is the minimum distance and avoids the normal hypoganglionic zone[2] and diagnostic confusion. The biopsy specimen should always be taken from the posterior or lateral rectal wall because of the increased risk of perforation into the rectovesical or rectovaginal pouch of the peritoneal cavity if the biopsy is full-thickness and anterior.

Suction is then applied to a maximum pressure of 300 mmHg (20–25 inches of water) by drawing on a 20 ml syringe attached to the suction tubing. After 2–3 s the knife is triggered and the instrument withdrawn. The end is cautiously unscrewed and the biopsy specimen removed with a needle. The specimen is usually about 3 × 1 mm and the critical submucosa can be recognized as a definite whitish layer (*Illustration 2*). The procedure may then be repeated at 3 cm and 4 cm above the anal verge.

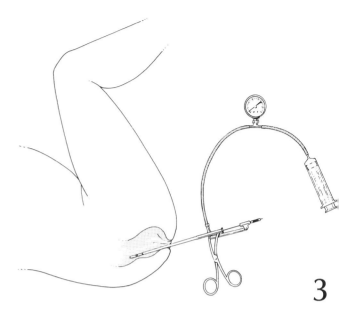

3

A rectal examination should be carried out after completing the biopsy to exclude active bleeding and the patient should be observed carefully for at least a further hour.

The method of processing suction biopsies must be ascertained before the procedure as dictated by specific laboratory requirements. Fresh specimens are, however, usually requested and the biopsy material should be placed on a piece of moistened filter paper marked with the level. It is essential to avoid drying out during transport. Although definitive diagnosis usually requires a combination of paraffin section histology and histochemistry (e.g. acetylcholinesterase activity), a diagnosis based upon frozen section of the biopsy is possible.

Postoperative care

Complications

Possible complications are:

1. Inadequate specimen retrieval. This can be avoided by meticulous attention to detail, ensuring that the biopsy instrument is always cleaned carefully after use and that the blade is sharpened at regular intervals.
2. Perforation. Full-thickness biopsies were identified histologically in 1.08% of 460 patients undergoing 1340 consecutive biopsies[3]. Although these perforations can generally be treated conservatively with antibiotics, nasogastric suction and intravenous fluids, a laparotomy may be needed.
3. Bleeding.
4. Pelvic sepsis, which occurs as a result of perforation into the perirectal tissues.

References

1. Noblett HR. A rectal suction biopsy tube for use in the diagnosis of Hirschsprung's disease. *J Pediatr Surg* 1969; 4: 406–9.

2. Aldridge RT, Campbell PE. Ganglion cell distribution in the normal rectum and anal canal. A basis for the diagnosis of Hirshsprung's disease by anorectal biopsy. *J Pediatr Surg* 1968; 3: 475–90.

3. Rees BI, Azmy A, Nigam M, Lake BD. Complications of rectal suction biopsy. *J Pediatr Surg* 1983; 18: 273–5.

Illustrations by Paul Richardson

Hirschsprung's disease

Daniel H. Teitelbaum MD
Assistant Professor of Pediatric Surgery, University of Michigan Medical School, C.S. Mott Children's Hospital, Ann Arbor, Michigan, USA

Arnold G. Coran MD
Professor of Surgery and Head of the Section of Pediatric Surgery, University of Michigan Medical School, and Surgeon-in-Chief, C.S. Mott Children's Hospital, Ann Arbor, Michigan, USA

Principles and justification

Recent advances in our understanding of the embryogenesis of Hirschsprung's disease have come about over the past several years. Despite our increased knowledge of the disease, significant complications continue to be associated with this process. One must maintain a high degree of suspicion for the disease. Suction rectal biopsy and anal manometry studies have allowed for easier and less invasive methods of establishing the diagnosis; however, the infant's history is the most important first step. Failure to pass meconium within the first 48 h of life, complaints of constipation and, finally, symptoms of enterocolitis should always be followed by a complete clinical examination for Hirschsprung's disease.

The classic approach to the neonate diagnosed with Hirschsprung's disease is to perform a leveling colostomy and to wait until 6–12 months of age to perform the definitive pull-through. Such an approach continues to be the standard practice, although this approach has been modified by performing a definitive endorectal pull-through operation in the neonatal period (*see* pp. 502–508). The three operations illustrated in this chapter — the Duhamel, Soave (endorectal pull-through) and Swenson procedures — are all still performed today. The techniques have been modified to correspond to the most current manner in which these procedures are performed.

Full-thickness rectal biopsy

Suction rectal biopsy, because of its relative ease and low morbidity, has become the most established manner in which Hirschsprung's disease is diagnosed. Nevertheless, full-thickness rectal biopsies are occasionally required, and the technique of full-thickness biopsy is presented here to assist surgeons who are not familiar with the procedure. Perhaps the most common indication for a full-thickness biopsy is in the child in whom there has been more than one indeterminate suction rectal biopsy.

Preoperative

No formal bowel preparation is required. The child's rectum is irrigated with saline or very dilute povidone-iodine solution. A sponge is placed into the proximal rectal vault to prevent stool from entering the operative field.

Operative technique

1   The patient is placed in the lithotomy position with the buttocks at the very end of the bed, supported with a folded towel. The feet are placed together (plantar surfaces adjoined) with a cotton roll, and both legs are suspended on an ether screen with the lower extremities flexed at the hips.

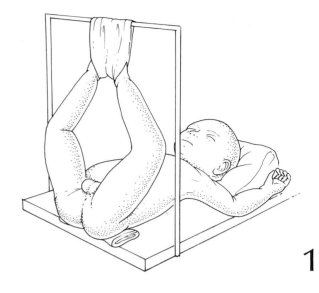

1

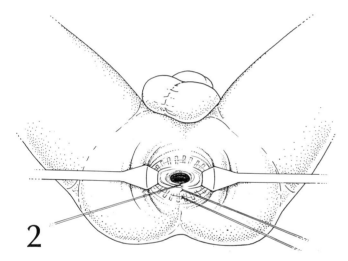

2

2   Digital dilatation is followed by placement of two narrow anal retractors. The posterior aspect of the dentate line is identified and marked with a silk suture (3/0) which is used for traction. Two additional silk sutures are placed on the posterior wall of the rectum at 1 cm and 2 cm proximal to the dentate line.

3   The surgeon's non-dominant hand holds the middle silk suture. Using a sharp curved scissors, a full-thickness incision is made along the lower half of the rectal wall, between the dentate line and the middle suture. Once this is done the scissors can be placed in the presacral space and gently spread. Bleeding can slightly obstruct the view at this point; however, by maintaining traction on the middle suture, the upper half of the rectum is incised with two smooth cuts of the scissors, each sweeping around one-half of the tissue suspended by the middle suture. The specimen is inspected and delivered off the table.

The rectal defect is closed in a single, running or interrupted layer with an absorbable suture (e.g. polyglactin (Vicryl). Hemostasis is achieved fairly quickly once this suture has been placed.

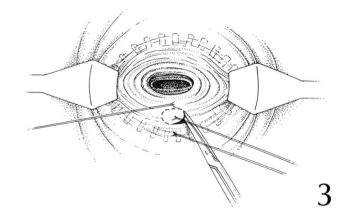

3

Leveling colostomy

Although a right transverse colostomy has been advocated by some surgeons as the initial procedure, the authors prefer a leveling colostomy. This allows for the determination of the aganglionic level at the time of the colostomy, facilitating the subsequent pull-through. In addition, placement of a leveling colostomy allows the proximal bowel to grow which will stretch the mesentery and simplify the subsequent pull-through procedure. Finally, this colostomy can be closed during the pull-through, thus avoiding a third operation. Placement of the ostomy is just proximal to the transition zone. The incision is generally an oblique one in the left lower quadrant. If the level of aganglionosis is not readily apparent, this incision can be extended transversely across the midline.

Preoperative

Essentially, only the diagnosis of Hirschsprung's disease is needed. Most diagnoses can be suspected based on the history alone but confirmation is required by histopathologic examination of a suction rectal biopsy. The infant should receive rectal washouts and be placed on broad-spectrum, intravenous antibiotics, but no formal bowel preparation is required or is effective.

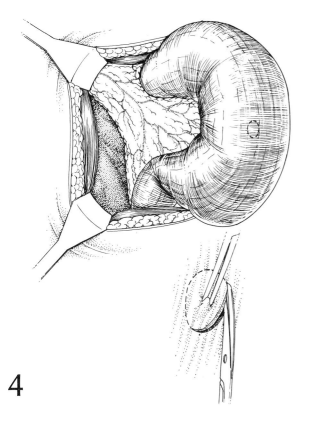

4

Operative technique

4 Once the peritoneum is entered, an attempt should be made to define a gross transition zone. The bowel proximal to the transition zone is normally dilated and has a diffuse hypertrophy of the muscular layer with no clearly distinguishable tenea. In neonates, such a transition often cannot be seen. If this is the case, a good starting point is just above the peritoneal reflection.

A pair of fine sharp scissors is used to make an incision only through the seromuscular layers. The muscular layer, which is fairly thick even in the aganglionic section, makes this dissection fairly easy. Blunt dissection is used to strip off the muscle. In general, a 1 × 0.5-cm biopsy specimen is taken and interrupted silk sutures are placed to close the biopsy site.

Each biopsy specimen is sent for frozen section, progressively moving more proximally until both ganglion cells as well as a loss of hypertrophied nerve bundles are seen. Hypertrophied nerve bundles, despite the presence of ganglia, suggest that one is still in the transition zone. Another biopsy specimen should be taken more proximally.

5 At this point a loop colostomy can often be created at one of the normal biopsy sites. Because of the relatively large caliber of the bowel, stomal prolapse and peristomal hernias are common complications. It is extremely important to begin the colostomy by placing numerous fine silk sutures to both the peritoneum as well as to the fascia. A stitch is placed between the proximal and distal loops of bowel, starting at the fascia, then to each limb of bowel, and finally back to the fascia.

If no transition zone is found and the first few biopsies are aganglionic, it is usually beneficial to perform an appendectomy. Aganglionosis of the appendix indicates the presence of total colonic Hirschsprung's disease.

Postoperative care

The stoma usually begins to act within 24 h and feeding can begin shortly thereafter. It is occasionally helpful to perform intermittent dilatations of the proximal ostomy. These dilatations will prevent narrowing of the opening and allow the dilated proximal colon to return to normal size.

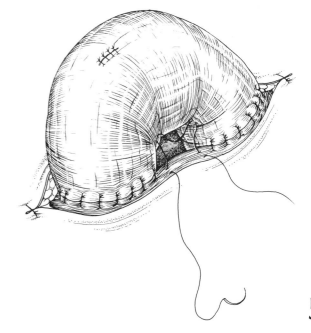

5

Operations

DUHAMEL

The Duhamel technique was advanced in 1956 to avoid the tedious pelvic dissection of the Swenson procedure. The procedure has undergone several modifications, the most important of which was by Martin, and included the use of an automatic stapling device. It is fairly straightforward and continues to be popular today. Despite its relative simplicity, several key technical points must be followed.

As with other pull-through procedures, ganglionic bowel is brought down to within 1 cm of the dentate line. To preserve the autonomic nervous plexus to the genitourinary system, very little manipulation of the rectum is performed anteriorly.

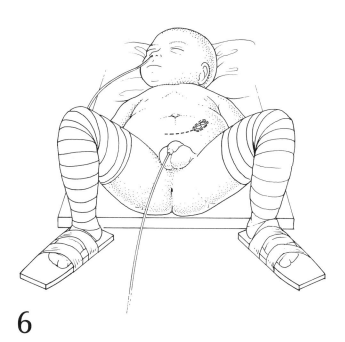

6

The child usually has a leveling colostomy, which was placed several months previously. This serves to decompress the bowel and return it to normal caliber. The operation is generally performed when the child is 6–12 months of age with a weight of 10 kg.

Preoperative

The child is admitted the day before the surgery for a mechanical bowel preparation as well as oral antibiotics. Care must be taken to give adequate rectal and colonic washouts as stool is often inspissated in the distal rectum. It is necessary to do a rectal examination on the child before the pull-through to ensure that no residual stool is present.

Operative technique

6 A nasogastric tube is placed after induction of anesthesia. The child is placed in a supine position and the patient is prepared circumferentially from the abdomen to the feet. Stockinets are placed around each foot and a Foley catheter is inserted in the bladder after the patient has been prepared and draped. Excellent exposure is obtained by assistants supporting and flexing the lower extremities at the hips during the anal anastomosis. Alternatively, the child can be placed in stirrups or on skis. A hockey stick or oblique incision is made incorporating the colostomy takedown. The bowel is mobilized proximal to the former colostomy and the splenic flexure is brought down, if necessary, to ensure adequate length for the pull-through. In general, the colon must reach the level of the perineum when drawn over the child's pubic symphysis with only modest tension. Occasionally, the mesentery is foreshortened and it is necessary to ligate the inferior mesenteric artery at the aortic root. By preserving the remainder of the arcades, the bowel should maintain its viability. The ureter is carefully identified and the peritoneal reflection between the rectum and bladder is incised. The distal rectum is mobilized for approximately 4 cm below the reflection. The colostomy site is removed with an automatic stapling device.

7 A retrorectal space is created, with dissection carried out directly in the midline. This dissection is carried down to the pelvic floor so that an assistant's finger can be felt when inserted no further than 1 to 1.5 cm into the anus. Dissection can be facilitated with a narrow clamp but is also very easily performed with the index finger.

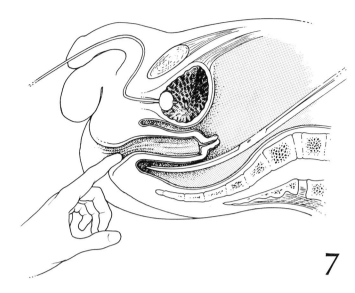

8 Once the retrorectal dissection is completed, redundant aganglionic bowel is resected down to the peritoneal reflection with an automatic stapling device. Tacking sutures are placed on both left and right sides of the bowel so that it can be retracted anteriorly during the pull-through procedure.

The ganglionic bowel is labeled mesenteric and antimesenteric with a separate polypropylene and silk suture. This allows the surgeon working on the pulled through segment to maintain correct orientation of the bowel as it is pulled into the anus.

At this point the surgeon's attention is directed to the perineum. Both legs are drawn upward allowing a clear view of the anus. Narrow anal retractors are placed and held in position by the two assistants still working on the abdomen. No separate field is created which allows improved communication and keeps surgeon and assistant on the same operative field. The authors have not found it necessary to have two completely different set-ups. However, all the instruments used in the perineal portion of the procedure are treated as dirty and gloves are changed at the end of the anastomosis.

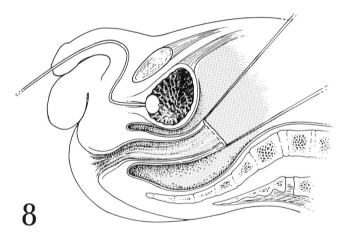

9 Using cautery, a full-thickness incision is made 1–1.5 cm proximal to the dentate line posteriorly. Care is taken to maintain this distance by curving the incision as one moves laterally in each direction. Three 4/0 undyed polyglactin sutures are placed on the inferior aspect of this incision, one in the midline and one each on both left and right sides. Three additional absorbable sutures (4/0 dyed polyglactin) are placed on the upper portion of this incision in similar positions. Each suture is held in position with hemostats. The different suture types prevent confusion of orientation once the ganglionic bowel is pulled through.

The surgeon operating on the anus inserts a long clamp into the retrorectal space towards the abdominal field.

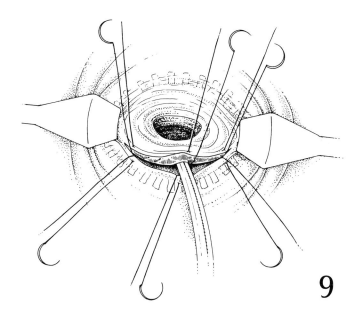

9

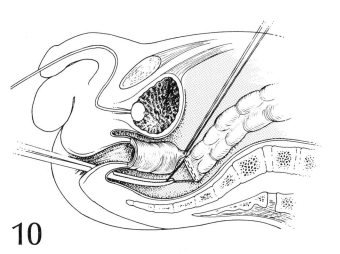

10

10 The two tacking sutures on the distal ganglionic bowel are fed into this clamp and pulled down. The surgeon remaining in the abdominal field makes sure that the bowel does not rotate as it is brought down.

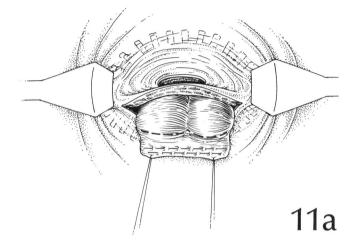

11a

11a, b Once the bowel is pulled through, the staple line is excised on the anterior half of the colon and a single-layered anastomosis is created, starting with the three previously placed polyglactin sutures. Care is taken with each stitch so that the anterior wall of the anus is not incorporated into any of the sutures.

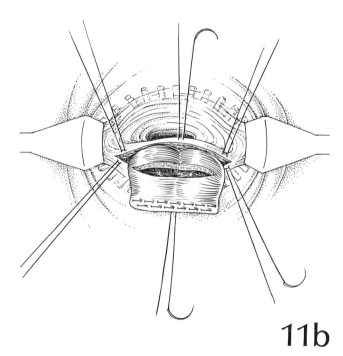

11b

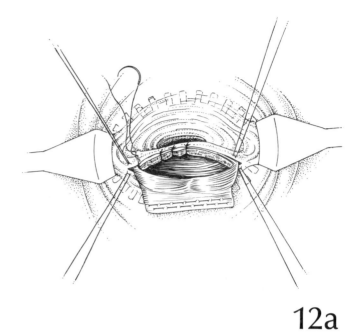

12a

12a, b Once the anterior half of the anastomosis is completed, the remainder of the staple line is excised and the anastomosis is finished.

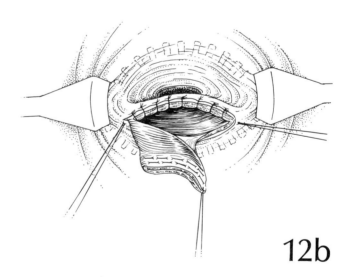

12b

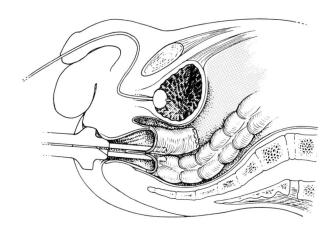

13a

13a, b

An extra long automatic stapling device is placed with one arm in the native anal canal and the other in the neorectum. The stapler is fired directly in the midline. Hemostasis along the suture line is checked.

In general, a complete anastomosis between the ganglionic and aganglionic bowel cannot be achieved with a single staple application from below. A second firing from the abdomen will be necessary.

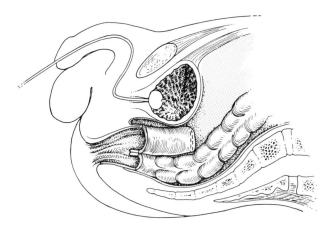

13b

14 The staple line of the remaining aganglionic rectum is opened and a small enterotomy is made in the ganglionic colon at a similar level. The abdominal surgeon places a reloaded automatic stapler between the two limbs of bowel to complete the anastomosis. This last step is critical. In the past, a proximal spur left between the bowel segments caused the eventual formation of huge fecalomas. It is critical for the surgeon to inspect digitally the anastomosis and make sure that the two limbs of bowel are completely anastomosed. The operation from below is completed at this point.

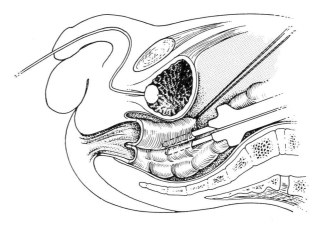

14

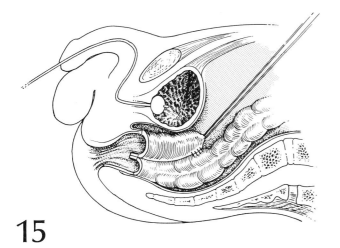

15

15 The anastomosis is completed by suturing the proximal end of the rectum to the enterotomy in the ganglionic colon in two layers. The neorectum may or may not be reperitonealized and the abdomen is closed.

MARTIN MODIFICATION FOR TOTAL COLONIC AGANGLIONOSIS

This procedure was originally described in 1972 by Martin. Children with total colonic Hirschsprung's disease may be plagued with large volume stool output and electrolyte losses after a conventional pull-through operation. In an attempt to correct this, Martin utilized the aganglionic left colon to recapture some of the absorptive capacities of the large bowel. The procedure is similar to the modified Duhamel, except that the ileum is used as the pull-through segment. The original description of the procedure utilized the entire left colon and the long anastomosis of colon to small bowel was performed as a secondary procedure. Currently, smaller sections of colon are used, comprising the rectum, sigmoid and a small portion of the descending colon. In addition, the entire anastomosis is performed at one operation.

After performing the rectal anastomosis and firing the automatic stapler, the remainder of the aganglionic colon is anastomosed to the small bowel with additional firings of the automatic stapler.

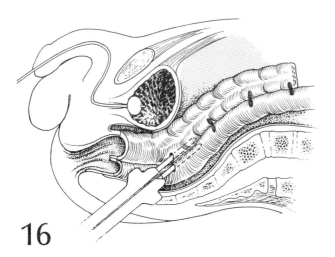

16 Using an enterotomy in both the small and large bowel, the stapler can be directed distally, and then refired proximally. The enterotomy is then closed with either a stapler or two rows of interrupted suture.

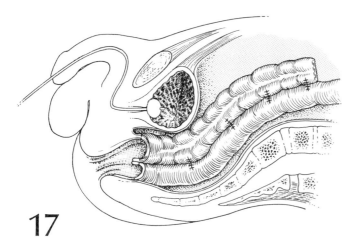

17 Usually two or three additional enterotomies must be made to complete the rest of the anastomosis.

AGANGLIONIC PATCH (KIMURA PROCEDURE)

Another technique that has recently become popularized is Kimura's utilization of a parasitized cecal patch. This procedure involves several steps.

18a–d The ganglionic ileum is first decompressed with an end ileostomy. Several weeks later the child is returned to the operating room for an extensive longitudinal ileocolostomy, approximately 10–25 cm in length. Anastomosis is created with a two-layered suture line. Staples are avoided because they may prevent sufficient vascular growth between limbs of bowel. The end of this is used as an end stoma. The child is left alone for 6–12 months, during which time the vascular supply of the two segments joins.

At the final operation the right colonic blood supply is taken down and an assessment of the blood supply to the colon is made (*Illustration 18c*). If the ileum has established adequate perfusion of the colon, the ileocolostomy is used for the pull-through (*Illustration 18d*) with either a Swenson or endorectal type pull-through. If the right colonic blood supply is inadequate, the ileocolostomy may be taken down and the ileum used with a Martin modification as described above.

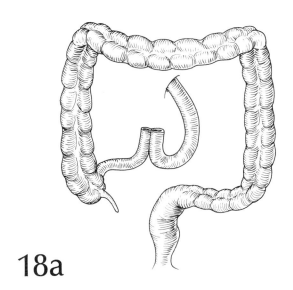

18a

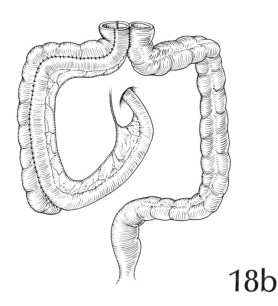

18b

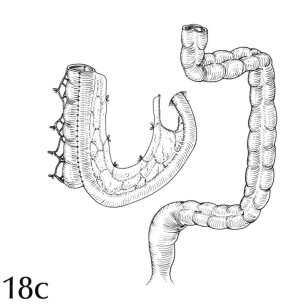

18c

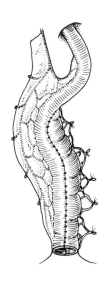

18d

ENDORECTAL PULL-THROUGH (SOAVE)

The Soave or endorectal pull-through was introduced by Franco Soave at the Institute G. Gaslini in 1955. The procedure was modified by Boley by performing a primary anastomosis at the anus and then further modified by Coran. This procedure is the most popular one used at the authors' institute and has been further modified to facilitate the suturing of the anal anastomosis. The operation has conventionally been performed on children at 6–12 months of age. However, the authors now have experience with 35 neonates undergoing the procedure within the first 1–2 weeks of life. The complication rate is identical to that seen with the standard two-staged approach. It is actually technically easier to perform the endorectal dissection at this age.

As with the Duhamel technique, this procedure avoids injury to the pelvic nerves and, by remaining within the muscular wall of the aganglionic segment, important sensory fibers and the integrity of the internal sphincter are preserved. Although one imagines that leaving aganglionic muscle surrounding normal bowel could lead to a high incidence of constipation, this is not the case.

Preoperative

Even in the neonatal period, serial rectal washouts and digital dilatations of the rectum are performed before beginning the pull-through, the last of the rectal irrigations containing 1% neomycin. Intravenous antibiotics are given before the beginning of surgery and are continued for 5 days.

Operative technique

The child is placed in a supine position, with the buttocks brought to the end of the operating table, and propped slightly up with a folded towel. The legs are carefully padded and placed on wooden skis extending off the end of the table. A Foley catheter is placed and the entire field is prepared and draped. The operating table is placed in a slightly Trendelenburg position. A hockey stick incision is made, incorporating the leveling colostomy. The same type of incision is made, however, for infants undergoing a primary pull-through operation.

The level of aganglionosis is established by frozen section.

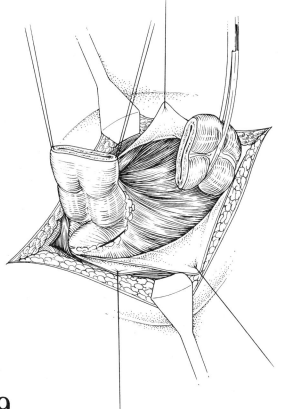

19 Ganglionic bowel is mobilized proximally and transected at the transition level with a stapling device. The distal colon is mobilized and resected to about 4 cm above the peritoneal reflection. Traction sutures are placed on either end of the distal bowel. The endorectal dissection is then started about 2 cm below the peritoneal reflection.

The authors have progressively shortened the length of the endorectal dissection because longer lengths of muscular cuff may lead to increased bouts of constipation and enterocolitis.

19

20 The endorectal dissection usually begins by completely clearing the serosa, mesentery and fat over a 2-cm length of bowel. The seromuscular layer is incised with either sharp dissection or Bovie cautery. Once the submucosal layer is reached the seromuscular layer is divided circumferentially using blunt dissection with hemostat or a Kitner dissector. In the neonatal period a cotton tip applicator is the most effective tool for this dissection.

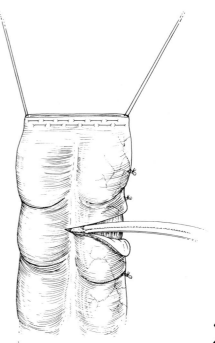

20

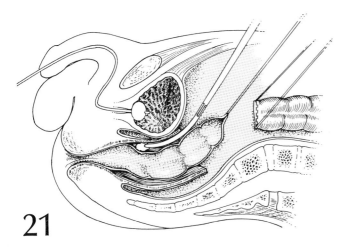

21

21 After the plane is established, it is continued distally and facilitated by an assistant pulling upward on the already dissected mucosal-submucosal tube for countertraction. As the muscular cuff begins to develop, traction sutures are also placed in the muscle, one in each quadrant. Larger communicating vessels are coagulated; however, the majority of these are not cauterized during the dissection without significant blood loss, particularly in the neonatal period. Dissection is carried down to within 1.5 cm of the anal opening in older children and less than 1 cm in a neonate.

Some have advocated performing part of the endorectal dissection from the transanal approach but the authors strongly advise against this. Once the endorectal dissection from above is started, it can proceed in a straightforward fashion. With appropriate traction and countertraction, the entire dissection can be performed in a child of almost any size (and adult). Dissection from the anus is less precise anatomically and adds considerable time to the procedure.

22 One of the surgeons then moves to the foot of the table. Narrow retractors (phrenic or army-navy) are placed at the anal-mucocutaneous junction and a ring or Kelly clamp is inserted into the rectum. An assistant at the abdominal field places the end of the mucosal-submucosal tube into the clamp. The segment is then everted onto the perineum. The end of the everted tube is placed in a clamp and held on traction by an assistant to facilitate the anastomosis.

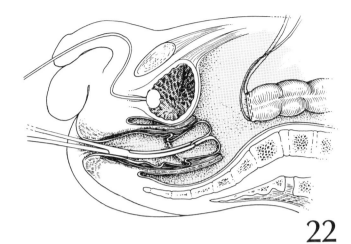

22

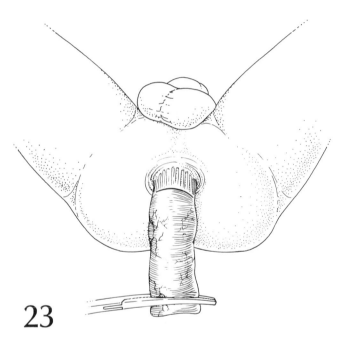

23

23 The mucosal-submucosal tube is incised on the anterior half, 1 cm above the dentate line.

24 A Kelly clamp is inserted into this opening and the ganglionic bowel is brought down to this point by grasping the two previously placed traction sutures. Great care is taken not to twist the bowel as it is brought through the muscular cuff. As with the Duhamel procedure, different colored sutures on each side of the bowel are helpful in maintaining orientation.

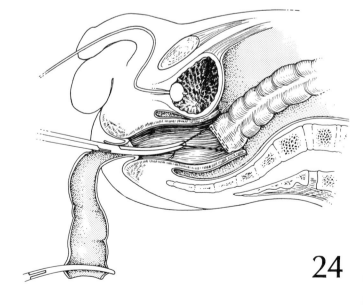

24

25 The anterior half of the ganglionic colon is incised and anastomosed to the anterior half of the anus with a 4/0 polyglactin (Vicryl) suture. The first sutures are placed at each corner and in the midline, followed by interrupted sutures in between.

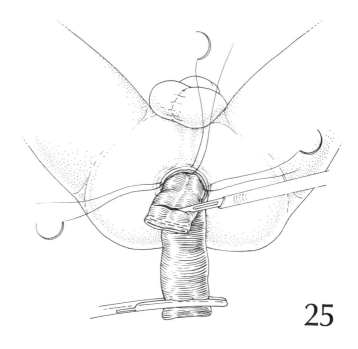

25

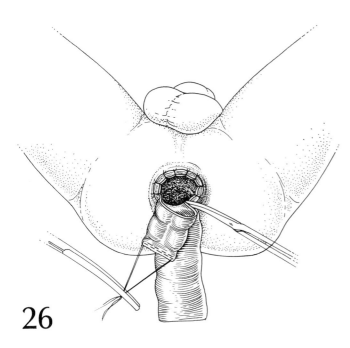

26

26 One-quarter of the remaining ganglionic colon and one-quarter of the everted mucosal-submucosal tube are opened. A suture is placed in the posterior midline and this quarter of the anastomosis is completed. Countertraction applied by an assistant on the everted tube will help with the exposure.

27 The final quarter of the colon and tube are removed and the anastomosis is completed and inspected.

The colon is pulled slightly upwards to invert the neorectum back into its correct position. Rectal examination at this point should reveal a well formed anastomosis 1.5–2 cm above the anodermal junction. Gloves are then changed and attention directed to the abdominal field.

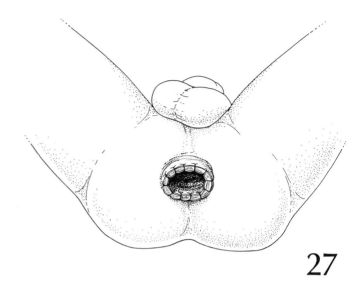

27

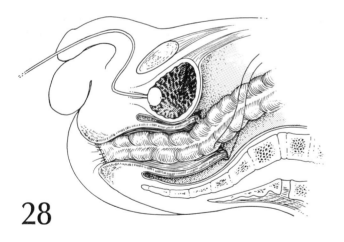

28

28 The pulled-through colon is attached with seromuscular bites to the muscular cuff to prevent the colon from prolapsing in the early postoperative period. No drain is placed either through the anastomosis or from above in the muscular cuff because there is rarely any significant oozing in the cuff (unlike the situation with ulcerative colitis in older patients).

This endorectal pull-through has also become the authors' standard approach for children with total colonic aganglionosis. The ileum is used for the pull-through segment and has given very satisfactory results.

SWENSON

This technique was originally described by Swenson and Bill in 1948 and was the first successful method of treatment for children with Hirschsprung's disease. They based their technique on the principle that the diseased portion of the bowel was the aganglionic distal rectum, and that removal of this segment was necessary to allow for normal stooling. The initial incidence of postoperative enterocolitis was fairly high (early 16% and late 27%), and this was attributed to leaving too much aganglionic rectum. The procedure has since been modified by resecting virtually all of the posterior rectal wall (and some internal sphincter).

The technique demands meticulous dissection of the rectum down to within 2 cm of the dentate line. If the dissection moves off the rectal wall a significant incidence of injury to the genitourinary innervation may occur. Properly performed, the results with this procedure are quite good; however, because of the technical difficulties of the dissection, it has fallen into relative disfavor.

Preoperative

The child is admitted the day before surgery for a routine bowel preparation. Assessment and preparation are similar to the other pull-through operations.

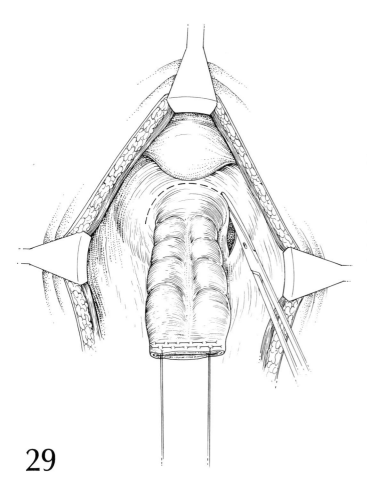

Operative technique

The child is positioned in a similar fashion as for an endorectal pull-through procedure. The incision was classically described as a left paramedian incision with takedown of the colostomy; however, the modified hockey stick incision will work equally well.

29 The redundant aganglionic rectum is excised and proximal ganglionated colon mobilized past the splenic flexure, if necessary, as in the other two techniques. At this point, the peritoneal reflection over the rectum is incised.

29

30 The operating surgeon then dissects the rectum caudally. This is a critical dissection which demands the surgeon to stay directly on the bowel wall. Dissection is facilitated by the first assistant applying upward traction on the end of the aganglionic rectum. Multiple blood vessels enter directly into the bowel wall; each must be dissected out and can usually be coagulated. Dissection is carried down toward the anal verge, but is not carried as far anteriorly in order to avoid autonomic nerve injury.

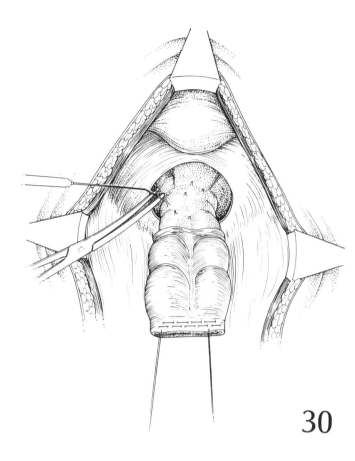

30

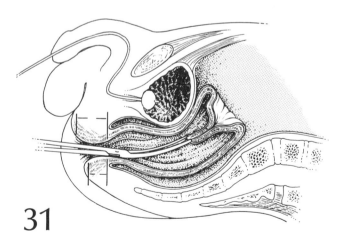

31

31 The perineal part of the operation is then started. The rectum is everted with the use of a long clamp. The anterior half of the everted rectal wall is cut 2 cm proximal to the anodermal junction. The posterior wall will be no longer than 1–1.5 cm in length. A gently curved incision which is shorter posteriorly is thus created along the anterior half of the bowel.

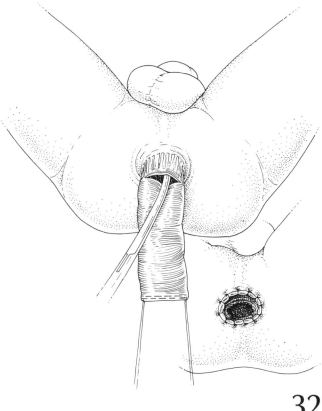

32 The ganglionic colon is pulled through and the anastomosis is virtually identical to that for the endorectal pull-through operation. Classically silk sutures have been used, but the authors have utilized polyglactin (Vicryl) sutures with good results.

The anastomosis is allowed to recede and is gently pulled upwards from the perineum. Closure is essentially the same as for the previous procedures.

32

SECOND PULL-THROUGH

A child with an initial unsuccessful pull-through operation may present with severe constipation or significant incontinence. These children should undergo a thorough investigation of the details of the initial operation as well as a review of the pathologic specimens. In most cases an appropriate pull-through has been performed and an aggressive bowel program needs to be instituted. It is essential to rule out a retained segment of aganglionic bowel. Should this be the case, a second pull-through operation will usually be necessary. Because of its relative ease, a Duhamel is generally the procedure of choice. We have, however, performed both an endorectal and Swenson pull-through as a second procedure. If the child has already undergone a Duhamel, one may resort to a Swenson procedure. For the child with debilitating incontinence, a detailed history and examination should be performed to rule out encopresis and to assess the degree of anorectal tone. Anal manometry is particularly helpful in

this group, as a lack of normal muscular control is generally felt to be a poor indicator of a successful outcome for a repeat pull-through operation. An occasional child in this latter group may best be served with a diverting colostomy.

ANAL/RECTAL MYECTOMY

A child with short segment Hirschsprung's disease may be a candidate for an anal/rectal myectomy. The advantage of this procedure is that it avoids an abdominal operation. The procedure must be confined to very short segment Hirschsprung's disease. One must be certain that the myectomy is extended beyond the level of aganglionosis. Because performing an inadequate myectomy may adversely affect the outcome of a subsequent pull-through operation, a myectomy should be avoided if there is any uncertainty as to the level of disease.

Operative technique

Transanal approach

The child is placed in an identical position as for the full-thickness rectal biopsy (*Illustration 1*).

33 Digital dilatation is performed and two narrow anal retractors are inserted and held by assistants. The posterior aspect of the dentate line is identified. A 2-cm transverse incision through the mucosa and submucosa starting 1 cm above the dentate line is made. Following this, a submucosal dissection is carried upward for several centimeters. The mucosal-submucosal flap is held up with silk sutures and can be extended proximally with vertical incisions on either side.

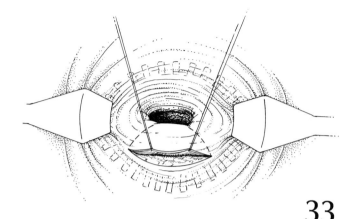

33

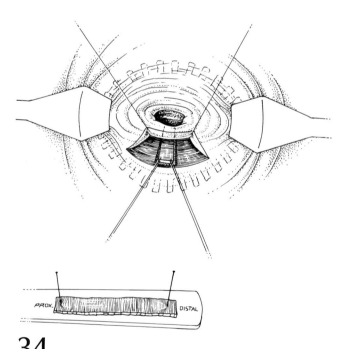

34

34 The myectomy is then performed by sharply incising the full thickness of the muscle layer and a 0.5–1-cm wide muscle strip is created in the midline using Bovie cautery. The initial strip removed should be at least 5 cm in length.

Before transecting this strip, two silk sutures are placed proximal to the point of transection so that, should further dissection be necessary, the proximal muscle will not retract beyond the view of the surgeon. The strip should be mounted on a tongue depressor with mounting pins or suture; proximal and distal orientation must be clearly depicted.

A frozen section confirming ganglion cells at the proximal margin must be obtained before the procedure can be terminated. The dissection can be carried out in this manner for approximately 8 cm. If the surgeon suspects that the level of aganglionosis is longer than this, it may be advisable to forego this approach.

Once a sufficient length of muscle has been removed, hemostasis is achieved with cautery. The wound is irrigated and closed with fine interrupted absorbable sutures approximating the mucosa/submucosal dissection.

Trans-sacral approach

A trans-sacral approach can also be used for the myectomy.

35 A vertical trans-sacral incision is made from the coccyx to within 1 cm of the anus and carried down to the levator muscle complex.

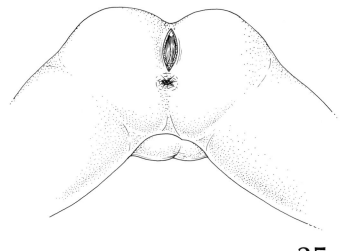

35

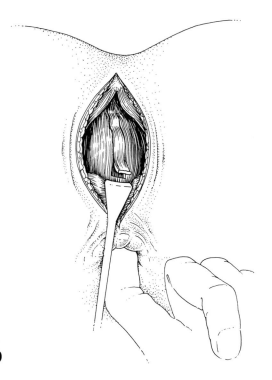

36

36 The levator muscles are retracted caudally with a retractor. With a finger in the rectum, the posterior rectal wall is exposed and a 5–6-cm strip of rectal muscle, 1 cm wide, is removed from the dentate line proximally. The mucosa and submucosa are not incised and the rectal lumen is not entered.

This approach is easier than the transanal approach and gives much better exposure of the posterior rectal wall.

Postoperative care

Following all of the pull-through procedures the nasogastric tube is removed once gastrointestinal activity returns. The Foley catheter can be removed on the second postoperative day following the endorectal and Duhamel procedures because bladder innervation has not been affected by the pelvic dissection. However, after the Swenson pull-through the Foley catheter should be left in for 5 days because of the possibility that there may be some bladder atony from the dissection. Antibiotics are continued for 5 days after the surgery.

Great attention is placed on examining the perineal region for the development of erythema or cellulitis, as this is an early sign of an anastomotic leak. Investigation of a leak consists of an enema contrast study or a computed tomographic scan with contrast medium. Although fairly uncommon, should a leak be found, the urgent placement of a diverting colostomy is needed.

For the endorectal pull-through, a gentle rectal examination with the small finger is performed to ensure patency of the rectal anastomosis before discharge. Parents are given thorough instructions on perineal care and the potential development of enterocolitis. To avoid perineal excoriation the parents are instructed to apply a thick coat of a zinc oxide based ointment with each diaper change. If a significant rash develops, more intensified applications are used.

Digital dilatations are performed starting on the third week after surgery. However, these are rarely needed after the endorectal pull-through procedure except in neonates. These dilatations are usually sufficient to prevent anastomotic stricturing.

Stool frequency is generally quite high (7–12 bowel movements per day) immediately after the pull-through operation, but this slowly decreases and is generally normal by 6–9 months.

Children should be followed up for several years. Occasionally some develop intermittent bouts of constipation, occasional soiling and enterocolitis. Most problems with constipation or soiling can be managed with changes in diet or enema regimens. Episodes of enterocolitis are managed with oral metronidazole; however, severe cases will necessitate admission, intravenous antibiotics and rectal washouts. Enterocolitis is so common after Martin's operation for total colonic aganglionosis that the authors have abandoned it in favor of total colectomy and ileoanal endorectal pull-through. Rarely, if episodes of enterocolitis or constipation are quite severe, additional surgical therapy may be needed (rectal myectomy). Before considering such additional surgery, however, one should be certain that all non-operative methods have been completely exhausted.

With regard to children with total colonic Hirschsprung's disease, large volumes of stool and electrolyte losses can occur after either a modified Duhamel or ileoanal endorectal pull-through. These losses must be replaced and are usually controlled with dietary changes and the addition of an opioid agent (e.g. loperamide). Perineal excoriation is very common in these infants and demands constant attention. Normalization of stooling will take much longer than in children with classic Hirschsprung's disease, and these children may sometimes require parenteral nutritional support for several months before full enteral feeding can be initiated.

Outcome

Controversy arises as to which procedure yields the best results. Long-term outcomes with the Duhamel, Soave and Swenson techniques are basically similar, provided they are performed with meticulous technique. Depending on the anatomy and history of the patient, the surgeon should be familiar with all of these techniques, but should use one as the primary procedure. This is the only way that consistently good results can be achieved.

Of equal importance is the need to follow such patients over long periods of time as many of the complications (e.g. enterocolitis, constipation and urgency) may not manifest themselves until much later in the patient's life.

Acknowledgments

Illustrations 19, 21 and *24* are reproduced from Coran and Weintraub, *Surgery, Gynecology and Obstetrics* 1976; 143: 277–82 with permission of the publishers.

Further reading

Boley SJ. New modification of the surgical treatment of Hirschsprung's disease. *Surgery* 1964; 56: 1015–17.

Coran AG, Weintraub WH. Modification of the endorectal procedure for Hirschsprung's disease. *Surg Gynecol Obstet* 1976; 143: 277–82.

Kimura K, Nishijima E, Muraji T, Tsugawa C, Matsumoto Y. A new surgical approach to extensive aganglionosis. *J Pediatr Surg* 1981; 16: 840–3.

Martin LW. Surgical management of total colonic aganglionosis. *Ann Surg* 1972; 176: 343–5.

Martin LW, Caudill DR. A method for elimination of the blind rectal pouch in the Duhamel operation for Hirschsprung's disease. *Surgery* 1967; 62: 951–3.

Swenson O, Bill AH. Resection of the rectum and rectosigmoid with preservation of the sphincter for benign spastic lesions producing megacolon. An experimental study. *Surgery* 1948; 24: 212–20.

Inflammatory bowel disease

Daniel H. Teitelbaum MD
Assistant Professor of Pediatric Surgery, University of Michigan Medical School, C.S. Mott Children's Hospital,
Ann Arbor, Michigan, USA

Arnold G. Coran MD
Professor of Surgery and Head of the Section of Pediatric Surgery, University of Michigan Medical School, and
Surgeon-in-Chief, C.S. Mott Children's Hospital, Ann Arbor, Michigan, USA

History

The evolution of surgical procedures for inflammatory bowel disease has been one of trial and error. Based on previous successful and unsuccessful outcomes, a variety of procedures has been developed which has allowed for maximal preservation of bowel length as well as function. These include proctocolectomy with end ileostomy, endorectal pull-through and stricturoplasty. The pediatric patient with inflammatory bowel disease presents with additional growth, nutritional and psychologic problems which may not affect the adult patient. All of these factors must be considered when determining the timing and type of procedure.

Over the past 15 years the use of the endorectal pull-through for ulcerative colitis has become increasingly popular. The operation was initially a modification of the endorectal pull-through technique for Hirschsprung's disease. The procedure has taken time to become accepted by the general surgical community, principally because of unfamiliarity with the endorectal dissection and the significant incidence of complications associated with many of the original cases.

Principles and justification

Protocolectomy with end ileostomy

This has been the standard procedure for children with ulcerative colitis and multiple polyposis, but can also be utilized in severe Crohn's colitis. The abdominal colectomy portion of the procedure may also be performed in conjunction with an endorectal pull-through. For patients with ulcerative colitis initial medical management is generally advised. In children with an acute exacerbation of ulcerative colitis, surgery is indicated in cases of severe hemorrhage or in those who fail to respond to intensive medical treatment after several weeks. The timing of an elective procedure is more difficult to establish. Some surgeons feel that resection is only indicated in those children who show mucosal atypia on colonoscopic biopsy. Detecting these changes is difficult because one cannot routinely biopsy the entire colon, and the incidence of carcinomatous changes increases as the duration of the disease increases. In fact, carcinoma can be found in many surgical specimens when only atypia was found on colonoscopic biopsy. Many surgeons therefore recommend a colectomy once the disease process has been present for 10 years. However, today many gastroenterologists recommend surveillance colonoscopy every year or every other year even if the disease has been present for more than 10 years. Surgery should be performed sooner if atypia is identified or in those children with significant growth failure, lack of sexual maturation, and in those on chronic high doses of steroids in whom significant changes and complications due to steroid use have occurred. In children with multiple polyposis the timing can also be controversial. If all the polyps can be removed from the colon and the child is followed every 6 months, then surgery can be delayed at least until the child is past adolescence. If the polyps are too numerous to be removed, surgery should be performed earlier.

Endorectal pull-through

The endorectal pull-through achieves a curative procedure for patients with ulcerative colitis as well as colonic polyposis, while eliminating the need for a permanent ileostomy. An additional advantage of this procedure is the elimination of the extensive pelvic dissection outside the rectal wall, which can be associated with a significant incidence of injury to the nerves supplying the genitourinary system.

Stricturoplasty

Strictures secondary to Crohn's disease of the small bowel do occur in children. Conventional approaches to their treatment have consisted of complete resections or side-to-side bypasses of the involved area. Multiple resections of these strictured areas have not uncommonly led to the development of the short bowel syndrome. Bypass of significant areas of the bowel usually results in bacterial overgrowth. Over the past 10 years the use of stricturoplasty has therefore evolved. The technique has enabled the patient to retain significantly greater lengths of bowel with adequate relief of the obstruction and is a modification of the Heineke–Mikulicz procedure for a pyloroplasty. Although the bowel length may appear shorter after the performance of multiple stricturoplasties, the functional length is the same. A few contraindications to this procedure exist, e.g. the occurrence of several small strictures very close together which could be more simply managed with a resection, although it is not uncommon for a patient to have multiple stricturoplasties during one operation. If the stricture is associated with fistula or abscess formation, the bowel segment should be excised.

Ileocolectomy

Although ileocolectomy is commonly performed in the pediatric patient for Crohn's disease, the procedure is reasonably straightforward and an operative description is not included in this chapter.

Preoperative

Proctocolectomy with end ileostomy

The child is admitted the day before surgery and undergoes a complete bowel preparation. Caution should be observed in those patients with severe colitis or Crohn's disease. Overly aggressive laxatives may cause a perforation of the colon or an exacerbation of the disease process. In general, a balanced electrolyte solution should be slowly administered orally. Oral antibiotics and gentle enemas are given the day before surgery. An enterostomal therapist should mark the skin site of the ileostomy with indelible ink the day before surgery.

Endorectal pull-through

Before performing the procedure, the diagnosis of ulcerative colitis must be as firm as possible. If Crohn's colitis is present instead of ulcerative colitis, recurrent disease in the pulled through ileum and fistula formation from this same segment of bowel are common. Repeat colonoscopy along with a series of small intestinal contrast studies should be performed to rule out Crohn's disease. If biopsies have been performed elsewhere they should be reread by pathologists at the center where the operation is to be carried out. Many of these children have been on steroids during the previous year and will need stress doses of steroids in the perioperative period.

Stricturoplasty

Suspicion of a stricture is usually initiated with the patient complaining of symptoms consistent with a partial bowel obstruction. Most patients complain of cramping abdominal pain, with obstipation and nausea. The diagnosis is made with a small intestinal contrast series. A thorough look for multiple strictures is necessary. No formal bowel preparation is needed, but intravenous antibiotics should be given.

Operations

PROCTOCOLECTOMY WITH END ILEOSTOMY

Position of patient and incision

1 The child is placed in the supine position with legs on popliteal rests (Lloyd-Davies type) for older children and skis for smaller children. Careful padding of the lower extremities is critical to avoid neurovascular injury. The procedure is best carried out through a large midline or left paramedian abdominal incision which extends from the pubis to a few centimeters above the umbilicus.

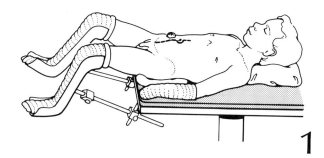

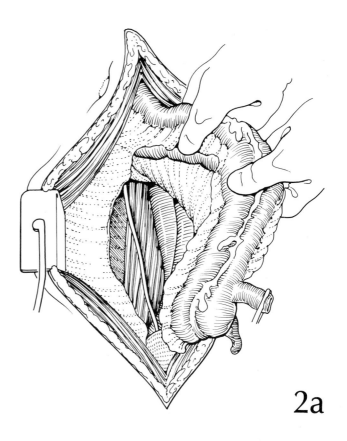

2a

Mobilization of colon

2a, b The abdomen is explored and the right colon is mobilized by incising the line of Toldt and by dividing the terminal ileum approximately 1 cm from the ileocecal valve. Identification of the ureters is performed on both sides of the abdomen. The hepatic flexure and splenic flexure are then divided without putting traction on the spleen. The omentum is included in the transverse colectomy specimen.

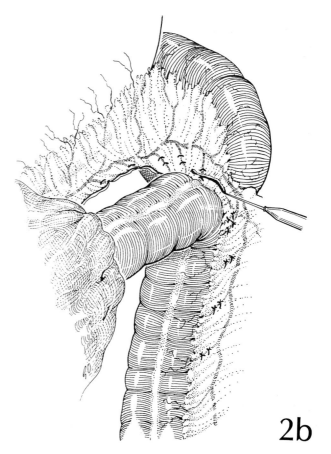

2b

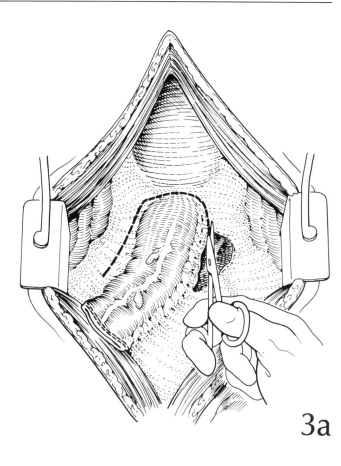

3a

3a, b The descending colon is mobilized in a similar fashion by dividing its retroperitoneal attachment. The mesentery of the colon is then divided and the vessels are suture ligated with 2/0 or 3/0 silk suture. The colon is then divided at the rectosigmoid junction with an automatic stapling device. The peritoneal reflection of the rectum is incised and the dissection is continued directly on the muscular rectal wall. Deviation from the rectal wall will increase the chances of injuring the pelvic autonomic nerves with subsequent impotence or bladder dysfunction. This portion of the operation is facilitated by countertraction on the remaining proximal rectum by the assisting surgeon (*Illustration 3b*). Each individual vessel is grasped with forceps and either cauterized or ligated. Dissection should continue down as far distally as possible from the abdominal approach.

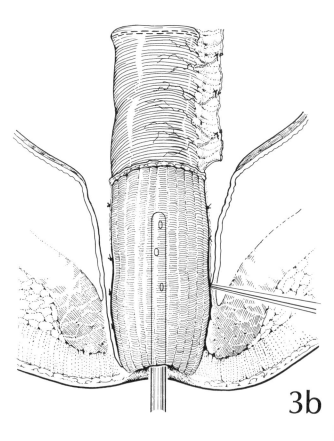

3b

Excision of rectum

4 The surgeon then moves to the foot of the table and an elliptical incision is made around the anus.

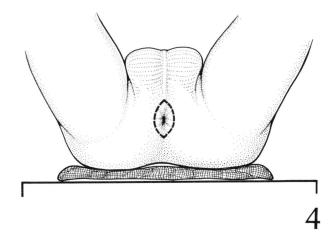

4

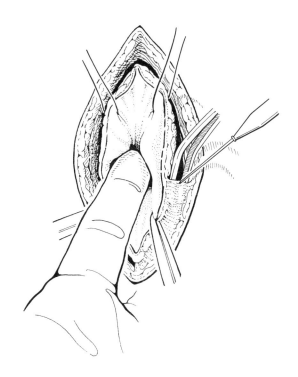

5

5 Dissection is carried upwards, remaining directly on the rectal wall. Skeletal muscles and the prostate should be avoided or considerable bleeding may arise.

6 Dissection continues until the presacral space is entered posteriorly. The remainder of the excision is carried out with the proximal rectum everted out onto the perineum. Sometimes, in a thin patient, the entire proctectomy can be performed transabdominally with the actual excision of the anus from the abdominal approach. The peritoneum is approximated from the abdominal side.

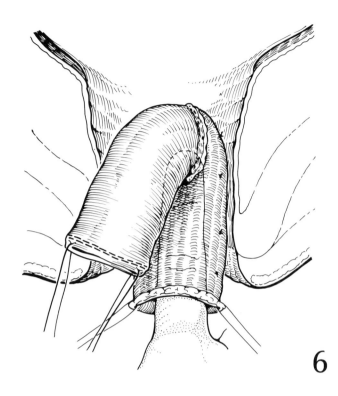

6

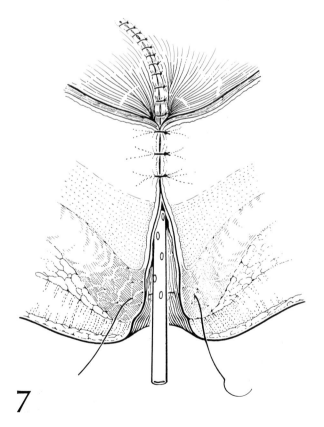

7

Tissue approximation

7 The levator complex and subcutaneous tissues are approximated through the perineal wound. A small, flat, closed suction drain is placed into the perineal wound.

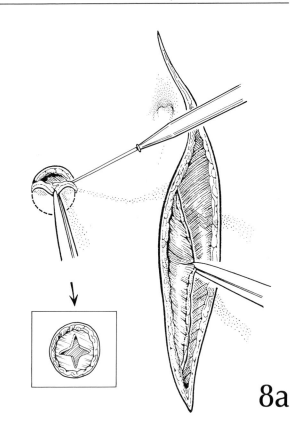

8a

Formation of stoma

8a, b The stoma is exteriorized at the previously marked site. The circle of skin about 1 cm in diameter is removed with cautery and the fascia is cruciated to allow the ileum to exit comfortably through it. The terminal ileum is prepared for creation of the ileostomy by ligating a few vessels along the most distal 3 cm of small bowel. The ileum is tacked to the peritoneum with interrupted sutures (silk or polyglycolic acid). Once the abdomen and skin are closed, a classic Brooke stoma is formed.

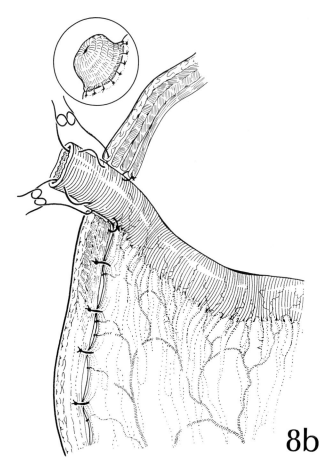

8b

ENDORECTAL PULL-THROUGH

Position of patient and incision

Positioning for this procedure is essentially identical to that for proctocolectomy; however, because of the longer procedure, very careful attention to padding of the lower extremities must be made to avoid neurovascular injury. A long midline or paramedian incision is made from the pubis to several centimeters above the umbilicus. The abdominal colectomy proceeds as already described.

Mobilization of ileum

The ileum is mobilized proximally to allow for an adequate length for the pull-through. In general, length is rarely a problem with a straight pull-through. With the J pouch and the lateral side-to-side reservoir more time must be spent in gaining bowel length. Adequate bowel length can also be difficult when the patient has had a previous ileostomy, as the mesentery may be scarred and foreshortened. In general, the main branch of the ileocecal artery can often be spared and the more proximal arcades ligated in the distal ileum. It is important to preserve the distal vascular arcade to the end of the ileum. If the ileocecal artery must be ligated, a bulldog clamp should initially be placed on this vessel to determine if a significant length of bowel will be lost.

Endorectal dissection

The authors prefer to do the entire endorectal dissection from the abdominal approach. It is technically more difficult to develop the correct plane from the perineum and, although the initial portion of the dissection can be quite difficult in children with ulcerative colitis, once this correct plane is found the dissection proceeds fairly smoothly.

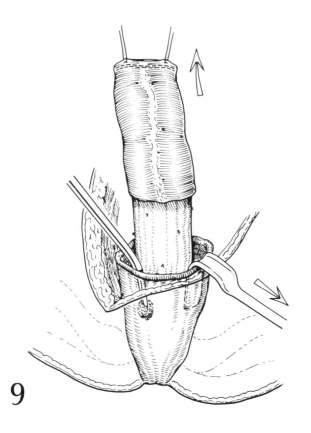

9

9 Countertraction of the dissected mucosal-submucosal tube, as well as traction in an upward and outward fashion on the muscular cuff, helps with the dissection.

The dissection involves greater blood loss than in cases of Hirschsprung's disease. Any large penetrating vessels should be cauterized but, once the dissection is completed, bleeding usually stops spontaneously. If the correct plane is lost the surgeon should turn to the opposite side of the bowel and work circumferentially until the dissection is distal to the area where the plane was lost. The level of the end of the dissection should be checked intermittently by feeling for an assistant's finger placed in the anus, just above the dentate line.

Formation of reservoir

The following description of the pull-through is applicable to all the different types of ileal reconstructions (straight and reservoir procedures). Construction of the J pouch, the lateral side-to-side ileal reservoir and the S pouch are subsequently described.

10 Once the endorectal dissection is completed one of the surgeons moves to the foot of the table. Narrow retractors are placed at the anal mucocutaneous junction and a clamp is inserted into the rectum. An assistant working in the abdominal field places the end of the mucosal-submucosal tube into this clamp. The segment is then everted outside the perineum. The end of the everted tube is placed in a clamp and held on traction by an assistant to facilitate the anastomosis.

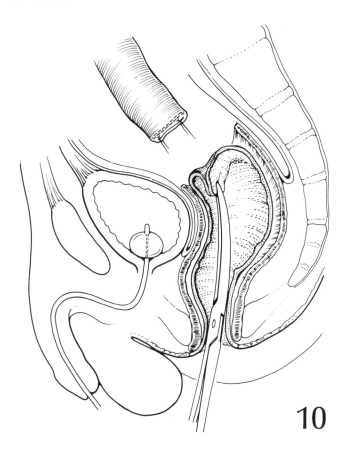

10

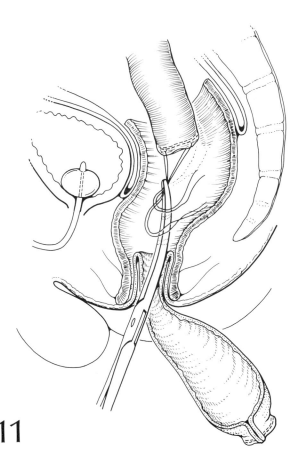

11

11 The submucosal-mucosal tube is incised on the anterior half, 1 cm proximal to the dentate line. A Kelly clamp is inserted into this opening and the ileum is brought down to this point by grasping two previously placed traction sutures. Great care must be taken not to twist the bowel as it is brought through the muscular cuff. Different colored sutures on mesenteric and antimesenteric sides of the bowel are helpful in maintaining this orientation.

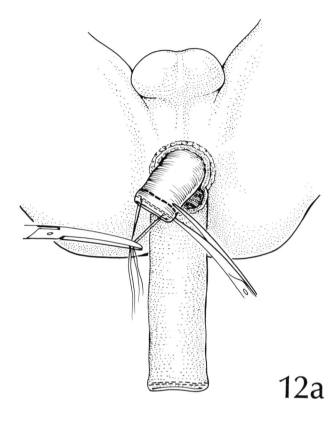

12a

12a, b The anterior half of the ileum is incised and is anastomosed to the anterior half of the anus with interrupted 3/0 or 4/0 absorbable sutures. The first sutures are placed at each corner and in the midline, and are followed by interrupted sutures placed in between.

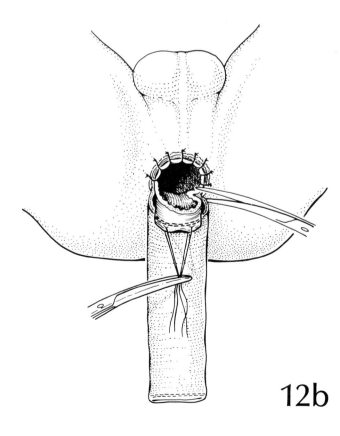

12b

13 One-quarter of the remaining ileum and one-quarter of the everted mucosal-submucosal tube are opened. A suture is placed in the posterior midline and this quarter of the anastomosis is completed. Countertraction, applied by an assistant on the everted tube and on the traction sutures on the ileum, will help with the exposure. The final quarter of the ileum and tube are removed and the anastomosis is completed and inspected. Before the last one or two sutures are placed a 3.5-mm closed suction drain is placed between the rectal muscular cuff and the pulled-through ileum and exits between the anastomotic sutures. The drain is placed most safely by advancing a small uterine sound retrograde through the anastomosis into the endorectal dissection. The drain can be secured onto this sound and then pulled through the anastomosis.

The ileum is pulled slightly upward, and this will invert the neorectum back into its correct position. Rectal examination at this point should show a well formed anastomosis 1.5–2 cm above the anodermal junction. Gloves are then changed and attention is directed to the abdominal field. The pulled-through ileum is attached with seromuscular sutures to the muscular cuff to prevent it from prolapsing in the early postoperative period.

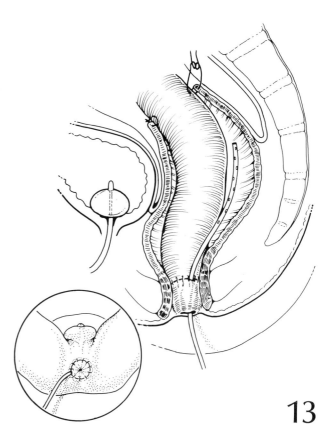

13

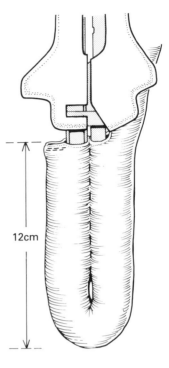

12cm

14a

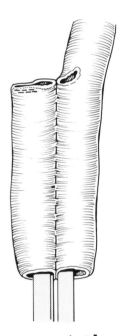

14b

14a–c For the J pouch the ileum is folded back on itself for a length of 12–15 cm. The bowel is opened at the stapled end and at an adjacent position in the proximal ileum. An automatic stapling device is fired to create the anastomosis. A small section of ileum will remain separated at the apex of the J. The apex is opened and the stapler is fired in the opposite direction to complete the anastomosis. This open end is brought down for the anal anastomosis. It is critical that a septum is not left between the ileal limbs as this will cause stasis, bacterial overgrowth and a fecaloma.

Although the J pouch is the most popular of all the reservoirs, some surgeons use other pouches such as the lateral ileal reservoir, the S pouch and the W pouch. The W pouch is rarely used in adults or children and will not be discussed here.

The lateral side-to-side ileal reservoir has been popularized by Fonkalsrud. The concept of this reservoir is similar to that of the J pouch except that both limbs of the lateral side-to-side reservoir are isoperistaltic which may improve emptying of the pouch and thus reduce the incidence of pouchitis.

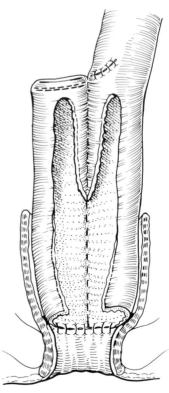

14c

Lateral side-to-side ileal reservoir

15a, b The ileum is divided 17 cm proximal to its stapled end. The proximal ileum is brought down, overlapping the distal ileum; both segments remain in an isoperistaltic direction. The two limbs are approximated along their antimesenteric sides. The distal 2 cm of the terminal ileum, in which there is no overlap, is used for the ileoanal anastomosis. The distal one-half of the pouch usually lies within the rectal muscular cuff. The two bowel segments are anastomosed using an automatic stapling device followed by a reinforced row of Lembert sutures.

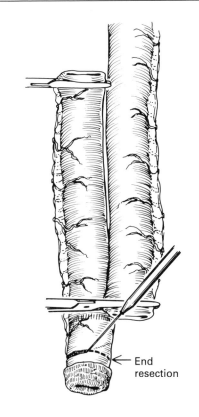

← End resection

15a

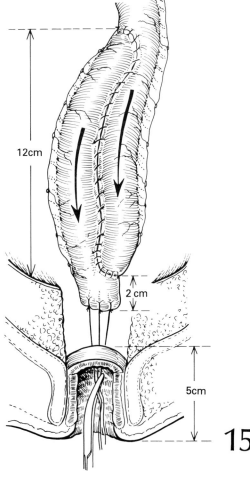

12cm

2 cm

5cm

15b

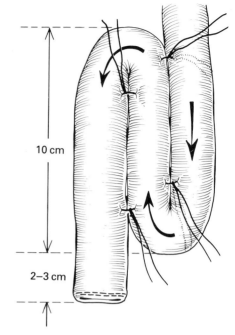

16a

S pouch reservoir

16a–c
The S pouch is created in a manner very similar to the J pouch except that there are two overlapping limbs of ileum. Each limb is 10 cm long with a 2–3-cm spout which is used for the ileoanal anastomosis.

For all four types of pull-through operations, a loop ileostomy is placed proximally. Care is taken to place this in an appropriate location marked before the operation. The ileum is carefully sutured to the peritoneum to prevent prolapse and twisting of the ileum at the site of the ileostomy.

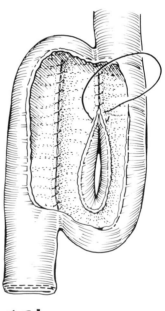

16b

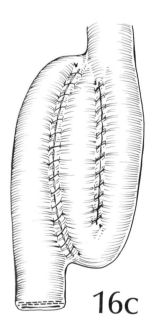

16c

STRICTUROPLASTY

The entire small and large bowel are mobilized and inspected. Each stricture is identified and marked with a silk suture. A typical short segment stricture is managed by placing traction sutures above and below the stricture on the antimesenteric surface of the bowel.

17 Using cautery the bowel is opened longitudinally along the antimesenteric surface. It is then approximated transversely using interrupted 4/0 absorbable or non-absorbable sutures and a second layer of silk Lembert sutures is placed.

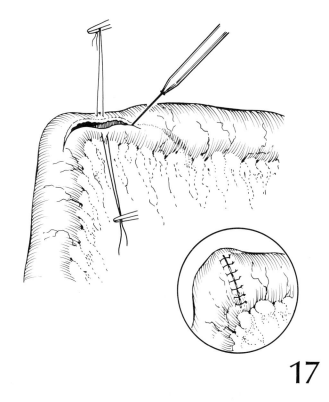

17

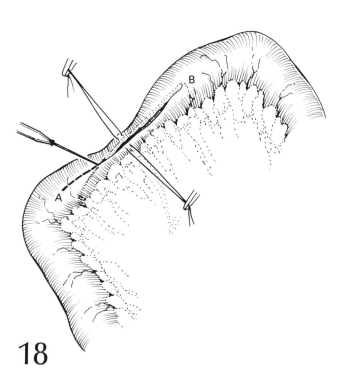

18

18 For strictures which are longer, the bowel is folded upon itself so that the stricture is at the apex and opened along a portion of both proximal and distal limbs.

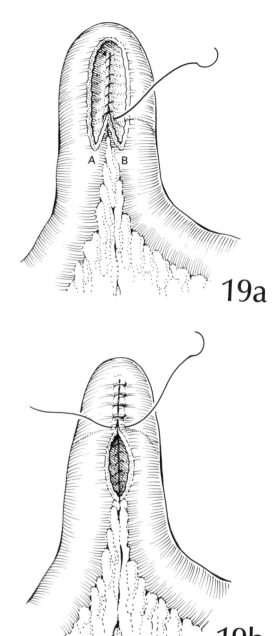

19a

19b

19a, b The limbs are anastomosed using an inner layer of running 4/0 absorbable sutures and interrupted Lembert sutures on the outside.

Postoperative care

Following proctocolectomy with end ileostomy a nasogastric tube is maintained until gastrointestinal activity returns. The Foley catheter can usually be removed in 3–4 days, but occasionally is left longer if the pelvic dissection was difficult. Steroids are tapered down to preoperative levels by the third postoperative day. Routine stoma care must be thoroughly learned by the family before discharge.

Postoperative care following endorectal pull-through is identical to that described for proctocolectomy. The ileostomy is generally closed after 3 months and a contrast study of the pull-through segment is usually performed before the closure

Postoperative care after stricturoplasty is routine. Nasogastric decompression is used until gastrointestinal activity returns. The child is given supplemental steroid therapy in the perioperative period. If the child has been malnourished for a prolonged period of time, consideration of perioperative parenteral nutrition should be given.

Complications

Complications associated with the endorectal pull-through are not uncommon. Diarrhea with 7–15 bowel movements a day initially after closure of the ileostomy is expected, and this should be explained to the child and family before the operation. Most patients slowly normalize their stooling pattern over the first several months after the pull-through. Major losses of fluids and electrolytes may occur at first, as well as excoriation of the perineum. Diarrhea is best controlled with Kaopectate (Upjohn, USA) and loperamide hydrochloride as needed. Occasionally, Metamucil (Proctor and Gamble, USA) may be added. Cholestyramine is occasionally added to this regimen.

Pouchitis is a well described complication of an ileal anal pull-through. The presumed etiology is stasis of stool in the ileal segment, with subsequent bacterial overgrowth. The incidence is around 25% if reservoirs are employed, but with a straight pull-through the incidence is lower (<5%). Treatment of this condition consists of serial washouts of the pouch, sitz baths and oral metronidazole.

The incidence of adhesive obstruction after any type of surgery for ulcerative colitis is 20–25%, irrespective of the type of procedure done. In the authors' series, however, adhesive obstruction occurred in 10% of cases, with only half of these requiring an enterolysis.

Acknowledgments

Illustrations 15a and *15b* are reproduced from *Annals of Surgery* 1988; 208: 50–5 with permission of the publishers, JB Lippincott Co, Philadelphia, Pennsylvania, USA.

Further reading

Alexander-Williams J, Haynes IG. Conservative operations for Crohn's disease of the small bowel. *World J Surg* 1985; 9: 945–51.

Coran AG. A personal experience with 100 consecutive total colectomies and straight ileoanal endorectal pull-throughs for benign disease of the colon and rectum in children and adults. *Ann Surg* 1990; 212: 242–8.

Fonkalsrud EW. Update on clinical experience with different surgical techniques of the endorectal pull-through operation for colitis and polyposis. *Surg Gynecol Obstet* 1987; 165: 309–16.

Martin LW, LeCoultre C, Schubert WK. Total colectomy and mucosal proctectomy with preservation of continence in ulcerative colitis. *Ann Surg* 1977; 186: 477–80.

Martin LW, Sayers HJ, Alexander F, Fischer JE, Torres MA. Anal continence following Soave procedure: analysis of results of 100 patients. *Ann Surg* 1986; 203: 515–30.

Vasilevsky CA, Rothenberger DA, Goldberg SM. The S ileal pouch–anal anastomosis. *World J Surg* 1987; 11: 742–50.

Rectal polyps

Richard C. M. Cook MA, BM, FRCS
Consultant Paediatric Surgeon, Royal Liverpool Children's NHS Trust, Alder Hey, Liverpool, UK

Principles and justification

Juvenile polyps may present throughout childhood and adolescence; the peak incidence is at 4–5 years, and boys are affected slightly more frequently than girls. While such polyps may develop in any part of the large intestine, the majority are found in the rectum and rectosigmoid region, i.e. they are within reach of a standard sigmoidoscope. In about 25% of these children more than one polyp (but not diffuse polyposis) is found, either at the initial examination or subsequently.

Juvenile polyps are hamartomas. They are usually 1–2 cm in diameter at presentation and have a smooth, ulcerated surface. The polyp is honeycombed with irregular cysts lined with mucus-secreting cells and separated by vascular connective tissue heavily infiltrated with inflammatory cells. About 70% of polyps are situated in the rectum (usually on the posterior wall), 15% occur in the sigmoid colon, and the remainder are scattered more proximally.

Clinical features

Local abrasion by the passage of stools often leads to a little bright red bleeding at or after defecation and a mucous secretion is often noticed. Polyps may also prolapse and be described by the mother as a 'dark red cherry' at the anus immediately after defecation. Digital rectal examination may reveal the polyp but, being soft and mobile, it is not easy to feel. The history makes it clear that sigmoidoscopy is needed so that rectal examination is unnecessary. Early admission as a day case for full examination under anesthesia is indicated.

Not uncommonly, a history is given of several small bleeds followed by a slightly larger one that precipitates a visit to the doctor. By the time of the hospital referral there has been no further sign of bleeding. Autoamputation of the polyp may have occurred with spontaneous cure. With such a clear history no investigation is warranted unless the symptoms recur.

Differential diagnosis

The possibility of an anal fissure, inflammatory bowel disease, or blood dyscrasia such as Henoch–Schönlein purpura, should be considered. A Meckel's diverticulum, duplication of the intestine or intussusception may cause bleeding, but it is generally more profuse and other related symptoms usually distinguish these conditions from the simple polyp.

A solitary adenomatous polyp is rare in childhood but, if found, familial adenomatous polyposis should be considered with appropriate examination of the rest of the colon.

Rectal polyps may occur in up to 30% of patients with Peutz–Jeghers syndrome, and a rare condition in which there is diffuse polyposis with a mixture of juvenile and adenomatous polyps has also been described.

Operation

The child is admitted as a day case without any bowel preparation, and a bisacodyl suppository is used for evacuating the rectum. Suitable premedication is given and general anesthesia induced. The child is turned into the left lateral position with the sacrum at the edge of the table and the pelvis raised on a small sandbag. The anus and perineum are inspected, the anus is lubricated and digital rectal examination performed. It may be possible to remove the polyp at this stage (*see Illustration 1*).

A suitably sized (and lubricated) proctoscope or sigmoidoscope held in the left hand is inserted through the anus towards the umbilicus. As soon as the anal canal is felt to have been passed, the tip of the instrument is directed more posteriorly and the obturator removed and replaced with the glass window. Only the minimum amount of air is insufflated to distend the rectum sufficiently to allow the instrument to be advanced gently up the rectum and into the sigmoid colon. Removal of feces with a moistened cotton wool swab, or by suction, may be needed. The bowel wall is observed during all maneuvers but a systematic search is easier on withdrawal rather than as the instrument is being advanced. As soon as the polyp is found it may be removed and sigmoidoscopic inspection then completed.

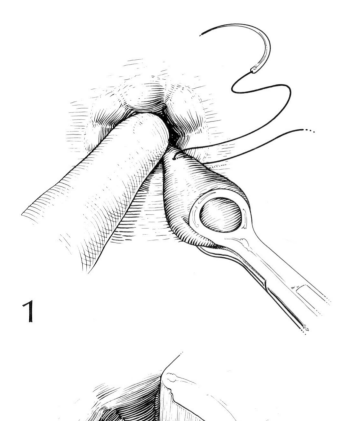

1 A polyp in the lower rectum can often be hooked out of the anus by the examining finger, and the stalk ligated, before its removal. It often breaks off spontaneously. Such a simple, deliberate avulsion is safely practised by some surgeons, as bleeding from the stalk is usually minimal and stops spontaneously. Persistent bleeding can be controlled by pressure from a cotton wool swab applied after identification of the site through the sigmoidoscope.

2 If bleeding is considerable, a Parks' or similar speculum is inserted. If the bleeding point is in view it can be grasped with a pair of artery forceps and ligated or cauterized.

If not in view, the speculum is left in place and the sigmoidoscope passed into the rectum through it to locate the 'lost' pedicle. This is grasped with forceps. Traction on these while withdrawing the sigmoidoscope will prolapse the mucosa into the view within the speculum, where it is grasped with another pair of forceps held outside the sigmoidoscope which is then removed. The pedicle may then be securely ligated or cauterized under direct vision.

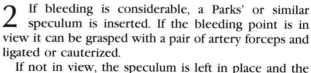

3 Polyps higher in the rectum are snared through the sigmoidoscope. A wire snare is looped over the polyp and either the polyp, the sigmoidoscope, or the patient is manipulated so that the stalk can be seen. It is not usually necessary to grasp the head of the polyp in order to snare it but it may be helpful. The snare is tightened nearer to the head of the polyp than to the intestinal wall. Using a suitably insulated snare, cautery can be used to coagulate and cut the stalk but simple traction on the snare to cut it seldom causes significant hemorrhage. The polyp must be recovered for histological examination.

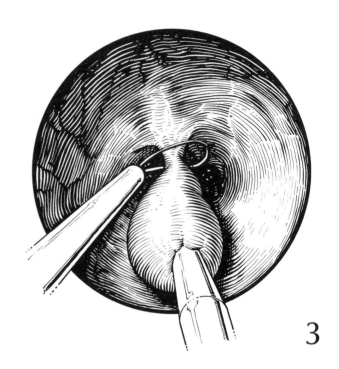

3

Postoperative care

Most children can return home as soon as they have recovered from anesthesia. Parents should be told to expect some old blood with the first bowel action but are warned to report any prolonged or large bleed. For solitary polyps a follow-up visit is not usually arranged, but parents should be asked to return if the symptoms recur and the surgeon should not close the case until he has seen that histology confirms a hamartomatous juvenile polyp.

Complications

Bacteremia, perforation and hemorrhage are all possible but are very rare. However, the surgeon should avoid rough handling, vigorous pulling on the polyp to tent the bowel wall, and excessive cauterization.

Outcome

Between 3% and 25% of children are said to develop recurrent juvenile polyps at different sites. As this is a benign and self-limiting condition, a prolonged search for more proximal polyps is unwarranted provided the histology of the distal, removed, polyp confirms the diagnosis. Such a search would involve full bowel preparation for double-contrast enema and colonoscopy. Easily accessible recurrent polyps should be removed as described if symptomatic.

Illustrations by Mark Iley

Anal fissure and anal fistula

R. C. M. Cook MA, BM, FRCS
Consultant Paediatric Surgeon, Royal Liverpool Children's NHS Trust, Alder Hey, Liverpool, UK

Anal fissure

Principles and justification

The relatively trivial complaint of anal fissure can be a source of severe symptoms for many years. It is often misdiagnosed, yet proper treatment is almost always effective[1].

Fissures are not uncommon in childhood, with a peak incidence in children aged between 6 and 24 months. Some are short-lived and heal spontaneously. An acute fissure causes pain on defecation, holding back when the call to defecate comes, the development of a large and hard stool, further trauma to the fissure, increasing pain and so on round the cycle. Unless this cycle is broken intractable bowel problems will follow, with a profound influence on the child's life. Long after a fissure is forgotten the psychiatrist may be struggling to help a family recover from serious disturbances of the child's behavior and of their relationships.

Diagnosis

1 The history of pain on defecation and of hard stools passed infrequently with a streak of blood is almost sufficient to make a diagnosis. Visual inspection of the anus by gentle separation of the buttocks will reveal the fissure together with a sentinel tag in the more chronic fissure. Digital examination or proctoscopy must not be undertaken except under anesthesia. Most fissures lie in the midline (at 12 or 6 o'clock) and (as in adults) posterior fissures are more usual in boys.

Anorectal abuse must always be borne in mind when examining even the very young child (of either sex) who presents with an anal problem[2]. Local features of buggery include fissures, very wide dilatation of the inspected anus, venous engorgement, perianal hematomata and edema.

Such a child usually exhibits other physical signs of abuse, and also behavioral abnormalities. The very early involvement of a pediatrician experienced in the diagnosis and management of child abuse is essential if the child is to be protected from further injury. Cessation of abuse usually allows healing of the anal pathology without the need for local therapy.

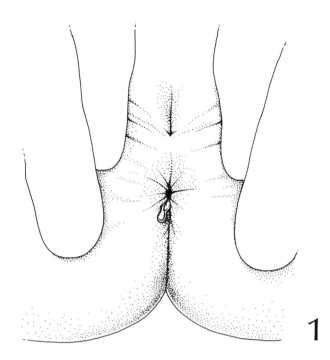

1

Differential diagnosis

Pruritis ani and inflammatory conditions of the perianal skin may lead to the formation of multiple, radial superficial cracks that do not extend into the anal canal.

Multiple fissures, or those lying laterally or extending above the dentate line, should raise the suspicion of Crohn's disease, ulcerative colitis or tuberculosis.

Medical management

The majority of acute fissures heal in a few weeks if regular defecation can be established and maintained. A mild stool softener and aperient (e.g. lactulose) should be prescribed and a diet adequate in vegetable and cereal fiber should be encouraged. To put only the child 'on a diet' is usually unsuccessful. The whole family should use wholemeal bread rather than white and join in other dietary adjustments that will also be to their advantage! Local anesthetic cream is not recommended since sensitization is common, it is painful to put it into the anal canal where it will be effective, and useful timing of its application is almost impossible.

Surgical management

The two procedures commonly used are anal dilatation and lateral sphincterotomy.

The reason for the effectiveness of anal dilatation is not certain, but it is assumed that it relieves spasm of the internal sphincter and allows drainage of infected

material from the base of the fissure. The lack of spasm permits the resumption of painless defecation and the re-establishment of normal bowel habits. The existence and cause of this spasm is not proven in adults and has not been tested in children[3,4].

Persistence of a symptomatic fissure after adequate dilatation, which may perhaps have been repeated once or twice, is an indication for lateral sphincterotomy. Such a fissure is usually accompanied by an inflamed or edematous sentinel skin tag, and is deep enough for the transverse fibers of the lower third of the internal sphincter to be seen. The edges will be undermined and indurated. Simple excision and midline sphincterotomy is not recommended because of the risk of 'keyhole' deformity of the anus with leakage and pruritus.

Preoperative

Digital examinations, enemas and suppositories are all forbidden. For anal dilatation the child is admitted as a day case, and must be suitably starved, but no oral or parenteral premedication is required. An anesthetic cream containing lidocaine (lignocaine) and prilocaine (EMLA) should be applied to suitable areas for venous access according to the anesthetist's preference. No special preparation is needed for lateral sphincterotomy.

Operations

ANAL DILATATION

2a, b Under general anesthesia (deep enough to prevent laryngeal spasm) digital examination is carried out with the child in the left lateral position (supine with a nurse flexing the hips is equally suitable for small children). A caudal block is a distinct advance in reducing postoperative discomfort. The position, extent and degree of induration round the fissure are noted. A biopsy sample should always be taken from fissures that appear atypical. The constricting ring described in adults with anal fissures is not so evident in children.

Dilatation is begun by gentle massage with the right index finger pushing mainly backwards; this hand is then pronated to pull anteriorly and the left index finger is inserted and gentle but firm stretching carried out anteroposteriorly.

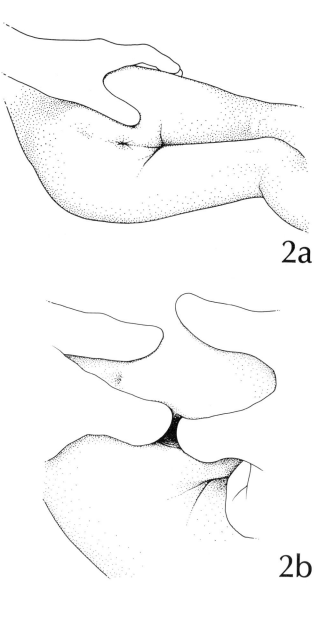

2a

2b

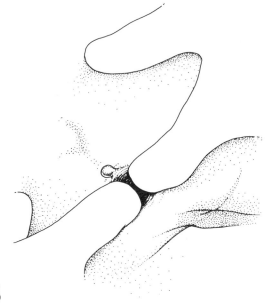

3

3 The surgeon's hands are rotated and the anal canal is stretched laterally. At this stage it is particularly easy to increase the depth and extent of a posterior or anterior fissure and the amount of force used must be limited in strength and direction. Most of the 'stretch' should be of the lateral components of the sphincter and, at the end of the procedure, although the hemorrhoidal plexus may appear congested, there should not be any additional mucosal or cutaneous tears or bruising. Hard feces should be evacuated digitally from the rectum. Local anesthetic gel may be applied at the end of the procedure.

LATERAL SPHINCTEROTOMY

Under general anesthesia a digital examination is performed to confirm the diagnosis; sigmoidoscopy is also necessary. The patient is placed in the lithotomy position and the perineum and anal canal are cleaned and draped. A well lubricated Park's retractor of suitable size is inserted and opened to stretch the anal canal slightly.

A fine needle is inserted in the 3 o'clock position through the palpable groove between the inferior border of the internal sphincter and the external sphincter; 1:250 000 epinephrine (adrenaline), with lidocaine (lignocaine) if desired, is then injected deep to the anal skin up to the dentate line and then outside the internal sphincter through the intersphincteric space.

4   A 2-cm circumferential skin incision is made just outside the anal verge.

A flap of anal skin is raised off the internal sphincter as far as the dentate line. Care must be taken not to button-hole the skin.

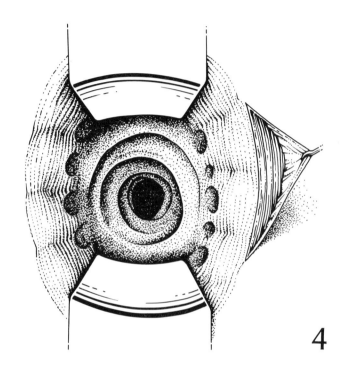

4

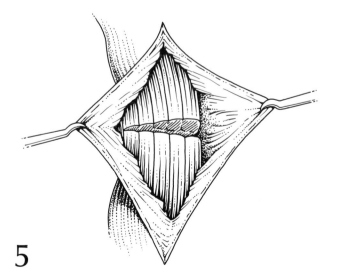

5

5   The intersphincteric space is opened for a similar distance on the other side of the internal sphincter, and the lower one-third or one-quarter of the sphincter is divided with scissors or a knife to the dentate line. The perianal skin is closed with two or three fine catgut sutures and, if a prominent skin tag is present, it is excised with sharp, pointed scissors after the speculum has been removed. Sufficient tissue is removed to prevent any overhang remaining at the external end of the fissure, but damage to the external sphincter or excessive skin removal should be avoided.

Postoperative care

Anal dilatation

Regular dilatation of the anal canal is ensured by regular passage of a normal stool. This requires: an aperient such as lactulose; a diet with adequate fiber; and parental support and encouragement.

At an outpatient review 3–4 weeks after dilatation the dietary and bowel history is checked. The abdomen should be palpated to search for loading of the pelvic colon. The anus can be inspected but digital internal examination is avoided. Aperients are gradually withdrawn and the child should be able to be discharged after a further visit 1–2 months later.

Lateral sphincterotomy

Mild analgesia may be required and should be given to ensure comfortable defecation. Attention to the diet and the administration of a mild aperient should continue. Cleansing after defecation is the rule.

Complications

A little bleeding may be noticed after dilatation and manual evacuation. The short period of incontinence and the bruising secondary to submucosal hemorrhages reported in adults have not been described in children.

Local infection is rare following lateral sphincterotomy. Hematoma formation has been described and some surgeons recommend the insertion of a petroleum jelly (Vaseline) gauze pack at the end of the operation to provide local compression: this is not usually necessary and adds to postoperative discomfort.

Outcome

Anal dilatation

No large series has been reported recently in children, but the majority seem to experience prompt pain relief. The skin tags usually shrink to insignificance with the passing years. Perhaps 5–10% have recurrence or persistence of symptoms and a further dilatation or sphincterotomy is indicated.

Lateral sphincterotomy

No large series involving children has been described but lateral sphincterotomy is generally considered to be a useful procedure. Careful follow-up is necessary for some months to ensure that good habits of regular defecation are maintained and that the bowel negativism that so easily develops in children who experience painful defecation does not occur.

Anal fistula

Principles and justification

6   Anal fistulas in infants usually present as recurrent small perianal abscesses. Their etiology is probably identical to that in adults, in that infection spreads from a crypt abscess tracking along the intersphincteric plane. The track of the fistula is usually straight, running radially from the affected crypt to the external site of the recurrent abscess. Boys are affected much more frequently than girls.

In the older child recurrent perianal sepsis or fistula cannot be assumed to be an isolated lesion. It is much more likely to be one of the features of inflammatory bowel disease or chronic granulomatous disease. A fistula as part of tuberculous enteritis is very rare in childhood. Fistulas in association with chemotherapy for leukemia in childhood are not uncommon. All perianal abscesses should be incised and drained early and antibiotic therapy has little place in their management. Because of their etiology, even after prompt drainage some 25% will go on to form a fistula.

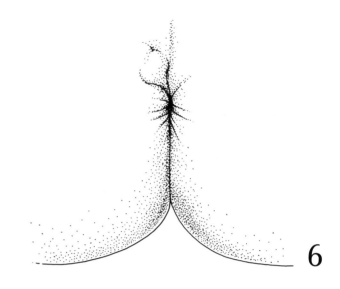

6

Preoperative

A recurrent perianal abscess is an indication for examination under anesthesia. No special preoperative preparation is necessary.

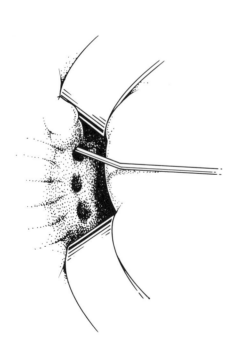

7

Operation

7   Careful digital examination of the perianal region and anal canal is done to define sites of induration and to exclude any other pathology. A well lubricated, self-retaining speculum (such as Parks') is inserted or an assistant may hold two malleable retractors of suitable width. A probe is gently inserted from one end of the fistula to the other with care being taken not to produce a false track.

8 A knife is used to cut down onto the probe to lay the fistula open. In many instances this is all that needs to be done, but if a lot of granulation tissue is present it may be curetted and, if there is a considerable amount of overhanging skin, it should be trimmed away to ensure that the track can drain freely.

If there is any suspicion of chronic inflammatory bowel disease a biopsy sample must be taken.

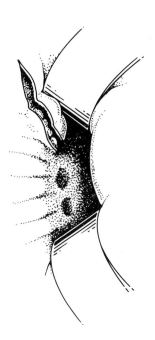

8

Postoperative care

Stool softeners should be given and a diet with adequate fiber encouraged. Careful anal hygiene is required and twice daily baths should be given.

Outcome

Such low fistulas in infants usually heal uneventfully. Recurrence should raise the suspicion of underlying disease and further appropriate investigation should be pursued.

References

1. Parks AG. The management of fissure-in-ano. *Hosp Med* 1967; 1: 737–8.

2. Hobbs CJ, Wynne JM. Buggery in childhood – a common syndrome of child abuse. *Lancet* 1986; ii: 792–6.

3. Abcarian H, Lakshmanan S, Read DR, Roccatorte P. The role of internal sphincter in chronic anal fissures. *Dis Colon Rectum* 1982; 25: 525–8.

4. Kuypers HC. Is there really sphincter spasm in anal fissure? *Dis Colon Rectum* 1988; 26: 493–4.

Colonoscopy

P. J. Milla MSc, FRCP
Reader in Paediatric Gastroenterology, Gastroenterology Unit, Institute of Child Health and Great Ormond Street Hospital for Children, London, UK

C. B. Williams FRCP
Consultant Physician, St Mark's Hospital for Diseases of the Rectum and Colon, St Bartholomew's Hospital and King Edward VII Hospital for Officers, and Honorary Consultant Physician, Great Ormond Street Hospital for Children, London, UK

Principles and justification

Indications

Limited colonoscopy is extremely well tolerated by children of any age, pediatric colonoscopes being thinner than an examining little finger. Without either sedation or bowel preparation it is possible to inspect, photograph and obtain biopsy or other specimens from the rectosigmoid as part of the initial assessment of symptomatic patients. Since more extensive colonoscopy requires both full bowel preparation and some form of sedation, it is reserved for selected patients, usually those with failure to thrive or weight loss, chronic diarrhea, anemia, bleeding, and when there is radiological abnormality (e.g. narrowed terminal ileal abnormality on small bowel follow through) or a need for therapy (e.g. Peutz–Jeghers polyposis).

Colonoscopy, where it is readily available, now supplants barium enema as the colonic investigation of first choice in children, not only because it can be performed without irradiation, but because high quality double-contrast films are not usually obtained by pediatric radiologists and radiography is, therefore, less accurate, and also a tissue diagnosis of a mucosal lesion will be obtained. When indicated it is feasible to perform both colonoscopy to the terminal ileum and gastroscopy to the duodenum at a single examination, a large proportion of the gastrointestinal tract thus being accessible to inspection, biopsy or instrumentation in one procedure.

Contraindications

There are few contraindications to colonoscopy in sensitive hands with appropriate instrumentation. Examination is likely to be difficult and unrewarding in simple constipation or megacolon unless adequate preparative precautions are taken, and the diagnostic yield is extremely low in abdominal pain unaccompanied by features to suggest systemic illness. There is a risk of septicemia in marasmic, immunodepressed or immunosuppressed subjects who should receive appropriate antibiotics; prophylactic antibiotics should also be given in the presence of any cardiac lesion. The danger of septic peritonitis contraindicates colonoscopy in the presence of ascites. The availability of immersible instruments and appropriate solutions (glutaraldehyde 2%) means that full sterilization of the colonoscope is possible between examinations, preferably with an automated washing machine, and there should, therefore, be no possibility of transmission of infective agents.

Preoperative

Bowel preparation

Half a phosphate enema may clear most of the colon of an infant or clear fluids can be given for 24 h for complete preparation. For older children oral bowel preparation (without enemas) is generally effective and better tolerated than older purge/enema regimens. Senna syrup and magnesium citrate are pleasant tasting and, accompanied by 24 h of fluid diet, give an adequately clean colon except in a few patients — paradoxically often those with colitis whose colon may not empty normally. The alternative is for the patient to drink a balanced electrolyte polyethylene glycol solution or isotonic (5%) mannitol, the latter being contraindicated before polypectomy because of the risk of forming explosive concentrations of hydrogen. Some children become nauseated and vomit before an adequate 1–3 litre volume has been ingested, resulting in failed preparation unless resort is made to large volume cleansing enemas.

Sedation or anesthesia?

Premedication is useful for apprehensive children in whom reassurance and explanation are often ineffective (antihistamine syrup orally, diazepam rectally, chlorpromazine or pethidine intramuscularly). In infants or older subjects premedication should be unnecessary, assuming a friendly atmosphere and supportive parents. Infants can be managed with surprisingly little medication, even during the examination, and older children are frequently more interested and less embarrassed by the prospect of internal examination than adult patients.

Colonoscopic examination is, however, frequently uncomfortable or painful for a short period as the instrument stretches the sigmoid colon mesentery or the visceral peritoneum, and adequate analgesia is, therefore, advisable to avoid traumatizing child or parents. There is no contraindication to the use of light general anesthesia, but this is usually unnecessary and tends to make colonoscopy a more serious procedure, more difficult to organize and less used; it also encourages heavy-handed instrumental technique. With appropriate intravenous medication, colonoscopy can be a routine day-case or side-room investigation. An indwelling venous cannula is inserted before the child is brought to the endoscopy room so as to avoid the trauma of venepuncture just before sedation for the endoscopic procedure. A combination of benzodiazepine (for amnesia) and opiate (for sedation and analgesia) is titrated by slow intravenous injection until the child is drowsy enough to accept introduction of the instrument through the rectum without protest. To avoid pain at the injection site, a lipid suspension of diazepam or water-soluble midazolam is preferred, and pethidine is diluted 1:5 with water. Initial dosage is based on midazolam 0.1 mg/kg and pethidine 0.5 mg/kg but, according to results, larger amounts may be needed and 50–100 mg intravenous pethidine is not unusual without over-sedation in an anxious adolescent. Pethidine is favoured for any incremental doses, since it is more effective in children and is reversible by naloxone. Flumazenil should be available to reverse benzodiazepines when required. Monitoring of heart rate and oxygen saturation by a portable oximeter during sedation and the procedure is mandatory. Appropriate use of oxygen as indicated by oxygen saturation level results in safer and more effective sedation.

Choice of instrument

In small children it is clearly preferable to have a suitable floppy 10–11-mm diameter instrument so as to pass small sphincters and variable colonic loops without undue stretching. In older children an adult colonoscope may be more appropriate. The length of the instrument is not usually a limiting factor, pediatric colonoscopes being at least 130 cm long, whereas the cecum of a baby may be reached using only 50 cm of instrument and shortened back to 25–30 cm as the colon straightens. As colonoscopes are more flexible than gastroscopes, if a pediatric colonoscope is not available an adult colonoscope is preferable to a pediatric gastroscope. With lubrication and slow dilatation the anus of even a baby will accept an instrument of 14–15-mm diameter.

Is radiographic control needed?

Most examinations do not require radiographic screening control and the majority of colonoscopists never use it. In the learning phase and for the less experienced, however, the extra information given can be invaluable. If radiographic facilities are available difficult procedures can be made quicker, safer and less traumatic. Radiography will also help in the localization of biopsy sites or lesions found unexpectedly at colonoscopy. Irradiation should be kept to a minimum, an occasional brief image being sufficient to demonstrate the position of the instrument and to explain and resolve any looping of its shaft. The best compromise is to avoid use of radiography in the majority of patients, but to have it available in case of need; if necessary the patient can be transferred to an X-ray table with the colonoscope *in situ*.

Operations

COLONOSCOPY

Position of patient

1 Infants are usually examined supine and this position is also appropriate if general anesthesia is used; otherwise most endoscopists commence with the patient in the left lateral position, and it is often possible to complete the examination without a change. If there are mechanical difficulties at any stage of the procedure a change in position may alter the configuration of the bowel and facilitate examination. Changing to the right lateral position will make the splenic flexure less acute and can also help to drain fluid from the descending colon and facilitate air distension within it if the view is poor. In addition, the prone position sometimes aids passage through the hepatic flexure.

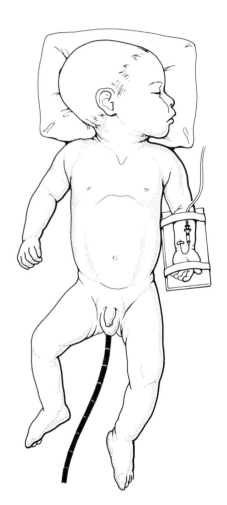

1

Insertion and passage through the rectosigmoid

The tip of the colonoscope and perianal region are lubricated with jelly, the anus being dilated if necessary with either the finger or tubes of increasing diameter until examination is possible. On insertion initially there may be no view because the tip is against the wall of the rectum. The instrument must be withdrawn slightly and air insufflated before a view is obtained, the tip then being angled and the instrument shaft rotated as necessary to follow along the lumen of the rectosigmoid.

In passing the many bends of the rectosigmoid, the object is to avoid distending or stretching the bowel so as to keep it short and pass almost straight to the descending colon. This is easier to suggest than to achieve, but is made more likely by observing the points set out below.

2a–c (1) As little air as possible should be insufflated to see; excess air should be aspirated from time to time. (2) The bowel lumen should be followed accurately. (3) If the view is lost, even for a few seconds, the control knobs must be released and the colonoscope withdrawn a short distance – the lumen will automatically reappear. (4) Blind pushing should be avoided, but on acute bends this may be necessary for a few seconds providing the mucosa continues to move and the general direction is known. (5) If the tip will not angle round a bend an attempt should be made to 'corkscrew' the instrument by pulling the shaft back straight and twisting it one way or the other. (6) The colonoscope should be pulled back repeatedly after passing each bend and before starting each inward push. A straight colonoscope and a shortened colon will result. (7) The instrument shaft should be held in the fingertips as far as possible – gripping in a clenched fist causes clumsiness.

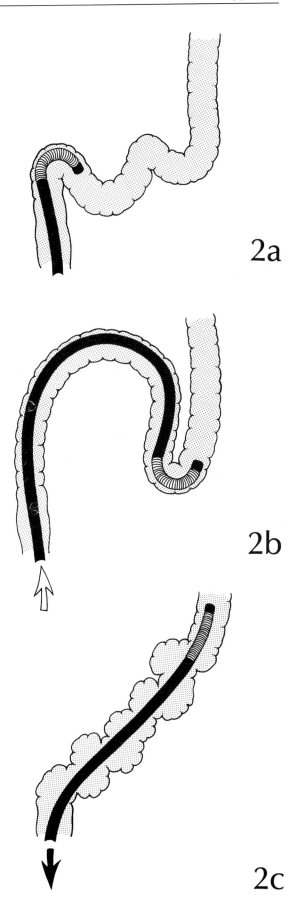

2a

2b

2c

Sigmoid N loop – hook and twist maneuver

The commonest situation on reaching the junction of the sigmoid and descending colon, in spite of all care, is for there to be an 'N loop' forming an acute tip angle which makes direct passage difficult or impossible. If the tip can be passed a short way around the bend, looking in to the retroperitoneal part of the descending colon, it can be held there without consciously hooking while the instrument is withdrawn 10–40 cm to reduce and straighten out the loop. Putting a clockwise twisting force or torque on to the shaft of the colonoscope while it is withdrawn will help to straighten out this loop and keep the tip in the descending colon.

Sigmoid 'alpha' loop

3   Often, if there is a redundant colon, a loop is obviously forming but the tip runs in easily without discomfort to the patient. This suggests that a spiral 'alpha' loop is forming (which can be confirmed if fluoroscopy is used). The correct thing to do is to continue pushing in as far as is comfortable for the patient, at least to the proximal descending colon and preferably to the splenic flexure. If there is little or no discomfort the instrument can be pushed round into the transverse colon before attempting to withdraw it and straighten it out.

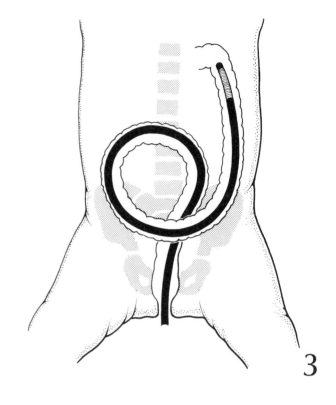

3

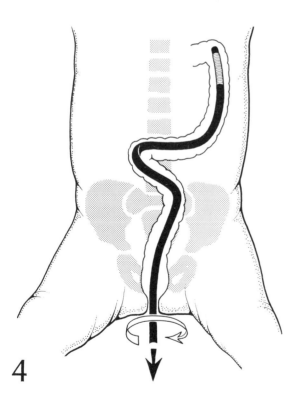

4

Straightening out loops

4   Having reached the upper descending or the transverse colon, the sigmoid colon loop should be removed, since loops create friction in the control wires and stress the instrument just as much as they stress the patient. To remove a loop, the instrument shaft should be withdrawn until the tip begins to slide past the mucosa or resistance to withdrawal is felt. Whilst pulling back the application of twist, usually in a clockwise direction, will be found to stop the tip slipping back excessively and facilitate the straightening of the instrument.

In the young child it is very likely that the colon will prove to be hypermobile, without conventional fixation of the descending colon and splenic flexure. In the 20–30% of patients having a mobile colon, unpredictable and sometimes uncontrollable loops may form which make it difficult or impossible to reach the proximal colon or terminal ileum. Such atypical loops (reversed 'alpha' loop, reversed splenic flexure) can sometimes be successfully removed by first pulling back to reduce their size and then twisting anticlockwise as the shaft is further straightened back.

Splenic flexure: keeping the sigmoid colon straight

5 With the colonoscope straightened in the proximal descending colon or splenic flexure, some care may be needed to prevent the sigmoid loop reforming. Continued clockwise (or sometimes anticlockwise) twist on the shaft during reinsertion is often enough to keep it straight. Shaft insertion without tip movement, or losing the 1:1 relationship between shaft and tip, indicate looping. The instrument is immediately pulled back again and the assistant pushes into the left iliac fossa to resist the tendency for the sigmoid loop to rise up from the pelvis. In the splenic flexure this tendency to reloop in the sigmoid colon results because the hooked instrument tip impacts in the splenic flexure. A combination of the following small corrective measures will usually overcome this: (1) the instrument shaft should be pulled back straight; (2) hand/finger pressure should be applied by the assistant over the left iliac fossa; (3) the instrument shaft should be twisted clockwise; (4) if necessary the instrument should be re-aimed toward the lumen, avoiding over-angulation; (5) it should be pushed slowly inwards, keeping on the clockwise twist.

Sometimes it is easier to reposition the child in the right lateral position to cause the splenic flexure to drop down and flatten out.

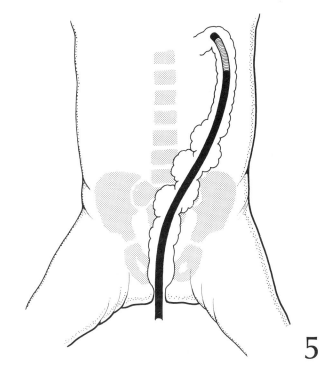

5

Redundant transverse colon

The transverse colon may sometimes be pushed down by the instrument into a deep loop which makes it difficult and painful to reach the hepatic flexure. Once again the correct procedure is to withdraw the instrument to shorten this loop. If necessary withdrawal may need to be repeated several times, the instrument advancing a few centimeters on each withdrawal ('paradoxical movement') until the loop is straightened. Keeping the colon deflated also helps to shorten the hepatic flexure region, making it easier both to reach and pass. In addition, an assistant pushing the transverse colon upwards and straightening this loop out is often helpful.

Difficulty in the transverse colon is often due to recurrent looping in the sigmoid colon, and the best corrective measures are abdominal pressure in the left iliac fossa and gentle clockwise twisting during reinsertion.

Passing the hepatic flexure

Having reached and deflated the hepatic flexure, and angled acutely around it into the ascending colon, the transverse loop may remain and make it difficult to pass the rest of the instrument into the ascending colon. By once again withdrawing the colonoscope and straightening out this loop it becomes easier to pass. Deflating the ascending colon by aspiration and simultaneously steering carefully to avoid haustral folds will often cause the colonoscope to descend spontaneously towards the cecum.

Reaching the cecum

Reaching the cecal pole can be facilitated by change of position (supine or prone), deflation, abdominal pressure and clockwise twist on the straightened instrument; aggressive pushing usually only results in looping. The colonoscope is seen to have reached the cecum when the bulge of the ileocecal valve is seen or, 2–5 cm

beyond it, the appendix orifice is identified. Brilliant transillumination in the right iliac fossa is usually apparent at this point. The depth of insertion of the straightened instrument is variable according to the age of the patient: 70–80 cm in a teenager down to 25 cm in a small infant. During withdrawal the splenic flexure or descending colon are found at appropriately shorter distances. During insertion, in mobile colons and if any loops have been formed, these distance rules may not apply, but if the room is darkened transillumination will show the position of the instrument tip.

To enter the terminal ileum it is necessary first to identify the bulge of the ileocecal valve, which may bubble or gush on deflation. The instrument tip is then pushed in just proximal to the bulge, angled in towards it and slowly withdrawn until a 'red-out' indicates embedding into the valve region, at which point air is insufflated to attempt to distend the ileum. Ileal mucosa is characteristically granular or nodulated by lymphoid hyperplasia, in contrast to the shiny surface and vascular pattern of the colon.

In infants under 1 year of age entry into the ileum may be impossible, either because the orifice is too narrow or because the dimensions of the cecum are too small to allow the instrument to make the necessary right-angle turn.

Examination

The colon is visualized to some extent during insertion of the instrument but active examination, biopsy or polypectomies are normally undertaken during withdrawal because the instrument is then straight and easy to maneuver, the view is better and the patient is more comfortable. At all stages during the examination, but particularly during withdrawal, it is best for the endoscopist to control the instrument himself, using a one-handed technique. Very active maneuvering of the controls, with rotation and to-and-fro movements of the shaft, allow a good view to be obtained of nearly all areas, although around acute bends and convoluted folds there may be some blind spots.

COLONOSCOPIC POLYPECTOMY

The principles of colonoscopic polypectomy are identical to those for proctosigmoidoscopic polypectomy, but it is particularly important that full coagulation of polyp stalk vessels is achieved before transection since any hemorrhage is difficult to control endoscopically. Most polyps in pediatric practice are hamartomatous, thin-stalked, and easy to coagulate. If a thick stalk (1 cm or more) is to be snared it may be wise to inject it with epinephrine (adrenaline) (1 ml of 1:100 000 solution), using a long Teflon sclerotherapy needle before applying the polypectomy snare.

6a–e Endoscopic snare wires are characteristically thick to guard against cutting too fast, but care should be taken not to apply excessive mechanical pressure before adequate electrocoagulation has occurred otherwise 'cheese cutting' of an uncoagulated stalk may occur with consequent hemorrhage. A low-power coagulating current (15–25 W) is employed until local whitening or swelling of the stalk indicates adequate coagulation, at which point tight strangulation should result in severance of the head. If bleeding does occur the stalk remnant can be quickly regrasped with the loop and strangulated for 15 min, after which bleeding will not normally recur.

The correct position of the snare is shown in *Illustration 6a*. Care must be taken to avoid contact of the polyp surface with the opposite wall leading to burns from dissipation of the current (*Illustration 6b*). Burns may also result if the active electrode or metal components of the colonoscope tip are in contact with the local tissue (*Illustrations 6c* and *6d*) or if the electrode is in contact with a pool of fluid (*Illustration 6e*).

Small polyps up to 6–7 mm can be destroyed using plastic insulated 'hot biopsy' forceps which simultaneously obtain a small biopsy specimen. The smallest hamartomatous polyps (1–3-mm diameter) can be numerous and frequently disappear spontaneously, so that it may be safer to ignore them. Retrieval of the larger polyps can be achieved by grasping them with the polypectomy snare or by aspirating them on to the tip of the instrument which risks missing any other polyps during withdrawal unless the instrument is reinserted. Small polyps may be retrieved by aspirating them through the suction channel into a bronchial mucus trap placed in the suction line. Large numbers of polyps in patients with polyposis can be washed out after suction by passing the colonoscope proximal to them and infusing 500 ml saline into the colon through the suction channel, followed by a phosphate enema or stimulant suppository after the instrument has been withdrawn.

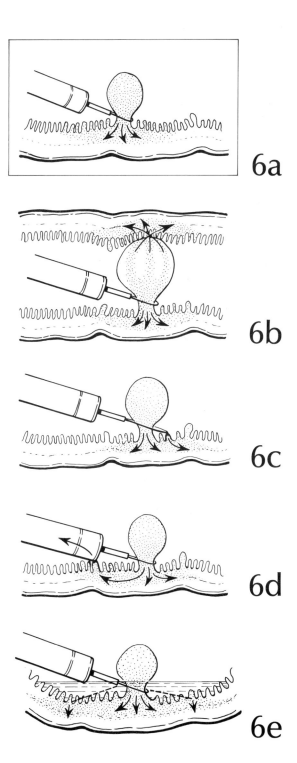

6a

6b

6c

6d

6e

OTHER THERAPEUTIC MANEUVERS

Electrocoagulation of telangiectases or cavernous hemangiomas (blue rubber-bleb nevus syndrome) is easy through the colonoscope. The use of laser photocoagulation for this purpose has been described but is probably unnecessary, since careful local electrocoagulation with hot biopsy forceps or judicious scleropathy of raised lesions, repeated as necessary, gives excellent results. Strictures, particularly anastomotic strictures after resection of Crohn's disease, can be successfully dilated with transendoscopic balloon dilators. The colonoscope can be used to introduce guide wires, tubes and other devices to any point in the colon, although this is rarely indicated in pediatric practice. The use of submucosally injected indian ink can be useful as a long-lasting marker. Surface irrigation with colorant (1:4 dilution of washable blue fountain pen ink is convenient) can be helpful in demonstrating the smallest lesions in conditions such as familial adenomatous polyposis.

Postoperative care

In most cases no special care is needed after colonoscopy, apart from a short period of rest until the after effects of sedation or anesthesia wear off. Food and drink can be taken immediately. When the patient appears and feels well normal activities can be resumed, many examinations being performed on a daycase basis.

Follow-up is probably unnecessary after colonoscopic polypectomy if only one to three juvenile polyps are present in the colon; larger numbers may suggest the possibility of juvenile polyposis which mandates follow-up because of the association with dysplastic foci. For subjects with Peutz–Jeghers polyposis colonoscopy is normally repeated every 2 years, often combined with gastroscopy as 'top and tail' endoscopy.

Complications

In normal children the elasticity of the colon means that the theoretical risk of bowel perforation during insertion of the instrument has not been observed in pediatric practice (in contradistinction to adult colonoscopy). The presence of severe acute inflammatory bowel disease with peritonism or deep ulceration, however, contraindicates examination because of the increased possibility of perforation; if unexpectedly severe ulceration is seen during colonoscopy it is wise to terminate the procedure as early as possible and to avoid excessive air insufflation. Even in a normal colon, if the procedure proves technically difficult common sense and humanity may nonetheless recommend abandonment of an examination; the percentage of failures to reach the cecum varies from 5% to 50% of all colonoscopies according to the skill and motivation of the examiner and whether or not there has been previous intra-abdominal surgery or sepsis. Neonatal examination is the most difficult. The highest percentage of complications occurs following therapeutic maneuvers such as snare polypectomy when both perforation and bleeding have been reported.

Rectal prolapse

Richard C. M. Cook MA, BM, FRCS
Consultant Paediatric Surgeon, Royal Liverpool Children's NHS Trust, Alder Hey, Liverpool, UK

Principles and justification

Children are said to be more susceptible than adults to rectal prolapse because of the vertical configuration of the pelvis and sacrum, but it remains a rare condition in the otherwise healthy child. Pelvic floor weakness due to neurogenic disorders leads to prolapse in many children with myelomeningocele or sacral agenesis. Prolapse is sometimes precipitated by straining at stool due to diarrhea, constipation, 'worms', rectal polyps, or too early and overzealous toilet training. Loss of weight (specifically perirectal fat loss) is blamed for prolapse in children with cystic fibrosis and other malabsorption syndromes, although the voluminous stools and the chronic cough of the former must also play a part. Pertussis and pulmonary tuberculosis are not uncommonly complicated by prolapse for similar reasons.

Assessment of children presenting with a prolapse must always include a general history and physical examination to exclude these etiologic factors. A sweat test or gene probe is strongly advised because rectal prolapse may be the presenting symptom of cystic fibrosis[1].

Rectal prolapse in the absence of systemic illness or specific abnormality has a peak incidence in the second and third years of life. Boys and girls are equally affected. The prolapse occurs only on defecation at first but may descend at other times later. The mother can usually reduce it easily, although this often happens spontaneously soon after defecation. If it remains outside it becomes edematous and there may be a discharge of blood and mucus.

Appearance

1 It is most commonly an incomplete mucosal prolapse protruding 2–3 cm from the anus and displaying radial folds.

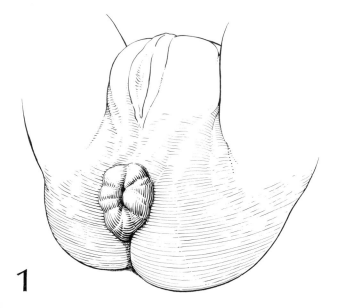

1

2 A complete prolapse of all the layers is more rare. The mucosal folds are said to be circumferential but this distinction is lost in both types of prolapse after about 1 h, when the mucosa become edematous, smooth and featureless. The size and palpable thickness of the wall of the prolapse will differentiate the two.

The distinction, however, is not necessarily important in planning treatment. After reduction of a prolapse, digital rectal examination usually reveals no abnormality but polyps should be felt for (even if not obvious on the prolapsed portion) and the sacrum checked for any deformity or agenesis.

Management

Management of rectal prolapse in childhood may be non-operative or the patient may undergo surgery.

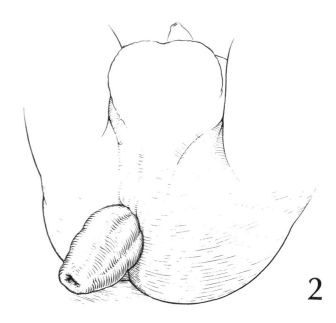

Non-operative treatment

In the absence of generalized disease that predisposes to prolapse, treatment should be supportive, optimistic and minimal. Efforts are directed at correcting bowel habits in the following ways: (1) by prescribing an aperient (e.g. lactulose); (2) by encouraging a diet containing more vegetable and cereal fiber; and (3) by ensuring that defecation is prompt, quick and performed in a sitting position. Prolonged straining and squatting must be avoided.

If this fails, support to the perianal region during defecation should be added to the above regimen. Most simply this consists of the mother holding the child out with her hands under the buttocks, fingers just inside the ischial tuberosities beside the anus.

3 More prolonged support can be given by strapping the buttocks together. A wide piece of strapping is stuck to each buttock and left for as long as possible. Two narrower strips are put across, stuck to the permanent pieces. These are left in position during defecation but removed afterwards to cleanse the perianal region before being replaced with new lengths.

Preoperative

Under general anesthesia initial digital rectal examination and proctoscopy are performed. If the rectum is loaded with hard stools these should be digitally evacuated. The perianal region and anal canal are then carefully cleansed with an aqueous agent.

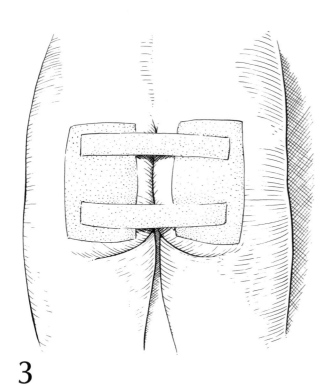

Operations

INJECTION OF MUCOSAL PROLAPSE[2]

4 With one index finger in the anal canal a long 23-gauge needle is guided in the submucosal plane to the lower rectum 4–5 cm from the anal verge, and 1–2 ml 5% phenol in almond oil is injected in each of the four quadrants.

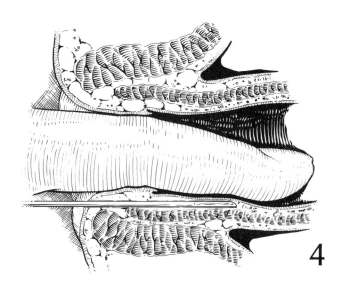

4

5

THIERSCH OPERATION (MODIFIED)

The rectum and lower colon must be cleared before operation by the use of suppositories and/or washouts. After induction of anesthesia, sigmoidoscopy is performed to rule out the presence of rectal polyps. The child is placed in the lithotomy position and the perianal region and the anal canal are cleansed.

5 Two small radial incisions are made, each 2 cm from the anal verge, at 12 and 6 o'clock. Using a fully curved aneurysm needle, a length of 1 catgut is threaded from posterior to anterior incisions around the anus just deep to the external sphincter muscle. The needle is rethreaded and the catgut pulled from anterior to posterior around the other side of the anal canal.

6   With an assistant's finger, or a no. 10 or 11 Hegar's dilator held in the anal canal, the catgut is pulled and tied inside the posterior incision. Fine catgut or other absorbable sutures are used to close the two incisions.

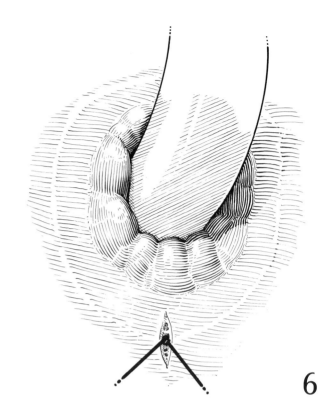

6

Postoperative care

After injection treatment the child can usually be allowed home on the same day and early resumption of normal bowel habits is encouraged as in non-operative management.

After the Thiersch operation mild aperients and appropriate dietary measures are used to ensure easy passage of a soft stool. The catgut will be absorbed within a few weeks but leaves sufficient reaction to support the bowel.

Complications

The injection treatment may be followed by infection and a perianal abscess if careful cleansing is not carried out, or if too much of the sclerosant is injected, if it is put too deeply, or if the rectal mucosa is perforated by the needle. Such infection usually settles without major problems but can cause serious scarring and deformity of the anal canal, allowing leakage of mucus, or may lead to the development of a fistula.

After the Thiersch operation breakdown of the skin wounds and exposure of the knots in the suture may occur if these are not buried deeply enough. If the Thiersch suture is tied too tightly and adequate bowel actions do not occur, stool retention and fecal impaction can follow.

Outcome

Recurrence is unusual, although about 5–10% of children will have further prolapse after injection therapy. The injection may be repeated 4–6 weeks later. Cauterization, rectosigmoidectomy and fixation of the rectum in the presacral space have all been advocated for persistent or severe prolapse in childhood, but in the author's experience have never proved necessary. They are well described in textbooks of adult surgery[3].

References

1. Stern RC, Izant RJ, Boat TF, Wood RE, Matthews LW, Doershuk CF. Treatment and prognosis of rectal prolapse in cystic fibrosis. *Gastroenterology* 1982; 82: 707–10.

2. Wyllie GG. The injection treatment of rectal prolapse. *J Pediatr Surg* 1979; 14: 62–4.

3. Fielding LP, Goldberg SM (eds). *Rob and Smith's Operative Surgery: Surgery of the Colon, Rectum and Anus*, 5th edn. London: Butterworths, 1993.

Management of portal hypertension

Frederick M. Karrer MD
Associate Professor of Surgery, The Children's Hospital and University of Colorado School of Medicine, Denver, Colorado, USA

Kennith H. Sartorelli MD
Instructor in Surgery, The Children's Hospital and University of Colorado School of Medicine, Denver, Colorado, USA

John R. Lilly MD
Professor of Surgery, The Children's Hospital and University of Colorado School of Medicine, Denver, Colorado, USA

1 Although portal hypertension is less common in children than in adults, the major clinical manifestations are identical, namely esophageal variceal hemorrhage, ascites and hypersplenism. The etiology is often different from adults in whom cirrhosis, most commonly due to alcohol abuse, is the predominant cause. Portal hypertension in children is commonly due to extrahepatic obstruction from portal vein thrombosis. If cirrhosis is present, it is usually caused by biliary atresia, chronic active hepatitis or metabolic liver diseases.

Management is related to the underlying cause of the portal hypertension. In children with intrahepatic disease, management is usually temporary, stabilizing measures until liver transplantation can be performed. Consequently, over the last decade the use of traditional shunts and non-decompressive operations has been increasingly replaced by endoscopic techniques followed by liver transplantation. The therapeutic options for children with extrahepatic portal vein obstruction must be tempered by the usual finding of normal hepatic synthetic function and by evidence that natural shunts develop over time, which often decompress the portal system. Management of the variceal hemorrhage in this group should provide long-term relief from bleeding with minimal long-term side effects. Extrahepatic obstruction in children has been treated successfully by both endoscopic techniques and shunts. In some circumstances, approaches directed at interruption of the varices (i.e. esophageal transection or Sugiura's procedure) are the only options but these procedures have had limited use in children.

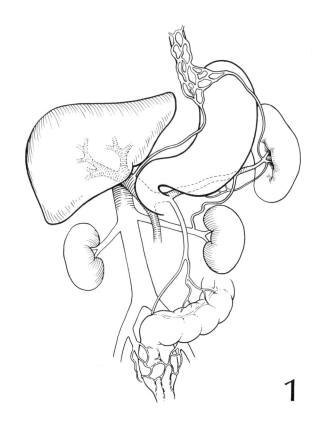

1

History

2   Injection of esophageal varices with sclerosant solutions was originally described in 1939, but was overshadowed by the widespread and successful application of portosystemic shunting. After Terblanche[1] published his impressive results in 1979, sclerotherapy was revived. Subsequent series of endosclerosis in children documented efficacy equal to that reported by Terblanche[2]. Initially, rigid esophagoscopy was used, but improvements in flexible endoscopic equipment have enabled most sclerotherapy to be performed using multichannel fiberoptic gastroscopes.

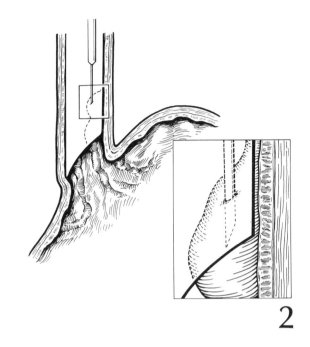

2

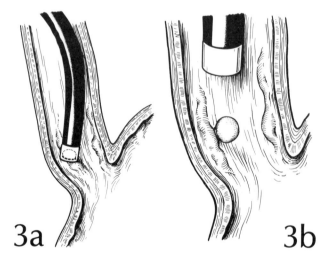

3a   3b

Endoscopic variceal ligation

3   Because of the occasional long-term complications of endosclerosis, endoscopic variceal ligation was developed by adapting techniques used for hemorrhoidal banding. Investigations in animals showed that the varices were eradicated by a process of strangulation, obliterating submucosal venous channels without involving the muscularis propria of the esophageal wall. Application of this technique in adults has resulted in good control of acute variceal hemorrhage and prevented recurrent bleeding with minimal treatment-related morbidity[3].

Portosystemic shunts

4 Operations designed to reduce portal pressure by diversion of blood from the portal to the systemic venous system were the mainstay of treatment for portal hypertension for over 30 years. Many different shunt procedures have been devised and a description of each is beyond the scope of this chapter. The two most commonly performed shunts in children are the mesocaval shunt and the central splenorenal shunt because they may be performed in children with portal vein occlusion (extrahepatic portal hypertension). Clatworthy's classic mesocaval shunt was designed specifically for children in whom the portal vein is not usable because of portal vein thrombosis. It is also easier to perform than some other shunts because the veins used are larger; occasionally, however, interruption of the inferior vena cava, which is necessary in the end-to-side type of mesocaval shunt, may result in venous stasis of the lower extremities. The interposition graft mesocaval shunt was developed to avoid this problem. Traditionally, the central splenorenal shunt was accompanied by splenectomy and exposed the patient to the risk of overwhelming postsplenectomy sepsis. More recently a side-to-side anastomosis of the splenic and renal vein has been used which avoids splenectomy and makes the procedure somewhat more attractive[4].

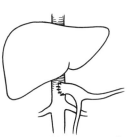
End-to-side portacaval

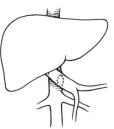
Side-to-side portacaval

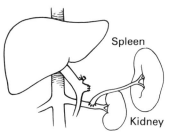
Distal splenorenal (Warren)

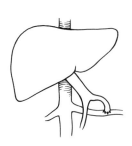
Proximal splenorenal

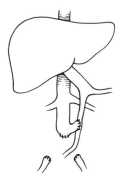
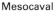
Mesocaval

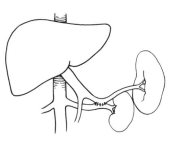
Side-to-side splenorenal

4

Principles and justification

Portosystemic shunts provide a means of decompressing the high-pressure portal system and thus esophageal varices. There is no question that shunt procedures are effective in reducing the incidence of variceal bleeding but the procedures have disadvantages: (1) hepatic encephalopathy may deprive the liver of trophic factors and develop as a consequence of diversion of portal venous blood into the systemic circulation; (2) a portoprival state, from diversion of portal blood flow from the liver, may accelerate hepatic deterioration; (3) the procedure or complications thereof may make future liver transplantation more difficult; and (4) in children, the small size of the portal, splenic and mesenteric veins increases the technical difficulty, resulting in a higher rate of thrombosis, shunt failure and rebleeding. The advent of endoscopic therapy and transplantation has reduced the role of shunts in treatment of portal hypertension in children. Shunt procedures are now generally considered only in cirrhotic patients who are *not* candidates for liver transplantation, in children with extrahepatic portal hypertension in whom endoscopic treatments have been tried and failed, or in those who have hemorrhage below the level of the esophagus (i.e. gastric, small intestine or colonic varices) for whom endoscopic control is not possible.

Transection and reanastomosis of the esophagus

Interruption of the submucosal esophageal veins responsible for variceal hemorrhage may be accomplished by transection of the lower esophagus and reanastomosis, usually using an end-to-end stapling device. This has the advantages of being quicker and simpler than transesophageal ligation of varices or division of the lower esophagus and reanastomosis using conventional surgical instruments and techniques, because the stapler divides and creates an anastomosis simultaneously, forming an inverted anastomosis approximated by a circular double staggered row of stainless steel sutures.

Esophageal transection is generally indicated for treatment of uncontrollable or massive recurrent variceal bleeding. Patients in whom endoscopic techniques have failed or are not feasible, and those in whom the major splanchnic veins (portal, splenic and superior mesenteric) are thrombosed and are therefore precluded from the option of portosystemic shunting, are also candidates.

Esophageal transection and reanastomosis interrupts the submucosal esophageal veins as well as the intramuscular venous collaterals and should always control esophageal variceal hemorrhage. Bleeding from gastric, duodenal or colonic varices is a contraindication for esophageal transection. Unfortunately, this procedure has a transient effect as portal pressure is not reduced and the rebleeding rate is high. In these circumstances liver transplantation is required.

Sugiura's procedure

Sugiura's procedure consists of lower esophageal transection and anastomosis, devascularization of the lower esophagus and stomach and splenectomy[5]. It was devised to avoid many of the complications of portosystemic shunts. However, Sugiura's excellent results have been difficult to reproduce worldwide, and experience in children is limited.

Sugiura's procedure remains an option for controlling esophageal varices due to intrahepatic or extrahepatic portal hypertension when endoscopic methods fail and portosystemic shunts are not possible.

Preoperative

The initial presentation of children with portal hypertension due to portal vein thrombosis is usually gastrointestinal hemorrhage – typically, sudden massive hematemesis. Occasionally, bleeding may be more insidious and melenic stools are observed. Conversely, in children with portal hypertension due to cirrhosis (e.g. biliary atresia) the diagnosis of liver disease is usually known and signs of liver disease (jaundice, ascites, splenomegaly) are present. In either case, initial management of gastrointestinal bleeding consists of volume resuscitation and stabilization. Two large-bore intravenous catheters should be placed for rapid administration of fluids and blood products as needed. A nasogastric tube is placed for evacuation of bloody gastric contents. Children rarely require balloon tamponade for control of variceal bleeding because most of these stop spontaneously. Cirrhotic patients may require replacement of coagulation factors and parenteral vitamin K. The upper gastrointestinal tract should be evaluated early using endoscopy to separate those bleeding from varices from those bleeding from unusual causes (peptic ulcer, gastritis, Mallory–Weiss tear).

Patients undergoing portosystemic shunt procedures should be stable and not actively bleeding. The source of hemorrhage from varices should be documented endoscopically. In addition to a complete blood count, liver function tests and coagulation studies, the patient should undergo radiologic studies to demonstrate the patency and adequacy of the portal, mesenteric and splenic veins.

Patients about to undergo transection and reanastomosis of the esophagus should undergo temporary control using gastroesophageal tamponade (with a Sengstaken–Blakemore tube). Adequate restoration of blood volume is essential.

Anesthesia

General endotracheal anesthesia is preferred. In adults, endosclerosis may be performed using intravenous sedation but the authors' experience in children has been entirely under general anesthesia. The endotracheal tube is fixed to the left side of the mouth.

Operations

RIGID ENDOSCLEROSIS

Position of patient

The patient is placed in a supine position.

5 The technique as originally described uses a slotted rigid esophagoscope. The esophagoscope is passed under direct vision through the cricopharyngeus into the stomach and withdrawn into the distal esophagus. The varix to be injected is identified and positioned in the slot. A long, 26-gauge injection needle is passed after purging with sclerosant. Sodium morrhuate (5%) is probably the most commonly used sclerosant in the USA; ethanolamine oleate is widely used in Europe.

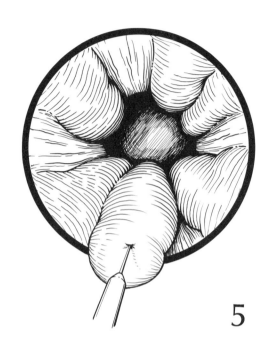

5

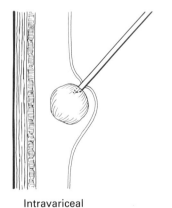

Intravariceal

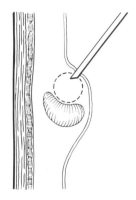

Paravariceal

6

6 Two techniques for sclerotherapy have been described: intravariceal and paravariceal. The authors prefer direct intravariceal injection because it is associated with better control of acute variceal bleeding. Paravariceal injection, designed to eradicate the submucosal space and compress the varix extrinsically, is more commonly used in Europe and Japan. After injection, the varix is immediately compressed by rotating the esophagoscope. Ordinarily, no more than three varices are injected at each session. If necessary, endosclerosis may be repeated 48 h later, but usually it should be repeated every few weeks until the varices are obliterated. The interval between the endoscopic sessions is gradually lengthened but continued surveillance at biennial or annual examinations is necessary because early recurrence is not uncommon.

FLEXIBLE ENDOSCLEROSIS

7 Flexible endoscopy has been used with equal success to rigid endosclerosis. Visualization is improved because the optical systems are superior. Flexible endoscopy also permits inspection of the stomach and duodenum, which is not possible with the rigid endoscope. The techniques are similar, except that the needle is flexible and sheathed.

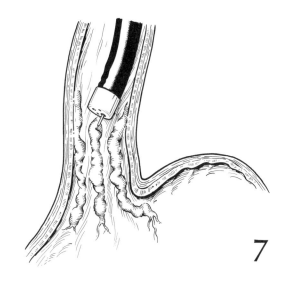

7

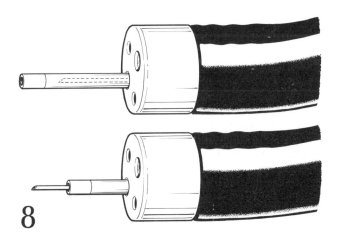

8

8 The needle is passed through the biopsy channel of the endoscope. The sheath is withdrawn, and the needle advanced under direct vision to the desired injection site (intravariceal or paravariceal) before sclerosant is injected. After injection the endoscope may be advanced into the stomach but the ability to compress the varix after injection is negligible.

ENDOSCOPIC VARICEAL LIGATION

9a–d The endoscopic ligating device consists of two fitted cylinders attached to the tip of a standard flexible endoscope. The inner cylinder has a small elastic O ring stretched over it which is released with a trip wire running through the biopsy channel of the endoscope. The inner cylinder has 1-mm calibrations which are visible through the endoscope. The endoscope is passed under direct vision into the distal esophagus. A varix is identified and tented into the cylinder by applying mild suction. When the varix is 2 mm within the cylinder the trip wire is pulled, withdrawing the inner cylinder into the outer cylinder and releasing the O ring to constrict the base of the varix. This results in strangulation of the varix and thombosis of the adjacent vein. Between one and three elastic band ligatures may be placed at each session. The bands and the varices slough off in 5–7 days.

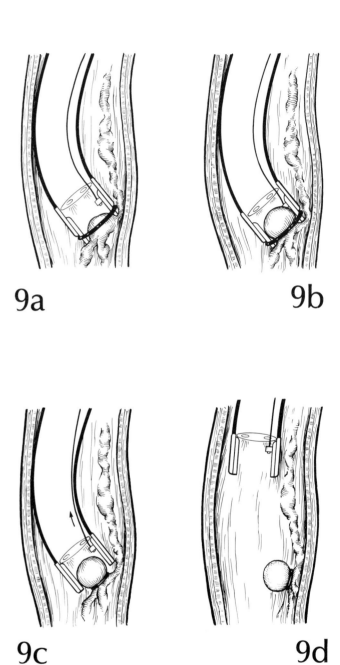

9a

9b

9c

9d

MESOCAVAL SHUNT

Exposure

10 A midline incision is preferred, to avoid interference with venous collaterals in the abdominal wall. The transverse mesocolon is retracted cephalad and the small intestine retracted inferiorly. A vertical incision is made in the mesentery of the small intestine over the superior mesenteric vein, which lies to the right of the artery. The veins in the transverse mesocolon may be followed to help identify the superior mesenteric vein, which is dissected free for about 5 cm inferior to the pancreas.

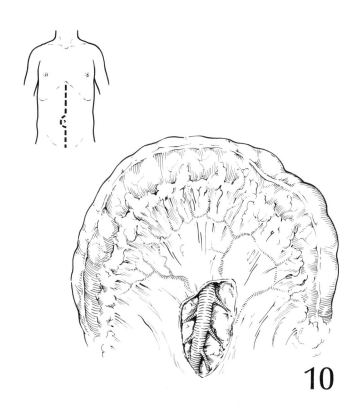

10

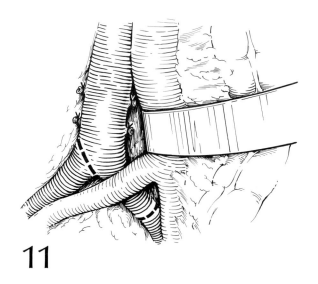

11

11 The inferior vena cava is exposed by mobilizing the right mesocolon. The duodenum is reflected by a Kocher maneuver. After exposure the inferior vena cava is mobilized from the renal veins to below the caval bifurcation. Individual ligation of several lumbar veins is often required. A tunnel is made in the retroperitoneum and posterior mesentery, often thick and edematous, to reach the superior mesenteric vein.

Anastomosis

12 At this stage, a critical decision must be made about the length of vein necessary to reach to the superior mesenteric vein. It is usually advisable to extend the inferior vena cava by dividing the right or left iliac vein at some distance below the junction with the inferior vena cava. The other iliac vein is oversewn flush with the bifurcation. The cava-iliac vein is fashioned to the appropriate length after passing it through the tunnel described previously.

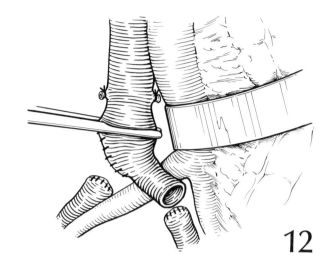

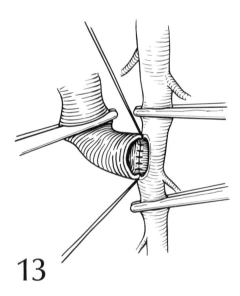

13 A small ellipse is cut in the superior mesenteric vein before anastomosis using fine continuous suture (6/0 polypropylene). The retroperitoneum and mesentery are reapproximated with a few absorbable sutures.

14 An alternative procedure utilizes an interposition graft between the superior mesenteric vein and the inferior vena cava. Although synthetic vascular grafts have been used, a graft of internal jugular vein appears to offer the best chance of long-term patency.

Wound closure

The abdomen is closed in a watertight fashion without drains.

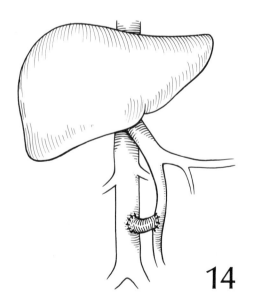

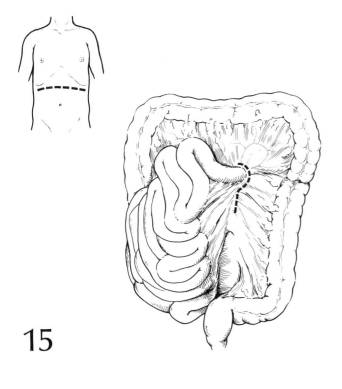

15

SIDE-TO-SIDE SPLENORENAL SHUNT

Exposure

15 A wide transverse upper abdominal incision is made. The transverse mesocolon is retracted cephalad and the small intestine to the right, to expose the duodenum. The ligament of Treitz is incised and the inferior mesenteric vein divided at its junction with the splenic vein. This allows the duodenojejunal junction to be swept cephalad and to the right. The renal vein is exposed from the kidney hilus to the inferior vena cava.

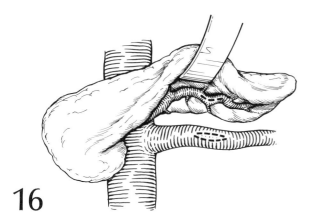

16

16 The left gonadal and adrenal veins are ligated and divided. At the base of the transverse mesocolon the pancreas is exposed and the inferior edge dissected transversely. In long-standing portal hypertension the retroperitoneum may be edematous and thick and may contain numerous small spontaneous collateral veins. Cephalad traction on the transverse colon will rotate the pancreas along its long axis to expose the splenic vein. The splenic vein is dissected and small tributaries divided for 4–5 cm. Numerous small pancreatic veins must be carefully and securely ligated and divided. The coronary vein is ligated and divided.

Anastomosis

17 Vascular clamps are placed on the splenic vein. The left renal vein is partially occluded using a Satinsky clamp. The splenic vein is opened transversely in its most dependent portion, if necessary extending the opening into the stump of the inferior mesenteric vein to create a larger anastomosis. The renal vein is opened in matching fashion. The anastomosis is performed with loop magnification using fine vascular suture (6/0 polypropylene). The posterior wall is completed first, then the anterior wall. The completed anastomosis should be 1.5–2.5 cm in length.

Wound closure

The retroperitoneum is closed with absorbable sutures and the incision closed in layers without drains.

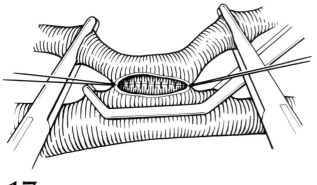

17

TRANSECTION AND REANASTOMOSIS OF ESOPHAGUS

Exposure

18 The abdomen is opened through a midline incision and the left triangular ligament of the liver divided to expose the gastroesophageal junction. The peritoneum of the anterior esophageal hiatus is opened, the vagus nerves freed and preserved and the lower esophagus encircled with a Penrose drain.

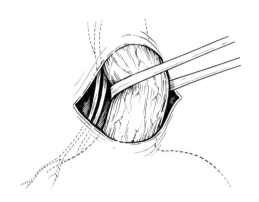

18

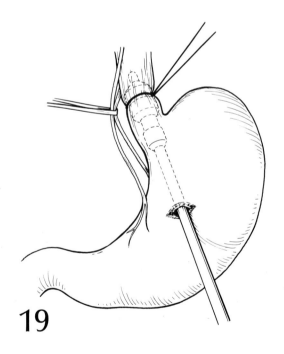

19

19 Through an anterior gastrotomy, the stapling instrument is positioned in the lower esophagus just above the gastroesophageal junction. A heavy suture is tied tightly between the instrument's cartridge and anvil. When the device is fired, the esophagus is simultaneously transected and stapled. If the stapler is used correctly, a complete ring of esophagus will be exicsed.

Wound closure

The anterior gastrotomy is closed in layers and the abdomen closed without drains.

SUGIURA'S PROCEDURE

Exposure

With the patient in a right lateral decubitus position, a left seventh interspace thoracotomy is employed to provide access to the lower esophagus and a left subcostal incision is used to expose the stomach and spleen.

Esophageal devascularization

20 Exposure of the esophagus from the hiatus to above the inferior pulmonary ligament is accomplished by dividing the mediastinal pleura anterior to the aorta. The vagal trunks are freed but not divided. Venous branches from the paraesophageal veins and all arterial and vagal branches to the esophagus are ligated and divided while preserving the paraesophageal veins. The mobilization and devascularization extends from the inferior pulmonary vein through the esophageal hiatus as far as possible. The diaphragm is opened radially, beginning 2–3 cm posterior to the phrenic nerve. Multiple suture ligatures are placed along the edge of the diaphragm to provide hemostasis and exposure.

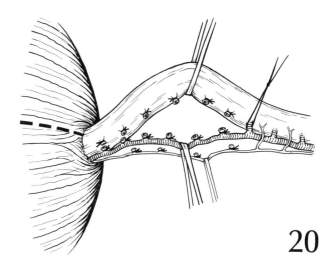

20

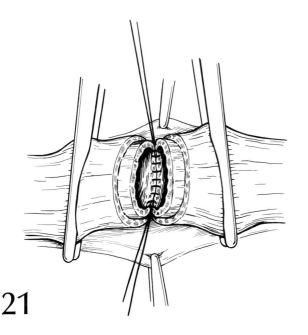

21

Division of the esophagus

21 Non-crushing clamps are applied across the esophagus 3 cm proximal to the cardioesophageal junction. The anterior muscular layer of the esophagus is divided. The posterior muscular esophageal wall is preserved. A mucosal and submucosal sleeve is developed circumferentially and is then divided and reapproximated. Anastomosis is accomplished by placing triangulating sutures followed by multiple closely placed, fine absorbable sutures which also ligate varices. The muscular wall is then reapproximated and the clamps removed.

Splenectomy and gastric devascularization

22 The abdomen is opened and the lateral segment of the left hepatic lobe mobilized by taking down the left triangular ligament. Splenectomy is performed. Proximal gastric devascularization is performed by interrupting all of the small vessels from the gastroepiploic artery to the proximal gastric greater curve. The proximal lesser gastric curve is devascularized by dividing branches from the coronary vein and the paraesophageal veins to the stomach. The devascularization extends 6–7 cm distally from the gastroesophageal junction.

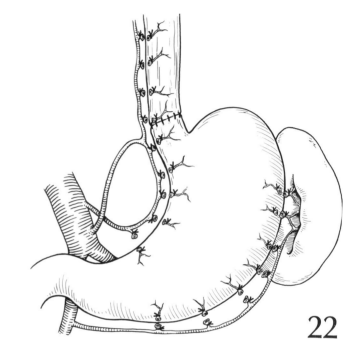

22

Wound closure

The mediastinal pleura is closed, and suction drains placed next to the esophageal anastomosis and brought out under the diaphragm. The diaphragm is closed in two layers with interrupted non-absorbable sutures. The thoracotomy is closed in the standard manner and a thoracostomy tube employed. The abdomen is closed in layers without drains.

Postoperative care

Children treated by endosclerosis for acute hemorrhage must be monitored closely for ongoing or recurrent bleeding. Once initial control has been achieved, follow-up endosclerosis may be performed on an ambulatory outpatient basis. Postoperatively, many patients experience low-grade fever and may have mild retrosternal discomfort. Severe chest pain and hyperpyrexia may indicate esophageal perforation (this is rare) and should initiate chest radiography and a contrast study. Ulceration at the injection site is common and is sometimes associated with mild self-limited hemorrhage a few days after the procedure.

If banding has been performed for acute variceal hemorrhage and bleeding persists, endoscopic variceal ligation may be repeated 24–48 h later. If there is no further bleeding, repeat endoscopy is delayed 2–4 weeks. Once the initial bleeding episode is controlled the patient enters a program of surveillance esophagoscopy and repeat endoscopic variceal ligation at intervals that are gradually extended to 6–12 months. If bleeding recurs the interval is shortened and the cycle repeated. Postoperative fever, chest pain and delayed bleeding are less common than with endosclerosis. The only perforation that has occurred in the authors' experience was caused by the use of an overtube which tore the cervical esophagus: the use of an overtube in pediatric patients has since been abandoned.

For all portosystemic shunt procedures, nasogastric decompression should be maintained until normal bowel function returns. Peptic ulcer prophylaxis is routine. Early ambulation and use of elastic stockings may prevent lower extremity edema which is seen occasionally after end-to-side mesocaval shunts. Vitamin K supplementation may be indicated based on prothrombin times. Dietary protein should initially be restricted and advanced only gradually to prevent hepatic encephalopathy. Ascites, which is common, may require salt restriction, diuretics and administration of exogenous albumin.

Following transection and reanastomosis of the esophagus or the Sugiura procedure, nasogastric suction is maintained until the adynamic ileus is completely resolved.

Broad-spectrum perioperative antibiotics are administered. Suction drains should be retained until there is no evidence of esophageal leakage.

Outcome

The authors' results and those of others have shown good control of variceal hemorrhage using endosclerosis in children, with regular surveillance sclerosis as needed to eradicate varices[2,6,7]. Especially in children with portal vein obstruction, the tendency towards variceal hemorrhage decreases with time, as spontaneous natural retroperitoneal shunts develop. Death is rare, except when related to cirrhosis and liver failure. Some authors have reported alterations in esophageal motility, esophageal strictures and even esophageal cancer after repeated endosclerosis.

The control of hemorrhage and eradication of varices obtained using endoscopic variceal ligation has been equal to or better than that obtained using endoscopic sclerotherapy. The authors have not encountered development of strictures or motility disturbances using endoscopic variceal ligation and now use the technique almost exclusively for endoscopic treatment of variceal hemorrhage.

A properly performed portosystemic shunt is almost invariably effective in controlling bleeding varices; however, because of the size of the vessels and therefore the propensity to thrombosis, rebleeding rates of 10–25% have been reported. The incidence of encephalopathy is difficult to estimate because different standards have been used to determine its presence and severity. In children with extrahepatic portal vein thrombosis the risk of encephalopathy is reported to be low, but in the cirrhotic group encephalopathy is directly related to liver synthetic function. The long-term prognosis for children undergoing portosystemic shunts also largely depends on the severity of hepatic dysfunction.

Recently, use of non-operative shunts has been gaining popularity in adults[8]. The transjugular intrahepatic portosystemic stent shunts have not yet been widely applied to children but avoid some of the surgical complications and should not interfere with future liver transplantation. Until these techniques have been miniaturized for children and clear benefits have been demonstrated, they should be considered investigational only.

Urgent or emergency esophageal transection is associated with a high mortality rate (related more to the underlying liver disease and poor preoperative condition of the patient than the procedure itself). Technical complications of leaks or stenosis are uncommon since the introduction of the EEA stapling devices but recurrent variceal hemorrhage occurs in 15–50% of patients.

Experience with Sugiura's procedure in children is limited. Control of variceal hemorrhage in 80% of patients with no operative mortality has been reported in one series[9]. Results in adults have been less gratifying, with recurrent variceal hemorrhage rates of up to 50% and morbidity and mortality rates of up to 33% having been reported.

Acknowledgments

The authors are supported in part by a grant (RR-69) from the General Clinical Research Centers Program at the Division of Research Resources, National Institutes of Health and the Pediatric Liver Center, University of Colorado/The Children's Hospital, Denver, Colorado.

References

1. Terblanche J, Northover JMA, Bornman P *et al.* A prospective controlled trial of sclerotherapy in the long term management of patients after esophageal variceal bleeding. *Surg Gynecol Obstet* 1979; 148: 323–33.

2. Lilly JR. Endoscopic sclerosis of esophageal varices in children. *Surg Gynecol Obstet* 1981; 152: 513–14.

3. Stiegman GV, Goff JJS, Michaletz-Onody PA *et al.* Endoscopic sclerotherapy as compared with endoscopic ligation for bleeding esophageal varices. *N Engl J Med* 1992; 326: 1527–32.

4. Orloff MJ, Orloff MS, Rambotti M. Treatment of bleeding esophagogastric varices due to extrahepatic portal hypertension: result of portal-systemic shunts during 35 years. *J Pediatr Surg* 1994; 29: 142–54.

5. Sugiura M, Futagawa S. A new technique for treating esophageal varices. *J Thorac Cardiovasc Surg* 1973; 66: 677–85.

6. Thapa BR, Mehta S. Endoscopic sclerotherapy of esophageal varices in infants and children. *J Pediatr Gastroenterol Nutr* 1990; 10: 430–4.

7. Howard ER, Stringer MD, Mowat AP. Assessment of injection sclerotherapy in the management of 152 children with oesophageal varices. *Br J Surg* 1988; 75: 404–8.

8. Richter GM, Noeldge, G, Palmaz JC, Roessle M. The transjugular intrahepatic portosystemic stent-shunt (TIPSS): results of a pilot study. *Cardiovasc Intervent Radiol* 1990; 13: 200–7.

9. Belloli G, Campobasso P, Musi L. Sugiura procedure in the surgical treatment of bleeding esophageal varices in children: long term results. *J Pediatr Surg* 1992; 27: 1422–6.

Surgery for biliary atresia

Edward R. Howard MS, FRCS
Consultant Paediatric and Hepatobiliary Surgeon, King's College Hospital, London, UK

History

Atresia of the extrahepatic bile ducts is the end result of a variable inflammatory process of unknown etiology which occurs before birth and which, if untreated, leads to death from cirrhotic liver failure. The incidence is between 0.8 and 1.0 per 10 000 births. Extrahepatic anomalies are associated with biliary atresia in approximately 20% of cases and the most common association (known as the polysplenia syndrome) comprises polysplenia, situs inversus and a preduodenal portal vein[1].

The patency of a proximal segment of the hepatic or common hepatic ducts is preserved in 10–15% of patients and bile may be aspirated from the duct during surgery. These rare variants were originally called 'correctable' cases because they could be treated with conventional biliary–enteric anastomoses such as hepaticojejunostomy.

Most cases, however, show obliteration of the extrahepatic bile ducts up to the capsule of the liver in the porta hepatis. Segments of the distal bile duct may remain patent, although without communication with the hepatic ducts, and in some cases injection of contrast material into the gallbladder may show free flow to the duodenum without filling of the proximal ducts. Occlusion of the proximal bile ducts was once believed to be surgically 'non-correctable' and the problems of treatment are reflected in reports of only 52 surgical successes between 1927 and 1970[2].

A new operation for biliary atresia was suggested by Kasai[3], who observed that excision of the obliterated bile duct remnants in the porta hepatis could result in bile drainage in a proportion of the patients with 'non-correctable' atresia. This operation is now known as portoenterostomy.

Classification

1 The historical division of biliary atresia into 'correctable' and 'non-correctable' types depending on the presence or absence of a residual segment of bile-containing proximal bile duct has been superseded by a classification which describes three major types of atresia. The Japanese Society of Paediatric Surgeons[4] has subdivided these main types to include details of the structure of the gallbladder and the distal bile ducts. These details have been omitted from the illustration as they have no influence on the results of surgical treatment.

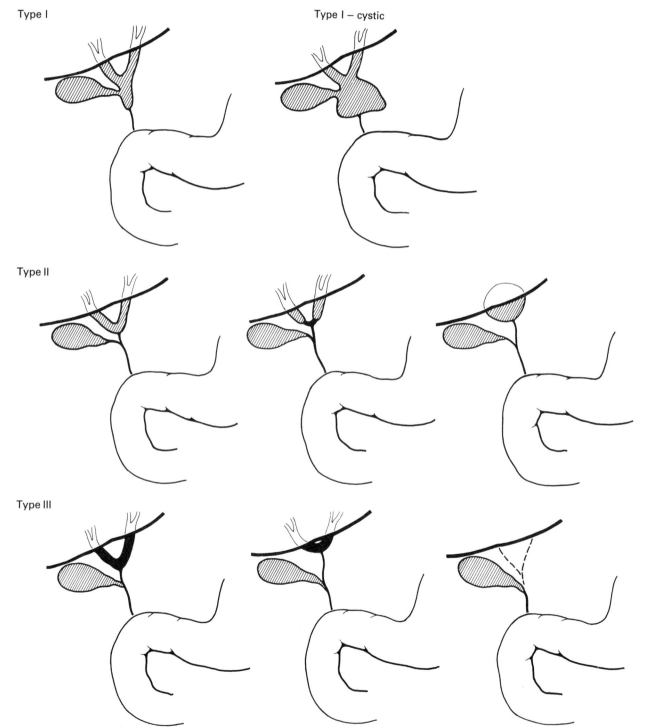

Type I

Type I – cystic

Type II

Type III

1

Diagnosis

The differential diagnosis of prolonged jaundice in neonates and infants includes giant cell hepatitis, intrahepatic bile duct hypoplasia, choledochal cyst, spontaneous perforation of the bile ducts and inspissated bile syndrome. Infection, metabolic abnormalities and α_1-antitrypsin deficiency may be detected as causes of neonatal hepatitis by appropriate screening tests, but the etiology is unknown in 70% of patients with intrahepatic cholestasis. These patients must be separated immediately from patients with surgical causes of jaundice.

Choledochal cysts, bile duct perforation and cases of obstruction from inspissated bile can be confidently diagnosed with ultrasonography and hepatobiliary scintigraphy using technetium-labeled iminodiacetic acid compounds. Liver function tests are of little value in differential diagnosis of atresia, but percutaneous liver biopsy is diagnostic in most cases. However, liver biopsies from patients with α_1-antitrypsin deficiency may be confused with atresia and it is essential to rule out this condition by α_1-antitrypsin phenotyping.

Other investigations useful for confirming the diagnosis of biliary atresia include laparoscopy combined with gallbladder cholangiography, endoscopic retrograde cholangiography and duodenal intubation (for the identification of bile). Unfortunately no single test is diagnostic in all cases, but two or more tests in combination usually differentiate biliary atresia from other causes of prolonged jaundice. Accurate preoperative diagnosis is imperative as the findings at laparotomy may be difficult to interpret or frankly misleading. It may be particularly difficult, for example, to identify small, proximal bile ducts in cases of biliary hypoplasia and the patency of such ducts may be difficult to determine even using operative cholangiography.

Preoperative

Vitamin K (phytomenadione, 1.0 mg/day) is administered intramuscularly for at least 4 days before surgery. Blood is cross-matched and oral neomycin (50 mg/kg/day) given, in six divided doses, for 24 h preoperatively. An adequate intravenous line is set up and a nasogastric tube inserted.

Antibiotics (cephalosporins) are given intravenously after induction of anaesthesia and should be continued for at least 5 days after surgery.

Operations

PORTOENTEROSTOMY

Originally the surgical management of suspected cases of biliary atresia was separated into two stages. The 'diagnostic' stage consisted of making a short transverse incision in the right hypochondrium, followed by operative cholangiography and liver biopsy. This was followed by definitive surgery a few days later. The author prefers to make the diagnosis using the techniques described above and to restrict surgery to only one procedure.

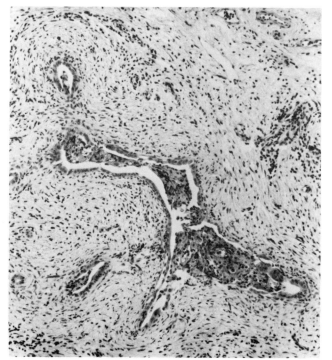

Haematoxylin and eosin, ×16. Courtesy of Dr M. Driver

2 Tissue excised from the porta hepatis during portoenterostomy shows epithelium-lined ductules which may measure up to 300 μm in diameter. Partial destruction and desquamation of the epithelium has occurred and the ductules are surrounded by fibrous tissue, which contains inflammatory cells.

3 Large ductules are often absent but serial section-
ing has shown that even small channels may
communicate with intrahepatic ducts. Biliary drainage is
achieved in the portoenterostomy operation by transecting these ductules and anastomosing a Roux-en-Y
loop of jejunum to the edges of the area of excision in
the porta hepatis. This operation is most effective in
patients under 6 weeks of age[5].

Position of patient

The patient is placed supine on a thermostatically
controlled heated operating table with facilities for
intraoperative cholangiography.

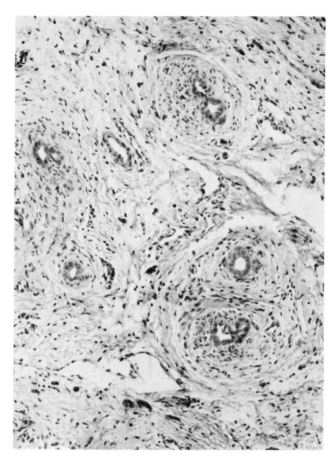

Haematoxylin and eosin, ×13. Courtesy of Dr M. Driver

3

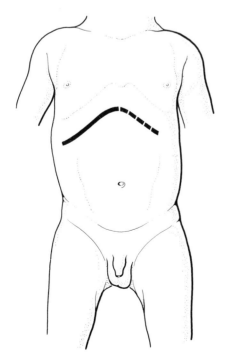

Incision

4 A bilateral subcostal incision, dividing the right and
left rectus muscles, exposes the inferior margin of
the liver. The appearance of the liver, and the presence
or absence of ascites and portal hypertension, are noted.
Associated anatomical anomalies (such as polysplenia,
asplenia, malrotation or preduodenal portal vein) will
be encountered in 15–20% of patients.

4

Cholangiography

5 Operative cholangiography via a gallbladder catheter is indicated either if the diagnosis remains in doubt following the preoperative examination or if bile is detected upon aspiration of the gallbladder. The presence of bile within the gallbladder is an absolute indication for radiographic studies of the biliary tract.

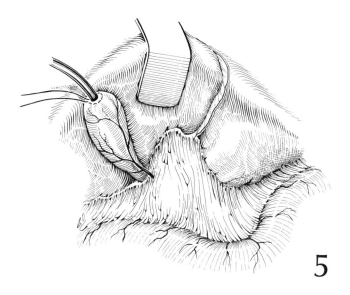

5

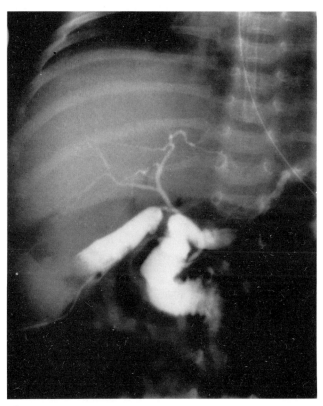

6

6 The demonstration of a patent common bile duct and a communication with intrahepatic ducts excludes a diagnosis of biliary atresia and terminates the operation.

7 In 20–25% of patients with biliary atresia the cystic and distal common bile ducts are patent and the duodenum will be opacified by injecting contrast material into the gallbladder. However, it is impossible to visualize the atretic proximal ducts even after occluding the supraduodenal portion of the bile duct with a soft clamp.

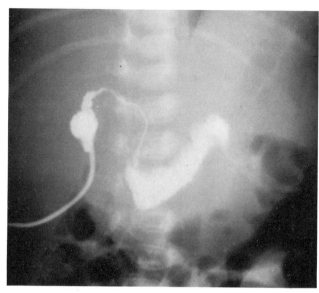

7

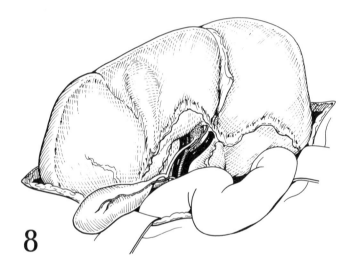

8

Mobilization of the liver

8 For accurate dissection in this operation it is imperative that the porta hepatis is clearly visualized. This is achieved by dividing the falciform and left and right triangular ligaments and completely mobilizing the liver. It is possible to evert the liver into the wound to expose the porta hepatis.

Mobilization of gallbladder and bile ducts

9 The remainder of the operation is more easily performed under magnification. The cystic artery, which is often enlarged, is ligated and divided and the gallbladder dissected from its bed. Care must be taken not to mistake the right hepatic artery for the cystic artery. The mobilized gallbladder is used as a guide to the fibrous remnant of the common bile duct, which may be partially obscured by thickened peritoneum and enlarged lymph nodes.

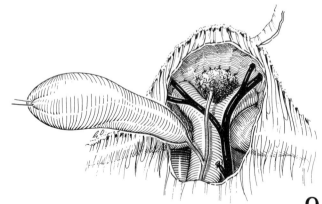

9

Dissection and exposure of porta hepatis

10 The lower end of the common bile duct is divided between ligatures at the upper border of the duodenum and the upper portion, with the gallbladder attached, is dissected upwards above the bifurcation of the portal vein. The portal vein and the hepatic arteries are exposed along their whole course until they disappear within the liver substance.

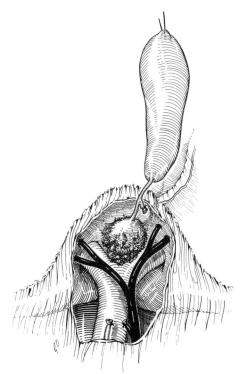

10

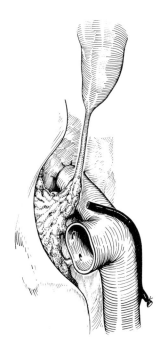

11

11 Clear identification and mobilization of the bifurcation of the portal vein is essential and may necessitate ligation and division of small venous radicles to the caudate lobe of the liver. Enlarged lymphatics should be ligated meticulously to prevent postoperative ascites caused by leakage of lymphatic fluid.

Excision of bile duct remnants

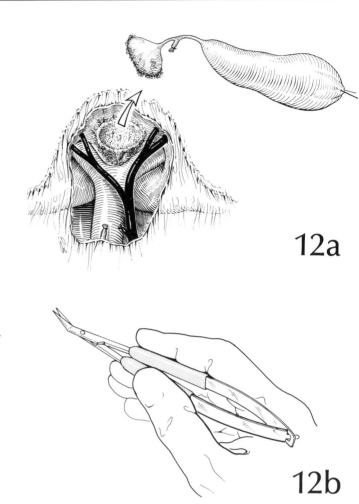

12a, b The remnant of the bile duct and the gallbladder are removed after transecting the fibrous tissue in the porta hepatis. The plane of transection is flush with, and outside, the liver capsule or 'portal plate'. All residual tissue is removed within the area bounded by the right and left branches of the portal vein and the accompanying hepatic arteries. The transection can be performed very accurately using angled scissors designed specifically for this stage of the operation[5].

Inferiorly the transection should extend behind the posterior surface of the portal vein. Bleeding points are controlled with direct pressure: diathermy could damage the small biliary ductules on the undersurface of the liver and should not be used.

12a

12b

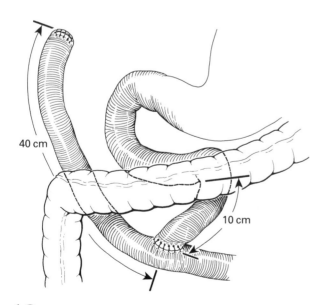

13

Preparation and anastomosis of Roux-en-Y loop

13 A 40-cm Roux-en-Y loop is prepared by transecting the jejunum approximately 10 cm distal to the duodenojejunal flexure. The distal end is oversewn and passed in a retrocolic position to the hilum of the liver. Continuity of the small bowel is established with an end-to-side enteroenterostomy.

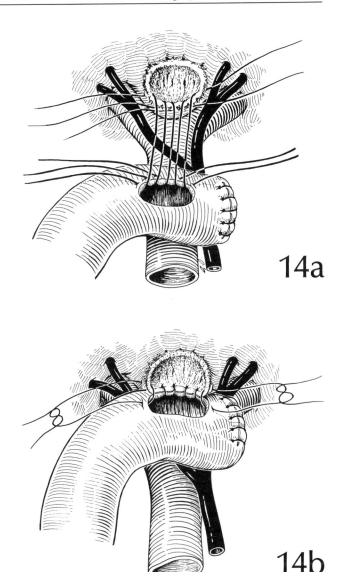

14a, b An anastomosis is fashioned between the edge of the transected area in the porta hepatis and the side of the Roux loop using sutures of 5/0 polydioxanone. The anastomosis is achieved by inserting the whole of the posterior row of sutures before tying them. The jejunal loop is then 'railroaded' into position and the sutures are tied in series. An anterior row of sutures completes the anastomosis. A small drain is placed down to the porta hepatis and a needle biopsy of the right lobe of the liver taken before closing the abdomen.

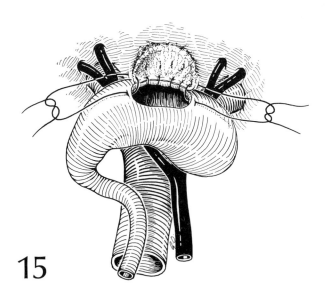

CHOLECYSTPORTOENTEROSTOMY

15 Presence of a patent gallbladder and distal common bile duct, demonstrated by operative cholangiography, may allow a more natural conduit for bile drainage to be constructed following anastomosis of the gallbladder to the transected tissue of the porta hepatis. This procedure may reduce the incidence of ascending cholangitis after operation but may be complicated by bile duct obstruction and leakage from kinking.

HEPATICOJEJUNOSTOMY

16 The rare finding of a large remnant of common hepatic duct may allow the construction of a hepaticojejunostomy as an end-to-side anastomosis between the bulbous end of the common hepatic duct and the side of the Roux loop.

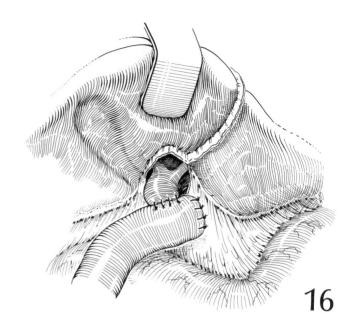

16

CUTANEOUS ENTEROSTOMY

Attempts to prevent attacks of ascending bacterial cholangitis following portoenterostomy have included fashioning cutaneous stomas and constructing a variety of 'valves' in the Roux loop conduit. However, there is no evidence that the incidence of cholangitis is lessened by these procedures, which do cause additional complications. For example, enterostomies tend to develop stomal varices and to hemorrhage repeatedly. Enterostomies also complicate liver transplantation, if it becomes necessary at a later date, and they are now generally avoided.

Postoperative care

Nasogastric drainage is continued until bowel activity returns and intravenous antibiotics (cephalosporins) administered for 5 days after surgery. An oral cephalosporin is then substituted for a further 3 weeks as prophylaxis against ascending bacterial cholangitis. The onset of any unexplained pyrexia, particularly if accompanied by a rise in serum bilirubin levels, suggests an ascending bacterial cholangitis, the cause of which must be identified with blood and liver biopsy cultures. Common organisms include *Escherichia coli, Proteus* spp. and *Klebsiella*.

The onset of effective bile drainage and an improvement in liver function tests are difficult to predict after portoenterostomy and may not occur for 2–3 weeks after surgery. Histological analysis of the tissue excised from the porta hepatis may aid prognosis, and early satisfactory bile flow may be expected if ductules with diameters greater than 150 μm are identified.

Phenobarbitone and cholestyramine are prescribed to encourage bile flow and vitamins D and K given routinely. At the time of discharge from hospital the parents and the referring physicians are given full information on the signs and hazards of any future episodes of cholangitis and the necessity for urgent treatment with intravenous antibiotics.

17 A Roux loop will occasionally become obstructed by adhesions and will require urgent surgical correction. Children who present with an episode of jaundice following a long trouble-free period should therefore be investigated with percutaneous cholangiography.

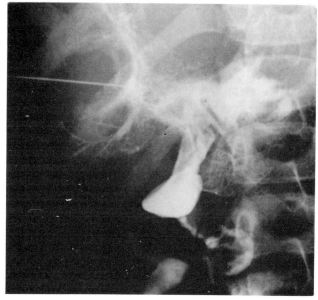

17

Outcome

Since the portoenterostomy operation was introduced more than 30 years ago, refinements in surgical technique and earlier referral for surgery have caused a steady improvement in the results for postoperative bile drainge. Children operated before 6 weeks of age have a much better chance of establishing effective bile drainage than older children. Bile drainage is achieved in more than 90% of patients under 6 weeks, but the success rate falls to less than 35% in infants over 12 weeks of age.

Although most patients continue to show some abnormalities in liver function after portoenterostomy, survival to adulthood is possible. Long-term complications include recurrent cholangitis, hepatic fibrosis, cirrhosis and portal hypertension. Injection sclerotherapy is the treatment of choice for hemorrhage from esophageal varices.

Current surgical techniques have increased the 10-year survival of patients with biliary atresia to more than 60%. Liver transplantation is reserved for those patients who either completely fail to respond to portoenterostomy or who develop liver failure at a later stage.

References

1. Davenport M, Savage M, Mowat AP, Howard ER. Biliary atresia splenic malformation syndrome: an aetiological and prognostic subgroup. *Surgery* 1993; 113: 662–8.

2. Bill AH. Biliary atresia – introduction. *World J Surg* 1978; 2: 557–9.

3. Kasai M, Kimura S, Asakura Y, Suzuki H, Taira Y, Ohashi E. Surgical treatment of biliary atresia. *J Pediatr Surg* 1968; 3: 665–75.

4. Hays DM, Kimura K. *Biliary Atresia: The Japanese Experience*. Cambridge, Massachusetts: Harvard University Press, 1980: 52–6.

5. Howard ER. Biliary atresia: etiology, management and complications. In: *Surgery of Liver Disease in Children*. Oxford: Butterworth-Heinemann, 1991: 39–59.

Choledochal cyst

R. Peter Altman MD
Professor of Surgery and Pediatrics, Columbia University, College of Physicians and Surgeons, and
Surgeon-in-Chief, Babies' Hospital, Columbia-Presbyterian Medical Center, New York, USA

Barry A. Hicks MD
Assistant Professor of Surgery, Division of Pediatric Surgery, The University of Texas Southwestern Medical Center, Dallas, Texas, USA

Principles and justification

Choledochal cyst was initially recognized by Douglas in 1852. In the clinical series reported over 100 years later, Alonso-Lej *et al.* described a classification system and suggested approaches to treatment[1].

1a–e Descriptions based on the anatomy of the cyst and distribution within the hepatobiliary tree have since been offered. The type I choledochal cyst predominates. Choledochal cyst is solitary and characterized by fusiform dilation of the common bile duct. The gallbladder and cystic duct, almost invariably dilated, enter the cyst. Choledochal cyst is not an isolated defect restricted to the bile duct, but is more appropriately regarded as part of a constellation of pathologic anomalies in the pancreaticobiliary system[2]. Types II (diverticulum of the common bile duct) and III (choledochocele) are less commonly encountered. In type IV, the second most common variant, both intrahepatic cysts and a choledochal cyst are present. Caroli's disease (type V) is characterized by intrahepatic biliary cystic disease with no choledochal cyst. The hepatic histology varies from normal in some patients to advanced fibrosis and cirrhosis in others.

Etiology

The etiology of choledochal cyst remains speculative. It has been proposed that the cause is distal narrowing of the bile duct originating *in utero*. A more commonly accepted explanation is that an abnormal junction of the bile duct with the pancreatic duct creates an anatomically common channel which allows reflux of pancreatic juice into the bile duct, thereby weakening its wall by enzymatic destruction resulting in inflammation,

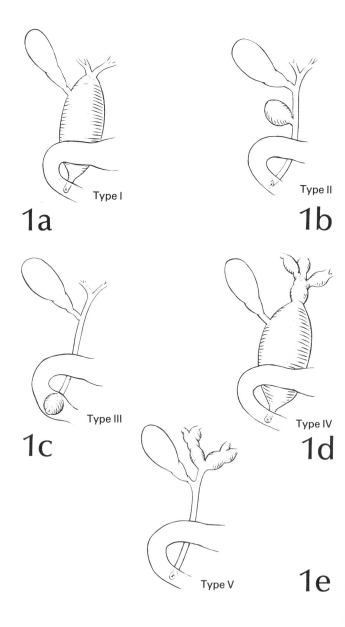

Type I   1a

Type II   1b

Type III   1c

Type IV   1d

Type V   1e

dilatation and cyst formation[3]. A 'common channel' is not found in all patients with choledochal cyst, however, and is found in some normal individuals. It is likely that multiple factors contribute to the formation of choledochal cysts and that the cysts are a component of the spectrum of anomalies within the pancreatico-biliary system. Regardless of the cause, the resulting dilatation and stasis leads to infection and hepatic cirrhosis unless remedied surgically.

Clinical features

Symptoms usually present during the first decade of life. Girls are more often affected than boys (ratio 4:1). The classic symptom complex of pain, abdominal mass and jaundice is, in fact, uncommon. With the wide use of prenatal ultrasonography, choledochal cysts are diagnosed or suspected in the antenatal period. In older patients the usual presentation is vague recurrent abdominal pain associated with minimal jaundice, which may not be readily apparent. Occasionally recurrent episodes of mild pancreatitis may predominate. In younger patients, and particularly in infants, the obstructive component predominates so that the common presentation is jaundice with an abdominal mass.

Diagnosis

2, 3 With contemporary imaging techniques confirmation of the diagnosis is now readily obtained. In previous years, an upper gastrointestinal contrast study demonstrating a mass effect and distortion of the duodenum was the standard test. This has been replaced by ultrasonography (*Illustration 2*) or computed tomography (*Illustration 3*). Both studies clearly define the dimensions of the cyst and the extent of intrahepatic ductal involvement.

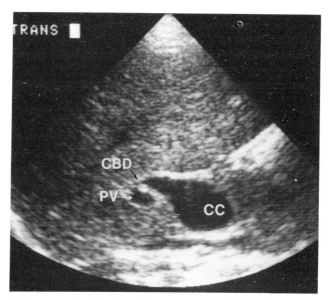

CBD = common bile duct; PV = portal vein; CC = choledochal cyst

2

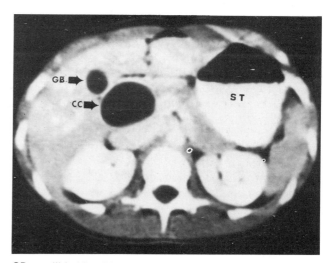

GB = gallbladder; CC = choledochal cyst; ST = stomach

3

4 Nuclear scanning with ^{99m}Tc-labeled IDA may demonstrate the extrahepatic biliary dilatation. In patients with high-grade distal ductal obstruction, no radionucleide is identified in the gastrointestinal tract.

If the regional anatomy remains obscure after these non-invasive studies, endoscopic retrograde cholangio-pancreatography is a useful adjunctive procedure. Routine use, however, is not advocated. Because of the risk of precipitating cholangitis, periendoscopic antibiotic cover is recommended.

Treatment

Internal drainage of the cyst by cystenterostomy was the traditional surgical approach. Resectional procedures were regarded as having an unacceptably high mortality rate. The long-term morbidity from cystenterostomy, however, has proved to be excessive. The cyst wall is composed of thick fibrous tissue devoid of mucosal lining, and even after drainage the cyst persists as a receptacle for stagnant bile. Anastomotic stricture and bile stasis result in cholangitis, stone formation and biliary colic, so that many patients will require subsequent surgery for management of these complications. Furthermore, it has been shown that cholangio-carcinoma may develop in the retained cyst wall[2,5]. The incidence of neoplasm in the remaining abnormal duct is reported to be between 3% and 20%.

Surgical resection of the choledochal cyst is the treatment of choice.

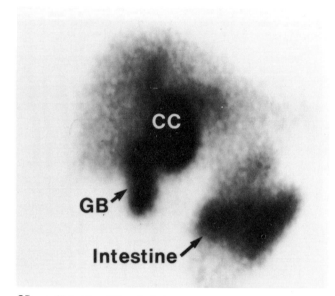

GB = gallbladder; CC = choledochal cyst

4

Operations

5 Accurate operative cholangiography is essential in planning the resection and reconstruction. After aspirating the gallbladder and cyst, contrast medium is instilled through a catheter placed in the gallbladder. The entire extrahepatic biliary ductal anatomy is thus visualized. It is important to identify the junction of the pancreatic and bile ducts in order to protect the pancreatic duct as the distal common bile duct is transected.

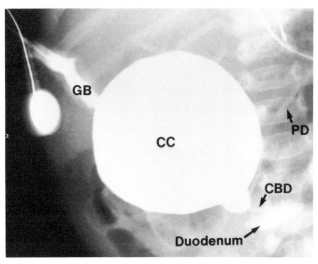

GB = gallbladder; CBD = common bile duct;
CC = choledochal cyst; PD = pancreatic duct

5

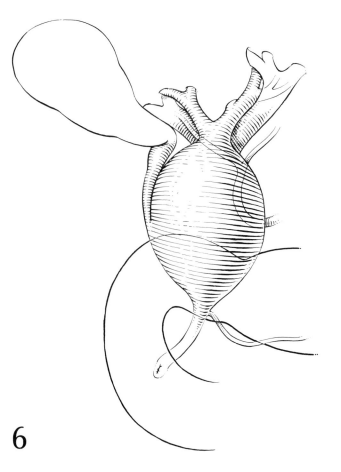

6

CIRCUMFERENTIAL DISSECTION

The choice of procedure depends on the degree of inflammatory reaction encountered at the porta hepatis. If the regional anatomy is readily defined, dissection of the gallbladder and choledochal cyst from the intimately associated vascular structures proceeds rather easily.

6 The cystic artery is divided and the gallbladder mobilized from its bed, leaving the cystic duct in continuity with the choledochal cyst from which it invariably arises.

As the dissection proceeds the cyst is mobilized by separating the medial and posterior aspects from the portal vein. When scarring and inflammation render dissection behind the cyst hazardous, an alternative technique for resection is proposed (*see below*). Once the distal extent of the cyst has been mobilized, the common bile duct is transected and secured by suture, taking care to ensure that pancreatic duct drainage is unimpaired should this duct enter the common bile duct to form a common channel.

7 The transition from abnormal cyst to normal-caliber hepatic duct is then identified as the distal cyst is elevated and the remaining posterior dissection completed proximally.

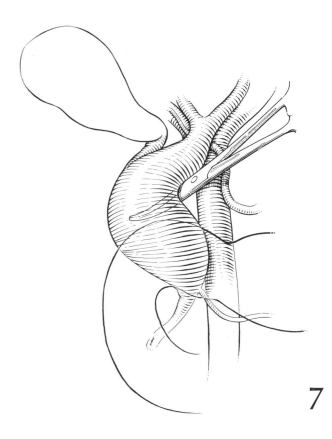

7

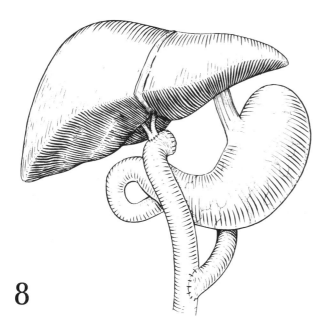

8

8 The hepatic duct is divided at this point, and biliary drainage is established with a retrocolic Roux-en-Y hepatic duct–jejunostomy.

An alternative conduit may be created with a valved jejunal interposition hepaticoduodenostomy, on the presumption that this more nearly approximates the normal gastrointestinal physiology[6].

ALTERNATIVE TECHNIQUES

If the pericystic inflammation obscures the anatomy, circumferential dissection of the cyst can be hazardous and may result in unacceptable blood loss, particularly if there is already established liver disease and portal hypertension. For such patients, Lilly[7] has described a technique of resection in which the plane between the posterior wall of the cyst and the underlying portal vein need not be disturbed.

9 The regional anatomy is defined by operative cholangiography. The gallbladder and cystic duct are then mobilized as described above. The anterior cyst wall is incised transversely and the cyst contents evacuated.

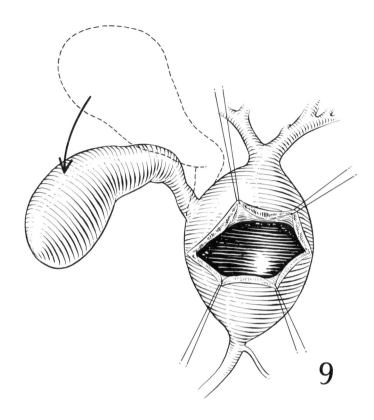

9

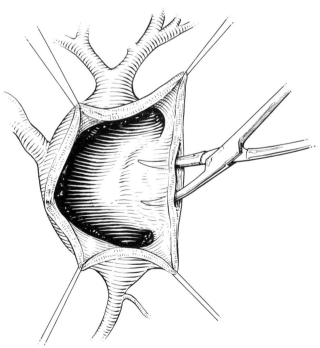

10

10 A plane is developed by dissection within the cyst wall in a posterior direction. This technique establishes an intramural separation of the thick inner cyst lining from the thinner exterior cyst wall, immediately under which lies the portal vein.

11 After developing the plane within the cyst posteriorly, the cyst lining is divided. Intramural dissection is continued cephalad and caudad as the remainder of the cyst is mobilized anterolaterally to the point at which the hepatic duct and common bile duct assume normal or near normal dimensions.

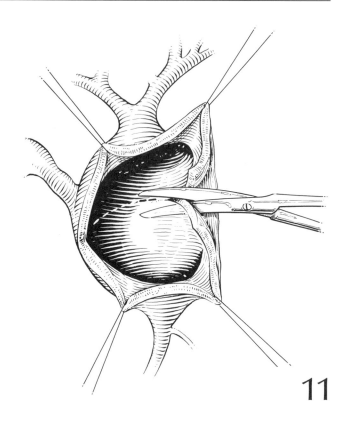

11

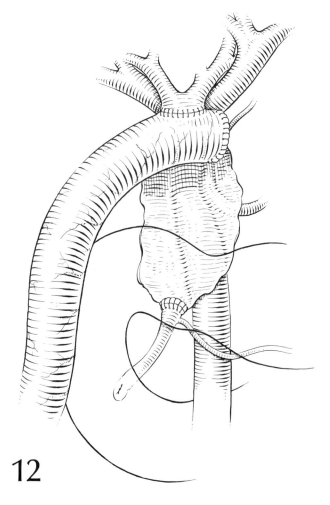

12

12 The cyst with attached gallbladder is resected and the distal common bile duct oversewn. By this technique, the cyst and its lining are removed but a portion of the outer posterior wall remains. This avoids the hazardous dissection between the densely inflamed back wall of the cyst and the portal vein. Biliary drainage is re-established with a retrocolic Roux-en-Y hepatic duct–jejunostomy.

If dilation of the choledochal cyst extends distally into the duodenum, it may be necessary to divide the distal cyst leaving some residual expanded common duct (cyst) cephalad to the duodenum. The cyst lining is readily stripped and removed before the walls are approximated and secured. Care should be taken to avoid injury to the pancreatic duct. Dilation may also extend proximally along the common hepatic duct to involve one or both of the hepatic ducts within the liver. In such patients the resection is extended, removing as much of the involved ductal structure as possible.

Outcome

The prognosis after choledochal cyst resection varies considerably. For some, particularly older patients operated on late and with established liver disease, the prognosis is doubtful. Further, cyst excision does not completely eliminate the risk of malignancy. None the less, the outcome is generally favorable and for the majority of patients the prognosis is excellent.

Acknowledgment

Illustrations 6, 7 and *9–12* have been redrawn from originals by J. K. Karapelou.

References

1. Alonso-Lej F, Rever WB Jr, Pessagno DJ. Congenital choledochal cysts, with a report of two and an analysis of 94 cases. *Int Abstr Surg* 1959; 108: 1–30.

2. Iwai N, Yanagihara J, Tokiwa K, Shimotake T, Nakamura K. Congenital choledochal dilatation with emphasis on pathophysiology of the biliary tract. *Ann Surg* 1992; 215: 27–30.

3. Babbitt DP. Congenital choledochal cysts: new etiological concept based on anomalous relationships of the common bile duct and pancreatic bulb. *Ann Radiol* 1969; 12: 231–40.

4. Young W, Blane C, White JJ *et al.* Congenital biliary dilatation: a spectrum of disease detailed by ultrasound. *Br J Radiol* 1990; 63: 333–6.

5. Ozmen V, Martin PC, Igci A *et al.* Adenocarcinoma of the gallbladder associated with congenital choledochal cyst and anomalous pancreaticobiliary ductal junction. Case report. *Eur J Surg* 1991; 157: 549–51.

6. Cosentino CM, Luck SR, Raffensperger JG, Reynolds M. Choledochal duct cyst: resection with physiologic reconstruction. *Surgery* 1992; 112: 740–8.

7. Lilly JR. The surgical treatment of choledochal cyst. *Surg Gynecol Obstet* 1979; 149: 36–42.

Splenectomy in childhood

Donald R. Cooney MD
H. William Clatworthy Jr. Professor of Pediatric Surgery, The Ohio State University, and Surgeon-in-Chief, Columbus Children's Hospital, Columbus, Ohio, USA

Principles and justification

Indications

Splenectomy may be used to treat a number of hematologic diseases, but each patient should be evaluated on the basis of the course of the disease, their response to medical therapy, and the relative merits of expected improvement following the splenectomy for that particular hematologic condition. It is most valuable in patients whose bone marrow has responded to a disease condition with an increased production of cellular elements.

Splenectomy is therapeutic for hereditary spherocytosis; the operation is usually delayed until the patient is 4 years old, and may be associated with cholelithiasis. It is indicated for children with idiopathic thrombocytopenic purpura treated with steroids who do not initially respond with an increase in the platelet count or if thrombocytopenia recurs during steroid therapy withdrawal.

Splenectomy may be used to reduce the degree of hemolysis and transfusion requirements in thalassemia.

Removal of the spleen usually corrects anemia caused by hereditary elliptocytosis; it may be associated with cholelithiasis.

Indications for splenectomy in sickle cell disease are not well established, but the procedure may be useful for patients with acute splenic sequestration. It may also be utilized, in conjunction with plasmapheresis and steroid therapy, in patients with thrombotic thrombocytopenic purpura.

Splenectomy may be indicated if the child does not respond to steroid therapy for idiopathic autoimmune hemolytic anemia.

Other hematologic conditions resulting in leukopenia, anemia, pancytopenia or thrombocytopenia, in which the spleen can be demonstrated diagnostically to play a major role in causing the deficiency of red/white cells or platelets, may be treated by splenectomy.

The procedure may also be used to treat life-threatening hemorrhage from splenic injury, splenic abscess or hypersplenism associated with portal hypertension, metabolic storage diseases, inflammatory or neoplastic conditions.

The spleen may be removed for diagnostic or therapeutic reasons related to such conditions as Hodgkin's disease, leukemia or lymphoma.

Miscellaneous other conditions for which splenectomy may be considered include Felty's syndrome, Gaucher's disease, sarcoidosis and porphyria erythropoietica.

Contraindications

Splenectomy should not be undertaken (1) if the patient has glucose-6-phosphate dehydrogenase deficiency anemia, (2) as the sole treatment for portal hypertension, (3) in most patients with sickle cell disease, or (4) for any condition in which it cannot be demonstrated that the spleen is responsible for removing cellular elements of the blood associated with the primary disease process.

Splenectomy for hematologic disease

Diagnostic studies

A bone marrow examination and reticulocyte count should be obtained to evaluate the potential for production of red/white cells and platelets. White cells, platelets, and particularly red blood cells should be labeled with isotopes to evaluate the rate of removal from the patient's bloodstream and the degree of localization of these cells in the spleen. These studies should be performed to evaluate the role of the spleen in removing cellular elements from the bloodstream. Additional specialized serologic tests may be indicated based on the specific disease for which the splenectomy is being considered.

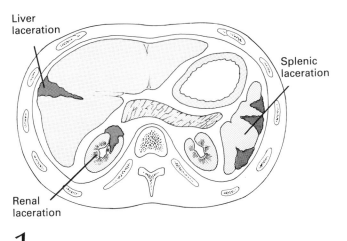

Liver laceration

Splenic laceration

Renal laceration

1

Splenectomy for trauma

Diagnostic studies

The spleen is one of the organs most commonly injured by blunt abdominal trauma. The major concern resulting from splenic injury is intra-abdominal hemorrhage. Although associated injuries may coexist, intra-peritoneal hemorrhage is the major determinant of mortality. Leukocytosis is characteristic in cases of splenic injury. Hematuria is also frequently encountered because of the high incidence of associated renal trauma. The hematocrit must be interpreted in the context of other clinical and historic findings. Sufficient time must pass from initial injury to determination of the hematocrit if the clinician is to rely on the hematocrit as an accurate predictor of the extent and rate of hemorrhage.

Radiographic evaluation

1 Radiographic findings suggestive of splenic injury include left sided rib fractures, displacement of the colon or stomach, a serrated appearance of the greater curvature of the stomach, and a loss of the splenic, renal, or psoas muscle shadows. Peritoneal lavage may be utilized when there is an urgent need to document the presence of life-threatening intra-abdominal hemorrhage or when computed tomographic (CT) scanning is not available. In the past it was considered appropriate for the child to undergo exploratory laparotomy if an intra-abdominal injury was suspected based on clinical, radiographic or peritoneal lavage findings. The present concepts of management are based on a recognition that a selective therapeutic approach results in the lowest morbidity and mortality rates. CT scanning techniques have enabled the clinician accurately to diagnose and serially evaluate intra-abdominal injuries.

Total splenectomy for trauma

Life-threatening splenic hemorrhage requires immediate operative intervention, whether as an initial measure or as a necessary step during non-operative management. Whenever multiple life-threatening injuries are encountered, total splenectomy should be the treatment of choice.

Non-operative management

If the patient's condition remains stable non-operative therapy should be undertaken. The patient should be observed in the intensive care unit for 48–72 h. A repeat CT scan or similar imaging study should be obtained 10–14 days after injury to assess healing. A predictable series of radiographic changes has been described:

Stage I (10–14 days) is characterized by the absorption of intra-abdominal blood and a cellular and morphologic reorganization of the injury.
Stage II consists of a coalition of the multiple lacerations into a larger single area of low density detected on the CT scan.
Stage III is characterized by an increasing density and decreasing size of the lesion.
Stage IV consists of the resolution of the injury, which occurs 2–6 months following the traumatic event, and is characterized by a diminution in the size of the lesion as well as possible calcification.

CT scans should be used to monitor healing and guide the clinician in giving appropriate recommendations to the parents and child regarding resumption of normal physical activities. Most children may be discharged from the hospital just before the second stage of the healing process, which occurs at 10–14 days

Adherence to a strict protocol for non-operative management cannot be over-emphasized. Close monitoring in the intensive care unit is essential and 24-h accessibility to the operating room is a prerequisite for non-operative therapy. Nasogastric decompression should be maintained during the period of intestinal ileus. Repeat physical examinations and serial hematocrits should be performed at frequent intervals. The onset of any hemodynamic instability, signs of increasing peritoneal irritation, or transfusion requirements

greater than 30–40 ml/kg (one-third to one-half of the estimated blood volume) are indications for exploratory laparotomy.

A decision-making algorithm for the management of abdominal trauma is shown in *Figure 1*.

Preoperative

Immunization

Immunization is the most important measure in preventing overwhelming postsplenectomy infection. Every child undergoing splenectomy or partial splenectomy on an elective basis should be immunized with commercially available meningococcal, hemophilus, and pneumococcal vaccines several weeks before the operation to ensure the best antibody response and to avoid any side effects which could cause confusing signs and symptoms during the immediate pre- or postoperative period.

Blood and platelet transfusion

Blood should be typed and cross-matched before surgery. Platelets are not infused for most children with idiopathic thrombocytopenic purpura because the platelets will usually be destroyed by the spleen before surgery. If the child is severely anemic, a preoperative blood transfusion may be necessary.

Age of the child at the time of elective operation

Elective operations should be performed with some consideration of the age of the child. Overwhelming postsplenectomy infection appears to be more common in the younger child. In general, operation should be delayed until the child reaches the age of 3–4 years. In addition, if there is not a well established indication for operation or a high expectation of elimination of signs, symptoms, or physiologic aberrations following splenectomy, the operation should be delayed until the child is older.

Other preoperative measures

For children undergoing exploration as a result of abdominal trauma, preoperative insertion of a nasogastric tube is extremely important to prevent the risk of aspiration and to facilitate the rapid exposure of the spleen. Broad-spectrum antibiotics are indicated for all children undergoing splenectomy, splenic repair, or partial resection, whether for an acute emergency or as an elective operation.

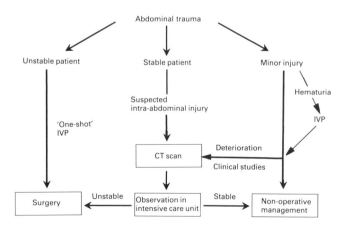

Figure 1 Decision-making algorithm for management of abdominal trauma

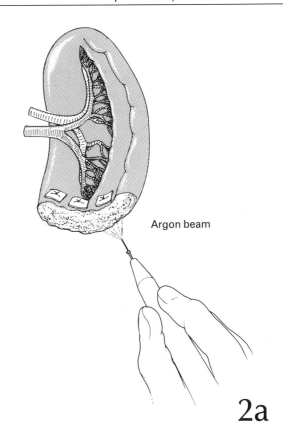

Argon beam

2a

Operations

SPLENIC REPAIR AND PARTIAL SPLENECTOMY

2a–c The spleen may be repaired or partially resected by first mobilizing the organ. The assistant should hold the spleen for the operator who will remove the injured portion of the spleen or resect that portion which is being excised using electro-coagulation, ultrasonics, laser or sharp dissection. Hemostasis is achieved by individually suture ligating the vessels and/or using the argon beam coagulator. Topical thrombin or microfibrillar collagen may also be applied to the cut surface of the spleen. Pledgets are used in conjunction with suture material to close the capsule or apply compression along the cut surface. Absorbable suture 'mesh' may be useful in achieving hemostasis in cases of 'shattered spleen'.

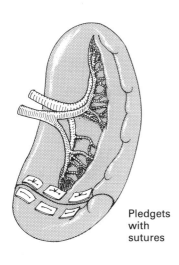

Pledgets
with
sutures

2b

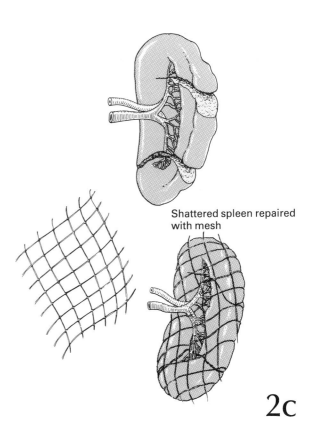

Shattered spleen repaired
with mesh

2c

SPLENIC ARTERY LIGATION AND SPLENIC REIMPLANTATION

Although splenic artery ligation and splenic reimplantation are safe procedures, they are experimental and do not provide adequate protection against overwhelming postsplenectomy sepsis.

TOTAL SPLENECTOMY

The operator should stand on the patient's right side. After adequate exposure has been obtained using either self-retaining or assistant-placed retractors, the dorsal margin of the spleen is grasped by the operator and pulled medially up and out of the incision. If possible, most of the operative procedure will take place outside the peritoneal cavity. Once the lateral attachments to the abdominal wall and splenorenal ligaments have been divided, the spleen is usually very mobile and may be delivered through the incision site. Exposure is facilitated by the surgeon placing several large sponges in the splenic fossa to prevent the spleen from retracting back into the abdomen. A careful inspection of all other organs is performed at the time of exploration and is particularly important in cases of trauma. Moreover, if the splenectomy is being performed for a hematologic condition, careful inspection and removal of any accessory spleens is also undertaken.

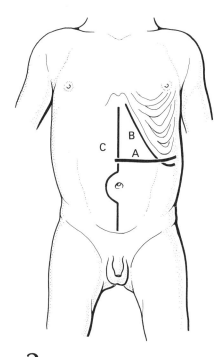

Incision and exploration

3   In small children a left upper quadrant transverse muscle-cutting incision is preferred for elective splenectomy (A). For older children with a narrow costal margin, a subcostal incision may provide better exposure (B). A midline abdominal incision should be utilized for all children with blunt abdominal or penetrating injuries of the abdomen (C). This incision provides quicker and more adequate exposure of possible multiple intra-abdominal injuries. During the initial stages of the operation an adequate exploration of the peritoneal cavity should be performed. The operator should carefully inspect the splenic hilum, the tail and caudal margin of the pancreas, the splenocolic ligament, the greater omentum, presacral area and adnexal region for accessory spleens. Surgeons should rule out the possibility of gallstones, particularly in children with hemolytic anemia.

3

Mobilization of the spleen

4a, b The spleen is grasped by the surgeon's non-dominant hand and gently retracted upward, medially and out of the incision. With an assistant retracting the lateral abdominal wall, the surgeon is easily able to visualize the splenorenal ligament and the lateral attachments to the abdominal wall. These attachments are incised using scissors and/or the electrocautery unit to control any bleeding. Large sponges are placed in the splenic fossa to control minor hemorrhage and to assist in maintaining the spleen in the best possible position for operation. The surgeon then divides the short gastric vessels between clamps. Each vessel is tied and suture-ligated to ensure hemostasis.

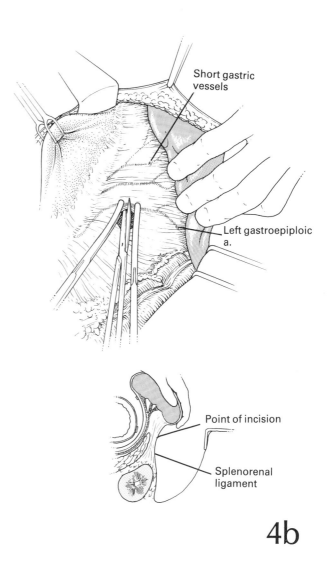

Short gastric vessels

Left gastroepiploic a.

Point of incision

Splenorenal ligament

4b

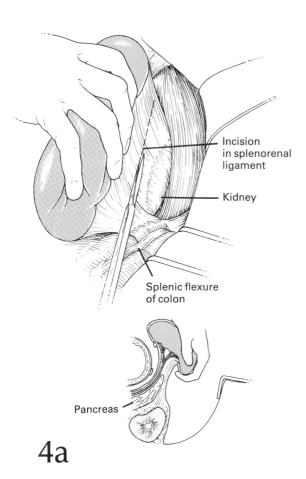

Incision in splenorenal ligament

Kidney

Splenic flexure of colon

Pancreas

4a

Ligation of the splenic artery and vein

5 With the gastrosplenic and splenorenal ligaments divided, the spleen is mobile and more easily delivered into the operative field. The assistant holds the spleen, exposing the hilum, and the surgeon identifies the pancreas and splenic vessels. Just before dividing the splenic artery and vein, the operator squeezes the spleen gently to return as much blood to the circulation as possible before clamping, first (if possible) the splenic artery and finally the splenic vein. The artery and vein are divided between clamps, tied and then suture-ligated. At the completion of this step, the surgeon inspects the area of the tail of the pancreas to ensure that it has not been damaged.

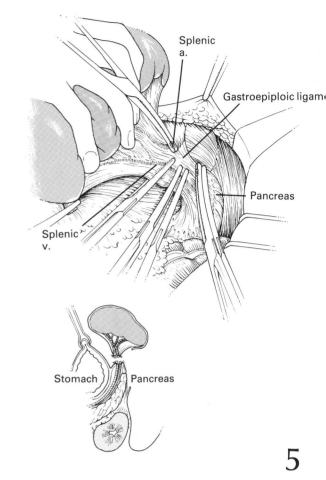

Re-exploration of the abdominal cavity and splenic fossa

The splenic fossa, the area of the ligation of the splenic vessels, greater curvature of the stomach, greater omentum, and all other areas of the abdomen should be carefully inspected for accessory spleens and adequacy of hemostasis.

Wound closure

For subcostal and transverse incisions the posterior peritoneum and fascia are closed with running absorbable sutures and the outer layers of the abdominal wall are closed with the same interrupted suture. If a midline incision is used for trauma, the fascia is closed with interrupted figure-of-eight sutures of appropriate size for the age of the child. Drains are not indicated unless there is an associated injury to the liver or pancreas, identified during the operations for trauma.

LAPAROSCOPIC SPLENECTOMY

Laparoscopic splenectomy may be an alternative for patients who do not have massively enlarged spleens. Standard laparoscopic techniques are utilized, which usually require 4–5 access ports. The splenocolic, gastrosplenic and splenic–peritoneal attachments and vessels are divided. The tail of the pancreas is dissected before ligation of the splenic artery and vein. The splenorenal ligament is usually divided just before morselizing the spleen inside an intraperitoneal bag before extraction from the abdominal cavity.

Postoperative care

Complications

Complications following the treatment of splenic injuries or operations on the spleen are rare. Postoperative hemorrhage following splenectomy or partial splenectomy is unusual. If the operator takes steps to ensure that no bleeding is present at the conclusion of the operative procedure, this complication can be avoided in almost all cases. Although there may be a sudden and marked rise in the platelet count following splenectomy or partial splenectomy, anticoagulation therapy is seldom indicated, particularly in young children. In older adolescent patients, particularly in young women, if concern develops regarding thromboembolic disease, aspirin therapy will usually suffice as appropriate prophylactic treatment. Leukocytosis is common following splenectomy but is not necessarily an indication of postoperative infection. If the child complains of abdominal pain, has fever and demonstrates leukocytosis, the surgeon should suspect an intra-abdominal or wound infection or pancreatitis. Pancreatitis is very rare in children undergoing splenectomy. If this complication occurs, conservative management with nasogastric decompression is adequate. Pulmonary complications such as atelectasis are also rare in children. If a pleural effusion develops, particularly on the left side, the surgeon should suspect that an intra-abdominal/subdiaphragmatic infection or pancreatitis may be causing the effusion. Measurements of the white blood cell count, serum amylase, and CT scanning of the abdomen may be useful in differentiating the cause of the pleural effusion.

Overwhelming postsplenectomy infection

The child's immunologic status is changed by removing a large portion of the spleen or the entire organ. Children may be more susceptible to intra-abdominal and wound infections as well as the other infectious complications following splenectomy or partial splenectomy. Major concern, however, relates mainly to the fact that children who undergo total splenectomy are at risk of developing overwhelming postsplenectomy infection. These infections vary in incidence as they relate to the age of the child as well as to the disease process for which the splenectomy is peformed. Although this complication occurs in only a small percentage of patients, these infections begin suddenly, progress rapidly, and are associated with a very high mortality rate. Controversy exists with regard to the use of long-term prophylactic antibiotics following splenectomy, but there should be no debate regarding the indication for antibiotics in the acutely injured and splenectomized child. During the perioperative period the patient is at greatest risk. Numerous potential portals of entry exist, and the child's host resistance is decreased following the traumatic event and operation.

The most common organisms causing overwhelming postsplenectomy infection are *Pneumococcus*, *Hemophilus*, *Neisseria*, *Escherichia* and *Pseudomonas*. Widespread antibiotic prophylaxis is appropriate for the immediate preoperative, postinjury and postoperative periods. Penicillin is recommended for long-term use because *Pneumococcus* (which accounts for approximately 50% of these infections) is exquisitely sensitive to the drug: ampicillin may be a good alternative. As most of these life-threatening infections occur in the first few months following operation, prophylactic antibiotics should be used during this period. Extended use of antibiotic prophylaxis is generally recommended for most children, although no epidemiologic data have proved the absolute necessity of such long-term antibiotic therapy.

Immunization

The most important measure in preventing overwhelming postsplenectomy infection is immunization. Splenectomized children respond well to vaccination. Each child undergoing splenectomy or partial splenectomy should be immunized with the commercially available meningococcus, hemophilus and pneumococcal vaccines. Children should not be immunized immediately after the operation or during the ensuing 2 weeks; instead, immunization should be performed during the preoperative period for elective splenectomy or delayed for several weeks following operation or treatment of the injuries to ensure the best possible antibody response. Vaccines will provide protection for approximately 5 years. Reimmunization is advised after this for most patients.

Further reading

Cooney DR. Splenic and hepatic trauma in children. *Surg Clin North Am* 1981; 61: 1165–80.

Cooney DR, Dearth JC, Swanson SE, Dewanhee MK, Telander RL. Relative merits of partial splenectomy, splenic reimplantation, and immunization in preventing postsplenectomy infection. *Surgery* 1979; 86: 561–9.

Ein SH. Splenic lesions. In: Ashcraft KW, Holder TM eds. *Pediatric Surgery*, 2nd edn. Philadelphia: WB Saunders, 1993: 535–45.

Schwartz SI. Spleen. In: Schwartz SI, ed. *Principles of Surgery*, 6th edn. New York: McGraw-Hill, 1994: 1433–47.

Zollinger RM, Cuttler EC. Splenectomy. In: Zollinger RM, Cuttler EC, eds. *Atlas of Surgical Operations*, New York: Macmillan, 1961: 164–7.

Illustrations by Patrick Elliott

Liver resections

R. M. Filler MD, FRCS(C)
Professor of Surgery, The University of Toronto, and Surgeon-in-Chief, The Hospital for Sick Children, Toronto, Ontario, Canada

History

The rate of success of partial hepatic resection increases as advances in preoperative preparation and surgical technique parallel refinements in diagnostic techniques and methods of postoperative management. The first partial hepatic resection was performed by Bruns in 1870 on a wounded Prussian soldier. The first resection in a child was performed by Konig, whose patient in 1889 recovered after excision of a large cystic adenoma. In 1894 Israel sucessfully excised a malignant tumor from a child's liver but no series of liver resections in children from one institution was reported until the 1950s. Techniques of hepatectomy in adults were published by Quattlebaum, Pack, Longmire, McDermott and others in the 1960s, and experience with infants then increased remarkably. In the early childhood series about 50% of tumors requiring hepatectomy were thought to be unresectable and even in patients for whom surgery could be curative, operative mortality was 15–25%.

Principles and justification

Indications

The presence of a malignant tumor is by far the most frequent indication for hepatic resection in childhood, accounting for approximately 90% of such operations. Hepatoblastoma is the most common hepatic neoplasm in children under 5 years of age; hepatocellular carcinoma accounts for most of the malignancies in older children. Metastatic tumors, most commonly Wilms' tumor and neuroblastoma, may be treated by hepatectomy in the absence of tumor at other sites but, because these situations arise only infrequently, resection for metastic disease constitutes only a small fraction of the hepatic resections performed.

Contraindications

Hemangiomas and hemangioendotheliomas of the liver are the most common benign neoplasms encountered in infants and children. Resection is not usually required for these lesions because they tend to undergo spontaneous regression or because their cardiovascular effects (due to arteriovenous shunting) can be managed by other means. The less frequently occurring benign neoplasms that are best treated by resection include cystic hamartoma and adenoma.

Hepatic resection is rarely employed for liver trauma because liver injuries in childhood may usually be treated conservatively. Even if surgery is needed for uncontrolled bleeding, techniques short of resection are usually sufficient for a satisfactory outcome.

The best results from surgery for cancer of the liver are obtained by total excision of the tumor without spill into the operative field. As most tumors arise from a site in one lobe and spread peripherally a complete lobectomy, or a complete lobectomy plus a partial lobectomy of the opposite lobe (extended hepatectomy), is necessary for cure. Traditionally no hope has been held out for those whose tumors have extended beyond these boundaries. Recent use of effective preoperative chemotherapy has modified this dictum; remarkable reductions in tumor have been achieved with preoperative chemotherapy, so that lesions which appeared at diagnosis to have progressed beyond the confines of resectability may be excised and other large but resectable masses may be removed with smaller resections than originally anticipated. The most effective chemotherapeutic agents are cisplatin and adriamycin.

Preoperative

Diagnostic evaluation should define the extent of hepatic involvement by tumor and, in the case of malignant tumors, the location and extent of metastatic disease. In the child with a hepatic mass the tests that most accurately describe the anatomic features which are most helpful in planning the operative approach are computed tomographic (CT) scanning and magnetic resonance imaging (MRI). These studies allow the surgeon to visualize the lobar anatomy of the liver and to determine with reasonable accuracy whether the lesion is amenable to resection, although at present surgical exploration is the most accurate way to make the final decision. Contrast injection is a useful adjunct to the CT scan; contrast injection which highlights the tumor vasculature results in patchy enhancement throughout the tumor mass in most malignant lesions. Vascular tumors may be difficult to differentiate on unenhanced scans. A specific pattern of enhancement may be seen, with initial dense peripheral enhancement and central low density and a gradual centripetal filling of the central low-density area from the periphery. MRI appears to be even more accurate than CT scanning in defining parenchymal involvement and tumor margins while providing a reliable definition of vascular structures, particularly the hepatic veins and the inferior vena cava.

Abdominal ultrasonography cannot be relied on to define the surgical anatomy. Similarly, radionuclide scanning is less accurate than the more sophisticated tests and yields little additional information.

The role of angiography is limited, and generally does not provide a more useful surgical 'road map' for the operation than CT scanning or MRI. However, angiography can be useful in evaluating a suspected or proven hemangioma, especially in patients with significant arteriovenous shunting and as a prelude to embolism of branches of the hepatic artery when this become an option.

The liver function of most children requiring hepatectomy is normal. Nevertheless, the surgeon must be certain that clotting parameters affected by liver function are not deranged. Abnormal partial thromboplastin or prothombin times must be corrected before surgery. A check of the platelet count is also necessary because portal hypertension may result in thrombocytopenia.

As most malignant hepatic tumors elaborate α-fetoprotein, the serum levels of this marker should be measured before surgery for diagnostic purposes and to establish a baseline to follow the progress of the child following surgery and/or chemotherapy.

Anatomy

1 The liver is divided into right and left lobes along the plane running from the gallbladder fossa inferiorly to the suprahepatic inferior vena cava superiorly. The right lobe constitutes about 70% of the hepatic cell mass and is the site of most hepatic neoplasms. The left lobe is divided into a medial and lateral segment by the midline falciform ligament or umbilical fissure. Each segment represents about 15% of the liver mass. Because of the liver's remarkable ability to regenerate, as much as 85% may be removed with the expectation that ultimately liver function will be adequate. Thus tumors that are contained in either lobe of the liver, and those that arise in the right lobe but do not extend beyond the medial segment of the left lobe, are amenable to surgical resection.

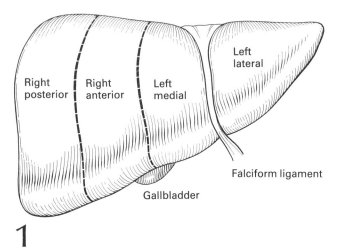

1

Right posterior

Right anterior

Left medial

Left lateral

Falciform ligament

Gallbladder

2 The liver comprises eight relatively independent segments, each supplied by a portal triad and draining into a hepatic vein running in its sector. Theoretically, each segment may be removed without adversely affecting any of the others. Segmental architecture is especially important if several tumor masses which are not in continuity need to be removed, a situation commonly seen with metastatic lesions and occasionally with primary neoplasms. The segmental anatomy of the liver also allows the surgeon to design resections short of a complete lobectomy for tumors that are localized (or become localized after chemotherapy) to one or two segments.

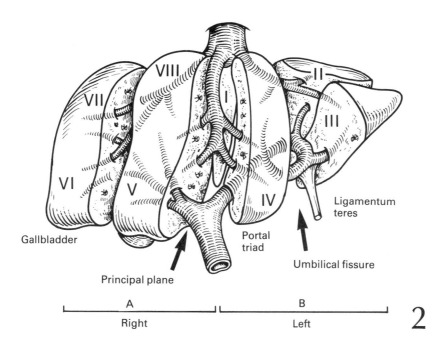

Gallbladder

Principal plane

Portal triad

Ligamentum teres

Umbilical fissure

A
Right

B
Left

2

Operation

Intraoperative management

The most common and serious intraoperative problem is hemorrhage: even in the absence of uncontrolled bleeding, the loss of one blood volume (up to 800 ml in a child weighing 10 kg) is not unusual. As a guide to proper replacement, precise measurement of blood loss and accurate assessment of intra-arterial blood pressure, central venous pressure, and urine output are necessary. An arterial line can be placed percutaneously in even the smallest infant. The central venous catheter should be placed through an arm or neck vein into the superior vena cava so that fluids and blood will enter the bloodstream proximal to the site of bleeding or obstruction. A Foley catheter is necessary for urinary output measurements.

Hypothermia tends to cause cardiac irritability, metabolic acidosis and abnormal blood clotting; therefore any blood administered during surgery should be warmed to 37°C. Unless the operation is performed with induced hypothermia (which is seldom advisable), the child's normal body temperature should be maintained by keeping the operating room warm and by using a warming blanket. Adjusting the pH of banked blood to 7.4 also decreases the risk of cardiac arrest, which can be triggered by the rapid infusion of large volumes of cold, acid blood.

The induction of profound hypothermia by cardiopulmonary bypass and the use of circulatory arrest has been used as an adjunct to surgery and may be considered in difficult cases in which massive bleeding might be anticipated. This maneuver should be prepared for before surgery commences, for it would be extremely difficult to initiate bypass and cooling during an operation in which uncontrolled hemorrhage suddenly occurred.

Position of patient

The child is positioned supine or with the right side elevated 45° on a sandbag if the tumor is located posterolaterally in the right lobe.

Incision

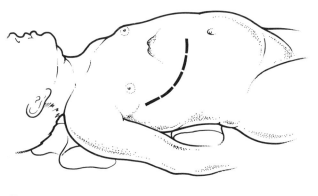

3

3 The author prefers a thoracoabdominal incision, although many surgeons believe this to be seldom necessary. Entering the thorax not only eliminates the possibility of air embolus when a hepatic vein or vena cava is opened, but also provides ready access to the suprahepatic inferior vena cava which can be encircled with a tape before lobectomy to provide vascular control should bleeding occur from branches of the vena cava or hepatic veins. In addition, exposure of the vena cava allows an internal venous shunt, which can be used to isolate liver blood flow in the event of catastrophic hemorrhage, to be placed.

For right hepatic resections the author opens the abdomen using an upper abdominal transverse incision through both rectus abdominal muscles and enters the chest by extending the incision across the costal margin into the seventh intercostal space.

For tumors that do not extend into the right lobe a transverse left upper abdominal incision with a vertical midline extension into the chest and median sternotomy is satisfactory. Extension into the thorax is not necessary if the tumor resides only in segments II and III. Exposure is important for safe and adequate liver resection and the surgeon should never hesitate to enlarge an incision to achieve this goal.

Resection

4 Once the abdomen has been opened and completely explored the ligamentum teres should be ligated and divided. Traction applied to the superior end of the ligament allows the falciform ligament to be divided to the region of the vena cava. The triangular ligament of the lobe to be removed is divided and the space between the bare area of the liver and diaphragm freed. The inferior vena cava below the liver is exposed and encircled with an umbilical tape superior to the entrance of the left renal vein; this aids dissection of the retrohepatic hepatic veins and facilitates control of any hepatic venous hemorrhage. Good control of venous bleeding can be achieved by occluding the vena cava above and below the liver in conjunction with clamping the porta hepatis (Pringle maneuver).

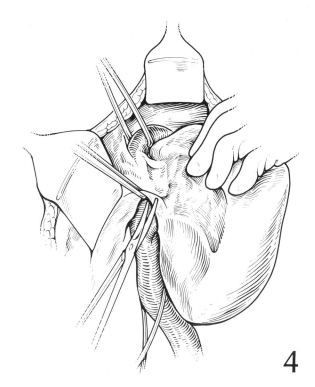

4

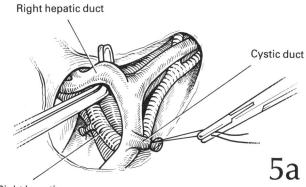

RIGHT HEPATECTOMY

$5a-d$ The common hepatic artery, common bile duct and portal vein are dissected in the porta hepatis. The cystic duct and cystic artery are divided between ties when the right lobe is to be removed. The hepatic artery and portal venous branches and the hepatic ducts to the lobe to be removed are ligated and divided between sutures. As an extra precaution the portal vein should also be suture ligated before or after division, or the open ends should be oversewn with a continuous vascular suture, because free ties alone on this large vessel tend to fall off during subsequent dissection.

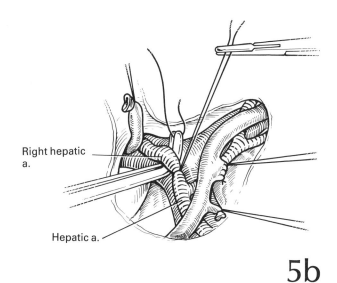

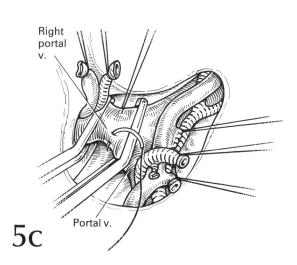

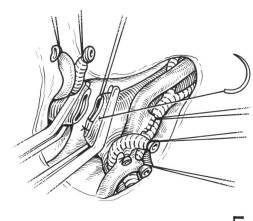

6 The main and accessory hepatic veins are now dissected and divided. In children the right hepatic vein usually has a very short extrahepatic course before it enters the inferior vena cava. The safe handling of this vessel is the greatest challenge of hepatic lobectomy, and the best way to approach it when the tumor is not located at the dome of the organ is through the liver substance. An incision is made in the liver capsule along the interlobar plane at the superior portion of the liver (the line of division is clearly evident because previous vascular interruption of venous and arterial inflow in the porta hepatis causes the right lobe to become cyanotic). The superior portion of the interlobar fissure is split using blunt finger dissection and vessels and ducts in the fissure are isolated, controlled with ligatures and divided, exposing the right hepatic vein. The hepatic vein should be surrounded by a right-angled dissecting clamp and doubly ligated. Suture ligatures are placed outside the ties for more secure control and the vein is divided. If the tumor occupies the superior portion of the interlobar fissure the hepatic vein should be freed and divided at a later stage in the procedure, as noted below.

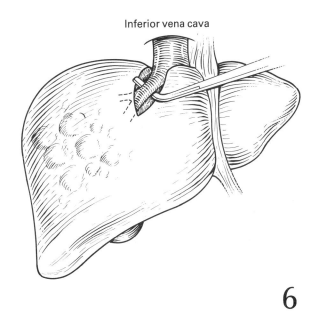

Inferior vena cava

6

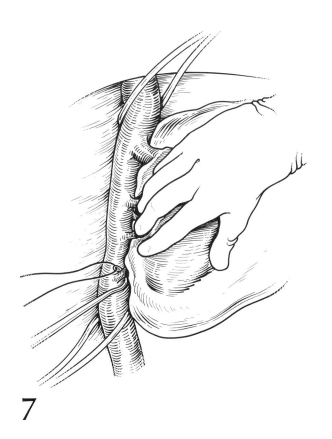

7

7 Next the unnamed hepatic veins issuing from the posterior aspect of the right lobe and entering the vena cava inferior to the main right hepatic vein are approached by rotating the liver to the left, ligated by passing fine silk ties around them and divided serially. The larger vessels should be suture ligated. It is important to divide all the accessory veins entering the cava below the right hepatic vein before proceding to complete division of the liver substance. These vessels can be numerous, especially when the primary tumor is highly vascular, and loss of control can cause troublesome bleeding so that meticulous care is necessary. In cases in which the right hepatic vein could not be divided earlier in the operation because of the location of the tumor, the hepatic vein is approached once these accessory veins are divided up to its entrance into the vena cava. The right hepatic vein is then completely exposed and when space permits a vascular clamp is applied to its caval end. The vein is cut between the clamp and a controlling ligature. A second clamp then is placed behind the first and after removal of the first clamp the open end of the vein is closed with a running vascular suture. When there is insufficient room to place the vascular clamp a suture ligature should be used for control of the caval side of the vein.

Use of controlling tapes around the vena cava above and below the liver is extremely important for this part of the operation, they should not be omitted, even if the pericardium must be opened to gain access to the vena cava above the diaphragm.

8 The portion of the interlobar fissure that has not yet been dissected is now divided by the finger fracture technique after incising the liver capsule with a scalpel. Use of a vibrating ultrasonic dissector to divide the liver is felt by some to reduce bleeding, but the author has found it to be more time-consuming than finger fracture, and no more efficient in reducing blood loss, although it is effective in demonstrating the vessels to be divided. The vessels and bile ducts that traverse the plane of fracture are cauterized, or clamped and ligated if they are large. This portion of the operation should procede quickly to minimize blood loss. Until the liver has been completely divided the surgeon should compress the liver on the surgeon's side of the fracture using his or her non-dominant hand, while the assistant compresses the other side. The porta hepatis may be clamped for periods of 10–15 min to aid hemostasis.

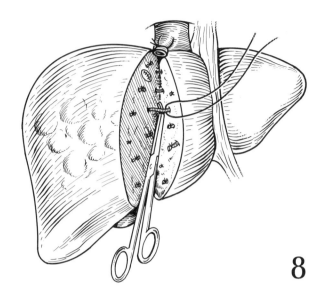

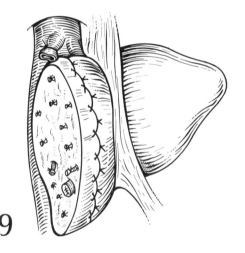

9 At the completion of the lobectomy or at stages during division of the liver substance, large mattress sutures of catgut on large curved blunt needles should be passed through the cut edge of the liver of the left lobe to control bleeding and potential bile leaks from the vessels and ducts which have not been individually ligated. It is not necessary to suture omentum to the raw edge of liver. There is rarely sufficient omentum available in a child to accomplish this. Use of fibrin sealant is recommended by some authors to enhance hemostasis and prevent bile leaks from the raw surface of the liver.

Wound closure

Before closing the wound a drain should be placed in the subdiaphragmatic space created by the hepatectomy. The author prefers a large flat Silastic drain with many holes which can be attached to a closed continuous suction device. The drain is brought out through a stab wound in the right side of the abdomen several centimeters from the main wound.

The wound is closed in two layers with continuous sutures after the diaphragm is repaired with interrupted non-absorbable sutures.

EXTENDED RIGHT HEPATECTOMY (TRISEGMENTECTOMY)

The initial steps in this operation are the same as for right hepatectomy but the medial segment of the left lobe of the liver (segment IV, quadrate lobe) must be devascularized and mobilized in continuity with the right lobe.

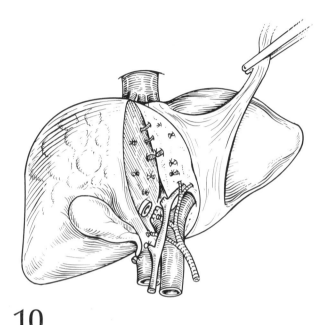

10

10 After dividing the right vascular and duct structures in the hilum, the main and accessory right hepatic veins should be exposed and secured if possible. The left portal triad is then separated from the undersurface of the medial segment of the left lobe, preserving the blood supply to the remaining left lobe. Any aberrant left hepatic artery arising from the celiac or left gastric arteries will enter the base of the umbilical fissure and will not be endangered by this dissection. The veins and arteries supplying segment IV feed back from the main trunks as they course through the umbilical fissure and, in order to avoid damaging the main trunks, the branches to segment IV should be divided just right of the falciform ligament as the umbilical fissure is being separated by finger fracture. This separation begins at the most inferior portion of the fissure at the hilum and extends superiorly and posteriorly. The middle hepatic vein is encountered close to the diaphragm and should be freed and ligated. If the right hepatic vein has not already been divided it should be approached through the liver substance at this stage of the operation and ligated as described previously.

The left hepatic bile duct must be visualized and protected from harm during the dissection and devascularization of the medial segment of the left lobe. It is a small structure in the young child and is easily injured at this stage of the procedure.

LEFT HEPATECTOMY

11 As with the right lobectomy, the liver is mobilized by dividing the triangular ligament of the lobe to be removed and the falciform ligament. The left hepatic artery, left portal vein and left hepatic duct are divided in the porta hepatis. The posterior vessels to the caudate lobe should be preserved unless this lobe is also to be removed. Following devascularization of the lobe a line of demarcation develops to the left of the gallbladder fossa along which the liver is divided by finger fracture. The bridging vessels and ducts are secured as described above. Ordinarily the left hepatic vein is most easily approached through the liver substance and suture ligated or oversewn at its caval end. If space at its entrance into the vena cava allows, a vascular clamp may be applied for control as described for division of the right hepatic vein during right lobectomy. This is not possible usually, but by encircling the vein with a right-angled clamp and securing it with a suture ligature safe control may be achieved. The middle hepatic vein is encountered in the liver substance during liver split and should be treated similarly. This vein often empties into the left hepatic vein rather than directly into the vena cava.

11

LESSER RESECTIONS

A lesion located in the periphery of the liver does not require formal lobectomy. Usually a metastatic tumor or even a primary tumor which has responded to preoperative chemotherapy can be completely removed by lesser resections. As a rule an operation will be successful if a lesion can be removed with a margin of normal liver of 1 cm around it.

12 The techniques of limited resections are relatively simple and safe and employ manipulations that have been described for lobectomy. A wedge resection is ideal for a lesion at the free edge of the liver. While the assistant applies manual compression to the liver on either side of the proposed line of resection, the normal liver is divided with a scalpel in a 'pie-shaped' fashion at least 1 cm from the mass. The resultant liver wound is closed with overlapping large catgut mattress sutures. If a large vessel has been transected bleeding can be controlled using a suture ligature before the mattress sutures are applied.

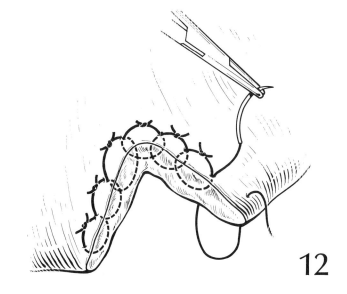

12

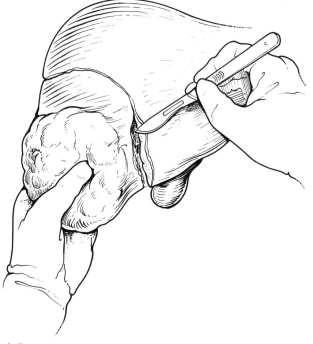

13

13 For larger lesions at the periphery of the liver, the capsule of the organ is scored with a scalpel, encircling the lesion which is to be excised. The liver is divided by finger fracture and the bridging vessels and ducts are controlled in the same fashion as those that are encountered in dividing the interlobar fissure during lobectomy. Hemostasis can be aided during the operation by manual pressure on the liver around the periphery of the incision.

Postoperative care

Young patients rarely have multisystem disease and their care after major hepatic resections is therefore less complicated than that for adults. The major problems encountered are related to the metabolic and physiologic derangements secondary to the loss of functioning liver tissue.

Maintenance of blood volume

Bleeding from small vessels which have not been completely controlled, or less commonly from a coagulopathy, means that maintenance of normal blood volume is the most immediate concern after surgery and judicious management is necessary. A single blood-stained dressing may represent a significant blood loss in an infant whose blood volume is only 800 ml, but an unnecessary 200 ml transfusion may result in pulmonary edema. The arterial blood pressure, hemoglobin and urine output must be monitored continuously, and central venous pressure monitoring may also be helpful.

Metabolic derangements

Possible metabolic derangements after extensive hepatic resections include hypoglycemia, hypoprothombinemia and hypoalbuminemia. To prevent hypoglycemia a 10% glucose solution should be administered intravenously until the child is able to feed orally. Administration of vitamin K for several days after surgery and daily monitoring of prothrombin times usually suffices to avoid hypoprothrombinemia. Albumin (25–50 g) is infused by vein daily to maintain serum levels above 30 g/l. Liver regeneration proceeds fairly rapidly after hepatectomy and, although not complete for several weeks, metabolic disturbances are rarely a problem for more than 3 or 4 days after surgery.

Chemotherapy

Chemotherapy required after surgery to treat real or potential residual tumor should be delayed until liver regeneration is complete. This is because normal liver function is necessary to metabolize most drugs and most chemotherapeutic agents limit liver regeneration.

Subphrenic abscess

Postoperative collections of blood, bile or serous fluid in the space produced by the liver resection are common complications even when appropriate drains are used and may result in subphrenic abscesses. This complication must always be considered when postoperative fever is prolonged. It is easily diagnosed by ultrasound imaging and is treated by percutaneous drainage. Drains inserted at the time of surgery should be left in place until drainage ceases, usually within 3 days in uncomplicated cases.

Outcome

With current perioperative and operative management mortality should be no more than 5%. The most common cause of death is uncontrolled hemorrhage, and this generally occurs in the region of the hepatic veins and the vena cava. Morbidity is due to infections in the subdiaphragmatic space and prolonged bile leak. Bile leaks may occur from the cut edge of the liver with or without a serious injury to the main hepatic duct or common duct in the porta hepatis.

The use of effective preoperative chemotherapy for the malignant lesions has helped to reduce the mortality and morbidity because the tumors to be resected are much smaller and less vascular than previously. As a result blood loss is lower, resections are less extensive and tumor spill is less frequent. Present cure rates for hepatoblastoma, the most common malignant neoplasm in children, approach 80% even when 'inoperable' tumors are included in the calculation; 15 years ago when patients were treated solely by surgery only 25% survived.

Surgical management of Wilms' tumor

Patrick G. Duffy FRCSI
Consultant Paediatric Urologist, Great Ormond Street Hospital for Children, London and Senior Lecturer in
Paediatric Urology, Institute of Urology, University of London, UK

Philip G. Ransley FRCS
Consultant Urological Surgeon, Great Ormond Street Hospital for Children, London and Senior Lecturer in
Paediatric Urology, Institute of Urology and Institute of Child Health, University of London, UK

In 1899 Max Wilms described a group of children with kidney tumors[1] and since that time his name has been applied to nephroblastoma of the kidney. The first nephrectomy for this malignancy was reported in 1877 by Jessop[2] and the first radiation treatment was recorded in 1915. Farber, in 1956, introduced actinomycin as a chemotherapeutic agent for nephroblastoma[3].

Surgical excision remains the cornerstone of the management of Wilms' tumor; however, a dramatic improvement in overall survival rate is a result of the coordinated use of surgery, multiple drug chemotherapy and radiation therapy (from 15% with surgery alone, to 85% with combination treatment). Thus the surgeon must be a member of an oncological team when managing a child with this disease.

Nephroblastoma is the most common solid abdominal tumor in childhood and usually presents as a painless abdominal mass in an otherwise well child. The peak age of presentation is approximately 3 years and the tumor is bilateral in 6% of cases.

Principles and justification

Indications for surgery

Radical nephrectomy is the primary treatment for unilateral Wilms' tumor. However, the presence of secondary deposits, caval tumor, bilateral disease or a tumor in a solitary kidney are indications for Tru-cut biopsy, chemotherapy and delayed partial or total nephrectomy.

Preoperative

Blood

Hemoglobin, creatinine, urea and electrolyte levels should be monitored, and liver function tests carried out.

Urine

A 24-h urine sample should be monitored to measure vanylmandelic acid, in order to exclude neuroblastoma.

Radiology

An ultrasonographic scan will demonstrate a solid tumor arising from a kidney and possibly extension of the tumor through the renal vein into the inferior vena cava. An intravenous urogram demonstrates the classical appearance of a space-occupying lesion within the kidney. Initial imaging must include the contralateral kidney to detect bilateral disease. Chest radiography (anteroposterior and lateral) is routinely performed, but computed tomographic (CT) scanning is more sensitive in detecting abnormalities of the contralateral kidney, lymphadenopathy, liver enlargement and lung secondaries.

Operation

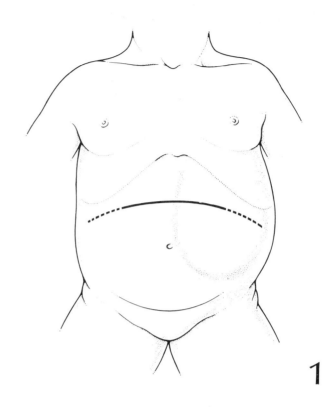

1 A generous transverse upper abdominal incision is required to facilitate complete exposure of both kidneys.

The rectus sheath is incised with diathermy. Both rectus muscles are completely divided. The falciform ligament is divided between ligatures. The peritoneum is entered with care to avoid breaching the anterior surface of the tumor and the incision is extended laterally under direct vision.

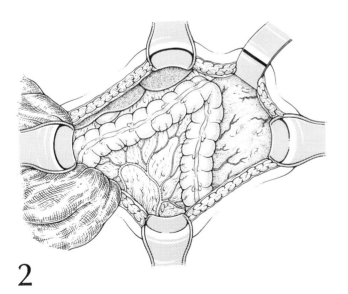

2 The abdominal contents are carefully examined for liver and peritoneal secondaries.

3 The contralateral kidney is fully mobilized and examined on both anterior and posterior surfaces in order to detect previously unsuspected bilateral disease. Biopsy of tissue only from the main tumor and contralateral lesion is performed under these circumstances.

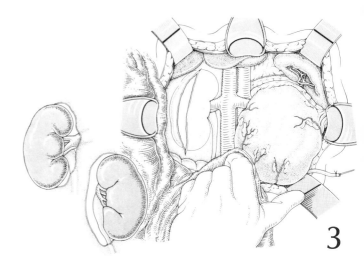

4 The colon with its mesentery is dissected from the anterior surface of the tumor.

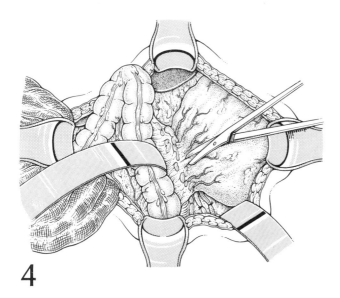
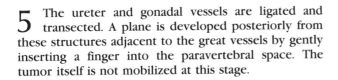

5 The ureter and gonadal vessels are ligated and transected. A plane is developed posteriorly from these structures adjacent to the great vessels by gently inserting a finger into the paravertebral space. The tumor itself is not mobilized at this stage.

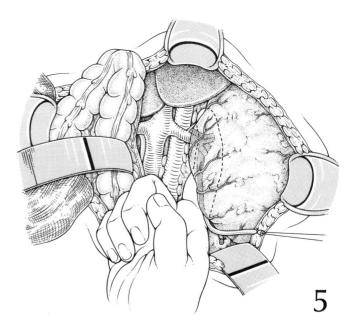

6 Dissection begins caudally, sweeping adventitial tissue and lymph nodes laterally off the great vessels. The renal vein and its branches are gently exposed. Careful palpation of the vein is performed to detect a venous extension of the tumor. Early mobilization of the inferior vena cava and renal vein may be required to prevent embolization of the tumor into the inferior vena cava, heart and pulmonary artery. On the right side the second part of the duodenum is encountered during this dissection.

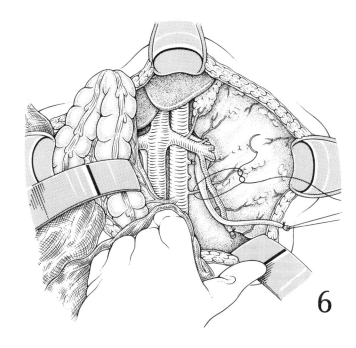

7 The renal vein is gently mobilized and elevated using a vascular sling to expose the renal artery, which should be ligated and divided before the renal vein to prevent swelling of the kidney with arterial blood.

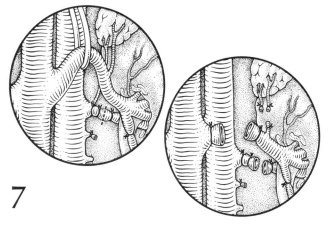

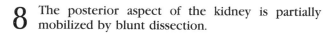

8 The posterior aspect of the kidney is partially mobilized by blunt dissection.

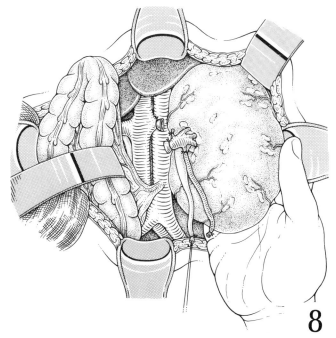

9 Superior dissection is hazardous on the left side, and damage to the spleen and tail of the pancreas must be avoided. The adrenal gland is removed if the tumor is in the upper pole of the kidney.

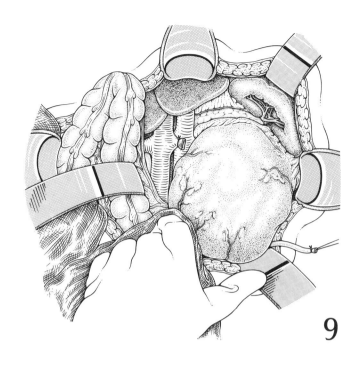

9

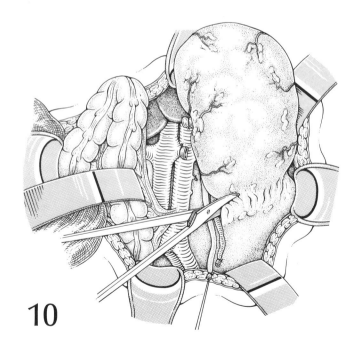

10

10 The kidney within Gerota's fascia is lifted out of the abdomen and the posterior dissection is completed under direct vision. The renal bed is inspected following removal of the kidney. Any remaining lymph nodes on the great vessels are removed.

Biopsy in unresectable tumor

11 With the patient in the lateral oblique position Tru-cut biopsy may be performed with ultrasound guidance.

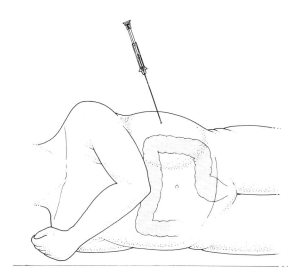

11

Postoperative care

Unilateral disease

Chemotherapy after surgery plays an integral part in the management of unilateral Wilms' tumor. However, if a tumor is exceedingly large chemotherapy may be administered before surgery to decrease the bulk of tissue. Intravenous chemotherapy is commenced within 24 h of operation. Subsequent adjuvant therapy in the form of radiotherapy and/or chemotherapy will be determined by the pathological stage and tumor type (favorable or unfavorable histology).

Bilateral disease

Biopsy[4] only is performed when bilateral disease is detected and chemotherapy administered. Subsequent surgical management may include a combination of total and partial nephrectomy, bilateral partial nephrectomy or bilateral nephrectomy with dialysis and subsequent renal transplantation. Such decisions are complex and require a team approach.

Conclusion

The management of Wilms' tumor consists of surgery combined with chemotherapy and radiotherapy. Chemotherapy has played a major role in decreasing mortality and morbidity. The surgeon should not embark on the management of Wilms' tumor without the aid of an oncology service.

References

1. Wilms M. *Die Mischgeschwuelste der Niere.* Leipzig: Arthur Georgi, 1899: 1–90.

2. Annotations. Extirpation of the kidney. *Lancet* 1877; i: 889.

3. Farber S, Toch R, Sears EM, Pinkel D. Advances in chemotherapy of cancer in man. *Adv Cancer Res* 1956; 4: 1–71.

4. Dykes EH, Marwaha RK, Dicks-Mireaux C *et al*. Risks and benefits of percutaneous biopsy and primary chemotherapy in advanced Wilms' tumour. *J Pediatr Surg* 1991; 68: 610–12.

Further reading

Mesrobian HGJ. Wilms' tumor: past, present, future. *J Urol* 1988; 140: 231–7.

Abdominal neuroblastoma

D. C. G. Crabbe MD, FRCS
Senior Registrar, Department of Paediatric Surgery, Great Ormond Street Hospital for Children, London, UK

E. M. Kiely FRCSI, FRCS
Consultant Paediatric Surgeon, Great Ormond Street Hospital for Children, London, UK

History

Neuroblastoma is the most common abdominal malignancy of childhood, the annual incidence being about six cases per million children. Neuroblastoma belongs to the group of embryonic tumors of childhood and, as such, presents in early life, with 50% of cases presenting before the age of 2 years. Most children have metastatic disease at the time of presentation. Although surgical excision is the mainstay of treatment for localized tumors, the place of surgery in children with advanced disease is uncertain. The biologic behavior of neuroblastoma is enigmatic and spontaneous regression, though rare, occurs more frequently than in any other human malignancy.

Much progress has been made in the last few years in understanding the biologic behavior of neuroblastoma at both the cellular and molecular level. This includes clarification of the role of growth factors and cell-surface receptors and demonstration of the activation of a specific proto-oncogene, N-myc, by genomic amplification. Mass screening for neuroblastoma is being studied by measurement of urinary catecholamines in infants. Despite all these advances the overall mortality rate is 40–50% with only modest improvement over the last 10 years.

Principles and justification

Clinical presentation

Abdominal neuroblastomas usually present with a palpable mass. There may be pain from tumor enlargement and compression of adjacent structures. Malaise and anorexia are common. Spinal cord compression is an important presentation, due to extension of the tumor through intervertebral foramina into the extradural space: the 'dumb-bell tumor'. Bony metastases are common in older children and present with local pain and swelling. Cutaneous metastases and massive hepatomegaly are a feature of stage 4S disease in infancy. Rare presentations include intractable diarrhea caused by secretion of vasoactive intestinal peptide by the tumor and the 'dancing eyes' syndrome of opsomyoclonus.

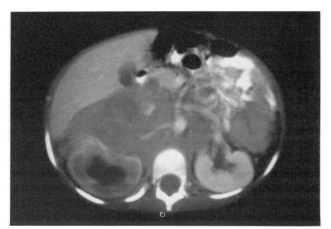

1a

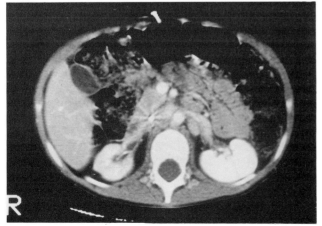

1b

Diagnosis

The clinical investigation of a child with a neuroblastoma is designed to confirm the diagnosis and stage the disease. The minimum criteria for diagnosis have been clarified by the International Neuroblastoma Study Group (INSG) and, in essence, this requires either an unequivocal pathologic diagnosis made from tumor tissue or the combination of tumor confirmed on a bone marrow aspirate or trephine biopsy and increased urine or serum catecholamines or metabolites. Pressure on surgeons to provide biopsies of the primary tumor in all cases, not only for histopathology but also for biologic studies, is increasing. The options for biopsy lie between Trucut needle biopsies or a formal open biopsy. Whichever method is chosen it is essential that the material is handled correctly; a sample of tumor should be placed aseptically in tissue culture medium for cytogenetic analysis, and tissue should be snap-frozen for molecular genetic studies and immunohistochemistry. Finally a small but representative sample should be fixed in buffered formalin for conventional histology.

1a, b Standard radiographic investigations of the child with a symptomatic abdominal mass include plain films, ultrasonography, computed tomography (CT) or magnetic resonance imaging (MRI) and radionuclide imaging. The tumor can often be seen on a plain abdominal film as a soft tissue shadow or paravertebral mass, which may be calcified. Ultrasonography will usually define the location of the mass and its relation to adjacent structures. However CT scanning and MRI have become the methods of choice for imaging the primary tumor. The typical appearance of an abdominal neuroblastoma on CT scan is an irregular mass arising in the suprarenal or paravertebral region which enhances after administration of intravenous contrast medium. Contrast enhancement is essential to evaluate vascular encasement and document excretion by both kidneys. Serial scans will demonstrate regression after chemotherapy but, in general, they underestimate disease and cannot dictate operability.

The contrast enhanced abdominal scan in *Illustration 1a* shows extensive disease in a 4-year-old-boy with stage 4 neuroblastoma. There are bilateral hydronephroses and the aorta is displaced forwards by tumor. The scan in *Illustration 1b* is of the same child after chemotherapy showing the tumor reduced in size and the hydronephroses resolved.

2a, b

Radionuclide imaging has an important place in the investigation of metastatic disease. Skeletal imaging with ^{99m}Tc-methylene diphosphonate is more accurate than conventional radiology for detecting skeletal metastases. Total body imaging with ^{131}I-meta-iodobenzylguanidine [^{131}I-MIBG] can be useful for localizing a primary tumor and metastases and is an essential prerequisite to therapeutic administration of ^{131}I-MIBG.

Excessive production of catecholamines is one of the most characteristic markers of neuroblastoma. Increased urinary catecholamine levels have been found in over 90% of children with neuroblastoma. Vanillylmandelic acid (VMA) and homovanillic acid (HVA) are measured most frequently and pretreatment values appear to correlate with tumor burden.

The ^{99m}Tc bone scan (*Illustration 2a*) and ^{131}I-MIBG bone scan (*Illustration 2b*) on the same patient as in *Illustration 1* both show metastases in the skull vault and upper humerus.

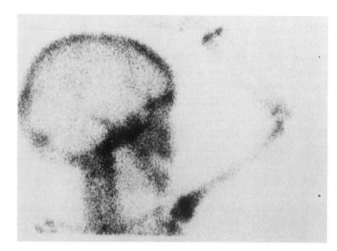

2a

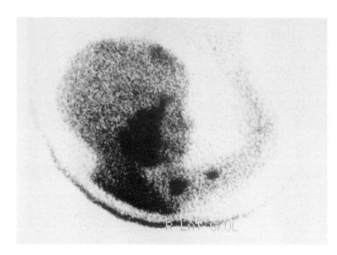

2b

Clinical staging

The International Neuroblastoma Staging System (INSS) has standardized the staging of neuroblastoma (*Table 1*). The definition of stage 3 has been revised extensively since its inception. A unilateral tumor was deemed to cross the midline if it invaded the spinal canal or extended to the midline anterior to the vertebral column, but such tumors differ clinically from massive tumors which infiltrate across the midline, encasing the great vessels. The vertebral column is now considered the midline and tumors originating on one side must infiltrate to or beyond the opposite side of the vertebral column to be considered stage 3.

Table 1   International Neuroblastoma Staging System

Stage	Description
1	Localized tumor with complete gross excision, with or without microscopic residual disease; representative ipsilateral lymph nodes negative for tumor microscopically (nodes attached to and removed with the primary tumor may be positive)
2a	Localized tumor with incomplete gross excision; representative ipsilateral non-adherent lymph nodes negative for tumor microscopically
2b	Localized tumor with or without complete gross excision, with ipsilateral nonadherent lymph nodes positive for tumor. Enlarged contralateral lymph nodes must be negative macroscopically
3	Unresectable unilateral tumor infiltrating across the midline, with or without regional lymph node involvement; or localized unilateral tumor with contralateral regional lymph node involvement; or midline tumor with bilateral extension by infiltration (unresectable) or by lymph node involvement
4	Any primary tumor with dissemination to distant lymph nodes, bone, bone marrow, liver, skin and/or other organs (except as defined in 4S)
4S	Localized primary tumor (as defined for stage 1, 2a, or 2b), with dissemination limited to skin, liver and/or bone marrow (limited to infants under 1 year of age). Bone marrow disease should be minimal, less than 10% total nucleated cells identified as malignant on bone marrow biopsy or aspirate

Treatment

The treatment of choice for stage 1 and 2a lesions is surgical excision. If the tumor is incompletely resected or recurs after surgery, the response to chemotherapy is usually good and radiotherapy is unnecessary. Stage 2b tumors with involvement of local nodes not adherent to it, despite complete extirpation of the primary lesion, have a significant chance of relapse and require chemotherapy.

The treatment of stage 3 and 4 neuroblastomas, considered 'high risk', is unsatisfactory: the mortality from disease progression and the morbidity from treatment are both high. Neuroblastoma is inherently chemosensitive and impressive initial responses to chemotherapy are common. However, relapses are common and invariably fatal. The most widely used regimen in the UK is OPEC (vincristine, cisplatin, etoposide and cyclophosphamide) alternating with OJEC (vincristine, carboplatin, etoposide and cyclophosphamide) administered at 21-day intervals. After five courses the tumor is restaged and, if distant metastases have regressed, surgical excision is undertaken. Children over 1 year of age with stage 4 disease are then given a myeloablative dose of melphalan with or without total body irradiation followed by rescue with a bone marrow transplant using autologous marrow harvested prior to surgery.

The number of children achieving complete responses has increased with this 'megatherapy', and the time to progression has been prolonged. Prolonged remissions have been obtained by this approach but the overall results are still poor and new therapeutic strategies are undergoing clinical trial. These include 'targeted' therapy with ^{131}I-MIBG, biologic response modifiers, including interferons and interleukins and differentiating agents (13-*cis*-retinoic acid).

Pathology

The typical untreated tumor is a rounded or lobulated soft mass of variable size with a reddish-gray cut surface, depending on the presence of hemorrhage. After chemotherapy the tumor is generally much firmer and less vascular. Flecks of calcification are often seen. The microscopic appearances are pleomorphic and multiple sections may reveal differences in cellularity and differentiation. The typical neuroblastoma is composed of small round cells with dense hyperchromatic nuclei and minimal cytoplasm in a background of eosinophilic stroma. Circumferential collections of cells with a central focus of eosinophilic filaments constitute the Homer Wright rosette, although these are relatively uncommon. Evidence of differentiation includes the appearance of ganglion cells (ganglioneuroblastoma) and, when neuroblasts are not visible, the term ganglioneuroma is used.

Prognosis

Age at diagnosis and disease stage at presentation are undoubtedly the two most important determinants of prognosis. Unpublished data from the European Neuroblastoma Study Group show 5-year disease-free survival of 80% for infants under 1 year of age, 38% for children 1–5 years of age and 21% for children over the age of 5 years. Data from the same series showing the

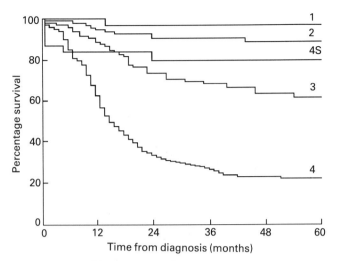

Figure 1   Neuroblastoma survival by disease stage

effect of stage are shown in *Figure 1*. Age is the only factor so far that has been shown to be of predictive value in patients with stage 4 disease.

The histologic grade of the tumor has been shown to correlate with prognosis. Serum ferritin levels reflect tumor burden and are of prognostic significance. Recently, several important biologic properties of the tumor have been shown to correlate with prognosis. These include DNA content (ploidy), growth fraction, the presence of cytogenetic abnormalities (particularly homogeneously staining regions, double minute chromosomes and deletions involving the short arm of

chromosome 1). Perhaps the most fascinating is the association of multiple copies of the *N-myc* oncogene with rapid tumor progression. These biologic studies require fresh primary tumor as post-chemotherapy specimens are usually too fibrous/necrotic for analysis.

Surgical management

Early surgery is appropriate for localized tumors, where resection can be completed without removing or permanently damaging the adjacent structures. In advanced cases chemotherapy facilitates surgery by shrinking large tumors and rendering them less friable and vascular, permitting a safer and more complete resection. Consequently with a systematic approach even very large tumors and associated nodal disease may be excised with relatively low morbidity. The use of a standard approach is also of value with less advanced tumors as the resection is more straight-forward when vital anatomy is displayed. The operation described here was developed to deal with the problem of vascular encasement. There are other ways of managing the problem but detailed accounts are infrequent. The use of the ultrasound dissector tends to result in a plane of dissection which is too superficial on the vessels and has not been found to be a great advantage.

The completeness of the procedure will depend on the attitude of the surgeon. Neuroblastoma rarely invades the tunica media of major blood vessels. Consequently a subadventitial plane may be entered and developed using sharp dissection. The procedure consists of three phases – vessel exposure, vessel clearance and tumor removal. In this section the excision of a localized, right-sided tumor and an advanced left-sided tumor are described.

Operation

3 The abdomen is opened through a long supra-umbilical transverse incision. For right-sided tumors the ascending colon and duodenum are reflected medially. The inferior vena cava below the limit of the tumor is exposed by incision of the adventitia longitudinally along the middle of the vessel.

3

4 The dissection advances proximally, exposing the anterior wall. The right renal vein is then encountered and displayed similarly. The right renal artery is sought posterior to the vein. Once these vessels are in view the caval dissection proceeds as before.

Reflection of the right lobe of the liver facilitates access to the superior aspect of the tumor and to the proximal inferior vena cava. Once the cava has been exposed as far as the liver both sides and posterior walls are cleared. The tumor may be quite strongly adherent to the lateral wall but a plane of dissection usually exists.

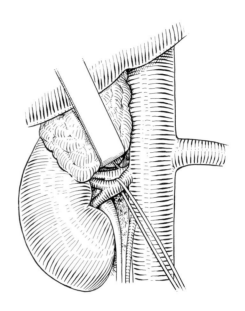

4

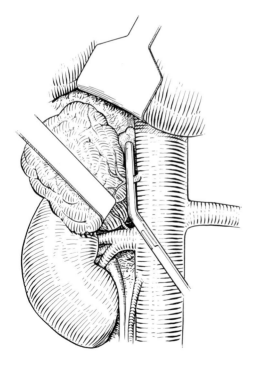

5

5 The blood supply and venous drainage are severed and the remainder of the dissection and tumor removal are straightforward.

6a, b The colon, spleen, pancreas and stomach should be reflected to expose extensive left-sided tumors. Dissection commences just beyond the inferior margin of the tumor along the middle of the common or external iliac artery to establish the correct subadventitial plane. The tumor is then incised vertically in 1–2-cm lengths down to the correct plane. In this way the aorta is approached and its anterior wall exposed.

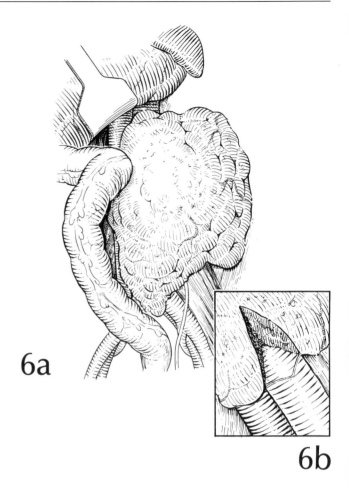

6a

6b

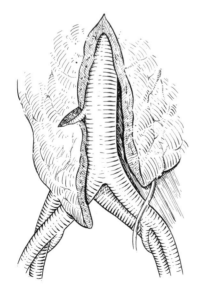

7

7 The origin of the inferior mesenteric artery is cleared in a similar fashion. The aorta is exposed up to the left renal vein, which is freed in turn over a 4–5-cm length.

8 Cautious dissection more proximally, exposing the left side of the aorta, will bring the left renal artery into view. At this stage the plane of the incision should move 45° so that the knife blade is cutting down onto the anterolateral wall of the aorta.

In this manner the diaphragm is reached and the incision continues until healthy tissue is encountered.

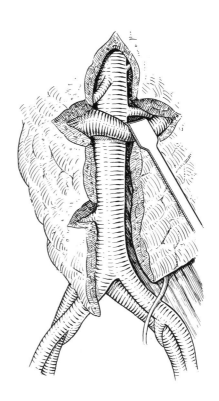

8

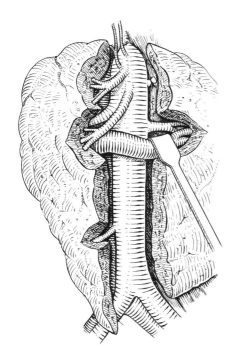

9

9 Once the upper limit of the tumor is visible a sling is placed around the aorta. The anterior wall of the aorta is then exposed and the proximal celiac and superior mesenteric arteries may be cleared of tumor. Each of these vessels is then dissected free from tumor in turn. The left renal artery and vein are cleared similarly.

Finally the distal aorta is completely freed of tumor on both sides as well as posteriorly. The origin of the right renal artery should be identified before the main tumor is removed. Once all the main vessels are in view and clear the tumor is removed in pieces. At the end of the procedure no macroscopic tumor should remain.

Postoperative care

Postoperative care follows the same principles as any other major laparotomy. Direct monitoring of arterial and central venous pressure continues for 24–48 h. Urine output should be monitored and blood glucose concentrations checked periodically. Effective pain relief is delivered in the form of epidural infusion or continuous intravenous opiate infusion. The postoperative ileus resolves after 3–4 days. Diarrhea is very common after extensive arterial clearance and frequently requires treatment.

Outcome

The authors have treated 129 children with abdominal neuroblastoma by radical surgery over the last 10 years. The average operation lasted for 4 (range 1–10) h and the mean transfusion requirement was 500 ml. There were five aortic injuries and one renal artery injury. Eleven nephrectomies were performed to achieve complete clearance of the tumor and a further patient lost function in a kidney that was noted to be swollen and congested at the end of the operation. There have been two postoperative deaths: one child died from complications of profound hypoglycemia before routine monitoring of blood sugars was undertaken; the second child died following an aortic rupture on the eighth postoperative day. The most common postoperative complication was diarrhea, which occurred in almost 20%. The adhesional intestinal obstruction rate was below 5% although presentation may be delayed: the extensive vascular dissection denervates the gut with the result that intestinal colic does not occur, hence the patient may experience no pain from the obstruction until peritonitis develops. Three children had marked chylous ascites and two subsequently required peritoneovenous shunting.

The effects of age, tumor stage and changes in adjuvant treatment confound attempts to analyse the influence of surgery on the long-term prognosis. The results of surgery for localized disease are good, although the numbers are small. Fifteen children had stage 1 or 2 disease and six received chemotherapy. Complete excision was not achieved in three cases because of intervertebral extension but despite this 14 of the 15 patients have survived. Complete resection was achieved in 18 of the 23 children with stage 3 disease. Of the 17 children who were followed for more than 30 months, eight of 12 who underwent complete excision are alive and free of disease, compared with three of five who underwent incomplete excision. Complete resection was achieved in 67 of 87 children with stage 4 disease; reasons for failure included adherence to vessels, invasion of the porta hepatis, obvious new growth of tumor, impenetrable periaortic calcification and gross involvement of the small intestinal mesentery. Of the 75 children followed for more than 2 years, 29% (22 of 75) are alive and free of disease but the the results of children who had complete resection were not significantly different from those whose resections were incomplete. The mean time to relapse was 7 (range 1–24) months. Distal relapse alone was a feature in 32, local relapse occurred in 12 and six had simultaneous local and distal relapse.

The role of surgery in the treatment of localized neuroblastoma is clear and the outlook is good. There does appear to be a modest survival advantage following complete excision in stage 3 tumors but the outlook of stage 4 disease is gloomy and the part surgical excision plays in its treatment is very uncertain.

Further reading

Brodeur GM, Pritchard J, Berthold F *et al*. Revisions of the international criteria for neuroblastoma diagnosis, staging, and response to treatment. *J Clin Oncol* 1993; 11: 1466–77.

Kiely EM. The surgical challenge of neuroblastoma. *J Pediatr Surg* 1994; 29: 128–33.

Matsumura M, Atkinson JB, Hays DM *et al*. An evaluation of the role of surgery in metastatic neuroblastoma. *J Pediatr Surg* 1988; 23: 448–53.

Nitschke R, Smith EI, Shochat S *et al*. Localized neuroblastoma treated by surgery: a Pediatric Oncology Group Study. *J Clin Oncol* 1988; 6: 1271–9.

Pochedly C, ed. *Neuroblastoma: Tumour Biology and Therapy*. Boca Raton: CRC Press, 1990.

Tsuchida Y, Yokoyama J, Kaneko M *et al*. Therapeutic significance of surgery in advanced neuroblastoma: a report from the study group of Japan. *J Pediatr Surg* 1992; 27: 616–22.

Rhabdomyosarcoma

Richard J Andrassy MD, FACS, FAAP
A. G. McNeese Professor of Surgery and Pediatrics, Chief of Pediatric Surgery, M.D. Anderson Cancer Center, and Pediatric Surgeon-in-Chief, Hermann Children's Hospital, Texas Medical Center, Houston, Texas, USA

Principles and justification

Rhabdomyosarcoma is the most common soft tissue sarcoma in infants and children and can arise from almost any site. The principles of surgical management are similar to those for sarcomas in adults, except that rhabdomyosarcoma is very responsive to chemotherapy, which thus allows for more conservative surgical management in many patients.

Survival in rhabdomyosarcoma was less than 10% until the late 1960s. In 1972 the Intergroup Rhabdomyosarcoma Study (IRS) was established, which has since studied large numbers of patients in a prospective fashion. This has led to tremendous advances in chemotherapy and survival. The excellent response to chemotherapy has allowed less aggressive surgery and the concept of delayed surgery and second-look surgery has been advanced.

Although the sites of presentation of rhabdomyosarcoma are ubiquitous, only a few selected surgical approaches will be discussed. Head and neck primaries are quite common, but generally only require biopsy initially, and further surgical management is beyond the scope of this chapter.

The practising surgeon may be asked to biopsy and/or surgically manage certain tumors such as extremity rhabdomyosarcoma, paratesticular and vaginal rhabdomyosarcomas, which will be discussed and surgical principles outlined. A clear understanding of the surgeon's role in the management of rhabdomyosarcoma is needed, as the surgeon plays a pivotal role in staging (preoperative clinical assessment) and in grouping (based on extent of surgical resection and intraoperative findings).

Preoperative

Evaluation and staging

Staging before treatment requires thorough clinical, laboratory and imaging examinations. Biopsy is required to establish the histologic diagnosis. Pretreatment size is determined by external measurement by magnetic resonance imaging or computed tomography, depending on the anatomic location. For less accessible sites computed tomography is also employed as a means of lymph node assessment. Metastatic sites require some form of imaging, but not necessarily histologic confirmation, except for bone marrow examination.

Pretreatment staging evaluates the primary site, tumor invasiveness, tumor size, lymph node status and metastases. The survival rate varies significantly with different primary tumor sites. Some tumor locations have a very favorable prognosis, e.g. orbit, vagina and vulva, and paratesticular. An intermediate prognosis is observed in cases of extremity, bladder, prostate, uterus, and non-parameningeal head and neck tumors. A relatively poor prognosis is observed with primary tumors at the parameningeal head and neck sites, retroperitoneum, buttocks, chest wall, trunk, perineal and perianal region. Poor prognosis is seen in patients with metastatic disease. The site of the tumor is, therefore, an important prognostic variable and has been taken into consideration in the pretreatment staging in IRS-IV as shown in *Table 1*. Site groups and primary anatomic sites are shown in *Table 2*.

Operations

Biopsy and general principles of operative resection

Clinical grouping is determined by the extent of biopsy and/or resection as well as of metastatic disease. Biopsy may be made by needle, incisional or excisional biopsy, depending on the site. Adequate tissue for biologic markers has been more of an issue in IRS-IV. Consideration of minimally invasive surgery should be made to allow adequate staging and sampling of tissue with minimal effect on the patient. Biopsy may be incisional in sites such as head and neck, or excisional in sites such as paratesticular. Most rhabdomyosarcomas are treated with biopsy followed by chemotherapy and then operative removal or cytoreduction with or without radiation to the primary site and positive regional nodes. Adequate sampling of regional lymph nodes is important, particularly if clinically positive (except perhaps in paratesticular tumors, *see below*). Positive regional nodes are treated with radiation to prevent local nodal recurrence.

Table 1   Tumour node metastasis (TNM) pretreament staging classification

Stage	Sites	T	Size	N	M
1	Orbit Head and neck (excluding parameningeal) Genitourinary (non-bladder/non-prostate)	T_1 or T_2	a or b	N_0 or N_1 or N_x	M_0
2	Bladder/prostate Extremity Cranial parameningeal Other (includes trunk, retro-peritoneum, etc.)	T_1 or T_2	a	N_0 or N_x	M_0
3	Bladder/prostate Extremity Cranial parameningeal Other (includes trunk, retro-peritoneum, etc.)	T_1 or T_2	a b	N_1 N_0 or N_1 or N_x	M_0 M_0
4	All	T_1 or T_2	a or b	N_0 or N_1	M_1

Definitions:
Tumor
  T (site)$_1$, confined to anatomic site of origin
  (a) ≤5 cm in diameter;
  (b) >5 cm in diameter.
  T (site)$_2$, extension and/or fixation to surrounding tissue
  (a) ≤5 cm in diameter;
  (b) >5 cm in diameter.
Regional nodes
  N_0, regional nodes not clinically involved;
  N_1, regional nodes clinically involved by neoplasm;
  N_x, clinical status of regional nodes unknown (particularly sites that preclude lymph node evaluation).
Metastasis
  M_0, no distant metastasis;
  M_1, metastasis present.

Biopsy of possible metastatic sites, such as the lungs, may also be warranted. Open or thoracoscopic techniques may be utilized. Solitary pulmonary nodules are usually not metastatic disease in rhabdomyosarcoma and should be biopsied to rule out an infectious focus.

The specific principles of surgical management vary with anatomic location, but in general the principle of wide local excision without destroying function is appropriate. The likelihood of gross or microscopic residual neoplasm when simple resection of an undiagnosed soft tissue tumor has been carried out is so high that reoperation is recommended as the initial definitive approach to management. Re-excision has been shown by IRS studies to improve disease-free survival. IRS grouping is shown in *Table 3*.

Table 2   Site groups and primary sites

Orbit	*Genitourinary*	Retroperitoneum
Eye	*bladder/prostate*	Pelvis, site
Orbit	Bladder	indeterminate
	Prostate	Retroperitoneum
Head and neck		
Cheek	*Extremity*	Trunk
Hypopharynx	Arm	Abdominal wall
Larynx	Buttock	Breast
Neck	Elbow region	Chest wall
Oral cavity	Foot	Paraspinal
Oropharynx	Forearm	
Parotid	Hand	Other
Scalp	Knee region	Adrenal glands
Thyroid	Leg	Bone
Other	Shoulder girdle	Brain, ventricles
	Thigh	and central
Parameningeal (PM)		canal
Infratemporal fossa	*Other*	Brain, general
Middle ear	Gastrointestinal and	Cerebrospinal
Nasal cavity/sinus	hepatobiliary	fluid
Nasopharynx	Esophagus	Lymph nodes –
Paranasal sinus	Gallbladder	distant
Parapharyngeal area	Intestine, colon/	Lymph nodes –
Pterygopalatine	cecum/rectum	regional
Cheek (with PM	Intestine, small	Marrow
extension)	and duodenum	Meninges
Larynx (with PM	Liver	Multiple sites,
extension)	Omentum	excluding lung
Orbit (with PM	Pancreas	Muscle
extension)	Peritoneum	Peripheral nerves
Oropharynx (with	Stomach	Pineal
PM extension)		Pituitary
Other head and	Intrathoracic	Skin
neck (with PM	Bronchi and	Spinal cord
extension)	bronchioles	Spleen
Parotid (with PM	Diaphragm	Subcutaneous
extension)	Heart	Unknown
Scalp (with PM	Hilum	Other
extension)	Lung and local	
	sites	
Genitourinary non-	Lung and other	
bladder/prostate	sites	
Cervix	Lung	
Epididymis	Mediastinum	
Kidney	Pericardium	
Ovary	Pleura	
Penis	Pleural effusion	
Spermatic cord	Thymus	
Testis–paratesticular	Trachea	
Urachus		
Ureter	Perineum–anus	
Urethra	Anus	
Uterus	Perineum	
Vagina		
Vulva		

Table 3   IRS clinical grouping classification

Group I   *Localized disease, completely resected*
Regional nodes not involved – lymph node biopsy or dissection is required except for head and neck lesions

   (a) Confined to muscle or organ of origin
   (b) Contiguous involvement – infiltration outside the muscle or organ of origin, as through fascial planes

Notation: This includes both gross inspection and microscopic confirmation of complete resection. Any nodes that may be inadvertently taken with the specimen must be negative. If the latter should be involved microscopically, then the patient is placed in group IIb or IIc (*see below*).

Group II   *Total gross resection with evidence of regional spread*

   (a) Grossly resected tumor with microscopic residual disease

(Surgeon believes that he has removed all of the tumor, but the pathologist finds tumor at the margin of resection and additional resection to achieve clean margin is not feasible.) No evidence of gross residual tumor. No evidence of regional node involvement. Once radiotherapy and/or chemotherapy have been started, re-exploration and removal of the area of microscopic residual does not change the patient's group.

   (b) Regional disease with involved nodes, completely resected with no microscopic residual disease

Notation: Complete resection with microscopic confirmation of no residual disease makes this different from groups IIa and IIc. Additionally, in contrast to group IIa, regional nodes (which are completely resected, however) are involved, but the most distal node is histologically negative.

   (c) Regional disease with involved nodes, grossly resected, but with evidence of microscopic residual histologic involvement of the most distal regional node (from the primary site) in the dissection

Notation: The presence of microscopic residual disease makes this group different from group IIb, and nodal involvement makes this group different from group IIa.

Group III   *Incomplete resection with gross residual disease*

   (a) After biopsy only
   (b) After gross or major resection of the primary (>50%)

Group IV   *Distant metastatic disease present at onset*

(Lung, liver, bones, bone marrow, brain, and distant muscle and nodes)

Notation: The above excludes regional nodes and adjacent organ infiltration which places the patient in a more favorable grouping (as noted above under group II).

The presence of positive cytology in cerebrospinal fluid, pleural or abdominal fluids as well as implants on pleural or peritoneal surfaces are regarded as indications for placing the patient in group IV.

PARATESTICULAR RHABDOMYOSARCOMA

1 A paratesticular mass should be resected by inguinal orchidectomy, with complete resection of the spermatic cord structures to the level of the internal ring. Resection of the scrotal skin is not necessary unless there is fixation or a trans-scrotal approach was used for biopsy. Recent IRS-III data suggest that retroperitoneal lymph node dissection is not necessary.

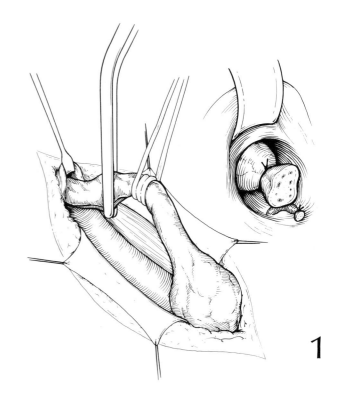

VAGINAL RHABDOMYOSARCOMA

2 Vaginal rhabdomyosarcoma presents with vaginal discharge, often bloody, or prolapse of a polypoid mass. The diagnosis is made by vaginoscopy and biopsy of the lesion. Treatment used to consist of extensive anterior pelvic exenteration, but since this tumor was found to be very chemosensitive, definitive surgery is delayed until after an initial course of therapy. Delayed tumor resection may consist of partial vaginectomy or vaginectomy with hysterectomy. Bladder salvage is possible in most patients. Vaginal tumors originate mainly from the anterior vaginal wall; they may invade the vesicovaginal septum or bladder wall due to its proximity. Cystoscopy is warranted during initial evaluation and at intervals during follow-up.

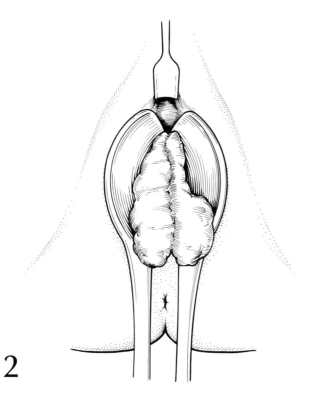

3 Treatment varies depending on the extent and location of the tumor. Tumors near the cervix are managed by hysterectomy and partial vaginectomy. Mid-vaginal tumors may occasionally be managed by sleeve vaginal resection with end-to-end vaginal repair, thus preserving the uterus and sufficient vagina. Tumors near the introitus can be managed by vaginectomy or occasionally by partial vaginectomy with flap or skin coverage to maintain vaginal patency and function. Occasionally anterior vaginal lesions will require a partial posterior cystectomy. Preservation of the bladder is possible in most cases without too high a risk of local recurrence. Patients with microscopically positive margins undergo local irradiation even with adequate resection. Local vaginal applicator radiotherapy has been recommended by some instead of vaginectomy.

Recent evidence has suggested that repeated biopsies and chemotherapy may be adequate for tumor evaluation in some patients.

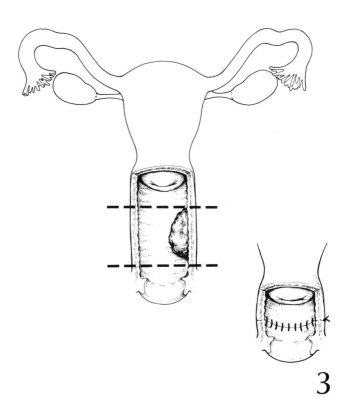

3

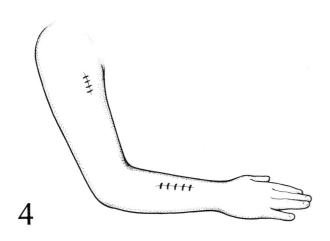

4

EXTREMITY RHABDOMYOSARCOMA

4 Biopsy of extremity lesions should take into consideration the need for reoperation and wide excision. Longitudinal incisions for biopsy are therefore preferable.

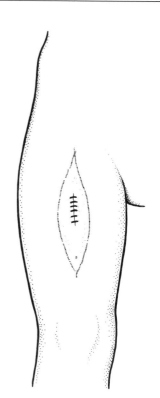

5   Wide local excision with clear margins is preferable for definitive surgery whenever possible. A limb-sparing operation is an important goal. Fewer than 5% of extremity tumors now require amputation. When biopsy is performed without knowledge of the diagnosis or when the margins are positive, re-excision of the primary site to achieve tumor-free margins improves survival. Regional nodes should be sampled so that appropriate local radiation may be given for positive nodes. Surgical removal of the primary site offers the best outcome.

Unfortunately, extremity rhabdomyosarcoma usually has alveolar pathology (poor prognosis) and the response to chemotherapy is not as good as for other sites; disease-free survival is therefore more clearly related to the completeness of initial excision of the primary tumor than is the case in patients with tumors in other locations.

5

Further reading

Grosfeld JL. Rhabdomyosarcoma. In: Ashcraft KW, Holder TM, eds. *Pediatric Surgey* 2nd edn. Philadelphia: WB Saunders, 1993: 875–89.

Hays DM, Lawrence W Jr, Wharam M *et al*. Primary reexcision for patients with 'microscopic residual' tumor following initial excision of sarcomas of trunk and extremity sites. *J Pediatr Surg* 1989; 24: 5–10.

Lawrence W Jr, Hays DM, Heyn R, Beltangudy M, Maurer HM. Surgical lessons from the Intergroup Rhabdomyosarcoma Study (IRS) pertaining to extemity tumors. *World J Surg* 1988; 12: 676–84.

Maurer HM, Ruymann RB, Pochedly C, eds. *Rhabdomyosarcoma and Related Tumors in Children and Adolescents*. Boca Raton, Florida: CRC Press, 1991.

Raney RB, Hays DM, Tefft M *et al*. Rhabdomyosarcoma and the undifferentiated sarcomas. In: Pizzo PA, Poplack DG, eds. *Principles and Practice of Pediatric Oncology*. Philadelphia: JB Lippincott, 1989: 635–58.

Weiner ES, Lawrence WH, Hays DM *et al*. Retroperitoneal node biopsy in paratesticular rhabdomyosarcoma. *J Pediatr Surg* 1994 (in press).

Sacrococcygeal teratoma

Daniel P. Doody MD
Associate Visiting Surgeon, Division of Pediatric Surgery, Massachusetts General Hospital, and Assistant
Professor of Surgery, Harvard Medical School, Boston, Massachusetts, USA

Samuel H. Kim MD
Visiting Surgeon, Division of Pediatric Surgery, Massachusetts General Hospital, and Associate Clinical
Professor of Surgery, Harvard Medical School, Boston, Massachusetts, USA

Principles and justification

Sacrococcygeal teratomas ('monstrous tumor') are complex neoplasms arising from totipotent cells of the yolk sac endoderm and contain tissues derived from the three embryonic layers: ectoderm, mesoderm and endoderm. The tumors are generally partly cystic and partly solid, consisting of a non-homogeneous mixture of hamartomatous connective tissue and tissues in varying stages of differentiation (glial tissue, dermal elements, pancreas, bone and/or muscle). These tumors occur in one in 35 000–40 000 births and are the most common neoplasms of the neonate.

Prenatal diagnosis

Increased application of antenatal ultrasonography has increasingly identified congenital lesions including sacrococcygeal teratomas. Infants with large tumors should be delivered by cesarian section as death could be caused by dystocia, tumor rupture, tumor avulsion or hemorrhage into the tumor. If the tumor is discovered before 30 weeks of gestation, the risk of fetal death appears to be greater. Placentomegaly or hydrops fetalis are particularly poor prognosticators, generally indicating fetal high-output cardiac failure; all fetuses showing these antenatal ultrasonographic findings have died *in utero*[1]. As the fetal evolution of sacrococcygeal teratomas becomes better defined and accurate predictors of fetal loss are delineated, certain tumors may benefit from *in utero* intervention.

Diagnosis in the neonate

1 The diagnosis of sacrococcygeal teratoma is generally made immediately after birth with the external appearance of the anomaly. Seventy-five percent of affected neonates are female. An important feature is the position of the anorectum, which is usually displaced anteriorly by the tumor but may be surrounded by it. The tumor typically has an external component although 10% of the lesions are completely internal.

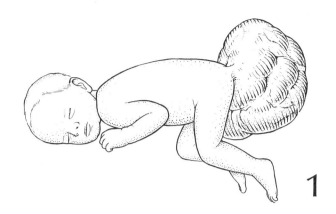

2a–c The anomaly has three basic forms (although four types have been defined by the Surgical Section of the American Academy of Pediatrics (AAPSS). These are: (1) pedunculated (AAPSS type I; 46%); (2) dumb-bell with pelvic or intra-abdominal extension (AAPSS types II and III; 44%); (3) sessile or intra-abdominal (AAPSS type IV; 10%)[2].

The tumor is always attached to the coccyx and projects to a varying degree into the presacral hollow. This upward extension into the pelvic space may compress and elevate the rectum, vagina, bladder and uterus; and the displacement of pelvic organs may cause urinary retention, hydronephrosis, or large bowel obstruction.

Neural deficit is not usually documented preoperatively. Additional anomalies are present in 20% of affected neonates, primarily affecting the musculoskeletal system including the spine. Differential diagnoses of this lesion include meningocele, lipomeningocele, hemangioma, lymphangioma, chordoma, pelvic neuroblastoma, hamartoma, cystic duplication of the rectum, neuroenteric cysts or perirectal abscess.

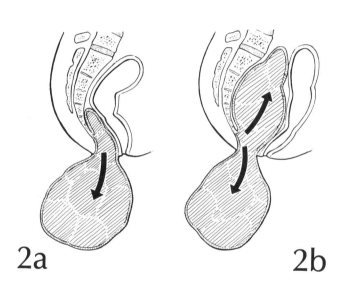

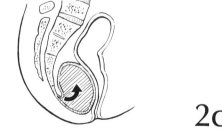

Indications for surgery

Of those children operated upon in the neonatal period, approximately 90% of the lesions are benign. In lesions removed after 6 months of life, 50% or more of the tumors are malignant, with the most common neoplasms being embryonal or yolk sac tumor. This natural history suggests a malignant transformation in a previously benign lesion. With this risk, these tumors should always be excised following discovery. In addition to the apparent malignant degeneration, spontaneous ulceration with exsanguinating hemorrhage may occur because of the tumor's rich vascular supply.

Preoperative

Radiographs of the abdomen and pelvis may reveal calcifications, which are seen in one-third of the lesions. Although ultrasonography may demonstrate a pelvic or intra-abdominal component to the tumor, computed tomographic scanning may be more helpful in defining the intra-abdominal extent of disease, which may dictate the surgical approach. Serum α-fetoprotein, a useful marker for malignant degeneration, is significantly elevated at birth and remains markedly elevated for 90–120 days after birth, decreasing to adult levels only at 6–12 months. None the less, this tumor marker should be assayed and compared to age-appropriate values[3].

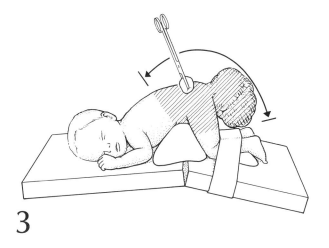

3

Anesthesia

General endotracheal anesthesia is mandatory. High-output cardiac failure secondary to arteriovenous channels in the tumor may limit the use of inhalation agents, which have known cardiodepressant effects. With the possibility of brisk blood loss during the procedure reliable venous access is necessary, and blood should be available in the operating room at the time of surgery. An arterial line for pressure monitoring is indicated; central venous monitoring is advantageous but not absolutely necessary. The stomach is emptied with a nasogastric tube, and an indwelling bladder catheter placed. Broad-spectrum antibiotics are given and adjusted for age and weight of the child.

Operation

Position of patient

3 In almost all cases the procedure is performed with the infant in an exaggerated prone jack-knife position. Rolled towels are used to support the pelvis and shoulders, allowing free movement of the chest and abdominal walls during assisted ventilation. A 1% solution of povidone-iodine (1:10 dilution in saline) is used as an enema to prepare the rectum for digital manipulation during the course of dissection. Other authors prefer to pack the rectum with a petrolatum-impregnated gauze and exclude the anus from the field.

Dorsal exposure

4 A chevron incision is performed with its apex over the sacrum, continuing around the dorsolateral surface of the tumor. The tumor capsule is usually well defined and separate from other tissues.

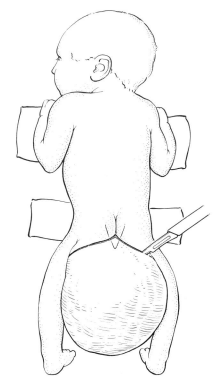

4

Coccygectomy and control of the middle sacral vessels

5 The sacrum and coccyx are identified and the coccyx is divided at the sacrococcygeal joint. The middle sacral vessels, located immediately beneath this landmark, are controlled in continuity and divided. Any collateral circulation from the lateral sacral vessels must be identified and ligated. Once this early control is established, the dissection becomes relatively bloodless. With an extensive intra-abdominal component, an initial transabdominal approach will be required to achieve vascular isolation.

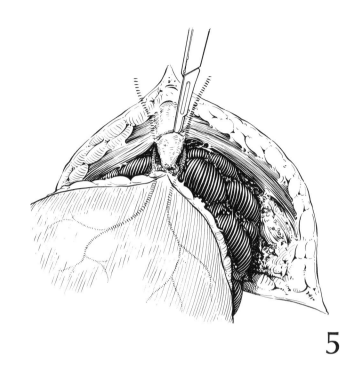

5

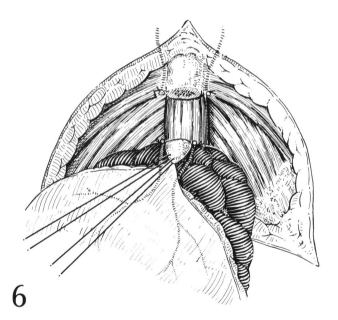

6

Exposure of the proximal rectum

6 The coccyx is always excised with the teratoma, but the muscles of the pelvic floor are preserved and carefully separated from the tumor during dissection. The coccyx is retracted with the neoplasm and with gentle tension the teratoma is separated from the inferior and medial aspects of the gluteus maximus muscles. The proximal rectum is identified at the base of the dissection during this portion of the procedure.

Ventral incision

7 A ventral chevron incision is made to allow the assistant to place upward traction on the tumor.

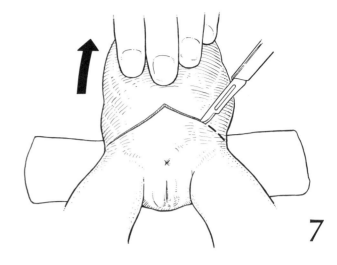

7

Ventral dissection and exposure of the distal rectum

8 An intrarectal pack or a finger allows the operator to identify the rectum and sphincter complex. Electrocautery is used to separate the fine attachments of the tumor from the anorectal sphincter complex, the levator ani muscles, and the gluteus maximus muscles. With gentle upward tension on the teratoma, the tumor is dissected free and removed.

8

Reconstruction of pelvic floor

9 The posterior and superior portions of the levator muscles are sewn to the presacral fascia using interrupted 4/0 silk sutures. This maneuver allows the anus to assume a near normal configuration and gives the best cosmetic outcome.

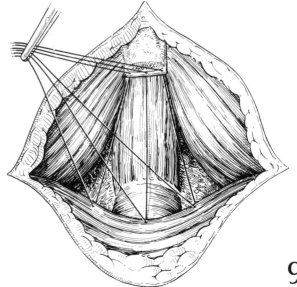

9

Approximation of gluteus maximus muscles

10 A Penrose drain, which is placed in the perirectal space, is brought out through a separate stab incision. The gluteus maximus muscles are then approximated in the midline using 3/0 silk or 3/0 polyglactin sutures.

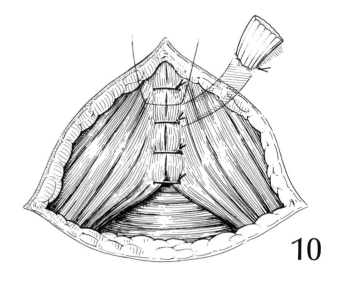

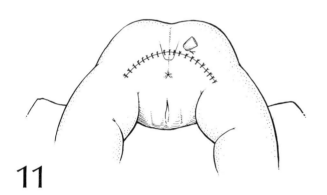

Skin closure

11 The anus returns to a near normal location. Any redundancy to the dorsal skin flap may be trimmed. The incision is closed with interrupted or running 5/0 nylon sutures.

Sacrococcygeal teratoma with bulky intra-abdominal disease

Extension of the tumor over the pelvic brim is unusual; it comprised 9% of the total lesions in the AAPSS survey but this is an important group because preliminary abdominal exploration precedes the pelvic excision[4]. The tumor is freed from the lower abdominal and pelvic viscera through a lower midline or transverse lower abdominal incision. By this preliminary dissection, the middle sacral vessels and collateral blood supply can be controlled. Transabdominal isolation of the tumor will prevent uncontrolled hemorrhage, which has been reported with a blind debulking of extensive pelvic or intra-abdominal disease through an isolated perineal approach. The laparotomy incision can be closed and the child placed in the prone position for the remainder of the procedure as described above.

Postoperative care

The child is maintained in a prone position to prevent soiling the surgical site with urine or feces for the first 3 postoperative days. The nasogastric tube is removed as bowel activity returns. The perirectal drain is generally removed 24–48h after the procedure. A pelvic neuropraxia may cause a poorly contracting, neurogenic bladder, which will require intermittent catheterization in the early postoperative period but this problem is usually temporary. Wound infections are infrequently seen despite the considerable rectal manipulation.

Long-term complications

Long-term complications occur frequently with approximately 40% of children experiencing mild functional bowel problems with soiling or constipation; 10% of infants will have urinary incontinence or neurogenic bladder, often associated with functional bowel impairment[5]. These problems do not appear to be related to the degree of pelvic tumor involvement, tumor size or the histology of the neoplasm. The tumor may recur if the coccyx is not removed, if malignancy is found at the initial excision, and in 5–10% of children who have excision of apparently benign lesions.

Pathology

Thorough histologic examination of the tumor is essential to define any malignant element. The risk of malignancy increases with age at the time of excision. Teratomas are classified as mature, immature with embryonic components or with malignant components. Immaturity is defined by the mitotic activity and the extent of neuroepithelium present. The cancers present in sacrococcygeal teratomas are germ cell in origin and almost exclusively embryonal carcinomas or yolk sac tumors (endodermal sinus tumors).

Chemotherapy

Cisplatin, bleomycin, vinblastine and/or VP-16 (etoposide) has had reported success as first-line therapy in the treatment of extragonadal germ cell tumors. This regimen may shrink the tumor, which may then be amenable to secondary resection. However, 4-year survival with extragonadal maligant teratoma is only 38% and the ideal chemotherapeutic regimen has not been defined.

Follow-up

Follow-up examinations, including a careful rectal examination, should be performed at monthly intervals for the first year, at 3-month intervals for at least 3 years, and then annually. Serial monitoring of serum α-fetoprotein levels has been found to indicate malignant recurrence, even following excision of histologically benign tumors[6]. Recurrent tumors should be approached surgically to remove or debulk any recurrent disease, although extensive disease may benefit from chemotherapy before definitive excision.

References

1. Flake AW, Harrison MR, Adzick NS, Laberge J-M, Warsof SL. Fetal sacrococcygeal teratoma. *J Pediatr Surg* 1986; 21: 563–6.

2. Altman RP, Randolph JG, Lilly JR. Sacrococcygeal teratoma: American Academy of Pediatrics Surgical Section Survey – 1973. *J Pediatr Surg* 1974; 9: 389–98.

3. Tsuchida Y, Endo Y, Saito S, Kaneko M, Shiraki K, Ohmi K. Evaluation of alpha-fetoprotein in early infancy. *J Pediatr Surg* 1978; 13: 155–6.

4. Hendren WH, Henderson BM. The surgical management of sacrococcygeal teratomas with intrapelvic extension. *Ann Surg* 1970; 171: 77–84.

5. Malone PS, Spitz L, Kiely EM, Brereton RJ, Duffy PG, Ransley PG. The functional sequelae of sacrococcygeal teratoma. *J Pediatr Surg* 1990; 25: 679–80.

6. Billmire DF, Grosfeld JL. Teratomas in childhood: analysis of 142 cases. *J Pediatr Surg* 1986; 21: 548–51.

Surgery for hyperinsulinemic hypoglycemia

Lewis Spitz PhD, FRCS, FRCS(Ed), FAAP(Hon)
Nuffield Professor of Paediatric Surgery, Institute of Child Health, University of London, and Consultant
Paediatric Surgeon, Great Ormond Street Hospital for Children, London, UK

Principles and justification

Hyperinsulinemic hypoglycemia (also known as nesidioblastosis, islet cell dysplasia) is a disease of the pancreas in which there is diffuse B cell and islet hyperplasia associated with fetal-type budding from the pancreatic ducts and disruption of cell ratios and cell-to-cell contact within the exocrine pancreas. It is a common cause of persistent hypoglycemia in infants and children and, if inadequately treated, can lead to permanent neurologic damage.

Hypoglycemia in the neonatal period is defined as a blood glucose concentration of less than 1.1 mmol/l (20 mg%) in preterm infants or less than 1.7 mmol/l (30 mg%) in term infants. The hypoglycemia may be *transient* (as in the 'stressed neonate', the infant of a diabetic mother or in Beckwith–Wiedermann syndrome) or *persistent*. In persistent hypoglycemia it is important to exclude leucin sensitivity and other endocrine disorders such as hypopituitarism and cortisol deficiency or inborn errors of metabolism such as glycogen storage disease.

Diagnosis

The diagnosis of hyperinsulinism is based on the following criteria: (1) inappropriately raised plasma insulin levels for the blood glucose concentration found; (2) a glucose infusion rate greater than 10 mg/kg per min to maintain a blood glucose level above 2 mmol/l (36 mg%); (3) low free fatty acids and blood ketone bodies during hypoglycemia; (4) glycemic response to glucagon despite hypoglycemia.

Special investigations such as ultrasonography, computed tomography, nuclear magnetic imaging and selective arteriography are of little value in the diagnosis of hyperinsulinism in infants, but may help to localize an adenoma in the older infant or child.

Indications

Surgical treatment is indicated if the patient remains dependent on intravenous glucose despite full dosages of diazoxide and chlorothiazide.

Medical treatment

Medical treatment consists of providing sufficient glucose (usually an intravenous infusion of 15% glucose solution) to prevent hypoglycemia. Diazoxide in doses of up to 25 mg/kg per day inhibits glucose-stimulated insulin secretion. The action of this drug is potentiated by the diuretic chlorothiazide. Somatostatin infusion may be useful as a short-term therapeutic adjunct in refractory cases.

Preoperative

A central venous catheter is essential to monitor blood glucose levels at regular intervals before, during and after surgery. Prophylactic antibiotics (flucloxacillin and gentamicin) should be administered to prevent wound sepsis.

Operation

1 The operative procedure consists of a 95% pancreatectomy. The lines of resection showing the extent of pancreatic resection are as follows:

$A–A_1$ = 99% resection
$B–B_1$ = 95% resection
$C–C_1$ = 80% resection
$D–D_1$ = 50% resection
$E–E_1$ = 30% resection

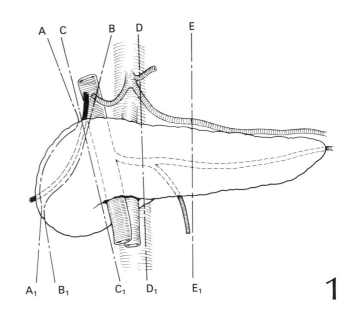

1

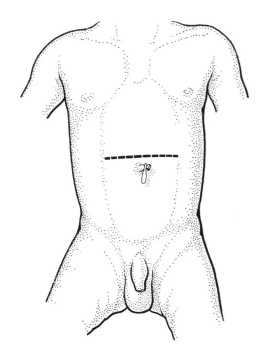

2

Incision

2 A laparotomy is performed via a generous supra-umbilical transverse muscle-cutting incision, extending through both rectus abdominis muscles. A thorough search must be made for sites of ectopic pancreatic tissue.

Exposure

3 The anterior surface of the pancreas is exposed by entering the lesser peritoneal sac via the gastro-colic omentum. Vessels in the greater omentum are ligated and divided, preserving the gastroepiploic and short gastric vessels.

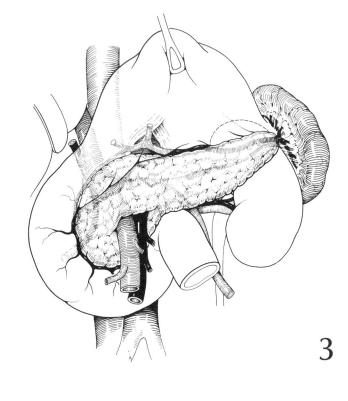

3

The hepatic flexure of the colon is reflected medially and a Kocher procedure used on the duodenum to expose the head of the pancreas. The entire pancreas is carefully inspected for the presence of an adenoma; this appears as a reddish-brown nodule on the surface of the greyish pancreas. Suspicious nodules should be excised and submitted for frozen-section histologic examination. The coexistence of a pancreatic adenoma and diffuse pancreatic disease (nesidioblastosis) is well recognized in early infancy. A generous biopsy of the tail of the pancreas should be performed to exclude nesidioblastosis before adenectomy alone is carried out.

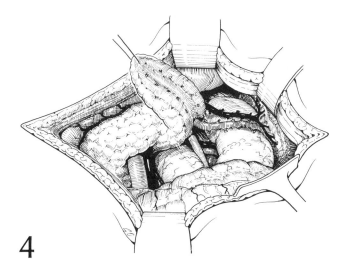

4

Mobilization of the body and tail of the pancreas

4 The tail of the pancreas is carefully dissected out of the hilum of the spleen, ligating and dividing short pancreatic vessels arising from the splenic artery and vein. Dissection proceeds medially from the tail towards the neck of the pancreas, which lies just to the right of the superior mesenteric vessels. It is essential to preserve the spleen for future immunologic competence by carefully exposing the short pancreatic vessels passing from the splenic vessels to the pancreas. These vessels, especially the veins, are extremely friable but with meticulous dissection they can be individually ligated or divided following the application of clips or bipolar electrocoagulation without traumatizing the main vessels. Should hemorrhage occur from damage to the splenic vein, the vein should be repaired directly, but if hemostasis cannot be achieved the main splenic vein can be ligated in the expectation that splenic function will be preserved by collateral supply from the short gastric vessels. Once the dissection has progressed to the right of the superior mesenteric vessels, attention should be directed to the head of the pancreas, particularly to the uncinate process.

Mobilization of the uncinate process

5 The uncinate process, which comprises up to 30% of the pancreatic weight, lies behind the superior mesenteric artery and vein. These vessels must be retracted to the left and the whole of the uncinate process should be carefully mobilized, coagulating numerous short feeding vessels. Failure to resect the uncinate process exposes the patient to the risk of recurrent hypoglycemia.

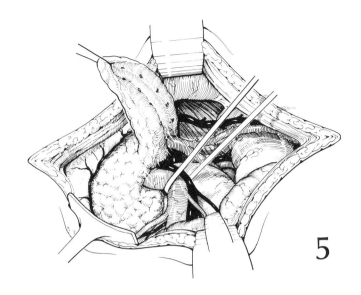

5

Exposure of the head of the pancreas

6 It is essential to define the course of the common bile duct accurately; it may course through the head of the pancreas or lie posteriorly on the posterior surface, in a groove between the pancreas and duodenum.

The head of the pancreas may now be mobilized without injuring the common bile duct. The superior and inferior pancreaticoduodenal vessels are ligated and divided to ensure hemostasis when completing the pancreatic resection.

For a 95% pancreatectomy, the head of the pancreas to the left of the common duct and in the concavity of the duodenal loop is excised, leaving a sliver of pancreatic tissue on the surface of the duodenum and on the left wall of the common duct. The pancreatic duct is identified and ligated with a non-absorbable ligature. Hemostasis is carefully and meticulously achieved. The remaining pancreatic tissue consists of that part of the gland between the duodenum and the common bile duct and the sliver of tissue on the medial wall of the second part of the duodenum. This represents approximately 5% of the total volume of the pancreas (white area on *Illustration 6*). A suction drain via a separate stab incision is left in the pancreatic bed.

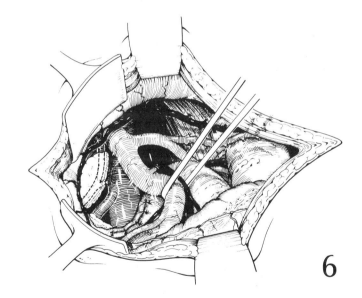

6

Wound closure

The wound is closed in layers or with an *en masse* interrupted suture of 3/0 polyglycolic acid (Dexon). The skin edges are approximated with a 5/0 Dexon subcuticular suture.

Postoperative care

Nasogastric decompression and intravenous fluids are continued during the period of postoperative ileus. Blood glucose levels are closely monitored postoperatively and soluble insulin administered as required. Rebound transient hyperglycemia is common in the early postoperative period. Occasionally more prolonged use of small amounts of insulin is required but adaptation usually occurs within 3–6 months.

Complications

Complications following surgery involve trauma to the bile duct, inadequate resection and wound sepsis.

Trauma to the common bile duct may be amenable to direct repair. If the duct has been transected, end-to-side anastomosis to the first part of the duodenum should be performed.

Inadequate resection will become evident within 48–72 h of surgery and a further resection is advisable at this early stage rather that later, when fibrosis can render the procedure extremely difficult. A review of the literature with references to recurrent hypoglycemia in relation to the extent of pancreatic resection is shown in *Table 1*.

Table 1 Extent of resection (literature review 1982–89)

Percentage resection	No. of patients (%)	Reoperation (%)
99	6 (3.0)	–
90–95	78 (40.0)	16.6
80–90	68 (34.0)	23.5
<80	41 (21.0)	26.8*

*Four of 11 patients required a third resection

Careful long-term follow-up is necessary to assess the adequacy of pancreatic exocrine function.

Acknowledgments

Illustrations 2–6 have been reproduced from *Operative Newborn Surgery* (ed. P. Puri) with permission from Butterworth–Heinemann.

Further reading

Aynsley-Green A, Polak JM, Bloom SR *et al*. Nesidioblastosis of the pacreas: definition of the syndrome and management of the severe neonatal hyperinsulinaemic hypoglycaemia. *Arch Dis Child* 1981; 56: 496–508.

Carcassonne M, DeLarue A, Le Tourneau JN. Surgical treatment of organic pancreatic hypoglycaemia in the pediatric age. *J Pediatr Surg* 1983; 18: 75–9.

Gough MH. The surgical treatment of hyperinsulinism in infancy and childhood. *Br J Surg* 1984; 71: 75–8.

Harken AH, Filler RM, AvRuskin TW, Grigler JF. The role of 'total' pancreatectomy in the treatment of unremitting hypoglycemia of infancy. *J Pediatr Surg* 1971; 6: 284–9.

Reyes GA, Fowler CL, Pokorny WJ. Pancreatic anatomy in children: emphasis on its importance to pancreatectomy. *J Pediatr Surg* 1993; 28: 712–15.

Spitz L, Buick RG, Grant DB, Leonard JV, Pincott JR. Surgical treatment of nesidioblastosis. *Pediatr Surg Int* 1986; 1: 26–9.

Spitz L, Bhargava RK, Grant D, Leonard JV. Surgical treatment of hypersinulinaemic hypoglycaemia in infancy and childhood. *Arch Dis Child* 1992; 67: 201–5.

Warden MJ, German JC, Buckingham BA. The surgical management of hyperinsulinism in infancy due to nesidioblastosis. *J Pediatr Surg* 1988; 23: 462–5.

Illustrations by Paul Richardson and Rachel Byron Moore

Pelviureteric junction obstruction

Julian Wan MD
Attending Pediatric Urologist, Children's Hospital of Buffalo, State University of New York at Buffalo, Buffalo, New York, USA

David A. Bloom MD
Chief of Pediatric Urology, Professor of Surgery (Urology), University of Michigan, Ann Arbor, Michigan, USA

Principles and justification

The pelviureteric junction is the most common site of obstruction in the upper urinary tract among pediatric patients. The pelviureteric junction is formed during the fifth week of embryogenesis and urine flows from the kidney and renal pelvis across it and down the length of the ureter by the 12th week. Flow occurs when renal pelvic pressure exceeds upper ureteric pressure. The pressure gradient is created partly by the hydrostatic force of the filtered urine but principally by peristaltic contractions originating in the region of the renal pelvis called the pacemaker and progressing across the pelviureteric junction and down the ureter. Hydronephrosis develops either when the pelviureteric junction is obstructed or when the normal peristaltic waves are impeded.

Obstruction more usually results from an intrinsic defect in the smooth muscle layer of the pelviureteric junction. External compression and blockage by aberrant renal vessels and adhesive bands occurs in one-third of cases. Murnaghan, using light microscopy, demonstrated abnormal smooth muscle architecture and increased fibrosis in obstructed pelviureteric junctions[1]. Hanna used electron microscopy to show disruption of the intercellular junctions that coordinate the transmission of peristaltic waves[2].

Incidence, signs and symptoms

The incidence of obstruction of the pelviureteric junction is 1:1000 to 1:2000 live births and is more common in boys than girls. The left side is affected in 60% and 5% of cases are bilateral. In duplex systems, the lower pole moiety is more likely to be obstructed, although both systems can be involved.

Before antenatal ultrasonography became common in the 1970s the common signs and symptoms of pelviureteric junction obstruction were abdominal mass, gross hematuria, urinary tract infection and pain. Now, antenatal ultrasonography allows pelviureteric junction obstructions to be identified before becoming symptomatic. Brown et al.[3] found a fivefold increase in detection of obstruction with antenatal ultrasonography, whereas the incidence of symptomatic obstruction remained the same.

Among older children and adolescents obstructions of the pelviureteric junction have protean manifestations, including failure to thrive, sporadic flank and abdominal pain (especially with diuresis), nausea, vomiting, hypertension and recurrent urinary tract infections. Hematuria or renal parenchymal injury may occur with disproportionally minor trauma.

Particular attention should be paid to infants with other congenital abnormalities. Conditions associated with pelviureteric junction obstruction include the VATER syndrome (vertebral defects, imperforate anus, tracheoesophageal fistula, radial dysplasia and renal dysplasia), contralateral multicystic kidney, esophageal atresia and vesicoureteric reflux.

Preoperative

Imaging studies

Clinically suspected obstruction should be confirmed by an imaging study. Ultrasonography is non-invasive, hazard-free and well tolerated. Characteristically, the pelviureteric junction produces a central lucency, which is the renal pelvis surrounded by communicating dilated calyces. A voiding cystourethrogram is advisable for all patients suspected of obstruction to rule out vesicoureteric reflux and other lower tract causes of hydronephrosis such as posterior urethral valves. Intravenous pyelography or urography provides excellent anatomic detail for identifying the region of obstruction and any other areas of narrowing. In severely affected patients delayed films are necessary to visualize the pelviureteric junction. The low glomerular filtration rate of neonates precludes the use of intravenous pyelography. Complex studies such as computed tomography offer little information beyond that which is more economically obtained, unless concomitant renal anomalies such as a horseshoe kidney need investigation.

Diuretic renal scintigraphy is particularly helpful in diagnosing the presence and the severity of obstruction. The most common radionuclides are DTPA (^{99m}Tc-diethylenetriamine pentaacetic acid) and MAG-3 (^{99m}Tc-mercaptoacetyltriglycine). A bladder catheter should be inserted in all patients undergoing a renal scan because a full bladder can exert back-pressure on the ureters and obscure the results. The scan produces two important findings: (1) it determines the percentage of total renal effort contributed by each kidney. A poor or non-functional kidney should be removed rather than repaired; (2) the time it takes for half of the radionuclide to wash out of the kidneys after administration of the diuretic ($t_{1/2}$) is calculated. A $t_{1/2}$ of more than 20 min is believed to be diagnostic of obstruction. A retrograde study will delineate the precise anatomy of the suspected obstruction, will aid detection of any distal ureteric strictures, and will aid in planning the specific incision. Retrograde pyelography risks infection, and must be performed under general anesthesia in children, so if it is necessary it should be performed at the time of pyeloplasty.

Alternatives to pyeloplasty

The aim of surgery is to improve drainage of the pelviureteric junction, which should relieve symptoms, correct the hydronephrosis, and prevent renal deterioration. For these reasons obstructions are generally promptly repaired.

The question of whether pelviureteric junction obstructions that are detected by antenatal ultrasonography but remain asymptomatic in the infant should be corrected surgically awaits an objective answer. Ransley et al.[4] found that 23% of neonatal kidneys with such an obstruction and good renal function ($\geqslant 40\%$ of total renal effort) deteriorated without treatment and ultimately required surgery in a modest period of surveillance. Koff et al. found that many newborn kidneys continue to grow and develop normally despite imaging studies consistent with obstruction[5]. These reports suggest gaps in our understanding of the natural history of obstruction of the pelviureteric junction and shake our confidence in the identification of those who will benefit from pyeloplasty. However, in the absence of hard evidence to the contrary, it is still recommended that all such obstructions be treated surgically.

Endourologic techniques used for removal of renal calculi have been adapted to the treatment of the pelviureteric junction. The obstructed segment is incised and dilated through a percutaneous nephrostomy and is left to heal over a stent. Initial reports suggest that this technique may be particularly useful in older children after previous pyeloplasty has failed[6]. Its utility in infants and neonates is constrained by the smaller diameter of the child's ureter and the relatively large size of the instruments currently available.

Operation

The technique described is dismembered pyeloplasty. Unlike methods using flaps and advancements, it excises the pathologic segment and may be applied to a variety of anatomic configurations.

Anesthesia

General anesthesia with endotracheal intubation is required.

Instruments and equipment

In addition to a pediatric major surgery tray, fine forceps, magnifying loupes, 5-Fr and 8-Fr feeding tubes, hooked and pointed scalpel blades, needle-point electrocautery, 3/0 to 6/0 synthetic or biologic absorbable suture with atraumatic needles should be available.

Position of patient

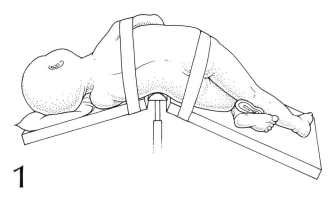

1 After intubation, a Foley catheter is placed in the bladder and the patient is turned on the side. The surgeon should stand facing the patient's back with the assistant opposite.

Incision

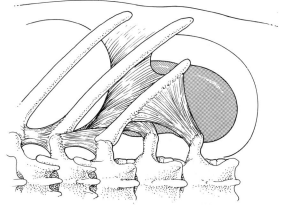

2 A flank incision is made using a supracostal extrapleural approach by the 12th rib[7]. The skin incision is made astride the 12th rib and extended anteriorly following the natural skin creases. The external and internal oblique, the latissimus dorsi, and the anterior edge of the serratus posterior muscles are divided until the periosteum of the rib is exposed.

3 Other approaches include dorsal lumbotomy, anterolateral muscle splitting, and anterior transperitoneal. Lumbotomy allows direct access to the renal pelvis but creates a scar which crosses normal skin folds[8]. The muscle-splitting approach is suitable in infants and young children. A transperitoneal approach is useful when accesss to the abdominal contents or the contralateral kidney is required.

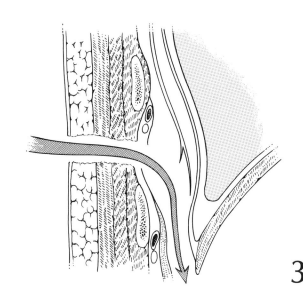

3

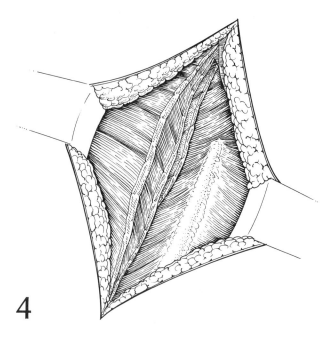

4

Releasing diaphragmatic fibers

4 Entry into the retroperitoneum is made at the rib tip and extended posteriorly along the superior edge of the rib.

5 The intercostal muscles should carefully be taken off the rib, keeping just above the rib to avoid the intercostal nerve and vessels.

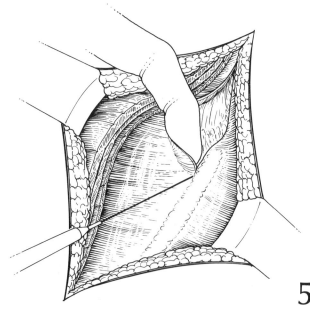

5

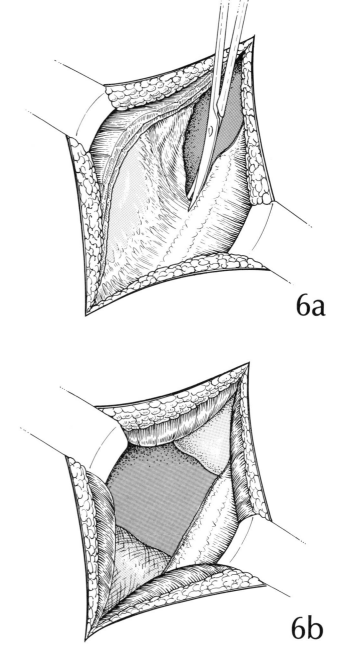

6a, b The diaphragmatic fibers are freed from their attachment to the rib using sharp dissection. The translucent pleura falls away as the diaphragmatic fibers are released. The assistant on the ventral side of the patient often has a better view of these fibers than the surgeon. The peritoneum is carefully peeled away from Gerota's fascia and retracted to allow more working room.

Kidney mobilization

A self-retaining retractor may be used to aid exposure. Gerota's fascia is opened longitudinally and the overlying fat dissected away from the kidney, taking care not to strip off the renal capsule which may be adherent because of previous pyelonephritis. Small blood vessels are coagulated. Branches and tributaries of the renal vessels around the anterior renal hilum pose added risk for injury but it is rarely necessary to skeletonize the hilar vessels. The kidney should be mobilized sufficiently to expose the renal pelvis (the kidney should be held in a padded retractor blade or an assistant's hand). Displacing the kidney out of the depths of the operative field may improve exposure but should be avoided because it can also stretch the renal vessels.

Identifying the ureter

7 The ureter should be located and traced towards the kidney to identify the pelviureteric junction. Care should be taken to ensure that the supporting adventitial vessels are not stripped away. A fine stay suture at the very proximal end will allow gentle manipulation. Aberrant vessels should be identified and teased away, not divided.

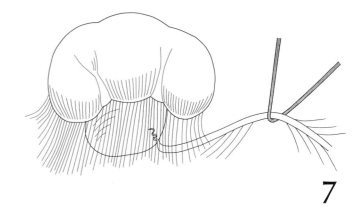

7

Pelvic stay sutures and division of pelviureteric junction

8 The pelviureteric junction is followed onto the renal pelvis and overlying fat cleared away. The type of pelviureteric junction (for example high insertion) encountered, presence of crossing vessels, or other findings causally related to the obstruction should be noted. The ureter should carefully be divided just below the pelviureteric junction. If cystoscopy and retrograde pyelography were not performed at the time of surgery the ureter should be intubated with a feeding tube to ensure that there are no other areas of narrowing. The surgeon must be sure the ureter has sufficient reach and, if further dissection is needed to gain adequate length, it should be done at this stage.

8

9 With the pathologic anatomy laid out, stay sutures are placed on the renal pelvis to correspond to lateral and medial corners of the intended anastomosis. These sutures will define the pyeloplasty.

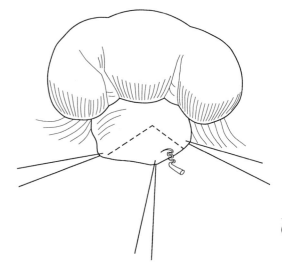

9

Excision of pelviureteric junction

10 Traction is applied to the stay sutures to splay the renal pelvis flat and one smooth cut made using sharp-pointed scissors; repeated cuts tend to result in a saw-tooth jagged edge. A sharp hooked or needle-tip scalpel may be used instead of the scissors. Any irregular tags should be carefully trimmed. Some additional pelvis may be excised if a giant pelvis will not reconfigure easily into a funnel-shaped pyeloplasty. Debris or calculi are irrigated from the kidney.

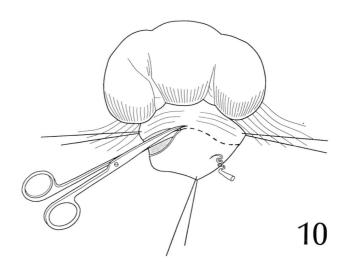

10

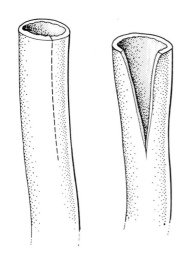

11

Spatulation of ureter

11 The course of the ureter is studied and then spatulated along the side that is most likely to fit the lower extent of the renal pelvis. The vascular supply to the proximal ureter enters its medial aspect. The decision must now be made whether to utilize a nephrostomy tube and ureteric stent; neither is necessary for an uncomplicated pyeloplasty, but intubation is a useful reassurance in difficult cases, floppy kidneys, revisions or giant collecting systems.

12 When intubating the authors prefer to use both a stent and a nephrostomy combined in a single nephrostent (which can be obtained ready-made or fashioned from a small feeding tube). A temporary intraoperative ureteric stent will help to position the ureter and minimize handling by forceps.

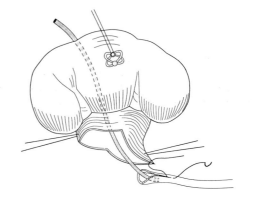

12

Anastomosis

13 The anastomosis should begin at the caudal end, where the lower lip of the renal pelvis meets the spatulated apex of the ureter. The first 6/0 stitch (5/0 in older children) is placed at the apex and one positioned on either side approximately 2 mm apart. A running or interrupted technique may be used.

Sutures should advance up the posterior wall and then up the anterior wall, keeping the suture bites even so that the tissue is evenly distributed and bunching does not occur. When the end of the ureter has been reached suturing should be continued until the pelvis is closed.

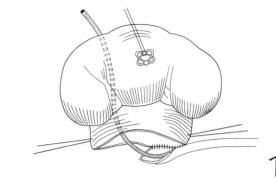

13

Fat wrap

14 A tongue of fat is freed from Gerota's fascia, carefully but loosely wrapped around the anastomosis and secured by stitching it to itself. A small drain should be placed in the region of the repair, and it and the other tubes brought out through separate stab incisions.

Wound closure

The wound is closed in layers, taking care to reapproximate the muscles. Local anesthetic is infiltrated along the intercostal nerves. All tubes and drains should be carefully sutured to the skin.

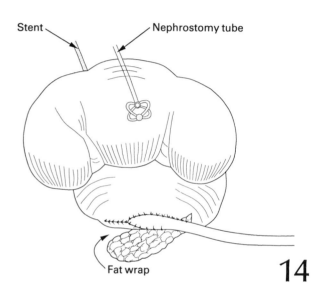

Stent   Nephrostomy tube

Fat wrap

14

Postoperative care

The patient should be fasted overnight. The bladder catheter is removed the following morning and diet advanced slowly. If the flank remains dry the drain may be removed on the third postoperative day. The patient is usually discharged on the fourth or fifth day after surgery. If the repair was intubated the tube should be left in place for 3 weeks after which the stent may be removed and nephrostography performed. If no drainage is seen flowing down the ureter the tube should be left to drain for a further 2 weeks and the test repeated. If contrast medium flows across the repair the tube may be removed. Follow-up renal scans and ultrasonography or intravenous pyelography are arranged 3 months after surgery.

Complications

The principal complication is stenosis of the anastomosis. Fortunately this is rare, and 90–95% of cases are successful. Although the repaired kidney may never look normal on ultrasound scan or intravenous pyelogram, it should function and drain normally on follow-up diuretic renal scintigraphy.

Special situations

Duplex systems

Obstruction is most commonly found in the lower pole moiety of duplex systems. The pyeloplasty technique described above may be used but the surgeon must be careful to identify and isolate the appropriate ureter. If a particularly long obstruction is found ureteropyelostomy or a pyelopyelostomy may be advantageous.

Horseshoe kidneys

In horseshoe kidneys the ureter often inserts high into the renal pelvis; a longer, more caudally placed anastomosis is needed. Division of the isthmus is usually not necessary. A Y–V advancement repair may be useful in some anatomic configurations.

Ureterocalycostomy

15a–c If the renal pelvis is too small or fibrotic to achieve dependent drainage a ureterocalycostomy is necessary[9]. The principal features of this are selection of the most dependent calyx and a thorough amputation of the lower pole of the kidney to prevent compression.

Ileal ureter

In some situations the gap is too long to bridge by mobilizing the kidney and distal ureter, usually in patients who have already undergone extensive surgery or trauma resulting in a long atretic ureter. In such patients interposition of a piece of prepared ileum from the renal pelvis to the bladder is an option.

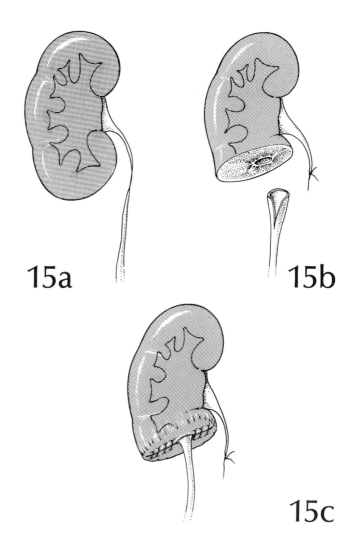

15a 15b

15c

Laparoscopic pyeloplasty

The technical feasibility of laparoscopic pyeloplasty has recently been demonstrated[10] but detailed comparison with the conventional methods is necessary before most surgeons are willing to perform it.

References

1. Murnaghan GF. The dynamics of the renal pelvis and ureter with reference to congenital hydronephrosis. *Br J Urol* 1958; 30: 321–9.

2. Hanna MK. Some observations on congenital ureteropelvic junction obstruction. *Urology* 1978; 12: 151–9.

3. Brown T, Mandell J, Lebowitz RL. Neonatal hydronephrosis in the era of sonography. *AJR Am J Roentgenol* 1987; 148: 959–63.

4. Ransley PG, Dhillon HK, Gordon I, Duffy PG, Dillon MJ, Barratt TM. The postnatal management of hydronephrosis diagnosed by prenatal ultrasound. *J Urol* 1990; 144: 584–94.

5. Koff SA, Campbell K. Nonoperative management of unilateral neonatal hydronephrosis. *J Urol* 1992; 148: 525–31.

6. Kavoussi LR, Meretyk S, Dierks SM *et al*. Endopyelotomy for secondary ureteropelvic junction obstruction in children. *J Urol* 1991; 145: 345–9.

7. Turner-Warwick RT. The supracostal approach to the renal area. *Br J Urol* 1965; 37: 671–2.

8. Novick AC. Posterior surgical approach to the kidney and ureter. *J Urol* 1980; 124: 192–5.

9. Ross JH, Streem SB, Novick AC, Kay R, Montie J. Ureterocalicostomy for reconstruction of complicated pelviureteric junction obstruction. *Br J Urol* 1990; 65: 322–5.

10. Vancaille TG, Schuessler WW, Preminger GM. Laparoscopic dismembered pyeloplasty. *J Urol* 1993; 149: 452A.

Partial nephrectomy

Michael L. Ritchey MD, FACS, FAAP
Associate Professor and Chief of Pediatric Urology, Department of Surgery, Division of Pediatric Surgery, University of Texas Health Science Center at Houston, Texas, USA

History

The first planned partial nephrectomy was performed by Kummell in 1889 for stone disease. Partial nephrectomy was initially performed predominantly for infectious problems and urolithiasis. Many patients in the early 1900s continued to have complete nephrectomy because of concerns of extensive bleeding following partial nephrectomy and the frequent occurrence of urinary fistula. Eisendrath reviewed the treatment of duplex kidneys in 1923 and found only 13 reports of heminephrectomy[1]. With improvements in radiographic diagnosis and surgical techniques, this operation became more routine even in younger children.

Principles and justification

Indications

The indications for partial nephrectomy for benign disease have diminished over the years. Treatment for urolithiasis has evolved from an open surgical approach to the use of endoscopic techniques and extracorporeal lithotripsy. Early recognition and treatment of vesico-ureteric reflux and urinary tract infections has lessened the risk of severe segmental renal damage.

1 The most common indication for partial removal of the kidney in a child is complete ureteric duplication with a non-functioning segment, usually involving the upper pole. These anomalies are increasingly diagnosed in the antenatal period. The upper pole moiety becomes dilated because of obstruction secondary to ureterocele or ectopic insertion of the ureter.

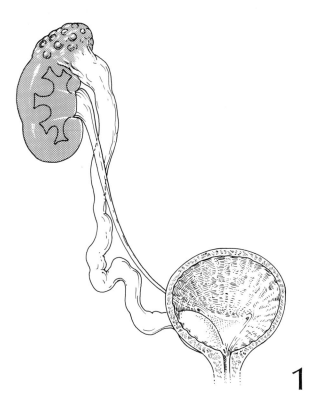

Evaluation of these patients consists of cystography, renal ultrasonography and radionuclide scans. In most cases this will provide the correct diagnosis and enable the clinician to decide upon the proper therapy. There are several treatment alternatives, including endoscopic incision of the obstructing ureterocele, ipsilateral ureteroureterostomy or pyeloureterostomy. The merits of each approach continue to be debated but, for non-functioning upper pole segments, partial nephrectomy with segmental ureterectomy is the favored approach.

Other less common indications for segmental resection of the kidney are trauma, renal cysts and calyceal diverticula. The last two problems are now frequently managed with endoscopic or percutaneous techniques.

Preoperative

Delineation of the anatomy of duplication anomalies can be readily accomplished in most cases by preoperative imaging. If the anatomy remains unclear, antegrade pyelography, retrograde ureterography or puncture of the ureterocele with retrograde injection of contrast medium can be performed. When the child is brought to the operating theater, endoscopic examination should be performed to assess the lower urinary tract.

Anesthesia

General anesthesia is used in all cases. Most centers now use caudal or epidural anesthesia to assist in pain control after operation. An intercostal nerve block can also be placed during the operation to assist in pain management.

Operations

Position of patient

2   The flank or lateral approach is preferred and the patient is placed in a full lateral position. For older children the break in the table is utilized, but in the neonate a small towel or pad under the mid section may suffice. A bladder catheter is placed to monitor urine output. Proper padding of all pressure points is important. The patient is secured to the table with tape to prevent motion during the procedure.

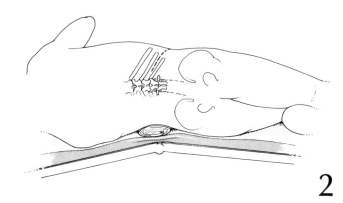

2

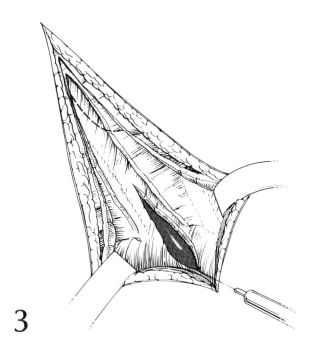

3

Incision

3   The incision will vary with the indication for surgery. Trauma patients are likely to be undergoing exploratory laparotomy, and therefore an intra-abdominal approach is utilized. For most elective patients, the incision is subcostal or above the 12th rib. For upper pole nephrectomy the higher incision affords better exposure and decreases the need for traction on the kidney to deliver it into the field of view.

With a subcostal incision, the muscles can either be split in the direction of the fibers or divided with cautery[2]. The neurovascular bundles are identified and preserved. The peritoneum is swept medially. With the approach above the 12th rib, it is important to free the diaphragmatic attachments to the lower rib carefully to avoid tearing into the pleural space when the self-retaining retractor is placed[3].

Gerota's fascia is entered posteriorly after palpating the kidney. The perirenal fat is then dissected by both blunt dissection and with the cautery. At this point the ureter and renal vessels can be identified. Mobilization and isolation of the renal vessels are generally not necessary, particularly in neonates where the vessels are prone to spasm. Infiltration of the hilar area with lidocaine (lignocaine) (0.25% solution) and papaverine, 15 mg, has been recommended to prevent this problem when performing renal surgery in infants[4].

The renal segment to be removed is generally readily identifiable, either due to atrophy and thinning of the renal parenchyma or because of a dysplastic or cystic appearance of the involved region. The upper pole moiety is generally small, representing less than 15% of the total parenchymal volume of the kidney. Occasionally a centrally located cyst or calyceal diverticulum may not be apparent on initial inspection. Intraoperative ultrasonography may be helpful to define the resection margin.

PARTIAL NEPHRECTOMY FOR DUPLICATION ANOMALY

4 In most cases the dilated upper pole ureter is readily identified. Caution must be used in that the lower pole ureter may also be abnormal; division of the ureter is not undertaken until the origin from the upper pole is assured. After transection of the ureter, the collecting system is decompressed. This allows the junction between the upper and lower renal segment to be readily identified. In most patients the ureters can be easily separated at the renal level. With careful dissection the upper pole ureter is freed from its mate and transposed above the renal hilar vessels. This maneuver allows access into the renal sinus between the two collecting systems. Traction on the upper pole ureter should be minimized to avoid injury to the renal vessels.

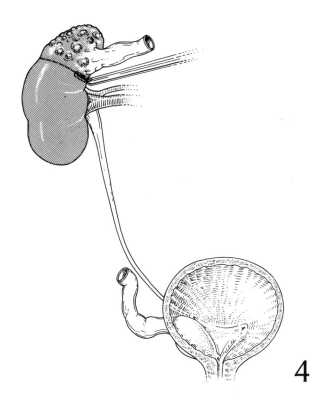

4

5 The author prefers to incise the renal parenchyma with the cautery in those cases where it is dysplastic and/or atrophied. If a branch of the renal artery is clearly seen to enter the parenchymal segment being removed, it can be ligated and divided. If there is question as to the region supplied by an upper pole arterial branch, a vascular clamp can be placed and the line of demarcation observed. Removal of the cystic non-functional upper pole segment can generally be accomplished with minimal blood loss. After the upper pole has been excised, suture ligation of bleeding points can be performed. Gentle manual compression of the parenchyma is all that is necessary to control bleeding. Mattress sutures are placed to approximate the cut edges of the renal parenchyma. Perirenal fat can be placed in this defect if it is too bulky to fold over.

When the upper resection is complete, the ureter is traced distally. Care should be taken to avoid devascularization of the lower ureter. The plane of dissection should be very close to the upper pole ureter. If the ureters are closely adherent, a strip of the upper pole ureter can be left attached to the lower pole ureter, but this is rarely needed. The ureter is removed as low as possible via the flank incision. This will be below the level of the iliac vessels in most infants and small children. The ureter is then transected and a catheter is passed into the stump of the ureter. This is irrigated with antibiotic solution and the catheter is aspirated. The ureter is left open except in rare cases of reflux into the upper pole moiety. Complete excision of the distal ureter or very low ligation is more appropriate in these patients. A drain is placed both in the renal bed and near the region where the ureter is transected in the pelvis.

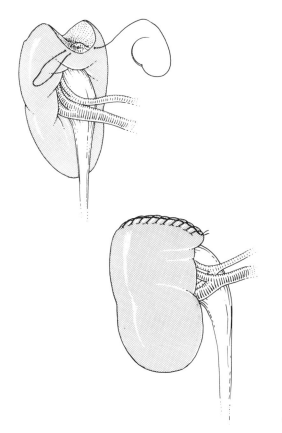

5

PARTIAL NEPHRECTOMY FOR OTHER CONDITIONS

6 Once the segment to be removed has been identified, the capsule can either be incised with a scalpel and peeled back (this may be adherent if the renal segment is diseased) or the cautery may be used to incise the renal parenchyma. Classic teaching is that blunt dissection with the back of a knife handle can be used to separate the parenchyma without disrupting the major blood vessels, which can then be ligated.

As mentioned, if the renal parenchyma is atrophied, it is divided with the cautery. If there is considerable renal parenchyma to be divided then the Cavitron Ultrasonic Surgical Aspirator (CUSA) is very effective in dividing the kidney[5]. The parenchyma is separated without dividing the vessels and this minimizes blood loss.

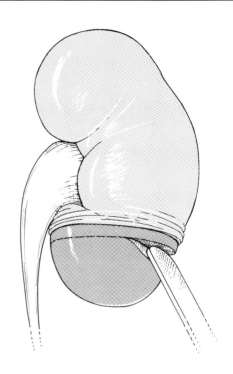

6

7a, b After partial resection of a kidney with a single collecting system, closure of the transected calyx or infundibulum is required. A watertight closure with fine absorbable suture (5/0 or 6/0 polyglycolic acid) is recommended. The renal capsule is closed over the cut surface of the kidney. If the capsule is not available, a patch of peritoneum is used.

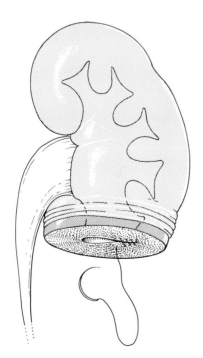

7a

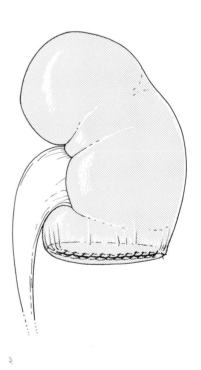

7b

Postoperative care

The majority of children will require only a short hospital stay after an uncomplicated partial nephrectomy for benign disease. The use of epidural catheters after operation can eliminate much of the postoperative discomfort. Most complications will be apparent before discharge from the hospital.

Complications

Pneumothorax

Before the wound is closed the flank is filled with saline and the anesthetist holds the patient in deep inspiration to check for air leakage. If the parietal pleura has been opened but the visceral pleura is intact a small catheter is placed into the pleural space and the air is evacuated. Closure of the pleural space and diaphragm is then performed and wound closure is accomplished. After closure of all the muscle layers the catheter is removed. A chest radiograph is obtained in the recovery room to ensure complete expansion of the lung.

Urine leak

The potential for urine leak exists in all patients, particularly if closure of the collecting system has been required. A flank drain is left for 4–5 days after operation to assess urine leakage. Persistent urine drainage can be managed by placement of a stent or percutaneous nephrostomy tube into the remaining collecting system.

Ischemia of the remnant kidney

This complication is most commonly due to spasm or traction injury to the renal vessels. Prevention is the most important factor, as recognition of this problem after surgery is difficult. Imaging studies to assess renal function are not routinely done in the early postoperative period. Unless the operation was performed on a solitary kidney the loss of function of the remaining renal segment will generally go unrecognized.

Outcome

Most children who undergo partial nephrectomy do very well. For those patients with duplication anomalies, careful follow-up is needed as approximately 20% of children will require secondary procedures on the lower ureter. Most of these operations are performed to correct vesicoureteric reflux into the ipsilateral lower pole ureter. Other indications for surgery include stasis of urine in the ureteric stump with recurrent infections and persistence or recurrence of the ureterocele. Renal function is generally well maintained, but patients with solitary kidneys should be followed throughout life as there are reports that these children are at increased risk for hypertension and renal insufficiency.

References

1. Eisendrath DN. Double kidney. *Ann Surg* 1923; 77: 531–57.

2. Gearhart JP, Jeffs RD. The use of topical vasodilators as an adjunct in infant renal surgery. *J Urol* 1985; 134: 298–300.

3. Turner-Warwick RT. The supracostal approach to the renal area. *Br J Urol* 1965; 38: 671–2.

4. Duckett JW Jr, Gibbons MD, Cromie WJ. An anterior extraperitoneal muscle-splitting approach for pediatric renal surgery. *J Urol* 1980; 123: 79–80.

5. Muraki J, Addonizio JC, Lastarria E, Eshghi M, Choudhury MS. New cavitron system (CUSA/CEM): its application for kidney surgery. *Urology* 1993; 41: 195–8.

Vesicoureteric reflux: endoscopic correction

Prem Puri MS, FACS

Consultant Paediatric Surgeon and Director, Children's Research Centre, Our Lady's Hospital for Sick Children, Dublin, Consultant Paediatric Surgeon, National Children's Hospital, Dublin, and Consultant Paediatric Surgeon, Children's Hospital, Dublin, Ireland

History

Primary vesicoureteric reflux is caused by congenital absence or deficiency of the longitudinal muscle of the submucosal ureter. This results in upward and lateral displacement of the ureteric orifice during micturition, thereby reducing the length and obliquity of the submucosal ureter. It is generally agreed that vesicoureteric reflux in a dilated system is unlikely to cease spontaneously in most cases, and is therefore a surgical problem. In 1984, reflux induced in piglets was corrected by subureteric injection of polytetrafluoroethylene (PTFE; Polytef; Teflon) paste[1]. This technique has since been used successfully to treat primary and secondary vesicoureteric reflux in children by endoscopic injection of PTFE paste[2–10].

The procedure consists of endoscopic injection of the paste into the lamina propria behind the submucosal ureter. The PTFE particles stimulate an ingrowth of fibroblasts at the site of injection, which helps to hold the particles within the tissues[11]. The subureteric PTFE mass is encapsulated by a thin layer of fibrous tissue, which provides a firm anchorage to the submucosal ureter and prevents it from sliding upwards and outwards during micturition, thus preventing reflux. PTFE paste has been used for 30 years by otolaryngologists to enlarge displaced or deformed vocal cords in patients with dysphonia[12,13], and by urologists to treat urinary incontinence[14,15]. No untoward side effects from these clinical uses of PTFE paste have been reported.

Principles and justification

Indications

The indications for endoscopic correction of vesicoureteric reflux are the same as for open antireflux operations. It is generally agreed that lesser grades of reflux (grade I or II international classification) can be managed conservatively. Grade III reflux is conservatively managed unless there are 'breakthrough infections' while on antimicrobial therapy, or poor compliance on medical management. Children with grade IV or V vesicoureteric reflux are generally considered candidates for surgery.

Preoperative

Material

The material used for injection (Mentor Polytef paste) is a suspension of biologically inert PTFE particles in glycerin. The glycerin is 50% of the paste by weight. After injection, the glycerin is absorbed into the tissues and the PTFE implant achieves a firm consistency, retaining its shape and position at the injection site.

Instruments

1 The disposable Puri catheter for PTFE injection (Storz) is a 4-Fr nylon catheter onto which is swaged a 21-gauge needle with 1 cm of the needle protruding from the catheter. Alternatively, a rigid needle can be used.

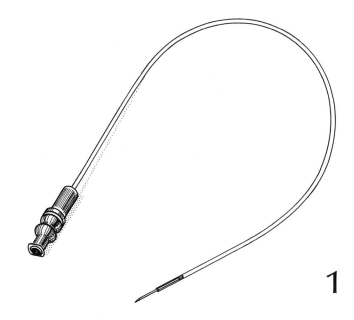

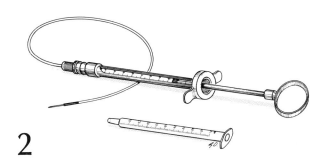

2 A 1 ml tuberculin syringe is filled with PTFE paste, and is then enclosed in the metal syringe holder, which ensures a secure connection between syringe and injection catheter. Using the metal piston which comes with the metal syringe holder the injection catheter is filled with PTFE paste.

3a–c All cystoscopes available for infants and children can be used for this procedure. The injection catheter can be introduced through a 10-Fr, 11-Fr or 14-Fr Storz cystoscope (*Illustration 3a*) or a 9.5-Fr Wolf cystoscope (*Illustration 3b*). A specially designed 11.5-Fr instrument called 'The Stinger' is available from Wolf through which a rigid needle or injection catheter can be used for injection (*Illustration 3c*).

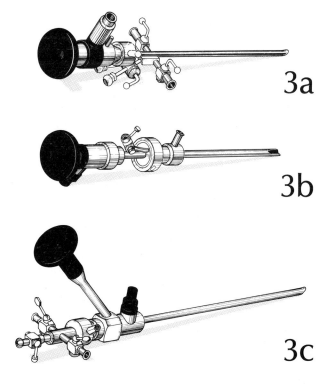

Operation

SUBURETERIC TEFLON INJECTION (STING) TECHNIQUE

The patient should be placed in a lithotomy position. The cystoscope is passed and the bladder wall, the trigone, bladder neck, and both ureteric orifices inspected. The bladder should be almost empty before proceeding with injection, since this helps to keep the ureteric orifice flat rather than away in a lateral part of the field.

4   The injection of PTFE paste should not begin until the operator has a clear view all around the ureteric orifice. Under direct vision through the cystoscope the needle is introduced under the bladder mucosa 2–3 mm below the affected ureteric orifice at the 6 o'clock position. It is important to introduce the needle with pinpoint accuracy. Perforation of the mucosa or the ureter may allow the paste to escape and may result in failure.

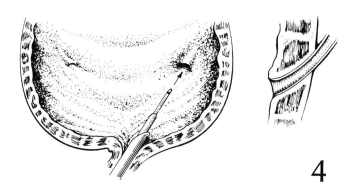

4

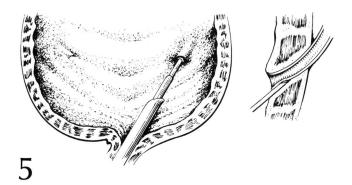

5

5   The needle is advanced about 4–5 mm into the lamina propria in the submucosal portion of the ureter and the injection started slowly. As the paste is injected a bulge appears in the floor of the submucosal ureter. During injection the needle is slowly withdrawn until a 'volcanic' bulge of paste is seen. The needle should be kept in position for 30–60 s after injection to avoid extrusion. Most refluxing ureters require 0.05–0.2 ml to correct reflux. Occasionally a little more than 0.4 ml of paste is needed, but the total amount should never exceed 0.5 ml.

6 A correctly placed injection creates the appearance of a nipple on the top of which is a slit-like or inverted crescentic orifice. If the bulge appears in an incorrect place, e.g. at the side of the ureter or proximal to it, the needle should not be withdrawn, but should be moved so that the point is in a more favorable position. The non-injected ureteric roof retains its compliance while preventing reflux.

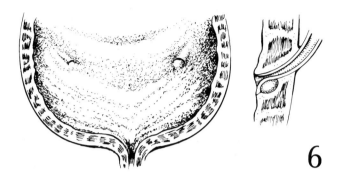

6

Postoperative care

Postoperative urethral catheterization is not necessary. Loose particles of PTFE paste in the bladder are harmless and are passed out painlessly. The majority of patients are treated as day cases. Co-trimoxazole is prescribed in prophylactic doses for 6 weeks after the procedure. Micturating cystography and renal ultrasonography are performed 3 months after discharge. A follow-up micturating cystogram and renal and bladder ultrasonographic scan are obtained 12 months after endoscopic correction of reflux.

Complications

Procedure-related complications are rare. The only significant complication with this procedure has been failure. This may be initial failure, i.e. the reflux is not abolished by the injection, or recurrence, where initial correction is not maintained. About 20% of refluxing ureters require more than one endoscopic injection of PTFE paste to correct the condition. Apart from failure to correct reflux, vesicoureteric junction obstruction is the only other reported complication following STING. A recent European survey of STING procedures in 6216 ureters in 4166 patients revealed vesicoureteric junction obstruction in 20 ureters (0.32%) requiring reimplantation of ureters[10]. No clinically untoward effects were reported in these 4166 children from the use of PTFE as an injectable biomaterial.

References

1. Puri P, O'Donnell B. Correction of experimentally produced vesicoureteric reflux in the piglet by intravesical injection of Teflon. *BMJ* 1984; 289: 5–7.

2. O'Donnell B, Puri P. Treatment of vesicoureteric reflux by endoscopic injection of Teflon. *BMJ* 1984; 289: 7–9.

3. Puri P, O'Donnell B. Endoscopic correction of grades IV and V primary vesicoureteric reflux: six to 30 months follow-up in 42 ureters. *J Pediatr Surg* 1986; 22: 1087–91.

4. Schulman CC, Simon J, Pamart D, Avni FE. Endoscopic treatment of vesicoureteral reflux in children. *J Urol* 1987; 138: 950–2.

5. Kaplan WE, Dalton DP, Firlit CF. The endoscopic correction of reflux by polytetrafluoroethylene injection. *J Urol* 1987; 138: 953–5.

6. Quinn FMJ, Diamond T, Boston VE. Endoscopic management of vesicoureteric reflux in children with neuropathic bladder secondary to myelomeningocele. *Z Kinderchir* 1988; 43(Suppl 2): 43–5.

7. Farkas A, Moriel EZ, Lupa S. Endoscopic correction of vesicoureteral reflux: our experience with 115 ureters. *J Urol* 1990; 144: 534–6.

8. Puri P. Endoscopic correction of primary vesicoureteric reflux by subureteric injection of polytetrafluoroethylene. *Lancet* 1990; 335: 1320–2.

9. Miyakita H, Ninan GK, Puri P. Endoscopic correction of vesico-ureteric reflux in duplex systems. *Eur Urol* 1993; 24: 111–15.

10. Ninan GK, Puri P. Subureteric Teflon injection (STING): results of a European survey. *Presented at the Annual Meeting of the British Association of Urological Surgeons*, Harrogate, UK, June 1993.

11. Stone JW, Arnold GE. Human larynx injected with Teflon paste. Histologic study of innervation and tissue reaction. *Arch Otolaryngol* 1967; 86: 550–61.

12. Arnold GE. Alleviation of aphonia or dysphonia through intrachordal injection of Teflon paste. *Ann Otol Rhinol Laryngol* 1963; 72: 384–95.

13. Lewy RB. Experience with vocal cord injection. *Ann Otol Rhinol Laryngol* 1976; 85: 440–50.

14. Schulman CC, Simon J, Wespes E, Germeau F. Endoscopic injections of Teflon to treat urinary incontinence in women. *BMJ* 1984; 288: 192.

15. Vorstman B, Lockhart J, Kaufmann, MR, Politano V. Polytetrafluoroethylene injection for urinary incontinence in children. *J Urol* 1985; 133: 248–50.

Illustrations by Peter Cox

Surgical treatment of vesicoureteric reflux

P. D. E. Mouriquand MD
Consultant in Paediatric Surgery, Addenbrooke's Hospital and Associate Lecturer, Cambridge University, Cambridge, UK

History

Pozzi first described the concept of vesicoureteric reflux at the end of the 19th century. The antireflux mechanism of the vesicoureteric junction was reported by Sampson in 1903 and in 1923 Graves and Davidoff stated that reflux does not normally exist[1].

Vesicoureteric reflux and its renal consequences ('chronic atrophic pyelonephritis') remained poorly understood until 1960. Children with recurrent urinary tract infections tended to be treated by surgical procedures to the bladder neck and urethra. Nephrectomy for recurrent unilateral symptomatic pyelonephritis was not uncommon. Hodson and Edwards in 1960 clarified the relationship between vesicoureteric reflux and renal damage and stressed the importance of pyelotubular backflow of urine into certain papillae[2]. In 1973 Bailey introduced the term 'reflux nephropathy'[3] and later Ransley and Risdon published an essential study of papillary morphology[4].

The concept of early damage of renal parenchyma ('big-bang') at the first urinary tract infection in infants with vesicoureteric reflux and the potential danger of intrarenal reflux of infected urine was proposed by Ransley and Risdon[4] and Smellie et al.[5] in 1975.

Surgical correction of vesicoureteric reflux was widely practised until it was documented that in many cases the reflux resolved spontaneously with growth of the child and the only treatment required was prophylaxis against urinary tract infections. Antenatal detection of urinary dilatation and reflux now provides an opportunity to commence prophylaxis soon after birth.

Principles and justification

Definition

Vesicoureteric reflux may be defined as a permanent or intermittent intrusion of bladder urine into the upper urinary tract owing to a defective ureterovesical junction. The defect in the ureterovesical junction may be a primary disorder or may arise secondary to bladder dysfunction (neuropathic bladder; unstable bladder) or bladder outlet obstruction (posterior urethral valve).

The refluxing urine can fill the upper excretory system (ureters and renal pelvis) between and/or during micturition, and can sometimes penetrate into the renal substance (intrarenal reflux). This latter event is due to a defective calycotubular junction. The volume of refluxing urine can vary in the same patient at different times. Attempts to classify the degree of reflux are therefore of limited interest and do not influence practical decisions.

Pathophysiology of vesicoureteric reflux

The pathophysiology of vesicoureteric reflux remains unclear but there is a general consensus that intrarenal reflux of infected urine can cause renal damage (reflux nephropathy). It is also likely that other disorders such as immune reactions, renal dysplasia, change of urine biochemistry, etc. can also be responsible for renal deterioration.

Spontaneous resolution of vesicoureteric reflux is common. Some cases are more severe than others, however, and two main groups of patients can be defined. The first group includes vesicoureteric reflux detected before birth (dilatation of the upper urinary tract), which is usually severe and mainly affects boys (80%). Spontaneous resolution of vesicoureteric reflux is possible but occurs in only one-third of these patients. The second group includes children more than 18 months old, mainly girls (75%) who present with recurrent urinary tract infections. In these cases, the vesicoureteric reflux is usually mild and can spontaneously disappear, which it does in more than two-thirds of patients, often before the age of 5 years.

Indications

As a consequence of the failure to reach a consensus on the precise indications for surgery, it is difficult to select the ideal treatment for each patient. The current policy is to prescribe prophylactic antibiotic treatment for prolonged periods (12–36 months) in expectation of spontaneous maturation of the ureterovesical junction (and a resolution of the vesicoureteric reflux). This policy involves repeated investigations to check if the vesicoureteric reflux is still present. The long-term side effects of prophylactic treatment are unknown and there are reservations regarding its effectiveness in preventing infection. If the patient suffers from recurrent breakthrough infections or if there are signs of continued deterioration of the renal substance, more radical treatment should be offered. Surgery consists of reimplanting the ureters into the bladder; endoscopic treatment consists of injecting a substance behind the intramural ureter to create an effective posterior backing which helps to restore the antireflux mechanisms.

The aim of these modalities of treatment is to stop the reflux. This does not necessarily mean that the progression of renal damage is halted or that further urinary tract infections are prevented. In cases where the reflux has caused severe damage to the kidney (relative function less than 15%), a nephroureterectomy may be the best option.

The choice between surgical or endoscopic correction of reflux is an individual matter, each technique having its own protagonists.

Preoperative

Assessment

Before planning operative correction of the vesicoureteric reflux, complete assessment of the urinary system is mandatory. The investigation should include the following:

1. Micturating cystography.
   (a) Direct contrast micturating cystography. This investigation is carried out during the first month of life where dilatation of the upper urinary tract is diagnosed by antenatal scanning. It is also recommended following diagnosis of the first urinary tract infection in boys or girls at any age.
   (b) Indirect radioisotope cystography is preferred in older girls as it is a less traumatic investigation.
2. Direct isotopic micturating cystography. This has the advantage of a considerably reduced radiation dose in centers where it is available.
3. DMSA (dimercaptosuccinate) or Mag 3 (^{99m}Tc-labeled mercaptoacetyl triglycine) renal scanning. This assesses the presence of renal scars and provides a measure of the relative function of each individual kidney.
4. Urodynamic study. This is important for detecting an underlying bladder dysfunction.
5. Ultrasonographic scanning of the urinary tract. Although a poor investigation to detect reflux this can be useful for assessing the size, shape and echogenicity of each kidney, the degree of dilatation of the ureter and bladder wall thickness.
6. Intravenous urography. This is only of use in detecting an associated anomaly such as a duplication of the excretory system.
7. Cystoscopy. Evaluation of the shape of the ureteric orifice or the length of the submucosal portion of the ureter is purely subjective and will not alter the therapeutic decision. It is, however, recommended if the vesicoureteric reflux is associated with a contralateral or ipsilateral ureterocele or if the reflux has occurred secondary to bladder dysfunction or bladder outlet obstruction.

Anesthesia

General endotracheal anesthesia is complemented by caudal anesthesia.

Operations

Transhiatal reimplantation of the ureter (Cohen's procedure; Glenn–Anderson's procedure) and suprahiatal reimplantation of the ureter are the two main surgical options. Their aim is to mobilize the distal segment of the ureter(s) (transmural ureter) and place it under a tunnel of bladder mucosa in order to restore the flap valve mechanism which is designed to prevent vesicoureteric reflux.

TRANSHIATAL REIMPLANTATION OF THE URETER

This is mainly represented by Cohen's procedure[6].

Position of patient

1 The patient lies supine on the operating table. A small sheet placed under the sacrum is useful to flatten the abdomen. A right-handed surgeon should stand on the left side of the patient, with the scrub nurse on his left. The two assistants should stand on the right side of the patient. A frame should be put between the surgeons and the anesthetist.

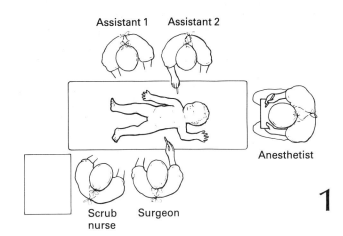

Incision

2 A transverse suprapubic incision is made, 2 cm above the pubic symphysis, in the low abdominal crease.

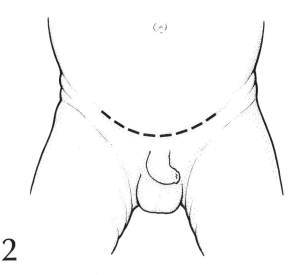

3 The subcutaneous tissues are incised, exposing the rectus sheath which is opened vertically in the midline. Both recti are separated and the peritoneum is gently pushed upwards, superiorly, providing good exposure of the bladder.

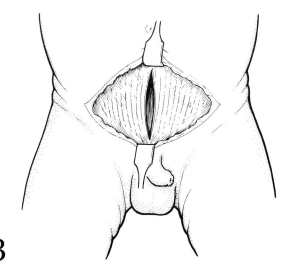

4 A Denis Browne retractor is inserted. The lateral blades retract the recti and the upper and lower blades retract the skin and subcutaneous tissues.

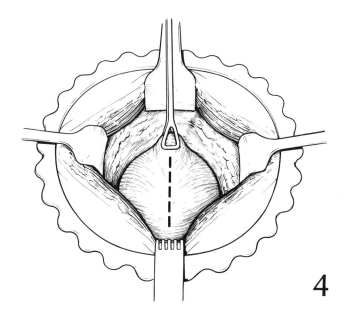

4

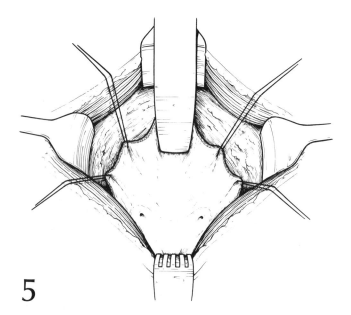

5

Exposure of the trigone

5 The anterior wall of the bladder is incised vertically and two or three stay sutures suspend each edge of the vesicotomy. One or several swabs are put inside the bladder and retracted upwards with a Deaver retractor held by the second assistant, in order to expose the trigone. A 3/0 or 4/0 absorbable suture is placed at the lowest point of the vesicotomy to prevent splitting of the incision downwards into the urethra.

The blades of the Denis Browne retractor should not be placed within the bladder for three reasons: (1) retraction is vigorous and may damage the bladder; (2) access to the laterovesical spaces may be difficult; and (3) the bladder wall loses its natural mobility rendering the procedure more difficult.

It is essential to avoid rigid retraction and to maintain the natural suppleness of the tissues.

The trigone is now well exposed and an infant feeding tube (3, 4, 6 or 8 Fr) is inserted into each ureter. A stay suture (5/0) is placed around each ureteric orifice and tied over the feeding tube. The first assistant holds this stay suture with mild traction.

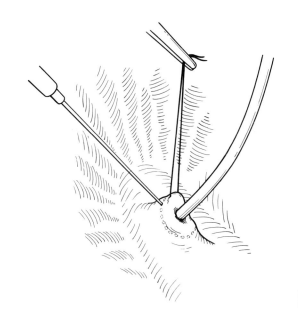

6

Transhiatal dissection of the ureter

6 The ureteric orifice is circumcised with diathermy (cutting and coagulation should be very low) and the mobilization of the distal 2 cm of ureter can be performed with diathermy alone (these 2 cm will be excised later).

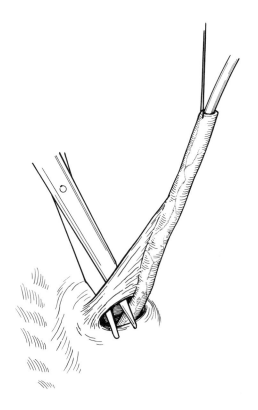

7

7 It is essential to enter the correct plane between the bladder and the transparietal ureter, commencing below the orifice. Sharp scissors should be avoided and Reynolds scissors make this procedure much easier. The tip of the Reynolds scissors elevates the muscle fibers that attach the ureter to the bladder musculature. These fibers are grasped with fine De Bakey forceps, coagulated and divided. The dissection continues progressively, circumferentially until the ureter is completely free. Coagulation of the fibers should be carried out some distance from the ureter to avoid damaging its blood supply.

The peritoneum is visible at the end of this dissection and should be teased away from the ureter. In boys the vas deferens may lie close to the ureter at this point and care must be taken to avoid damaging it.

A similar procedure can be used for the opposite ureter. In cases of ureteric duplication both ureters are dissected together and should not be separated thus avoiding damage to their blood supply.

Cohen or trigonal reimplantation of the ureter

In some cases the ureteric hiatus is wide and should be
narrowed by one or two absorbable sutures. This is
done to prevent the formation of a diverticulum. These
sutures should narrow the hiatus, but still allow the free
movement of the ureter and not restrict or constrict it.

8 The submucosal tunnel is then constructed. It is
usually a horizontal tunnel, crossing the midline of
the posterior surface of the bladder, just above the
trigone. Its length should represent at least five times
the ureteric diameter (Paquin's rule)[7] and, if this
condition cannot be fulfilled, trimming or remodeling of
the ureter should be considered (*see below*).

The site of the new ureteric orifice is selected and the
bladder mucosa is lifted from the underlying bladder
muscles with a pair of Reynolds scissors, starting either
from the hiatus or from the new ureteric orifice. Again,
sharp scissors should be avoided (especially Potts
scissors) and Reynolds scissors are ideal. The tunnel
should be wide enough to allow easy insertion of the
ureter, without constriction.

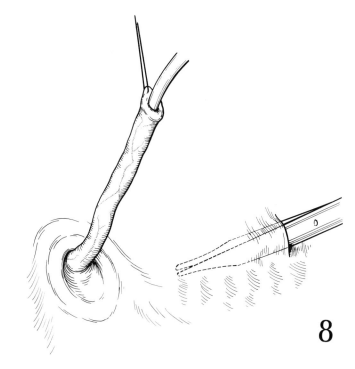

8

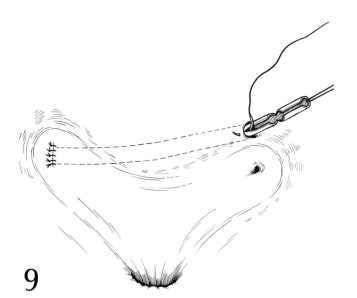

9

9 A similar procedure can be carried out for the
opposite ureter in cases of bilateral reimplantation.
The construction of the lowest tunnel which crosses the
trigone can bleed a little and the lifting of the mucosa is
slightly less easy.

A pair of artery forceps or right-angled forceps is
inserted through the tunnel, the stay suture is grasped
and gently pulled to draw the ureter into place, taking
care not to twist or kink it in the process.

10 The last 2 cm of ureter are excised and the ureteric opening is spatulated with a pair of angulated Potts scissors. The 5/0 absorbable suture anchors the ureter to the bladder muscles and the ureterovesicostomy is completed with interrupted 6/0 absorbable sutures.

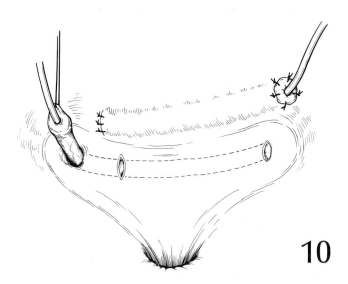

10

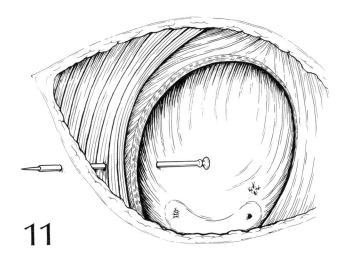

11

Closure and drainage

11 An infant feeding tube is inserted into the reimplanted ureter and exteriorized through the bladder wall, the rectus muscle and the skin, using the punch of a suprapubic catheter. The feeding tube is left in position for 2 days, or for 10 days if the ureter has been remodeled.

There is no consensus on the efficacy of drainage of the reimplanted ureter and some authors do not leave any drain. The bladder is drained either by a transurethral catheter which is left *in situ* for 5 days or by a suprapubic catheter.

The bladder is closed with a 3/0 or 4/0 suture (interrupted or continuous). The prevesical and subcutaneous spaces are drained by a suction drain. The abdominal wall, the subcutaneous tissues and the skin are then closed.

SUPRAHIATAL REIMPLANTATION OF THE URETER

Megaureters are the principal indication for this technique which should be performed by an experienced pediatric urologist. It is a difficult procedure which carries a significant complication rate.

The approach to the bladder, the retraction with the Denis Browne retractor and the exposure of the bladder mucosa are as in the transhiatal procedure.

The extravesical approach to the ureter is the main step in this procedure.

12 The peritoneum covering the dome and the lateral face of the bladder should be pushed upwards which involves ligation of the obliterated hypogastric ligament. It is then easy to mobilize the peritoneum upwards and to expose the full length of the iliac vessels. The vas deferens and its pedicle are easily located and should also be freed before the ureteric reimplantation.

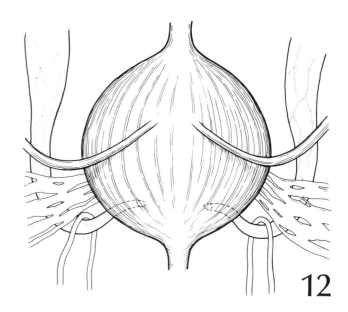

Identification of the ureter

The ureter is now identified passing over the iliac vessels close to their division into the external iliac and hypogastric arteries. The ureter is progressively mobilized from this point down to the bladder, preserving its blood supply and the vascularity of the bladder. There is, in fact, a plethora of small vessels and nerves arising from the pelvic pedicles to the bladder which cross the distal part of the extravesical ureter and should be preserved.

In severe megaureters the ureter is grossly dilated and kinked, and its dissection should be very meticulous to straighten it and maintain enough tissue around it to preserve its vascularity and innervation. The ureter is divided at its entrance into the bladder and a stay suture facilitates its mobilization. The ureter which normally passes under the vas deferens should be redirected over it to straighten it out.

Excision of the distal segment of ureter and remodeling

The distal segment of the ureter is usually narrowed and its excision allows urine to flow out freely. The ureteric diameter rapidly contracts and it is then possible to decide whether ureteric reimplantation can be achieved with or without remodeling or trimming. This decision is dictated by Paquin's rule: the length of the submucosal tunnel should represent at least five times the ureteric diameter.

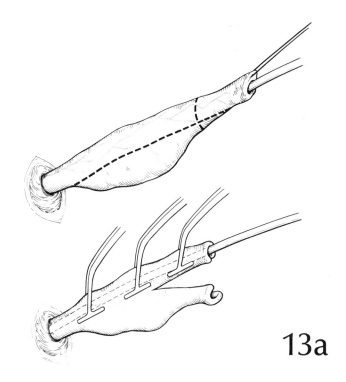

13a

13a, b If the ureter remains too large after excision of its distal end, the caliber of the ureter should be reduced either by excising a strip of ureter (Hendren's technique)[8] or by infolding the ureter (Kalicinski's technique)[9].

Excision of a strip of ureter may threaten ureter vascularity whereas ureter infolding can create a degree of obstruction. Whichever technique is chosen, the length of the remodeled or trimmed segment of ureter should not need to exceed the length of the submucosal tunnel.

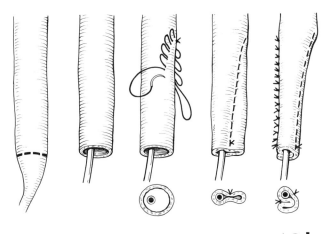

13b

Reimplantation of the ureter creating a new hiatus of entrance

14 The hiatus of entrance into the bladder of the ureter should be medial and high at the top of the posterior surface of the bladder. The ureter should not be constricted at this level and it is necessary to excise a disk of bladder to allow free passage of the ureter. The submucosal tunnel is fashioned as described above and should be vertical. Its distal end should open on the trigone. The passage of the freed ureter through the tunnel is the most difficult step of this procedure. The ureter should not be twisted or kinked, especially at the entrance into the bladder, and its pelvic course should be smooth. A few absorbable sutures are placed at its entrance into the bladder and sometimes the bladder itself is tacked down on the psoas muscle to maintain the smooth course of the ureter. The ureterovesicostomy is as described above.

A bilateral procedure may be performed. Some authors prefer to perform a transureteroureterostomy to avoid bilateral suprahiatal reimplantation.

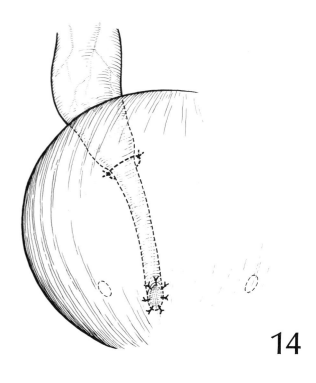

14

Closure

Closure and drainage are as described above except that the ureteric stent is maintained for at least 10 days if the ureter has been remodeled.

Postoperative care

The child is hospitalized for 5 days. The ureteric stent is removed after 2 days (or 10 days if the ureter has been remodeled). The bladder catheter is removed on the fifth postoperative day. Both suction drains are usually removed on the second day. Bladder spasms are common and administration of oxybutinin can be useful to reduce the discomfort. Antibiotic prophylaxis with gentamicin (48 h) and amoxicillin (10 days) is one possible option, followed by 3 months of trimethoprim–sulphamethoxazole (co-trimoxazole). Pain is controlled with diclofenac suppositories (12.5 mg).

The child should stay away from school for 2 weeks and avoid sport for 1 month.

A Mag 3 scan is repeated after 6 months in order to detect indirect signs of reflux. Ideally a repeat micturating cystogram should be performed but this is usually poorly accepted by the patient. Repeated isotopic renal scans are useful to detect the possible progression of existing or new scars.

Outcome

It is essential to reiterate that these procedures only aim at stopping vesicoureteric reflux. Their effects on the renal damage and on the recurrence of urinary tract infections are questionable.

Transhiatal procedures resolve vesicoureteric reflux in more than 95% of cases. Suprahiatal procedures are more difficult and have a significant incidence of complications (around 10%), including persistent reflux, secondary dilatation of the upper tract and stenosis.

References

1. Barrou B, Bitker MO, Chatelain C. Réimplantations urétéro-vésicales antireflux. *Urologie–Gynécologie. Encyclopaedia Médical Chirurgie: Editions Techniques* Volume 41133. Paris, 1990: 20 pp.

2. Hodson CJ, Edwards D. Chronic pyelonephritis and vesico-ureteric reflux. *Clin Radiol* 1960; 11: 219–31.

3. Bailey RR. The relationship of vesico-ureteric reflux to urinary tract infection and chronic pyelonephritis – reflux nephropathy. *Clin Nephrol* 1973; 1: 132–40.

4. Ransley PG, Risdon A. Renal papillary morphology and intra-renal reflux in the young pig. *Urol Res* 1975; 3: 105–9.

5. Smellie J, Edwards D, Hunter N, Normand ICS, Prescott N. Vesico-ureteric reflux and renal scarring. *Kidney Int* 1975; 8 (Suppl. 4): S65–72.

6. Cohen SJ. Ureterozystoneostomie: eine neue antirefluxtechnik. *Aktuel Urol* 1975; 6: 1–8.

7. Paquin AJ Jr. Ureterovesical anastomosis: the description and evaluation of a technique. *J Urol* 1959; 82: 573–83.

8. Hendren WH. Operative repair of megaureter in children. *J Urol* 1969; 101: 491–507.

9. Kalicinski ZH, Kanzy K, Kotarbinska B, Joszt W. Surgery of megaureters – modification of Hendren's operation. *J Pediatr Surg* 1977; 12: 183–8.

Ureteric duplication

Claude C. Schulman MD, PhD
Professor of Urology, University Clinics of Brussels, Erasmus Hospital, Brussels, Belgium

Principles and justification

Indications

Ureteric duplication is one of the most common malformations of the urinary tract. In many patients it is discovered as an incidental finding without clinical symptoms and does not require any surgical correction. With the advent of prenatal ultrasonography an increasing number of uropathies are discovered before clinical manifestations. Duplication can be associated with other anomalies, however, such as reflux, mega-ureter, ectopic ureter, and ureterocele.

Duplication can be complete or partial, when the two segments unite with one another somewhere between the renal pelvis and the intramural ureter above the bladder.

Partial duplication

Bifid ureters (incomplete duplication) may join at any level from the bladder to the ureteropelvic junction. The presence of a bifid ureter does not predispose toward vesicoureteric reflux, and surgical correction is based on the same indications as for a single refluxing ureter. When reflux occurs, the urine goes up through the short common stem and affects both ureters.

Peristaltic incoordination between the two ureters at their point of junction is a disorder associated with incomplete duplication. Antiperistaltic contractions propelling the urine from one ureter to the other rather than down into the common branch (the 'yoyo' phenomenon) may result in variable, but seldom important, dilatation of the ureters associated with flank pain, which will be the main indication for operative correction.

Surgery consists of converting the bifid ureter into the bifid pelvis by pyelopyelostomy or ureteropyelostomy, anastomosing the upper ureter to the lower pelvis, and excising the remaining length of the upper ureter.

Complete duplication

Reflux

Two operative possibilities exist for reflux in ureteric duplication, depending on whether reflux affects the lower pole ureter or both ureters. As reflux into the lower pole ureter is the more common presentation when associated with duplication because the intra-vesical segment is shorter and opens higher in the bladder, pyelonephretic lesions affect the lower pole of the duplex kidney selectively. When both ureteric orifices open into the bladder one next to the other, like a double-barrelled gun, reflux may affect both ureters. The therapeutic considerations for surgical correction of reflux associated with duplication are similar to those for reflux in a single ureter, though spontaneous resolution is less likely to occur with growth of the child when reflux involves the lower pole only. When reflux affects only the lower pole and the patient has severe pyelonephretic lesions as demonstrated by urography and quantitative scintigraphy, heminephrectomy should be considered. Removal of the remaining ureteric stump is not routinely necessary.

Megaureter

Primary megaureter associated with duplication occurs only in the upper pole ureter, which has a longer intravesical course than the lower pole ureter. Mega-ureter can be either segmental or complete. Symptoms are related to urinary tract infection and hydro-nephrosis.

The upper pole parenchyma related to the anomaly still has enough function to warrant preservation and ureterovesical reimplantation should be considered. The stenosed segment of megaureter is removed, and if dilatation is confined to the terminal portion of the ureter, both ureters are treated as a single unit and are reimplanted (see Illustrations 3a, b). If dilatation related to the megaureter is appreciable, however, remodeling is required, and both ureters are separated and reimplanted into the bladder individually. For segmental megaureter limited to the pelvic portion of the ureter, ureteroureterostomy is another alternative.

Ectopic ureter

An ectopic ureter exists when the ureteric opening is located outside the bladder. In approximately 80% of cases it is associated with duplication, particularly in girls. In boys, however, the ectopic ureter is more often a single ureter than related to a duplex system. Duplication in boys may be observed in a relatively high ectopic ureter (bladder neck, urethra). The upper pole parenchyma related to the ectopic ureter in a duplex kidney is commonly of little functional value, and dysplastic lesions are usually present. It is therefore pointless to try to preserve a structure that does not contribute to total renal function and is likely to maintain a source of infection. Prenatal ultrasonography may sometimes demonstrate upper pole dilatation in an ectopic ureter in a kidney that is worth preserving, and in these rare cases reimplantation should be considered.

The question of how complete the excision of the ectopic ureter should be is often raised during heminephrectomy in ureteric duplication. If no reflux is present in the ectopic ureter and the terminal portion is not too dilated, it may be preferable not to undertake total excision because this is likely to jeopardize the delicate neighbouring structures, in particular the ipsilateral ureter and the urinary sphincter. Simple removal of the lumbar ureter during heminephrectomy should be sufficient. If reflux is present in the ectopic dilated ureter, however, which is usually the case when it opens in the bladder neck or urethra, complete excision might be necessary.

Ureterocele

Ureterocele associated with duplication is a common anomaly in pediatric urology, with a great predomi-nance in girls. In a duplex kidney, a ureterocele is always related to the upper pole, and the position of the ureteric orifice allows for distinction between an intravesical ureterocele and an ectopic (extravesical) ureterocele. In the intravesical form, the opening of the ureterocele is located between the normal position of the ureteric orifice and the bladder neck. In the extravesical ureterocele, the opening is located at the bladder neck or in the urethra. This anatomic distinc-tion is important because both presentation and treatment of the anomalies are different. With the advent of prenatal diagnosis, asymptomatic ureteroceles are being encountered more often, allowing appropriate evaluation and management before infection aggravates the obstructive uropathy.

Intravesical ureterocele associated with duplication is similar to simple ureterocele without duplication, which is more common in adults. An intravesical ureterocele is relatively small, causing only mild, or no, obstruction and hydronephrosis. It may be symptomless until complicated by stasis, infection or stone formation.

In most cases of intravesical ureterocele, the upper urinary tract changes are not severe and kidney function is preserved; thus treatment should focus on the ureterocele only. In some small, uncomplicated cases in adults, no treatment is needed. Endoscopic resection of ureteroceles was widespread in the past, but it invariably resulted in reflux, necessitating further surgery in children. There remains, however, a place for minimal endoscopic incision of a small adult ureterocele complicated by a stone or infection and minimal dilatation. In neonates and young infants, there is also a place for cystoscopic incision of asymptomatic ureteroceles discovered by ultrasonography. A small careful horizontal incision is made at the base of the ureterocele, which does not seem to lead to reflux. This allows good drainage of the obstructed but otherwise salvageable kidney with a single or duplex system. In older children with large intravesical ureteroceles with dilatation, the treatment is usually operative. The recommended operation is excision of the ureterocele with ureteric reimplantation, using one of the advance-ment techniques or the Politano–Leadbetter procedure. When the involved ureter is massively dilated, tapering of the lower ureter should be considered.

In the uncommon situation of a small intravesical ureterocele associated with a duplication, the renal parenchyma related to the ureterocele maintains satisfactory function, and the ureter is minimally dilated or undilated, the condition being similar to a uretero-cele with a single ureter. Reflux may be present in the lower pole ureter. Treatment is similar to that used when there is a single ureter, namely removing the ureterocele with a common sheath and reimplantation of both ureters using an antireflux procedure. Occasion-ally, gentle endoscopic incision may be considered in selected cases if there is no reflux in the lower pole ureter.

Extravesical (ectopic) ureterocele is almost always

associated with ureteric duplication. The renal parenchyma drained by these ureteroceles is usually small and dysplastic, whereas the ureter is grossly dilated. The lower pole ureter often refluxes, and the associated parenchyma presents with pyelonephritis. In other cases, the lower pole ureter is dilated from obstruction by the ureterocele, which may also affect the contralateral ureter.

The patient often presents during early childhood with symptoms of urinary infection or failure to thrive. The ureterocele may sometimes appear as a genital deformity in girls, if it prolapses into the vulva. Very occasionally a flank mass is palpated during physical examination. Since the introduction of prenatal fetal ultrasonography, a new patient population is encountered: the uninfected neonate with asymptomatic obstructive uropathy caused by a ureterocele.

Management of a large, infant-type extravesical ureterocele depends on the child's age and clinical condition, presence of renal failure or sepsis, presence of associated lesions of the lower pole and contralateral kidney or bilateral ureteroceles, and expertise of the surgeon. No general agreement exists on the optimal treatment for an ectopic ureterocele. Of importance to the surgeon is the extravesical extension of the ureterocele, which causes bladder outlet obstruction, and the strength or weakness of the underlying detrusor muscle backing, which might appear as an extensive defect after excision of the ureterocele.

With few exceptions, a conservative approach cannot be justified, as dysplastic lesions or severe damage to the upper pole parenchyma are associated with the ureterocele, and such procedures as ureteropyelostomy should only be considered in a solitary kidney or when both kidneys are damaged. Thus, in most patients, heminephrectomy is the procedure of choice. It is accomplished easily through a retroperitoneal flank incision with resection of the proximal portion of the involved ureter.

The controversial question is whether excision of a ureterocele is necessary after upper pole nephrectomy. Complete excision with extensive reconstruction of the floor of the bladder and reimplantation of the ipsilateral and sometimes contralateral ureter is advocated as the standard procedure by several pediatric urologists. This approach is considered when the ureterocele is large, when detrusor backing is weak, when ipsilateral and even contralateral reflux is present, and when the ureterocele extends down into the urethra. Complete dissection of the ureterocele may be difficult, particularly at the lower end where it may adhere closely to the bladder neck and urethra. In these patients, a combination of intravesical and extravesical approaches is useful for complete downward dissection of the ureterocele with mobilization of the entire bladder. During dissection of the ureterocele, care should be taken not to injure the external sphincter area. When the ureterocele is unroofed, it is important to remove the entire wall of the ballooning, particularly near the

bladder neck and in the posterior urethra, to avoid having a retained lip of incised ureterocele acting as a valvular fold and causing obstructive problems. After the ureterocele has been excised completely, the urethra and trigone should be reconstructed with reimplantation of the lower pole ureter, and sometimes the contralateral lower pole ureter, following the Politano–Leadbetter technique or Cohen's advancement procedure.

An essentially extravesical dissection has been advocated to avoid potential damage to the urethra or vagina. Individual skill and experience remain essential for the choice of approach.

In the last decade, an increasing number of authors has advocated a more conservative approach, consisting of heminephrectomy with removal of the upper pole ureter to the level of the iliac vessels, if excision of the ureterocele is not considered mandatory. Complete decompression of the ureterocele, as well as disappearance of mild to moderate reflux in the ipsilateral lower pole ureter, can be anticipated in a significant number of cases. This approach avoids the risk and potential complications of extensive surgical reconstruction at the bladder level, because the bladder is never entered. The procedure is completed entirely through a single retroperitoneal flank incision. The ureteric stump is left open and drained so that urine remaining in the ureterocele and distal ureter empties in a retrograde fashion when the child voids and intravesical pressure rises.

If reflux was noted in the obstructed system or if the ureterocele was incised causing reflux, the distal stump is ligated. This more conservative approach gives satisfactory results in about two-thirds of cases. If the ureterocele fails to collapse and remains obstructive or if reflux persists in the lower pole ureter, however, it is likely to result in recurrent infection, bladder outlet obstruction, bladder diverticulum or reflux, all of which necessitate an additional operation through a suprapubic incision in a second stage some time later in one-third of cases. This expectant approach also allows total reconstruction at a separate time, and usually in easier and safer conditions, in naturally selected cases that really need it.

Endoscopic horizontal incision, which is advocated for neonates with asymptomatic intravesical ureteroceles, may also be considered in severely ill neonates or those with sepsis, when preliminary drainage is dictated by the poor clinical situation and endoscopic incision of the ureterocele provides temporary internal drainage of the obstructed bladder and upper pole. After the condition has improved, one-stage or two-stage repair is undertaken at a later date, with upper pole nephroureterectomy of the non-functioning or minimally functioning dysplastic parenchyma and complete removal of the incised ureterocele with reimplantation of the associated lower pole ureter.

There is no unanimity on how to manage surgically complex ureteroceles in children; all points of view have certain advantages and drawbacks. For the surgeon who is not familiar with the condition and seldom operates on infants, upper pole nephrectomy alone is the safest initial procedure. In neonates with sepsis and in poor general condition, preliminary decompression may be necessary and simple endoscopic incision of the ureterocele is advisable, because these neonates are poor candidates for a major procedure. In neonates with an uninfected ureterocele discovered by prenatal ultrasonography, minimal endoscopic meatotomy may have merit in allowing recovery of satisfactory renal function. For older children in good general condition, the experienced surgeon should consider a total,

single-stage complete reconstruction. Very occasionally, total nephroureterectomy is indicated when the lower pole is also destroyed by obstruction or reflux. Alternatively, complete excision of an ectopic uretero-cele with reimplantation of the lower pole ureter and sometimes of the contralateral ureter may be performed. Upper pole nephroureterectomy is performed first, during the same operative session, through a retroperitoneal flank incision. Cautious extravesical dissection separates both ureters; great care must be taken to preserve the periureteric adventitia of the lower pole ureter with its blood supply.

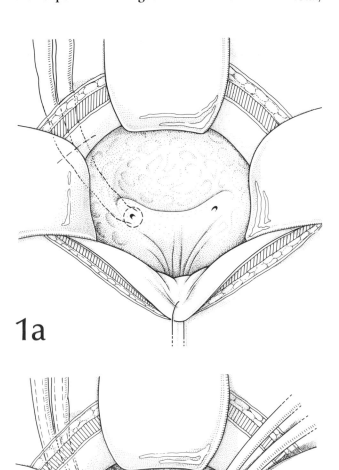

1a

1b

Operations

REIMPLANTATION FOR REFLUX IN PARTIAL DUPLICATION

1a, b
Through a Pfannenstiel incision, the bladder is opened and a self-retaining retractor is placed. Intravesical and extravesical dissection will liberate the ureters, which should be sectioned above their point of junction, the common trunk is excised and both ureters are reimplanted as a single unit in a common submucosal tunnel using the classic antireflux procedure. Stenting of both ureters is usual for a few days, with bladder drainage.

URETEROPYELOSTOMY IN PARTIAL DUPLICATION

2a–c A flank incision is made, the kidney is left *in situ*, and the ureters are liberated from the renal sinus up to their point of junction. The dilated upper pole ureter is excised exactly where it opens into the lower pole ureter. It is important not to leave any ureter that could act as a diverticulum. The excess abnormal ureter is removed, and the incision in the remaining ureter is closed with interrupted polyglycolic acid sutures. A large end-to-side anastomosis between the upper ureter and the renal pelvis is created so that the end result mimics a bifid renal pelvis without functional obstruction.

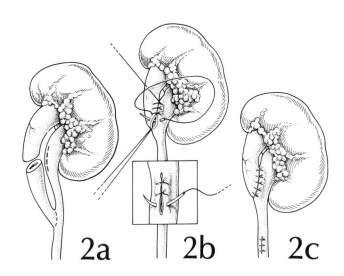

OPERATION FOR REFLUX IN COMPLETE URETERIC DUPLICATION

3a, b As both ureters are bound together in a common sheath at their lower end, they are treated *en bloc* as a single unit as the two elements may be devascularized in an attempt to separate them.

Any of the procedures to correct reflux may be used, either by intravesical advancement or by extravesical ureteroneocystostomy. The classic Cohen reimplantation is most widely used.

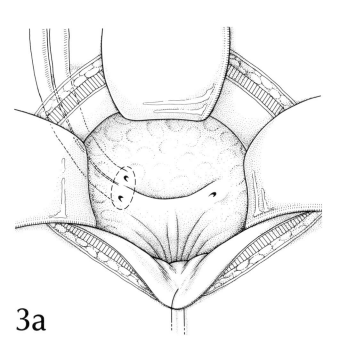

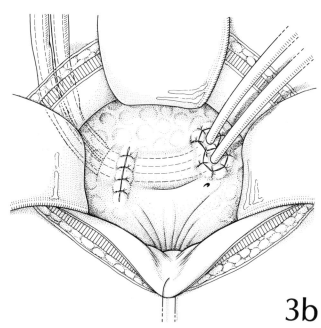

OPERATION FOR MEGAURETER IN COMPLETE URETERIC DUPLICATION

$4a, b$ The extravesical space is entered and the upper pole ureter is anastomosed to the lower pole ureter at a level where little or no dilatation is present. The terminal portion of the megaureter can either be left in place or split widely and its edges cautiously removed, being careful to avoid damage to the blood supply of the lower pole ureter.

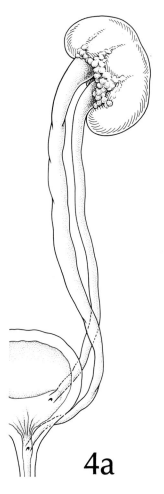

4a

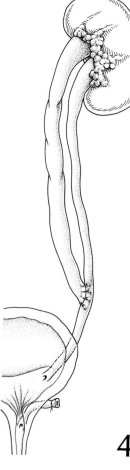

4b

HEMINEPHRECTOMY

5a–c
Through a subcostal lumbotomy or through the last intercostal space, the atrophied and dysplastic upper pole with the corresponding dilated ureter is removed. The renal capsule on the upper pole is incised to be used later to suture over the renal parenchyma. As vascularization of the upper pole often varies and some arterial branches are likely to separate from the main artery close to the renal sinus, it may sometimes be hazardous to clamp and ligate these vessels because this could cause ischemic lesions of the remaining parenchyma.

A clear demarcation is often visible between the destroyed upper pole and normal lower pole, and it is preferable to follow the cleavage plane which is less vascularized and to achieve hemostasis as necessary, and to complete the procedure by suturing the parenchyma of the remaining lower pole and then closing the capsule.

It is also advisable to undertake simple nephropexy of the lower pole, for example, by fixing it to the posterior muscular wall, to avoid its rotation around a long pedicle that has been stretched severely because of ureteric dilatation.

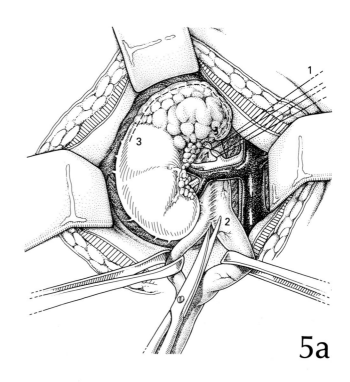

5a

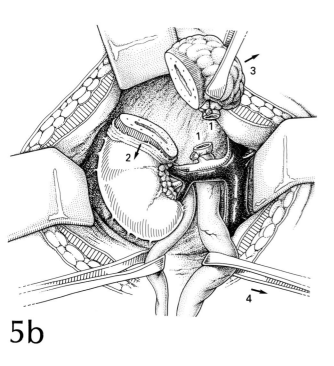

5b

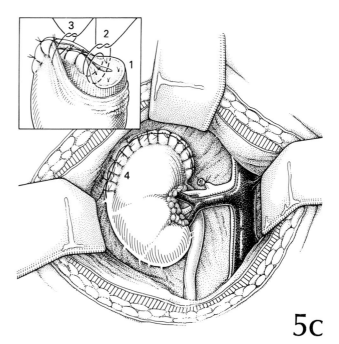

5c

REMOVAL OF ECTOPIC URETER

6a–d Complete extravesical mobilization of both ureters is carried downward to the bladder adventitia. For complete removal, the ectopic ureter is approached through a transvesical incision and pulled through the bladder. The ectopic ureter is dissected by freeing it from the trigonal mucosa down to its opening.

After the ectopic ureter is removed, the trigone is reconstructed, and the lower pole ureter is reimplanted into the bladder as in a standard antireflux procedure.

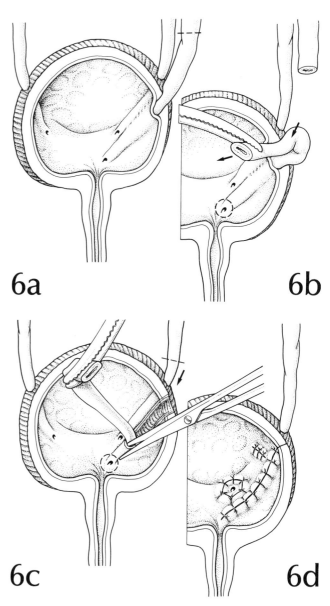

6a

6b

6c

6d

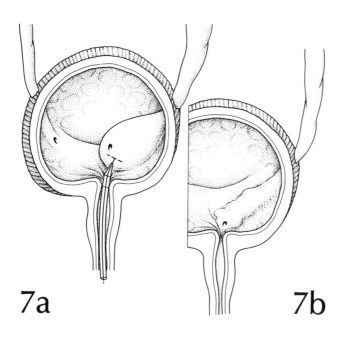

7a

7b

ENDOSCOPIC INCISION FOR INTRAVESICAL URETEROCELE

7a, b Simple ureteroceles, if complicated by stasis, infection, or stone formation, may be treated by endoscopic incision. A small knife electrode, simple stylet, or a Bugbee electrode is introduced into the ureteric orifice, preferably cutting horizontally, which leads to less (or no) reflux than unroofing with a conventional loop electrode. This approach may also be considered for decompression in neonates with an uninfected ureterocele or in acute conditions.

INTRAVESICAL URETEROCELE REMOVAL AND REIMPLANTATION

8a–d Ureteric dilatation is usually moderate, and treatment is similar to that used for simple ureterocele with a single ureter, consisting of excision of the ureterocele with common sheath ureteric reimplantation.

The bladder is opened, and a circumferential incision is made at the base of the ureterocele. Previous injection of saline into the ureterocele is helpful for its dissection from the trigone.

After excision of the ureterocele, the hiatus may be quite large and it is closed, treating the two ureters as a single unit.

The ureters are reimplanted, using one of the advancement techniques or the Politano–Leadbetter procedure. A transverse submucosal tunnel, as is used in the Cohen reimplantation procedure, is illustrated.

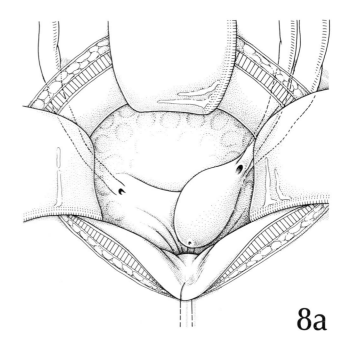

8a

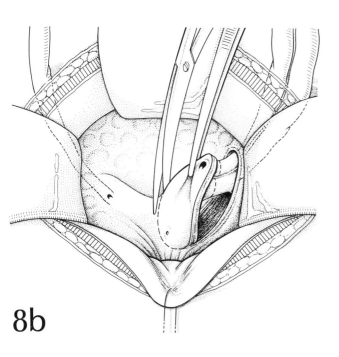

8b

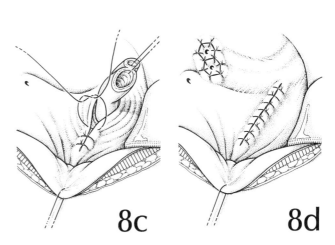

8c　　8d

OPERATION FOR EXTRAVESICAL URETEROCELE

9a–f The bladder is opened through a long median incision, or better, by a T-shaped incision to expose the entire bladder and bladder neck. The ureterocele is dissected from the trigone by incision of the vesical mucosa, which includes the lower pole ureteric orifice. The entire ureterocele is removed down to the bladder neck.

Extravesical mobilization and dissection of the ureterocele facilitate its removal. Previous complete mobilization of the bladder is necessary to allow easy access.

Extravesical extension of the ureterocele is difficult to remove where it is fixed to the bladder neck and urethra. This excision is facilitated by opening the upper wall of the ureterocele extension in the bladder neck and urethra.

The lateral and posterior walls of the ureterocele extension are dissected from the bladder neck and urethra and removed.

The urethra, trigone and posterior bladder wall are reconstructed to ensure a strong backing to the bladder. Reimplantation of the lower pole ureter (*Illustration 9e*) is done by advancement (solid arrow) or by a transverse submucosal tunnel following Cohen's procedure (broken arrow).

The lower pole ureter is covered by the vesical mucosa.

The contralateral ureter, which may be refluxing, obstructed, or sectioned during dissection of the ureterocele, is reimplanted by a standard antireflux procedure.

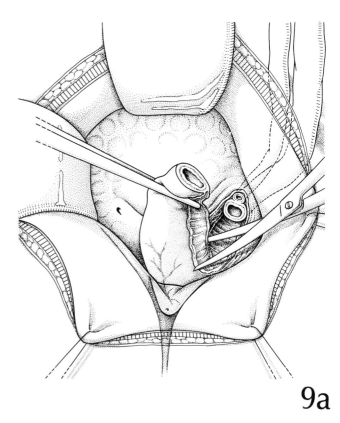

9a

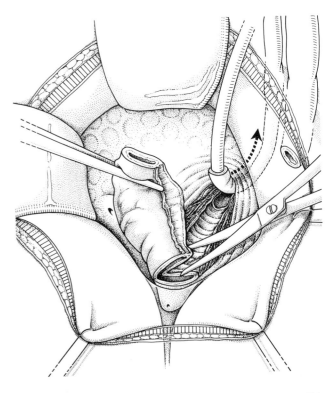

9b

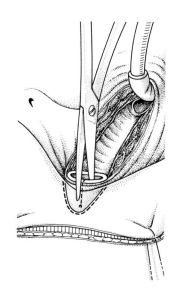

9c

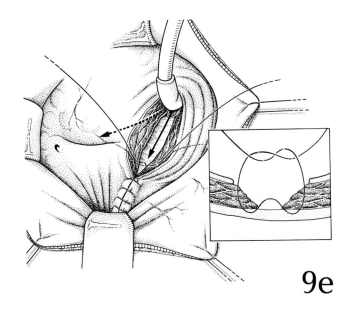

9e

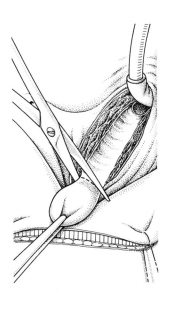

9d

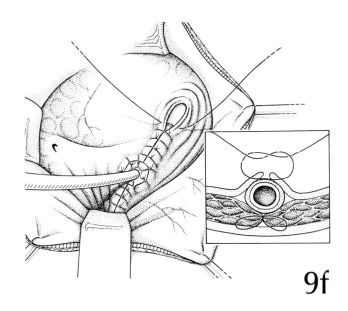

9f

Postoperative care

Following ureteropyelostomy in partial duplication drainage of the collecting system is usually not necessary, but if the anastomosis is not very large a nephrostomy tube is placed in the dilated upper pole for a few days.

After intravesical ureterocele removal and reimplantation ureteric cathers are usually left *in situ* for a few days with bladder drainage.

Illustrations by Paul Andriesse

Urinary diversion and undiversion

W. Hardy Hendren MD, FACS, FRCSI(Hon)
Chief of Surgery, Children's Hospital, and Robert E. Gross Professor of Surgery, Harvard Medical School,
Boston, Massachusetts, USA

Principles and justification

Urinary diversion is carried out much less often today than it was 20–30 years ago because better methods of treating children with urinary malformations have been developed. For example, a child with myelodysplasia and a neuropathic bladder was formerly treated by urinary diversion to stop wetting and/or deterioration of the urinary tract. Today, if there is vesicoureteric reflux, ureteric reimplantation will be performed. If the bladder is small and non-compliant, augmentation cystoplasty will be done[1]. If there is incontinence from inadequate outlet resistance, bladder neck narrowing will be done, often together with augmentation cystoplasty. Intermittent self-catheterization is commonly used if the patient cannot empty the bladder. If a ureter is grossly enlarged, it can be tapered in caliber and reimplanted with a tunnel to avert reflux. None of these procedures was in common use 30 years ago.

Several types of diversions will be described because some surgeons still use them. However, most problems can be repaired today, so that diversion in general can usually be avoided.

Operations

URINARY DIVERSION

Ileal loop urinary diversion

1 This was used widely in children for about 20 years, beginning in 1955. The ileal loop, however, has no mechanism to prevent reflux. Infected urine from the external appliance and the intestinal segment can reach the kidneys. This often causes renal deterioration in the long term, even when the urinary tract is normal initially. Therefore, the author believes that an ileal loop should never be performed in a young patient with a good prognosis. The ileal loop continues to be an acceptable procedure for adults with malignant disease who will not live long enough to suffer the possible consequences of reflux.

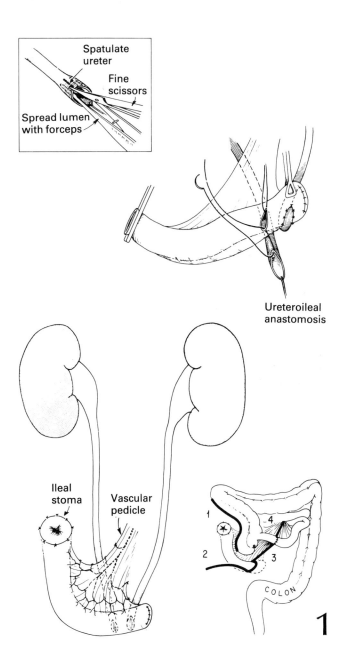

Spatulate ureter

Fine scissors

Spread lumen with forceps

Ureteroileal anastomosis

Ileal stoma

Vascular pedicle

COLON

1

Colonic conduit urinary diversion

This has the advantage of draining the upper urinary tract without reflux. Therefore, in the rare case today where a continent diversion into an appliance on the abdominal wall is used, this technique is applicable. In a laboratory study using dogs an ileal loop was used to divert one ureter and a non-refluxing colonic conduit was used to divert the other ureter. There was a marked difference in the incidence of pyelonephritis, 84% on the side of the ileal loop and only 7% on the side with a non-refluxing colonic conduit[2]. Bowel preparation for all reconstructive surgery utilizing bowel consists of a clear liquid diet for 2–3 days and preoperative bowel lavage with a polyethylene glycol electrolyte solution which passes quickly and is not absorbed.

2a–e
A colonic segment is selected with an ample mesenteric blood supply. The mesentery should be kept as broad as possible. The segment selected should be long enough. Other segments of colon can be used if the sigmoid colon is not suitable because of previous pelvic irradiation or anatomic variations.

The proximal end of the conduit is closed with two layers of inner chromic catgut and outer non-absorbable sutures. Silk or braided suture material should be avoided in case a suture should enter the bowel lumen where it could be a nidus for stone formation. The conduit is rotated 180° clockwise and is anchored at the aortic bifurcation when the ureters are both of normal length. It can be anchored higher if they are short.

Saline is infiltrated to facilitate creating a seromuscular flap beneath which the ureter is placed to create a non-refluxing valve.

The completed conduit is shown in *Illustration 2d*. Mesenteric traps are closed, but no attempt is made to close the space on either side of the conduit. The author usually makes a midline laparotomy incision, placing the stoma on the left, on the belt line. The stoma is fashioned as a turn-back stoma, which protrudes slightly.

Sometimes the patient does not have two good ureters. The better ureter can be used to create the non-refluxing anastomosis, draining the second ureter as a transureteroureterostomy or transureteropyelostomy. In that case, the butt end of the conduit is placed high in the appropriate gutter near the lower pole of the kidney. If a ureter is dilated, it can be tapered in caliber to obtain a ureter caliber:tunnel length ratio of 1:5 which will usually prevent reflux.

Implantation of the colonic conduit into the colon (*Illustration 2e*) is suitable in some patients who have normal rectal control, normal renal function, and no way to construct a bladder. Examples in which it could be a reasonable option include patients who have undergone anterior pelvic exenteration for malignancy and bladder exstrophy deemed unsuitable for primary

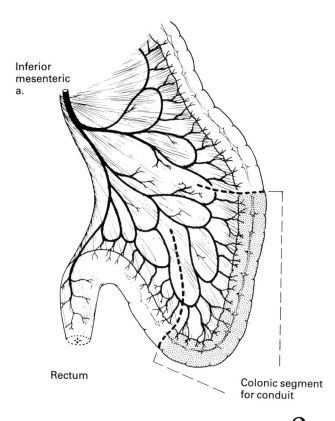

Inferior mesenteric a.

Rectum

Colonic segment for conduit

2a

reconstruction. It would not be suitable for patients with myelodysplasia. Primary one-stage ureterosigmoid diversion should not be performed, in the author's opinion, simultaneously with anterior exenteration for cancer, because recurrence in the pelvis can present a serious problem. Furthermore, radiation therapy can cause proctitis, a contraindication to diversion of urine into the fecal stream. Also, primary diversion of the urine to the colon should be avoided in young infants, because it can lead to several years of malodorous incontinence of both urine and feces. It is better to wait until bowel control is well established before diverting urine to the rectosigmoid colon. It is well recognized that ureterosigmoidostomy carries a 10% risk of colon carcinoma. Whether the staged technique will offer protection from cancer remains to be seen. The author's patients are routinely followed with colonoscopy every 2 years, or sooner if blood appears in the excreta.

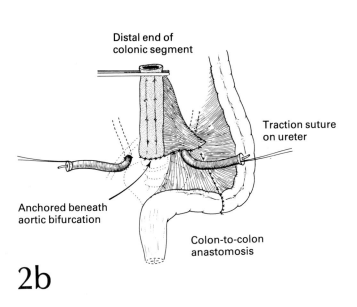

Distal end of
colonic segment

Traction suture
on ureter

Anchored beneath
aortic bifurcation

Colon-to-colon
anastomosis

2b

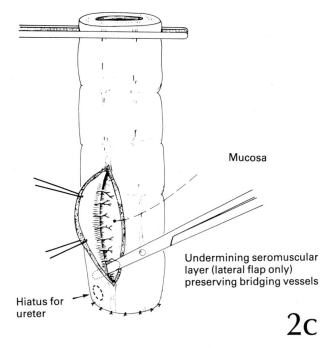

Mucosa

Undermining seromuscular
layer (lateral flap only)
preserving bridging vessels

Hiatus for
ureter

2c

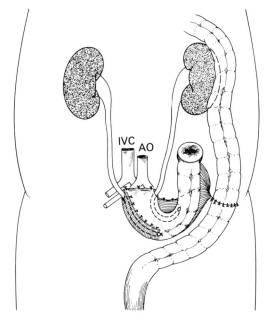

IVC AO

2d

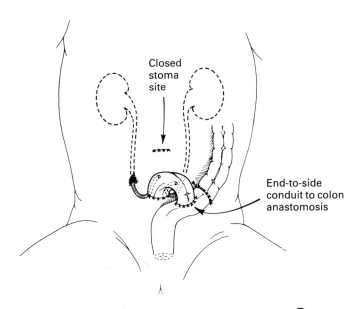

Closed
stoma
site

End-to-side
conduit to colon
anastomosis

2e

Ileocecal conduit

3 This can be used for cutaneous diversion, creating a non-refluxing nipple by intussuscepting the terminal ileum. The ileum must be sutured to the cecal wall to maintain the intussuscepted nipple. The ileocecal conduit can prolapse through its stoma unless the base is well anchored in the abdominal gutter.

When retrograde filling of an ileocecal conduit shows that its non-refluxing mechanism is effective, the stoma can be implanted into the colon or joined to the bladder. The bladder must be bivalved, however, to give a large anastomotic union so that the cecum will not behave as a diverticulum.

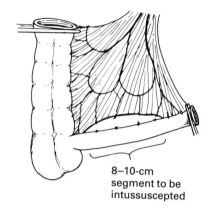

8–10-cm
segment to be
intussuscepted

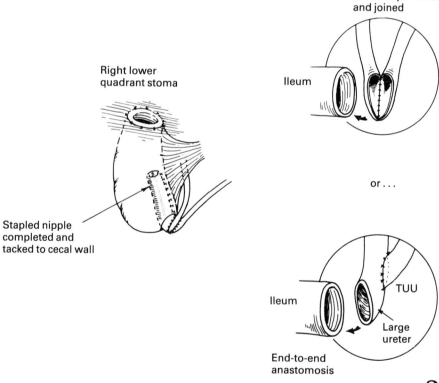

Right lower
quadrant stoma

Stapled nipple
completed and
tacked to cecal wall

Ureters spatulated
and joined

Ileum

or . . .

Ileum

TUU

Large
ureter

End-to-end
anastomosis

TUU = transureteroureterostomy

3

Ureterostomy

Much has been written about diversion of the urinary tract by ureterostomies, especially for temporary diversion of the urine with a plan for a reconstructive operation at a later age. It is the author's opinion that this has been greatly overused in the past and that ureterostomy can cause certain complications, making ultimate reconstruction more difficult than if diversion had been avoided in the first place[3].

End-ureterostomy should be avoided if there is any likelihood of a subsequent reconstructive operation. End-ureterostomy often does not drain effectively and commonly develops stomal stenosis. Similarly, mid-ureteric loop ureterostomy can greatly complicate subsequent reconstructive surgery by tethering the mid-ureter and interfering with the blood supply of the lower ureter.

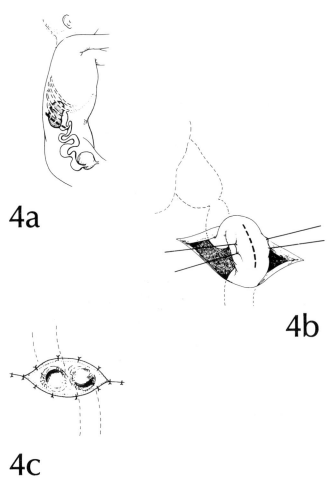

4a

4b

4a–d When ureterostomy is used it should be a high loop ureterostomy (*Illustrations 4a–c*) if there is enough ureteric length below that point to allow subsequent reconstruction and ureterostomy closure, or loop pyelostomy (*Illustration 4d*) at the ureteropelvic junction.

When closure of a high ureterostomy or pyelostomy is performed, both limbs should be mobilized widely and joined with a spatulated anastomosis. Minimal mobilization and simple closure of the ostomy can leave a kinked segment which does not drain well. The author has seen many such examples which required resection of the former ureterostomy site to obtain good drainage.

4c

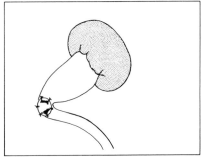

4d

Vesicostomy

Vesicostomy has been widely used by many surgeons for temporary diversion of the lower tract, especially in young infants with severe urethral valve pathology, massive vesicoureteric reflux and myelodysplasia. The author believes that many of these diversions can be avoided. For example, in boys with valves, modern 7.5-Fr endoscopes allow transurethral cutting of valves in all but the smallest infants. Massive reflux can be treated by ureteric reimplantation even in small infants if the surgeon is experienced and familiar with surgery of infants. Patients with myelodysplasia can be treated by intermittent catheterization if the bladder is not emptying properly. Vesicostomy can fail to provide good lower tract drainage because there can be secondary obstruction at the ureterovesical junction.

5a, b In the rare case where temporary vesicostomy is used, it is performed as illustrated. The urachal ligament is divided and the peritoneum is dissected from the dome of the bladder to make the incision high. The bladder muscle is tacked to the fascia and the skin is sutured to the edge of the opened bladder. If the vesicostomy is placed too low (*Illustration 5b*) it can be blocked by prolapse of the posterior wall of the bladder.

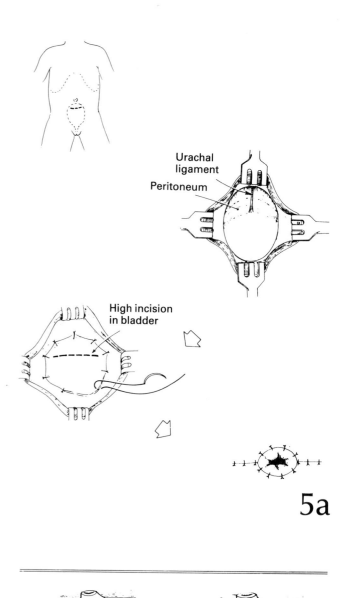

Urachal ligament

Peritoneum

High incision in bladder

5a

5b

CONTINENT URINARY DIVERSION

In the past few years there has been a trend toward creating an intra-abdominal urinary reservoir which can be catheterized through a continent abdominal wall stoma, avoiding a bag on the abdominal wall. These methods are used much more often in adults to provide a catheterizable reservoir following cystectomy for bladder cancer. The author believes that fewer children should be considered candidates for continent diversion, as most pediatric problems can be solved by a direct reconstructive operation if the surgeon is willing to invest the required time and effort. Many methods have been used, and those shown illustrate the principles involved.

Kock pouch

6 A long segment of ileum is used to create this continent reservoir. The two limbs are sewn together and folded over into a reservoir pouch. At each end an intussusception is created to prevent reflux from the pouch. One is the surface stoma, which will be catheterized to empty the pouch. The other nipple prevents reflux from the pouch to the kidneys. There is a 30% incidence of postoperative complications in these patients, including incontinence of the mechanism designed to prevent leaking on the abdominal wall, difficult catheterization, parastomal hernia, stoma complications and electrolyte disorders. Many of these patients have asymptomatic bacilluria, but pyelonephritis is unusual when there is no reflux.

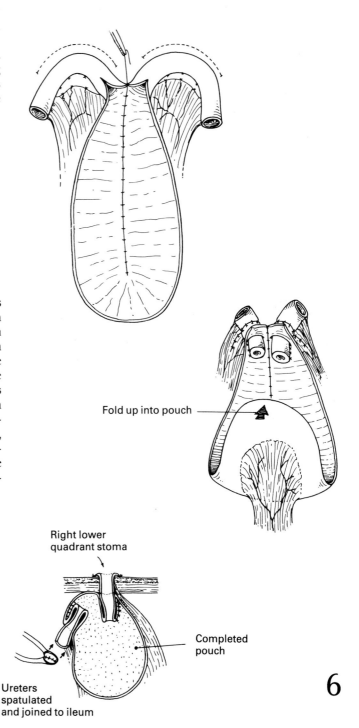

Fold up into pouch

Right lower
quadrant stoma

Completed
pouch

Ureters
spatulated
and joined to ileum

6

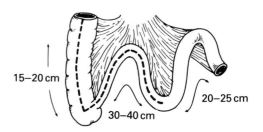

Mainz pouch

7 The ascending colon and terminal ileum can be fashioned into a reservoir[4]. The ureters are joined by a tunneling technique. Often, this is done most easily by working inside the lumen of the bowel using the technique described by Goodwin[5]. The terminal ileum is intussuscepted as a nipple and is sewn to the wall of the reservoir to prevent it from unravelling. If staples are placed in bowel used as urinary tract, they are subject to stone formation if they are bathed with urine. Therefore, staples should not be placed in a position which cannot be viewed endoscopically in case stones form and need to be plucked out endoscopically with foreign body forceps while they are still small.

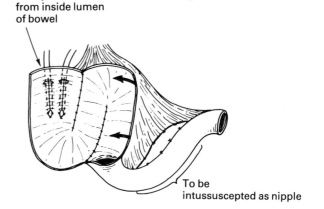

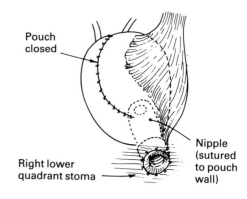

7

Right colonic pouch

8 The colon is opened widely and laid back on itself to form a reservoir of high capacity and low pressure. Bowel should always be detubularized to prevent it generating high contractile pressures in the system. A nipple is created to prevent leakage through the stoma, as in the Mainz pouch. The Indiana pouch[6] is an alternative technique in which the ileum is not intussuscepted, but is tapered in caliber and brought to the surface as an ileostomy of reduced size. Tapering is accomplished by applying a stapler parallel to a catheter in the ileum, excising the excess ileal diameter along its antimesenteric border.

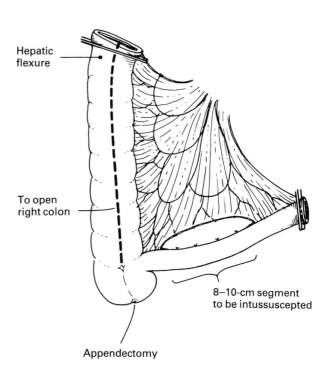

Hepatic flexure

To open right colon

Appendectomy

8–10-cm segment to be intussuscepted

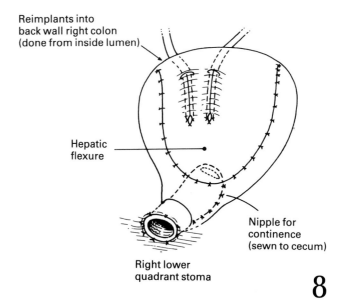

Reimplants into back wall right colon (done from inside lumen)

Hepatic flexure

Nipple for continence (sewn to cecum)

Right lower quadrant stoma

8

Mitrofanoff technique

9 This has gained considerable popularity in the past decade as a means for creating a catheterizable stoma which does not leak urine from a reservoir of either bladder or bowel[7]. The appendix is detached from the cecum, preserving its blood supply. The base of the appendix with a small patch of cecal wall is brought to the skin as a catheterizable stoma. The end of the appendix is tunnelled into the wall of the reservoir to prevent reflux. If the appendix is not available, or is too short, a tapered segment of ileum can be used. Alternatively, a lower ureter can be used as a conduit, draining its kidney to the opposite side by transureteroureterostomy.

Regarding all types of diversions, continent or otherwise, the author believes that the surgeon should seek ways to reconstruct the urinary tract whenever possible, instead of turning to a diversion procedure. Three decades ago the ileal loop was in vogue. Two decades ago the non-refluxing colonic conduit became very popular. Both of these techniques passed from fashion as better methods were devised. The present decade is, perhaps, the era of continent diversions, but greater emphasis should be placed on functional reconstruction whenever possible.

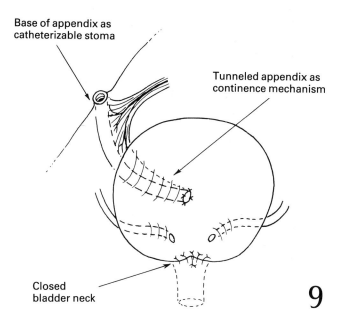

Base of appendix as catheterizable stoma

Tunneled appendix as continence mechanism

Closed bladder neck

9

BLADDER AUGMENTATION

Much of the reconstructive surgery that is performed today depends on enlarging a bladder that is too small. The following methods are in current use.

Ileocecal augmentation

10a–h The ileocecal segment is selected, maintaining its pedicle as wide as possible to ensure a good blood supply. Mesentery is removed from the terminal ileum for 8–10 cm to facilitate intussusception of that segment. A good vascular arcade is preserved at each end of this bowel segment.

The intussusception is created by a combination of pulling with a Babcock clamp and pushing with blunt forceps. Sutures are placed between the bowel wall and cecum to maintain the intussusception. This nipple will not persist, however, if it is not sewn to the adjacent wall of the cecum. Two or three rows of staples are placed through the nipple to help to hold it. These can be used only when it will be possible to endoscope the segment later to retrieve any small stones which can form on staples that do not become covered by mucosa. In the author's experience, however, stapling a nipple will not prevent it from unravelling, so it is better sewn to the adjacent wall of the cecum (*Illustration 10f*).

Using cautery, an incision is made from the full length of the nipple, through the ileocecal valve, and along the back wall of the cecum for a corresponding distance. The nipple is then sewn to the adjacent wall of the cecum with two running sutures. If a nipple is not fixed in this manner it can become loose, allowing the intussuscepted bowel to evert, which results in reflux.

The ileocecal segment is rotated clockwise and joined to the bladder. The bladder is opened widely like a 'clamshell', so that the cecum does not behave as a diverticulum. A long segment of tubular-shaped bowel should be prevented. A generous Heineke–Mikulicz plasty to the anterior wall can prevent that. An onlay patch of ileum can do the same.

The completed augmentation is shown in which the ileocecal junction is used to prevent reflux. This technique is used only when ureters are too large or too short to tunnel into the bowel wall. The author prefers direct tunnel implantation of ureters into the colon wall to prevent reflux.

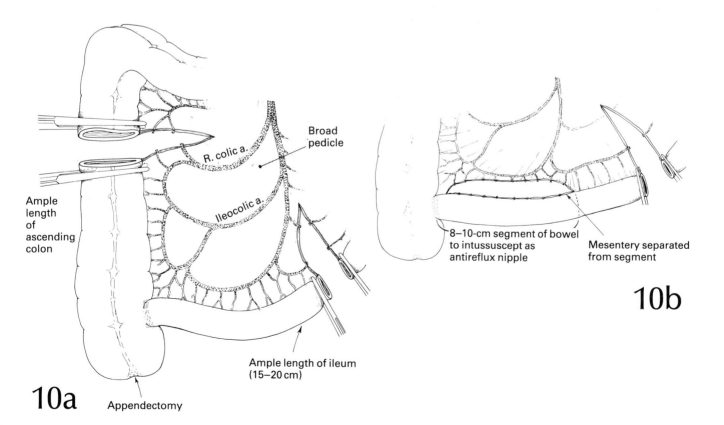

10a   Ample length of ascending colon

R. colic a.

Ileocolic a.

Broad pedicle

Ample length of ileum (15–20 cm)

Appendectomy

10b   8–10-cm segment of bowel to intussuscept as antireflux nipple

Mesentery separated from segment

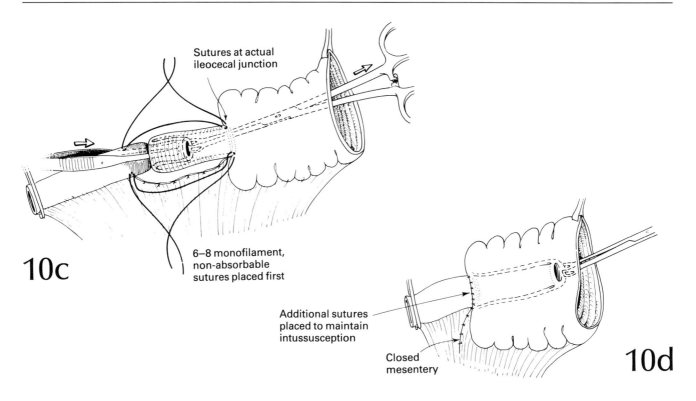

Sutures at actual
ileocecal junction

6–8 monofilament,
non-absorbable
sutures placed first

10c

Additional sutures
placed to maintain
intussusception

Closed
mesentery

10d

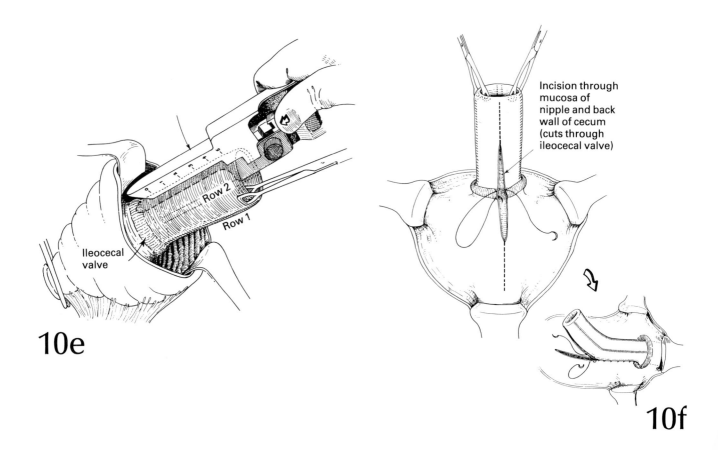

Row 2

Row 1

Ileocecal
valve

10e

Incision through
mucosa of
nipple and back
wall of cecum
(cuts through
ileocecal valve)

10f

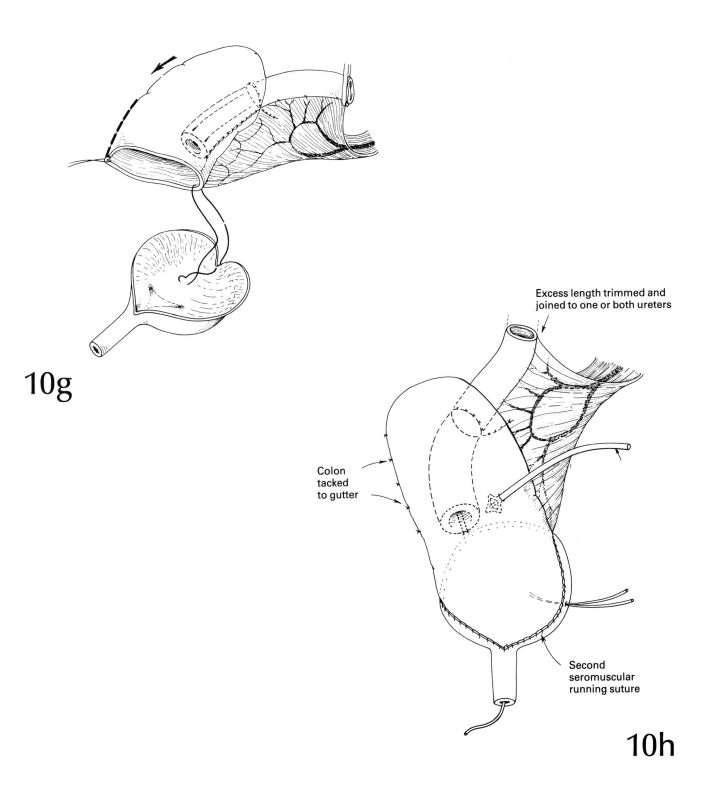

10g

Excess length trimmed and
joined to one or both ureters

Colon
tacked
to gutter

Second
seromuscular
running suture

10h

Bowel ureter

11 When ileal intussusception is impossible or there are no ureters, another piece of small bowel can be tapered and tunneled to create a non-refluxing union of the upper urinary tract to the cecum.

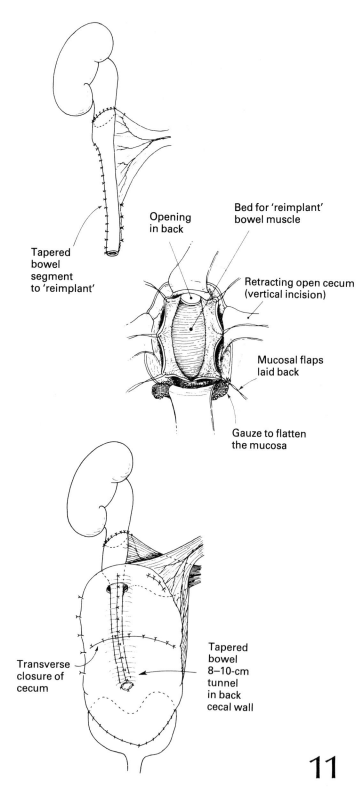

Tapered bowel segment to 'reimplant'

Opening in back

Bed for 'reimplant' bowel muscle

Retracting open cecum (vertical incision)

Mucosal flaps laid back

Gauze to flatten the mucosa

Transverse closure of cecum

Tapered bowel 8–10-cm tunnel in back cecal wall

11

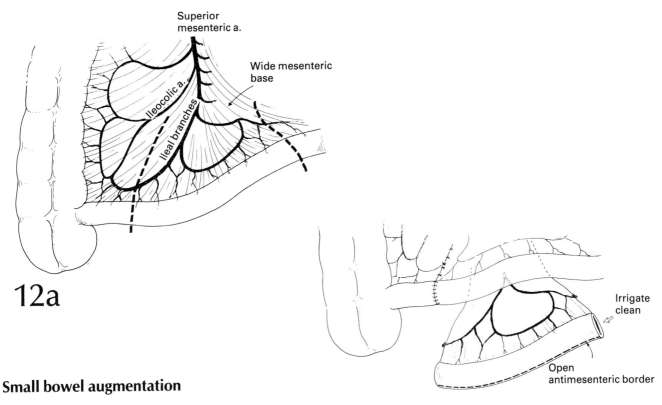

Small bowel augmentation

12a–e Often small bowel is used to augment the bladder. It should be detubularized to increase its volume and ablate high-pressure peristalsis. Even though bowel is detubularized, in some patients urodynamic testing after augmentation can show persistence of intermittent spontaneous contractile waves.

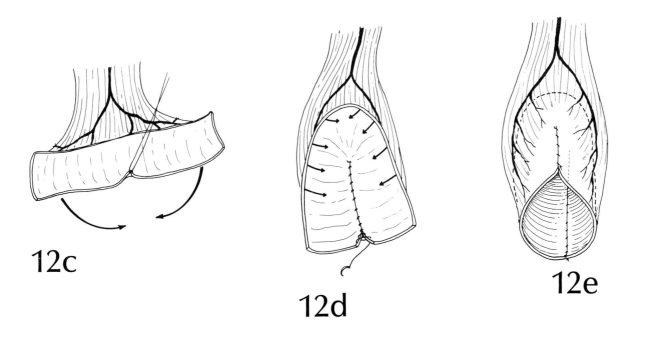

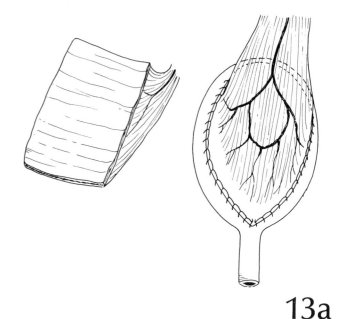

Augmentation with colon

13a, b When a small augmentation is needed it can be used as a patch (*Illustration 13a*). More often the native bladder size is very small and a larger reservoir is needed similar in capacity to the cecum and right colon. Sigmoid colon can be fashioned in the manner shown in *Illustration 13b*. The choice of bowel segment used for augmentation will depend on what is available, the blood supply to the bowel, and what must be accomplished. The cecum is ideal when large ureters must be joined to it, providing a non-refluxing mechanism.

The sigmoid colon is ideal when simple augmentation is needed. Its mesentery lies next to the bladder on the left side. Small bowel mesentery may be too short in some cases, and it has a pedicle which can trap bowel if not carefully tacked to prevent this. The sigmoid and left colon may be unavailable in cases where a pull-through operation has been performed for imperforate anus. When cecum is used loss of the ileocecal valve can change the bowel flora and interfere with bile salt resorption in the terminal ileum.

13a

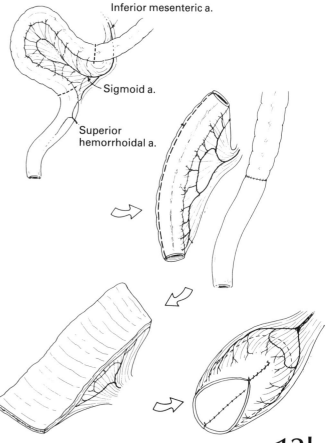

13b

Gastrocystoplasty

<big>14a–d</big> The operation is performed as shown. The stomach has some outstanding advantages as a means for augmentation[8]. It is metabolically advantageous regarding chloride absorption and base loss which is seen when segments of small bowel, and especially colon, are used. These segments tend to lose bicarbonate and potassium, and to a lesser extent sodium, while resorbing chloride. If potassium loss is replaced as potassium chloride, bicarbonate loss can be accelerated, aggravating acidosis. In contrast, gastric mucosa secretes chloride ions and, therefore, is preferred in patients with poor renal function who cannot tolerate increased solute resorption with resulting acidosis. The urine is more often sterile postoperatively after gastrocystoplasty because its pH is not so alkaline. Ureters can be tunneled and implanted easily into the stomach wall. Finally, the stomach is durable and compliant. Some patients will complain of pain in the bladder which can be relieved by taking a drug to block hydrogen ion production, e.g. cimetidine. In those patients who empty by intermittent catheterization, instillation of sodium bicarbonate solution can prove helpful. If a patient with a gastrocystoplasty develops vomiting and diarrhea, severe electrolyte depletion can occur rapidly because the gastric segment continues to excrete chloride. The patient may require intravenous replacement.

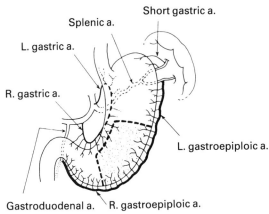

14a

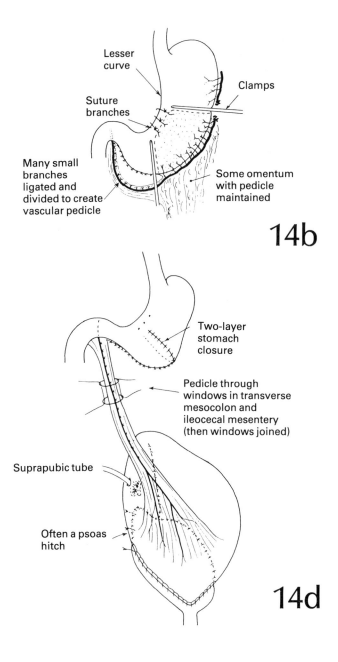

14b

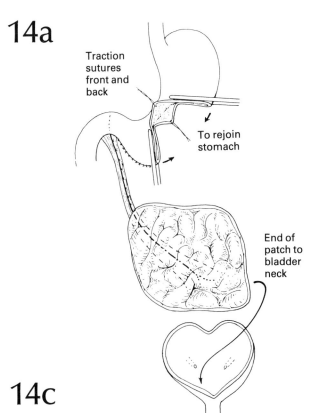

14c

14d

UNDIVERSION

The advances in reconstructive urology in the past two decades mandate reconsidering patients who underwent various types of urinary diversion in the past. Some can be switched from a refluxing ileal loop to a non-refluxing colonic loop. Others can be altered to a continent-type diversion, and still others can have late refunctionalization of a long-diverted bladder[9]. Since 1969 the author has performed urinary undiversion in 200 patients (*see Table 1*). The bladder in these patients is usually small from long disuse. This precludes preoperative urodynamic testing for bladder function. These bladders can be fragile and, during preoperative evaluation, instillation of contrast medium using only mild pressure can cause rupture and extravasation.

Percutaneous insertion of a small catheter during cystoscopy can allow instillation of saline to cycle the bladder. This can give information concerning sensation, continence and the ability to empty. It can also show whether a small bladder will increase its capacity towards normal when refunctionalized. If there is incontinence when the bladder is filled, an operation may be required to correct this. In actual practice today, however, the author relies more often on augmentation than prolonged cycling of the bladder.

Undiversion operations are usually long and difficult. Meticulous surgical technique is required to avoid potentially disastrous complications, e.g. leakage, stricture, reflux, or loss of a kidney[10]. A high standard of anesthetic care is mandatory. In ordinary pediatric surgery, fluid volume replacement is generally in the range of 5 ml/kg body weight/h. In undiversion surgery where there is mobilization of the bladder, extensive retroperitoneal dissection and long exposure of the intestine, fluid replacement can be in the range of 20–25 ml/kg/h. The urinary output should be carefully followed intraoperatively, placing catheters in the ureters and measuring urinary production hourly.

Operative exposure is always a long vertical midline incision, usually from the pubic symphysis to the xyphoid process, using a large self-retaining ring retractor. When mobilizing the ureter, all periureteric tissue should be kept with it, including the gonad vessels which are divided at the internal ring in boys, or close to the ovary in girls. The author has not seen loss of a gonad. Transureteroureterostomy or transureteropyelostomy is often used, joining the better ureter to the bladder and entering the contralateral ureter into it. The psoas hitch is an important tool in these reconstructions. After the ureter or tapered bowel segment is reimplanted, the bladder is hitched to the psoas muscle to fix the point of entry of the ureter so that it will not angulate when the bladder fills. Bladder augmentation is often required. A cardinal principle in undiversion surgery is to defer the decision of what to do until all anatomy is laid out at the operating table, and the various options can be considered based on what is available.

Table 1   Urinary undiversion, 1969–1994 (200 cases)*

	No. of patients		*No. of patients*
Ileal loop	71 (14 pyeloileal)	Permanent diversions	135
Colonic conduit	15 (3 had been ileal loops)	Temporary diversions	65
Loop ureterostomy or pyelostomy	40		
End-ureterostomy	17	Females	77
Cystostomy or vesicostomy	46	Males	123
Nephrostomy	8		
Ureterosigmoidostomy	2	Patients with one kidney	50 (3 had a transplant)
Continent diversion	1	Patient anephric (later transplanted)	1

*13 operations performed by author, 187 performed elsewhere

Ileal loop undiversion

15 This has been the most common type of reconstruction of the long-diverted urinary tract in the author's experience. Various options are available. Tapering a bowel segment and implanting it into the bladder as a 'ureter' should not be attempted if the bladder is small and scarred. It can be done with success only in the unusual circumstance where there is a large pliable bladder which allows achieving a long tunnel length: bowel diameter of at least 5:1.

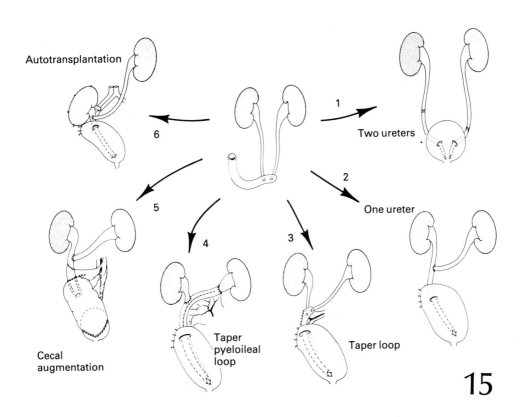

15

Conclusion

Major changes have taken place in diversion and undiversion techniques in recent years. Urinary diversions in children are needed less often than previously because improvements in reconstructive surgery have obviated the need for the majority of diversions.

In those children for whom a diversion is required, it should be performed by a method which does not allow reflux, thereby preventing damage to the kidneys. If there is sufficient bowel, and if renal function is sufficient to cope with solute reabsorption, a continent diversion technique should be considered. Patients are happier with a small stoma which they can empty by intermittent self-catheterization rather than a bag worn over a stoma which drains continuously.

There are many patients with various types of urinary diversion who should be re-evaluated for the possibility of undiversion by refunctionalizing a long-diverted urinary tract.

References

1. Hendren WH, Hendren RB. Bladder augmentation: experience with 129 children and young adults. *J Urol* 1990; 144: 445–53.

2. Richie JP, Skinner DG, Waisman J. The effect of reflux on the development of pyelonephritis in urinary diversion: an experimental study. *J Surg Res* 1974; 16: 256–61.

3. Hendren WH. Complications of ureterostomy. *J Urol* 1978; 120: 269–81.

4. Thuroff JW, Alken P, Riedmiller H, Jacobi GH, Hohenfellner R. 100 cases of Mainz pouch: continuing experience and evolution. *J Urol* 1988; 140: 283–8.

5. Goodwin WE, Harris AP, Kaufman JJ, Beal JM. Open transcolonic ureterointestinal anastomosis: new approach. *Surg Gynecol Obstet* 1953; 97: 295–300.

6. Mitchell ME, Rink RC. Pediatric urinary diversion and undiversion. *Pediatr Clin North Am* 1987; 34: 1319–32.

7. Duckett JW, Snyder HM. Use of the Mitrofanoff principle in urinary reconstruction. *World J Urol* 1985; 3: 191–3.

8. Adams MC, Mitchell ME, Rink RC. Gastrocystoplasty: an alternative solution to the problem of urological reconstruction in the severely compromised patient. *J Urol* 1988; 140: 1152–6.

9. Hendren WH. Urinary tract re-functionalization after long-term diversion. A 20-year experience with 177 patients. *Ann Surg* 1990; 212: 478–95.

10. Hendren WH, McLorie GA. Late stricture of intestinal ureter. *J Urol* 1983; 129: 584–90.

Surgery of renal calculi

Patrick G. Duffy FRCSI
Consultant Paediatric Urologist, Great Ormond Street Hospital for Children, London, and Senior Lecturer in Paediatric Urology, Institute of Urology, University of London, UK

Philip G. Ransley FRCS
Consultant Urological Surgeon, Great Ormond Street Hospital for Children, London, and Senior Lecturer in Paediatric Urology, Institute of Urology and Institute of Child Health, University of London, UK

Principles and justification

The majority of renal calculi in children are of infective origin. Boys are more commonly affected than girls and the peak incidence occurs between the ages of 2 and 3 years. The most commonly associated organisms are urea-splitting *Proteus* or *E. coli*. The finding of a *Proteus* organism in urine should raise the index of suspicion. The calculi are soft, containing a large amount of organic matrix, and are often poorly opacified. They contain magnesium ammonium phosphate (struvite) and varying quantities of calcium phosphate (apatite), oxalate, carbonate and urate. They may be discrete or form an extensive cast of the pelvicalyceal system. Soft matrix may be passed via the urethra. The kidneys are often normal, but pyonephrosis, perinephric abscess or progressive pyelonephritis may occur.

Metabolic calculi are rare in children. Hypercalcemia may be idiopathic or due to vitamin D overdosage or hypophosphatasia, and usually results in nephrocalcinosis. Hyperparathyroidism is extremely rare in children. Hypercalciuria is defined (in the UK) as greater than 4 mg/kg per 24 h or as a urinary calcium:creatinine ratio of greater than 0.25. Hypercalciuria also occurs in some children with infective stones, especially following a milk load. Renal tubular acidosis results in an alkaline urine, hypercalciuria, and recurrent urinary calculi in addition to nephrocalcinosis. Hyperoxaluria also produces nephrocalcinosis and recurrent oxalate stones, which may require removal if there is urinary obstruction. Uric acid calculi occur in children with leukemia and are usually sufficiently calcified to be visible on radiography. Cystinuria results in recurrent cystine stones which are radiopaque but not very dense, and rib shadows are clearly visible through them. Surgical intervention will be required for large calculi or obstructing stones prior to establishing an effective regimen of high fluid intake with or without D-penicillamine. Xanthine and dihydroxyadenine stones are radiolucent.

Preoperative

Radiology

The plain abdominal radiograph must include the whole urinary tract and may need to be repeated following bowel preparation.

The intravenous pyelogram and/or ultrasonographic scan will reveal urinary obstruction and demonstrate the renal anatomy, including any associated anomaly. A degree of ureteric dilatation is often seen in the ureter draining a kidney containing infected stones, and does not necessarily indicate the presence of obstructing calculi.

A micturating cystogram is essential to detect vesicoureteric reflux, but may be usefully postponed until the stones have been removed and the urine rendered sterile for some weeks, provided that by doing so it is not overlooked.

Urinalysis

Microscopy and culture are performed. pH determination is carried out on an overnight urine. A pH of less than 5.3 in a sterile urine excludes renal tubular acidosis.

Twenty-four hour urinary calcium and oxalate excretion tests are performed. It is essential that these investigations are carried out before surgery or very much later when the child is ambulant and eating a normal diet.

A screening test for amino acids is carried out.

Plasma

Creatinine, urea, electrolytes, calcium, phosphate, and uric acid tests are performed.

The findings of nephrocalcinosis or recurrent calculi demand more extensive biochemical investigation.

Operations

The more traditional forms of surgery for renal calculi
are being superseded by extracorporeal shock wave
lithotripsy (ESWL), and percutaneous disintegration and
removal of the stones. In the adult population routine
open renal calculus surgery is being replaced by the
lithotripter and the percutaneous approach to the pelvis
of the kidney. It is foreseen that, as the instruments
improve, more children will be treated by these modern
techniques

EXTRACORPOREAL SHOCK WAVE LITHOTRIPSY (ESWL)

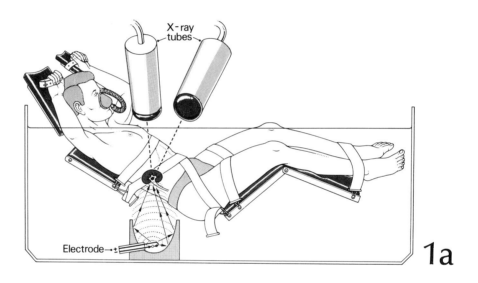

1a

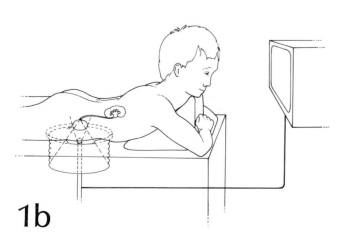

1b

1a, b The principle of shock wave lithotripsy is
to disintegrate a stone with a mechanical
stress wave. The stress wave was originally produced by
discharging electrical energy into a water bath, and
subsequent focus of the shock wave onto the stone
(*Illustration 1a*). The patient is placed in a water bath.
Two X-ray cameras detect the position of the stone and,
using a computer, the shock wave from the probe is
directed through the water onto the stone. Other
methods of inducing shock waves include rapid changes
of multiple piezoelectric crystals using an electric
current or with an electromagnetic diaphragm. The
newer, second generation machines do not require a
large water bath and the pediatric patient may be
treated under local analgesia instead of general anesthesia because of improved accuracy of focusing of the
waves onto the stone (*Illustration 1b*). In practice,
however, it is difficult to maintain the child in one
position during treatment. The long-term effect of ESWL
on the developing kidney is unknown.

PERCUTANEOUS REMOVAL

2 Percutaneous removal of calculi has yet to find a clearly defined place in pediatric surgery. There is a limited application in (1) debulking large stones before ESWL; (2) surgery on patients with gross spinal deformities where focusing the shock waves onto the stone is difficult; and (3) possible removal of a moderate sized calculus without disintegration and risk of residual fragments. Indications for surgery increase as the child grows and enters adolescence as the main advantages of these non-invasive techniques are to avoid large muscle-cutting incisions.

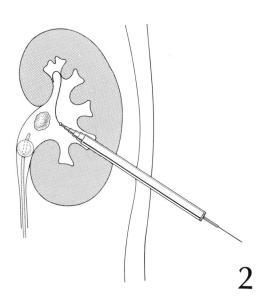

2

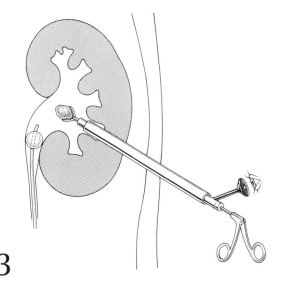

3

3 A nephroscope in a sheath with a stone grasper can be used.

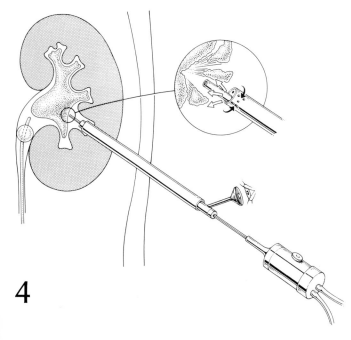

4

4 A staghorn calculus can be disintegrated under direct vision using an ultrasound-guided probe.

Suitable endoscopic equipment for approach to the kidney and ureter in the pediatric population has not yet been fully developed.

OPEN SURGERY

For those centers which do not have this sophisticated equipment the traditional surgical approach to the kidney in children is given.

Preparation of patient

If possible the urine should be rendered sterile before the operation. Whether or not this is successfully achieved, an appropriate antibiotic should be given with the premedication.

Anesthesia

General anesthesia with an endotracheal tube, relaxation, and artificial ventilation are required. Excessive respiratory movement should be avoided to reduce the movement of the kidney and the intrusion of the pleura into the operative field.

Position of patient

The surgeon should personally supervise the positioning of the patient on the operating table.

The patient is placed in a full lateral position with the lower ribs positioned over the table break or adjustable bridge. The degree of break or bridge elevation will vary with the size of the child. In infants and small children a loosely packed sandbag or foam rubber pad may be more suitable. (Note that if a foil diathermy plate is used the sandbag should go beneath it.) A degree of head-down tilt is convenient and aids venous return. The patient is secured to the table with non-elastic zinc oxide strapping passed over the pelvis and secured to the table on either side. Further strapping of the shoulder may be required in older children, whilst in smaller children a foam pad or sandbag under the dependent side of the chest may aid stability. The child should be held firmly with the back vertical while the strapping is applied, following which a little lateral roll of the table towards the surgeon may be helpful.

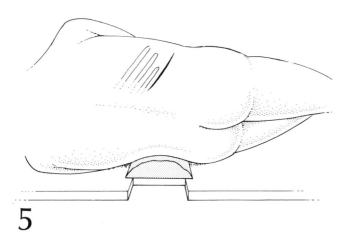

5

Incision

5 A subcostal incision is suitable in most cases. In older children a supracostal approach or an approach via the bed of the 12th rib may give better access. The incision extends forwards from just below the tip of the 12th rib and is continued down to the muscle layer. Bleeding is controlled by diathermy.

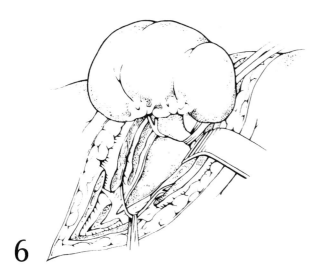

6

Exposure of the kidney

6 The incision is deepened using cutting diathermy, the peritoneum being pushed forwards with the fingers before completing the anterior portion. The subcostal nerve is identified and preserved. Gerota's fascia is incised longitudinally and a finger swept over the kidney surface to free it from surrounding fat. The ureter is identified and secured with a sling. In most children the kidney may now be delivered into the wound and the posterior surface exposed.

Incision into renal pelvis

7 The surface of the pelvis is freed of fatty tissue and the parenchyma retracted. Formal dissection of the renal sinus is not usually required in children. With a large extrarenal pelvis a vertical incision may be employed. If the pelvis is small, an oblique incision extending up towards the infundibulum of the upper calyx gives better access and may be continued into the lower calyx to raise a triangular flap. Stay sutures are applied to the margins of the incision.

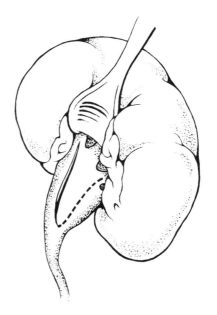

7

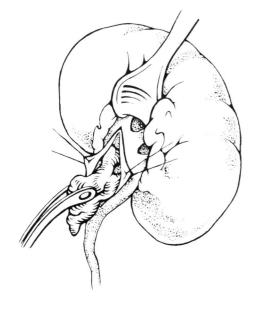

8

Removal of stones

8 A stone in the renal pelvis will now be visible and can be lifted out gently with stone forceps.

Irrigation of pelvicalyceal system

9 Gauze swabs are now placed around the pelvis to catch small stones and debris and to allow suction without fatty tissue occluding the sucker. A soft catheter with an end hole rather than side holes is introduced, and the calyces are irrigated systematically with normal saline. Stones and debris are carefully removed and any lost into the wound must be retrieved to prevent confusion on later radiographs. A radiograph of the exposed kidney is then taken to confirm complete clearance. A marker should be included in the film to assist orientation.

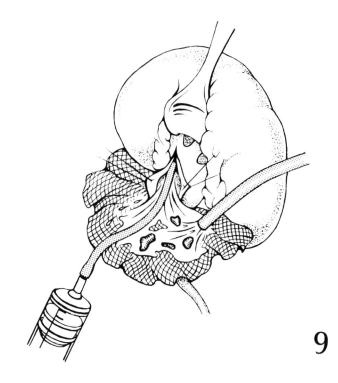

9

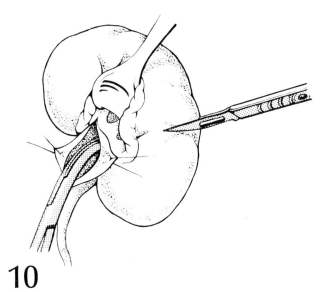

10

Removal of calyceal stones

10 Calyceal stones may be removed via the renal pelvis with curved stone forceps. If a calyceal stone can be identified using the stone forceps or by palpation, a nephrotomy incision directly onto the stone or the tip of the forceps may be simpler, quicker and less traumatic.

Exposure of several calyces

11 Extensive staghorn stones may require the exposure of several calyces. A bulldog clip is applied to the renal artery, or the whole renal pedicle is occluded with a soft intestinal clamp. A longitudinal incision of the posterior surface parallel to the lateral margin of the kidney gives good access. Following removal of the stones the clamps are released intermittently to allow identification and under-running of major vessels. The calyces are approximated with interrupted 3/0 catgut stitches and the kidney parenchyma is apposed with loosely tied horizontal mattress sutures through the capsule. The kidney swells on removal of the clamps, and if these sutures are too tight they will cut out.

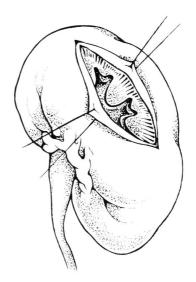

Lower pole calculi

12 The lower branch of the renal artery is readily identifiable and may be occluded with a bulldog clip. Intravenous methylene blue following occlusion may aid demarcation.

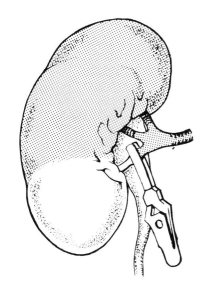

Incision into lower pole

13 Simple incision into the lower pole calyx may then be performed. Lower pole partial nephrectomy is rarely required in children.

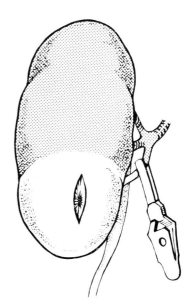

Closure

14 Following radiographic confirmation of complete clearance, the incision in the renal pelvis is closed with interrupted 4/0 catgut sutures. A drain is positioned adjacent to the renal pelvis and Gerota's fascia is reconstructed using 3/0 catgut. The wound is closed in layers with absorbable sutures.

The stones should be sent separately for analysis and culture.

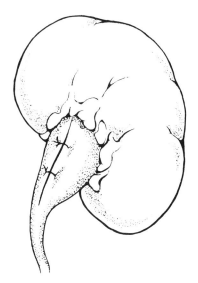

14

Postoperative care

Intravenous fluids are administered for 24 h. If the peritoneal cavity has been opened during the course of the operation fluids may be required for a longer period.

The drain may be removed after 48 h if there is no urine leak, or shortened at 5 days if urine leakage has occurred.

Antibiotics are administered throughout the postoperative period and continued prophylactically if vesicoureteric reflux is present. Where a delayed cystogram is planned reflux must be assumed to be present until the examination has been performed.

Follow-up

Monthly urine cultures should be carried out and a follow-up pyelogram obtained at 6 months. Further plain radiographic films of the urinary tract are taken at 6-monthly intervals for 2 years. Provided the urine remains sterile, recurrences are rare. Further surgery may be required for the correction of vesicoureteric reflux.

Further reading

Smith LH, Segura JW. Urolithiasis. In: Kelakis PP, King LR, Belman B, eds. *Clinical Paediatric Urology.* Vol 2. 3rd edn. Philadelphia: WB Saunders; 1992: 1327–52.

Posterior urethral valve

Ian A. Aaronson MA, FRCS
Professor of Urology and Pediatrics and Director of Pediatric Urology, Medical University of South Carolina, Charleston, South Carolina, USA

Principles and justification

1 A posterior urethral valve is a single structure that takes origin from the inferior margin of the verumontanum. Although its embryology is uncertain, it lies in the position of the infracollicular folds, which can often be discerned in the normal posterior urethra running downwards from the verumontanum towards the bulb on either side of the midline.

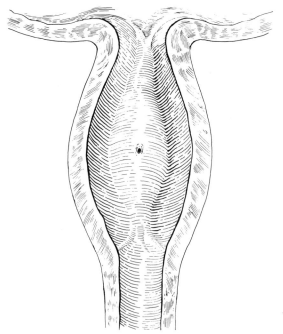

1

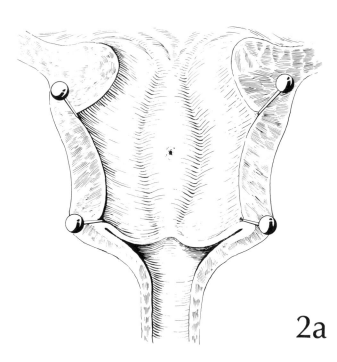

2a

$2a-b$ When exposed at autopsy through the anterior urethral wall, a posterior urethral valve appears as two separate leaflets, but on endoscopy these are seen to fuse anteriorly to form a curtain where most of the obstruction occurs.

Most valves are thin filmy structures that balloon downwards during voiding, but a few are thicker and more rigid, forming a transverse obstruction in the mid posterior urethra. As all true valves originate from the inferior aspect of the verumontanum, Young's classification should be regarded as only of historic interest.

Minor degrees of valve are sometimes encountered, in which the two leaflets blend with the lateral urethral wall. They are more properly regarded as prominent infracollicular folds. It is unlikely that they ever cause symptoms or obstruction, and they do not require treatment.

Above the valve, back pressure effects are nearly always present; these are a widely dilated posterior urethra, a thick-walled and usually trabeculated bladder, widely dilated tortuous ureters and bilateral hydronephrosis which is usually symmetrical. Vesicoureteric reflux is common and often associated with a varying degree of dysplasia of the affected kidney.

The bladder neck is always thickened as part of detrusor hypertrophy, but this hardly ever causes obstruction or requires treatment.

Nowadays, the diagnosis is usually made either before birth as a result of antenatal ultrasonography, or immediately afterwards because of a persistently palpable bladder. Urinary ascites is an occasional presentation in the first weeks of life.

Infants in whom the diagnosis has been missed usually present with urinary infection and acute-on-chronic renal failure. This is generally accompanied by hyperkalemia and a severe metabolic acidosis, which may lead to respiratory arrest. Water and sodium balance are often also profoundly disturbed. Septicemia is common and may be complicated by a consumptive coagulopathy. Older boys may also present with urinary infection, but often the main complaint is of a poor stream with straining or urinary incontinence.

The diagnosis will usually be suspected on clinical grounds and will be supported by the ultrasonographic findings of a widened posterior urethra, distended bladder, and dilated upper urinary tract.

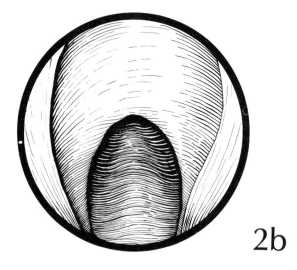

2b

Preoperative

On suspicion of the diagnosis, an 8-Fr plastic infant feeding tube should be passed transurethrally and secured for continuous bladder drainage. Self-retaining catheters should be avoided, as the hypertrophied bladder tends to clamp down around the balloon and obstruct the ureters.

It is essential that the bladder drains well, and failure to do so is usually because the catheter has curled up in the dilated posterior urethra. Withdrawing the catheter for a few centimeters and repassing it with a finger in the rectum will usually ensure its passage through the hypertrophied bladder neck. Persistent difficulty can usually be resolved by injecting a few milliliters of contrast medium through the catheter and manipulating it under fluoroscopic control.

A full blood count including platelets, plasma electrolytes, creatinine and acid–base status should be determined, and severe derangements, particularly hyperkalemia or a severe metabolic acidosis, should be corrected as a matter of urgency. An assessment should also be made of the infant's state of hydration. In difficult cases the aid of a pediatric nephrologist should be sought.

When the urine appears to be infected, both a blood sample and a urine sample should be sent for culture, following which ampicillin and an aminoglycoside or a third-generation cephalosporin should be started intravenously. When septicemia is suspected, blood coagulation studies should also be carried out.

All infants with any respiratory distress should undergo chest radiography to exclude a pneumothorax secondary to pulmonary hypoplasia.

In most cases the above actions will result in a rapid improvement in the infant's metabolic state and general condition. Those infants who remain in a toxic state or whose plasma creatinine does not begin to fall within 24 h, despite correction of other metabolic abnormalities, should be considered for percutaneous drainage of both kidneys.

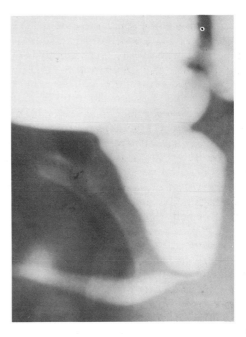

3a

3a, b The presence of a posterior urethral valve should be confirmed by micturating cystourethrography, but this should be delayed until urinary infection has been brought completely under control and metabolic disturbances have been corrected.

A voiding film taken in the steep oblique projection during full micturition is necessary to demonstrate the valve, which appears like a spinnaker sail billowing out before the stream. Distal to this a thin stream will be seen emerging from the posterior margin of the obstruction (*Illustration 3a*). Dilatation of the urethra proximal to the valve is essential to the diagnosis, and signs of bladder wall hypertrophy are usually also present. A very lax valve may occasionally prolapse down as far as the bulbar urethra (*Illustration 3b*). Here the posterior run-off may not be readily apparent, but the filling defect caused by the valve leaflets can usually be made out running down from the verumontanum.

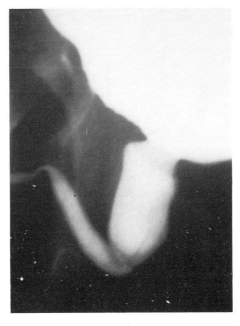

3b

4a–h

A variety of other conditions may masquerade as a posterior urethral valve on the cystogram, and failure to recognize them often leads to inappropriate treatment. Among these are prominent infracollicular folds, which can sometimes be made out on a good quality study in normal children (*Illustration 4a*).

Hesitant voiding in a normal baby may cause an abrupt change in caliber of the posterior urethra, while extrinsic compression by the pelvic floor may cause one or more concentric indentations in the urethral contour (*Illustration 4b*). Neither of these is associated with evidence of obstruction above the lesion, however, and both should be regarded as normal variants.

A neuropathic bladder may closely simulate a posterior urethral valve (*Illustration 4c*), but the thin stream below the obstruction will be seen emerging from the center of the external urethral sphincter rather than from the posterior margin as seen with a valve. In such cases, the spine should be carefully examined and other evidence sought of a neurologic deficit in the perineum or lower limbs.

A posterior urethral stricture may cause a similar appearance (*Illustration 4d*), but this will invariably be associated with a history of urethral or pelvic trauma.

The prune-belly syndrome may closely mimic a posterior urethral valve (*Illustration 4e*) but the correct diagnosis should be suspected from the appearance of the bladder, which lies horizontally and is invariably smooth walled, and the dog-leg configuration of the posterior urethra, which often bears a utriculus masculinus.

A distended, non-visualized ectopic ureter opening into the ejaculatory duct may distort and partially obstruct the posterior urethra and thus simulate a valve (*Illustration 4f*), while dilatation of the posterior urethra may also be caused by a prolapsed ectopic ureterocele (*Illustration 4g*) or posterior urethral polyp (*Illustration 4h*). Careful examination of these films, however, will usually reveal a filling defect, leading to the correct diagnosis.

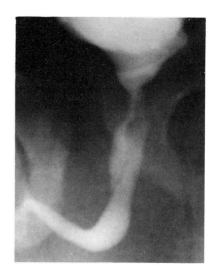

4a

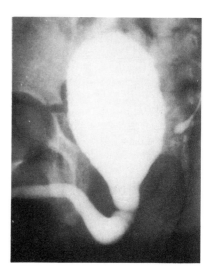

4b

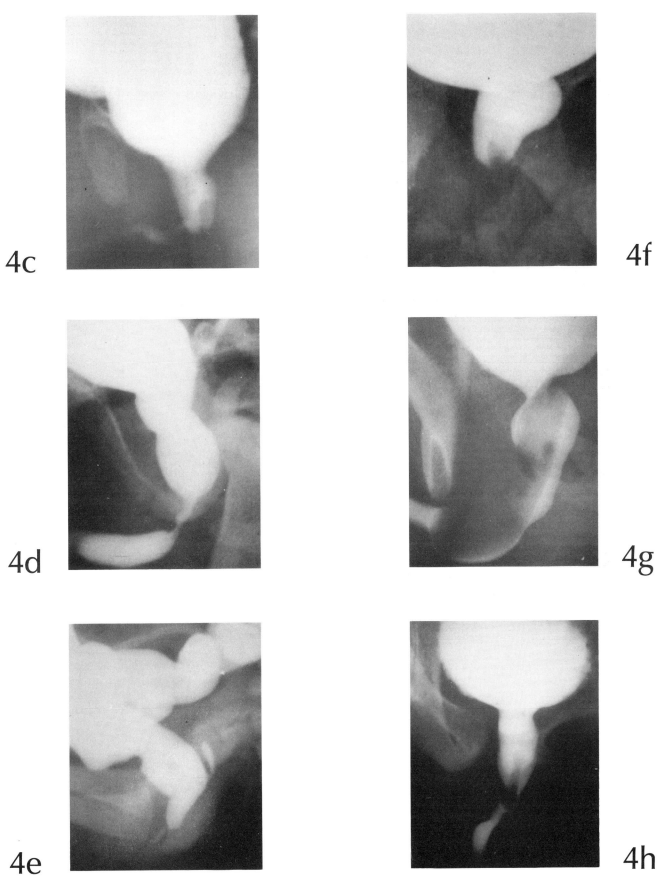

4c

4d

4e

4f

4g

4h

Operation

RESECTION IN FULL-TERM INFANTS AND CHILDREN

Under endotracheal anesthesia, the intubated infant is placed supine with the buttocks brought well down to the end of the operating table. The legs should be well protected with cotton wool and fixed with crepe bandages, either to pediatric stirrups or in the frog-leg position, taking care to provide ample support to the thighs. The skin is prepared and drapes applied, taking care to exclude the anus from the operative field. Fixing the posterior towel to the perineal skin with three staples or 4/0 nylon sutures will ensure that the anus does not become exposed during subsequent manipulations.

The calibre of the penile urethra should first be checked with a well-lubricated 10-Fr sound, which should be introduced only for 1–2 cm. If necessary, a meatotomy can be performed, but no attempt should be made to dilate the urethra. The diagnosis is then confirmed using a well-lubricated 9.5-Fr or 10-Fr cystoscope introduced under vision.

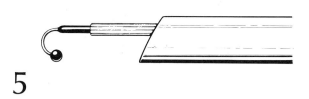

5

5 Resection of the valve is undertaken using a 10-Fr Storz resectoscope fitted with a hooked ball electrode.

The instrument is first assembled and the alignment of the working parts checked using the 0° telescope. The sheath is then dried and thoroughly coated with a water-soluble lubricant, and with its introducer in place is gently inserted through the meatus. The introducer is removed and the instrument reassembled and gently advanced under vision towards the bladder neck. It is often necessary to angle the eyepiece end of the instrument downwards to allow the beak to move anteriorly to pass through the bladder neck. Once in the bladder, the shape and position of the ureteric orifices are noted and the presence of any periureteric diverticulum recorded.

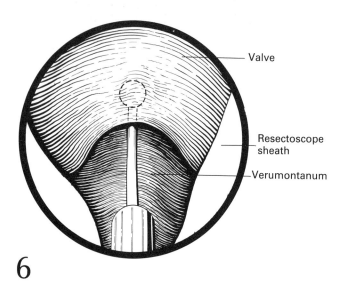

Valve

Resectoscope sheath

Verumontanum

6

6 The instrument is now rotated through 180°, and with the irrigation fluid flowing in under low pressure, it is progressively withdrawn. Once through the bladder neck, the ball is run down along the anterior wall of the posterior urethra until, just beyond the verumontanum, the valve will suddenly snap across the anterior portion of the field of view like a curtain. Further withdrawal of the instrument and manipulation of the trigger will cause the ball to engage the valve in the 12 o'clock position. A short burst of cutting current is then applied.

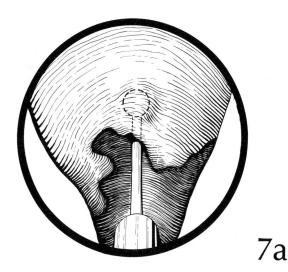

7a

7a, b The instrument is returned to the normal position and advanced under vision back into the bladder. It is again rotated 180° and withdrawn into the posterior urethra to engage the now partially disrupted valve in the 12 o'clock position, where it is further disrupted. This maneuver should be repeated until it is certain that the anterior portion of the valve has been completely ablated.

The instrument is again returned to the bladder and is rotated to engage residual valve tissue in the 10 o'clock, 2 o'clock, 8 o'clock and finally the 4 o'clock positions. Any remaining freely floating tags do not require treatment.

The resectoscope is removed and the presence of an unobstructed urethra confirmed by manual expression of the bladder. Finally, an 8-Fr feeding tube is passed, placing a double-gloved finger in the rectum if necessary to ensure that it is not curled up in the dilated posterior urethra. This is retained in place with a 4/0 nylon suture passed through the prepuce or glans and connected to a sealed drainage bag. The tube is removed after 48 h.

If any significant bleeding occurs, attempts at valve ablation should be immediately discontinued and the situation reassessed after 2–3 days of catheter drainage.

In older children a 13-Fr resectoscope may be used, employing a similar technique.

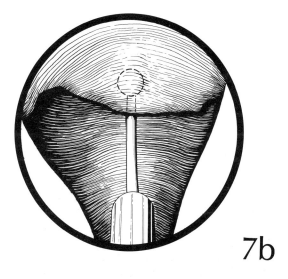

7b

RESECTION IN PRETERM INFANTS

It is inadvisable to attempt to pass a 10-Fr resectoscope in infants weighing less than 2.5 kg. For those weighing between 2.0 and 2.5 kg a few days of bladder drainage with an 8-Fr catheter will often have the effect of gently dilating the urethra so that the 10-Fr resectoscope can be safely used. Alternatively, the newly available 8-Fr operating cystoscope (Storz) may be employed. A 3-Fr ureteric catheter with its tip cut off is introduced through the working channel and the exposed end of a metal stylet used to coagulate the valve in a circumferential fashion.

Other techniques are also available for resecting the valve in a very small infant but all have some disadvantages. The Whitaker hook electrode is a slender, well insulated metal instrument that can be introduced through the urethra under fluoroscopic control and withdrawn to engage the valve. Short bursts of cutting current may relieve the obstruction, but the procedure is essentially blind and carries the risk of urethral trauma.

A Fogarty catheter can be passed into the bladder where the balloon is inflated with 0.1–0.3 ml of water. It is then withdrawn until the balloon is felt to engage the valve. Disruption may be achieved by a further short sharp pull on the catheter. If undue resistance is encountered, however, the procedure should be abandoned to avoid possible avulsion of the urethra.

Access to the valve with an 8-Fr or 10-Fr resectoscope sheath can usually be achieved via a perineal urethrotomy. The small caliber of the urethra and the friable nature of the urothelium, however, render the operation difficult in the neonate and may be complicated by bleeding, a persistent urinary fistula, urethral diverticulum or stricture.

An alternative approach is to create a suprapubic cystotomy through which the valve can be resected in an antegrade fashion. Using a 10-Fr sheath and the hooked ball electrode, the valve is first engaged in the 12 o'clock position and coagulated. However, the hypertrophied bladder neck sometimes closes across the telescope lens so that the procedure has to be carried out blindly.

VESICOSTOMY

In very small infants it is the author's preference to carry out a vesicostomy rather than attempt to disrupt the valve by the above methods. A few months later, when the infant has reached an adequate size, the valve is coagulated through the urethra using the hooked ball electrode in the standard fashion. The vesicostomy is closed at the same visit, and the urethral catheter removed 1 week later.

UPPER TRACT DRAINAGE

Following relief of the urethral obstruction, correction of metabolic derangements and eradication of infection, the plasma creatinine will in most cases rapidly fall to within the normal range for the patient's age. When it remains elevated, the possibility of obstruction of the dilated flaccid ureters as they pass through the hypertrophied bladder wall must be considered. In most cases this phenomenon is transient and, provided that the infant remains well and the plasma creatinine is showing some improvement, an expectant policy may be adopted.

When the plasma creatinine shows no sign of falling in spite of adequate bladder emptying, a percutaneous nephrostomy should be carried out and a Whitaker test performed. If obstruction is confirmed, Sober Y cutaneous ureterostomies should be undertaken. Alternatively, the ureters may be remodeled and reimplanted, but this operation is rendered difficult by the thickness of the bladder wall and trabeculation, and in inexperienced hands complications are common.

A persistently raised plasma creatinine level in infants with gross bilateral vesicoureteric reflux is usually caused by severe renal dysplasia.

Postoperative care

Following removal of the urethral catheter, adequate emptying of the bladder should be confirmed clinically or by ultrasonography. Postoperative antibiotic prophylaxis, usually with trimethoprim-sulphamethoxozole, is continued for 1 month to guard against infection in the healing posterior urethra. In infants in whom cystography reveals the presence of vesicoureteric reflux this should be continued for 6 months. Sodium bicarbonate supplements are also often necessary to correct a persistent metabolic acidosis, and these may need to be given for 1 year or more. Polyuria is also common, and the parents should be advised to give supplementary clear feeds early in the event of a diarrheal illness.

At 3 months the glomerular filtration rate of each kidney is measured by the slope clearance method using ^{99m}Tc-DTPA (diethylenetriaminepenta-acetate), and intravenous urography is carried out. Both of these will serve as a baseline for any future studies. A blood sample is also taken to check the plasma creatinine, electrolytes, and acid–base status.

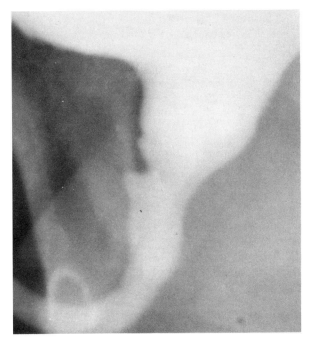

8

8 At 6 months, micturating cystourethrography is repeated to confirm adequate resection of the valve and the absence of any stricture of the urethra, and to determine whether any previously noted vesicoureteric reflux is still present. In about one-third of cases it will be found to have disappeared. When reflux is persistent and unilateral, renal scanning using ^{99m}Tc-DMSA (dimercaptosuccinic acid) is carried out to determine the contribution of the kidney on the refluxing side to total renal function. When this is negligible, nephroureterectomy should be carried out through two incisions to ensure safe ligation of the ureteric stump.

All infants and those older children with impaired renal function at presentation will require close supervision until adult life is reached. A progressive rise in plasma creatinine is often seen during childhood, and in the most severe cases renal transplantation may be required before puberty. Persistent urinary incontinence is an indication for cystometrography. Bladders showing severe hyperreflexia or very poor compliance generally require augmentation, which should be carried out before transplantation.

Further reading

Aaronson IA. Posterior urethral valve: a review of 120 cases. *S Afr Med J* 1984; 65: 418–22.

Crombleholme TM, Harrison MR, Langer JC et al. Early experience with open fetal surgery for congenital hydronephrosis. *J Pediatr Surg* 1988; 23: 1114–21.

Kaneti J, Sober I. Pelvi-uretero-cutaneostomy en-Y as a temporary diversion in children. Soroka experience. *Int Urol Nephrol* 1988; 20: 471–4.

Parkhouse HF, Barratt TM, Dillon MJ et al. Long term outcome of boys with posterior urethral valves. *Br J Urol* 1988; 62: 59–62.

Hypospadias repair

John W. Duckett MD
Professor of Urology, School of Medicine, University of Pennsylvania, Children's Hospital of Philadelphia, Philadelphia, USA

The surgeon dealing with hypospadias must be equipped with a variety of techniques, knowledge of past variations, experience with delicate, precise, optically enhanced surgical technique, and be fully aware of the pitfalls in order to avoid them.

Incidence and classification

1 One in 300 boys has hypospadias; 8% of their fathers will also have hypospadias while 14% of male siblings are affected. Apart from undescended testes (9%) and inguinal hydroceles and hernias (9%), the incidence of other anomalies is not significant in isolated hypospadias. When other systems are involved, evaluation of the upper tracts and bladder is indicated. Utricles are present in perineal and penoscrotal varieties (15%).

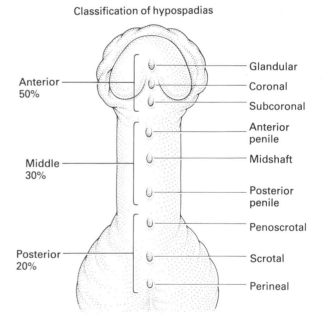

Classification of hypospadias

Anterior 50%
Glandular
Coronal
Subcoronal
Anterior penile
Middle 30%
Midshaft
Posterior penile
Penoscrotal
Posterior 20%
Scrotal
Perineal

1

Preoperative

The best age for surgery is between 6 and 18 months. The infants are amnesic of the procedure and management in a diaper is less stressful for the parents and permits outpatient surgery.

Ophthalmic instruments are necessary, including Castroviejo forceps and needle holders and iris scissors. Optical magnification is essential, although low magnification will suffice ($\times 1$–2); some prefer to use an operating microscope.

Epinephrine (adrenaline) (1:100 000) in 1% lidocaine (lignocaine) helps to reduce operative and postoperative bleeding. A tourniquet is optional but should be released every 20 min. Hemostasis with cauterization needs to be more aggressive if a tourniquet alone is used. A compressive dressing is required for the first few hours after surgery to avoid hematoma and edema formation. This should be easily removed at home by the parents in 48 h. The author prefers to compress the penis on the lower abdomen with gauze and a bio-occlusive dressing. Urinary diversion is accomplished with a 6-Fr Silastic stent placed into the bladder and sutured to the glans. This drips into the diaper at a continuous rate and is removed in 7–10 days. Oxybutynin or suppositories containing methanthelinium bromide and opium are prescribed for bladder spasms.

Operations

MAGPI (MEATAL ADVANCEMENT AND GLANULOPLASTY)[1]

The majority of cases are caused by inadequate canalization of the glans urethra. This leaves the meatus at the subcoronal area, frequently stenotic, with a dorsal lip which deflects the urinary stream downwards at 30–45°. The bridge of tissue distal to the meatus in the glanular groove needs to be wedged out. The dorsal meatal edge can be advanced up to the end of the urethral groove with fine sutures (meatoplasty).

2a–j

The glanuloplasty is accomplished by elevating the ventral edge of the urethral meatus forwards and rotating the flattened glanular wings around to the ventrum in a conical shape. Excess skin on the ventral V is excised in order to bring together the glanular wings. It is important to reapproximate glans tissue in a two-layer fashion with a deep closure of glans mesenchyme and a superficial layer of glans epithelium. This exaggerated rotation of glans tissue on the ventrum prevents the meatus from regressing back to the subcoronal area.

Several modifications of this technique have been described[2–7].

Complications

A secondary operation is required in 1% of cases; meatal regression is the most common complaint; fistulas should not occur.

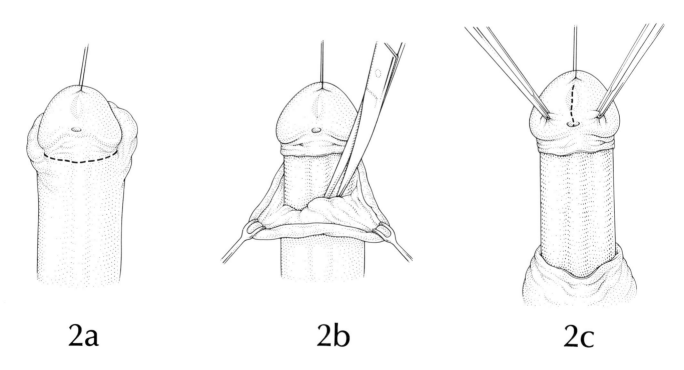

2a   2b   2c

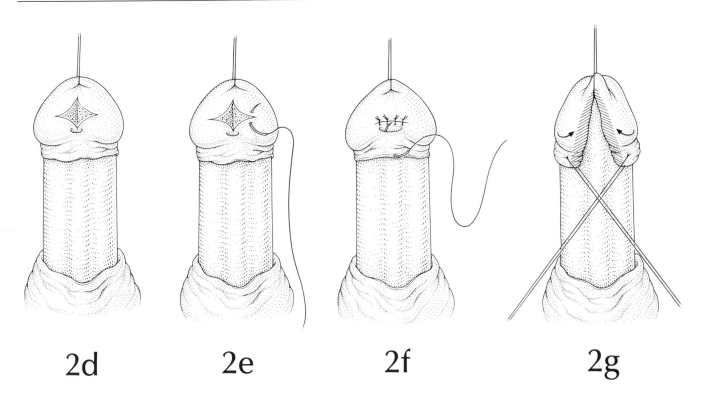

2d   2e   2f   2g

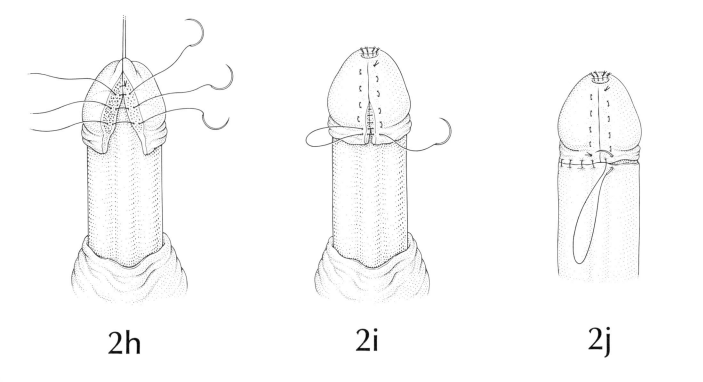

2h   2i   2j

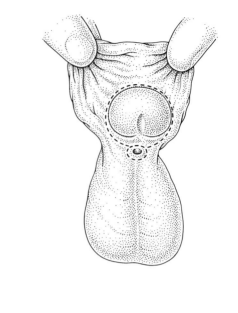

3a

TRANSVERSE PREPUTIAL ISLAND FLAP[8]

3a–i The curvature must be released, leaving a gap between the proximal meatus (peno-scrotal or perineal) and the tip of the glans. A full tubed urethra may be formed from the transverse preputial island flap, dissected from the undersurface of the two layers of dorsal prepuce. Holding sutures are placed in a rectangular fashion on the undersurface of the prepuce, measuring to make the width 12–15 mm. The length, however, must suffice to bridge the gap and can always be obtained by going down onto the penile skin in a horseshoe fashion on either side. The inner shiny skin with its blood supply is dissected free of the outer prepuce and penile skin by taking the axially orientated subcutaneous tissue free from the outer skin. The plane usually dissects very neatly and the vasculature is obvious in the pedicle (*Illustrations 3a–d*).

The pedicle is rotated in order to bring the rectangle of skin to the ventrum. This is tubularized over an 8-Fr catheter as a template and after careful suturing should calibrate at 12 Fr with a bougie à boule (*Illustrations 3e, f*).

A proximal oblique anastomosis is made to the native urethra after all the skin has been removed from the urethral meatus. The dorsal edge is fixed to the tunica albuginea (*Illustration 3g*).

The glans is channeled, staying close to the tunica albuginea of the corpora cavernosa. A tip of glans epithelium is excised; glanular tissue must be removed in order to make an adequate glans channel (18–20 Fr). Splitting the glans may be appropriate in certain cases, with approximation around the neourethra (*Illustrations 3h, i*).

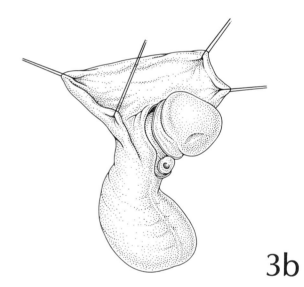

3b

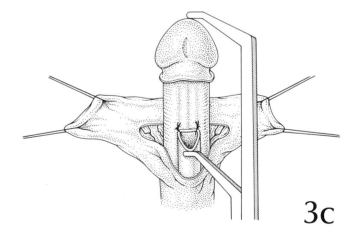

3c

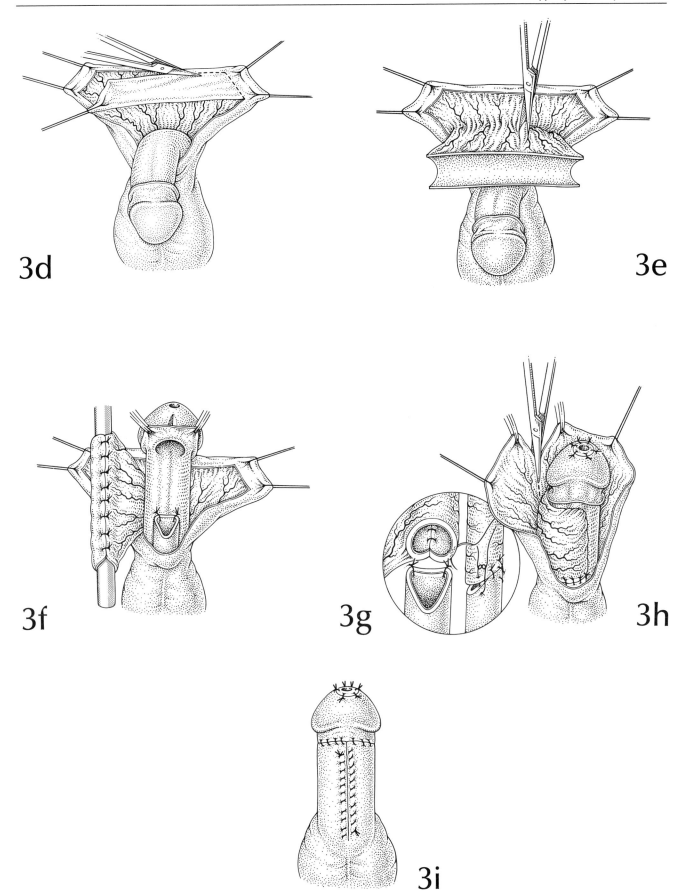

3d

3e

3f

3g

3h

3i

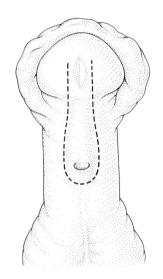

4a

ONLAY ISLAND FLAP[9]

4a–f For the mid-shaft meatus without curvature, the urethral plate may be preserved with a parallel incision into the glans similar to that in the Mathieu procedure[7]. Straightness is checked by means of an artificial erection. Ventral urethral construction is effected using a transverse preputial onlay flap, which is sized after one edge has been sutured to the urethral plate, taking care to avoid redundancy that could lead to a diverticulum or ballooning of the neourethra.

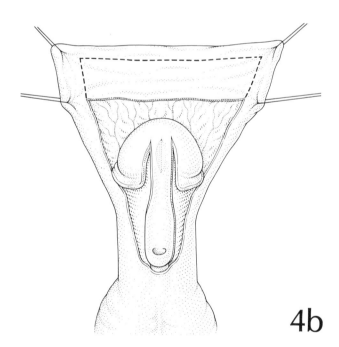

4b

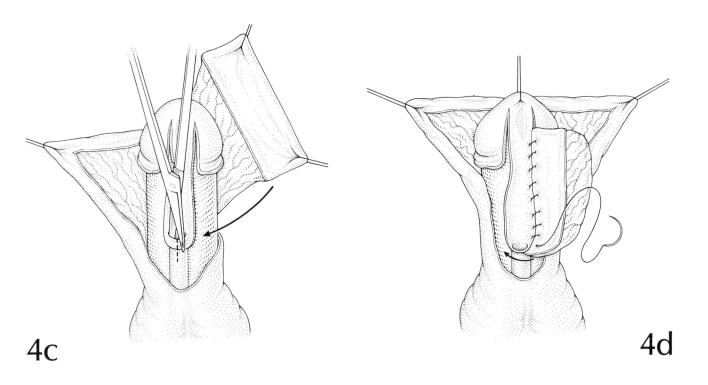

4c

4d

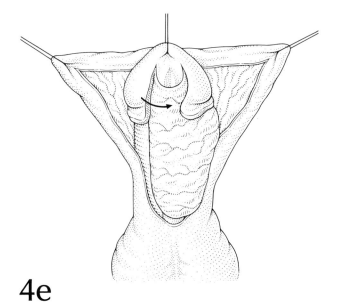

4e

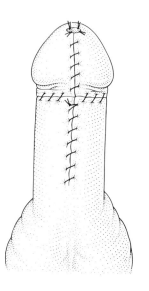

4f

BLADDER/BUCCAL MUCOSA[10]

5a–k In repeat operations it may be necessary to excise the previous urethroplasty and to replace it with new epithelium. A free graft of bladder mucosa or buccal mucosa, depending on the length of the urethra to be replaced, has been the most successful modern urethroplasty.

As the graft must be revascularized, perfect cover of viable tissue must be assured and drained appropriately so that no hematoma occurs.

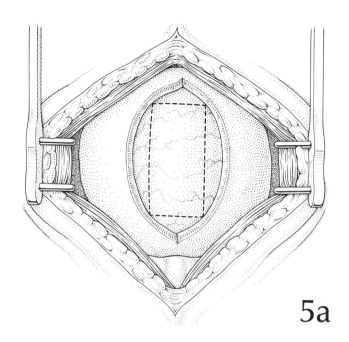

5a

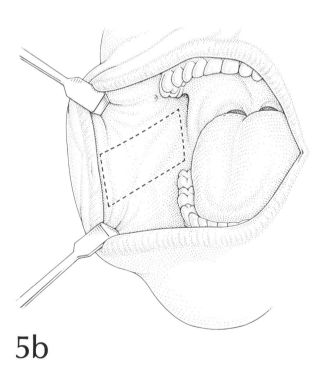

5b

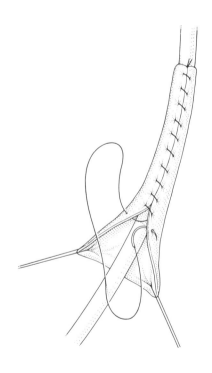

5c

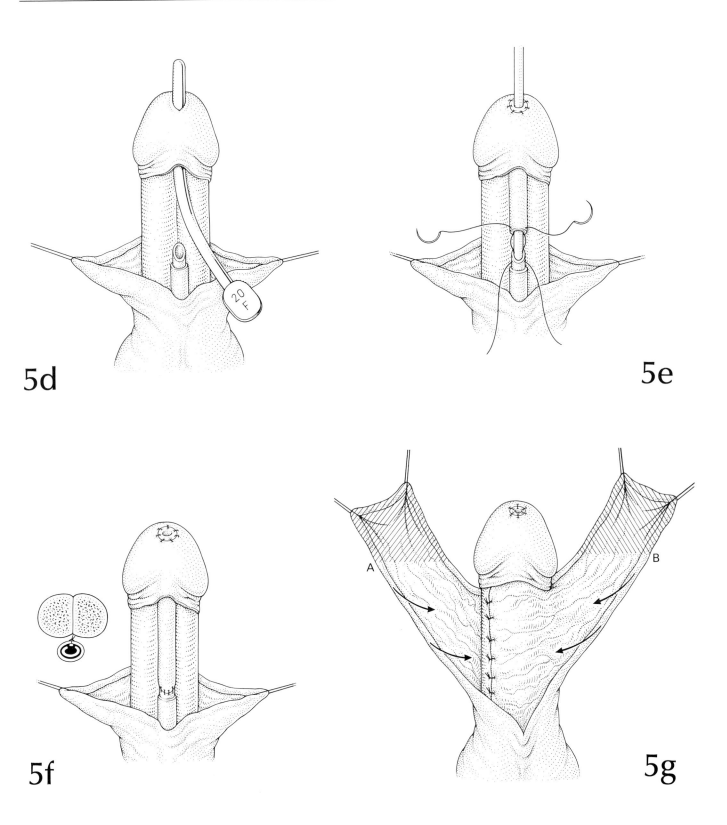

5d

5e

5f

5g

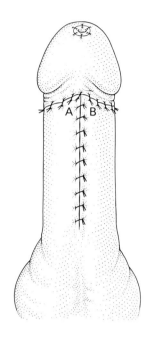

5h

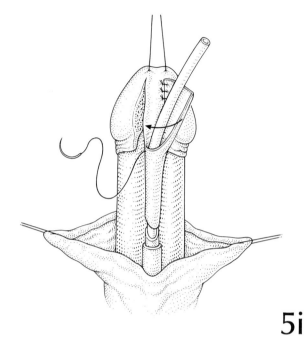

5i

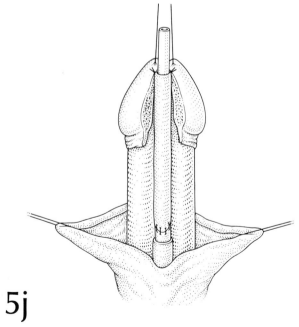

5j

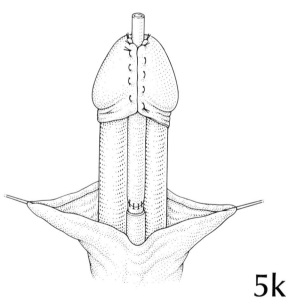

5k

ADJUNCT PROCEDURES

Orthoplasty

6 Straightening of curvature may require several maneuvers. In many cases the urethral plate may be left intact while skin takedown proceeds and straightness is assessed by artificial erection; frequently only minimal curvature will remain. The next step is to resect all fibrous tissue on the ventrum if it is tethering the penis ventrally.

Imbrication of the dorsal tunica albuginea may be performed to straighten the penis. Two parallel incisions are made at 10 and 2 o'clock on the dorsal lateral aspects away from the neurovascular bundles in Buck's fascia at the apex of maximal bend. The outer edges of these two parallel incisions are sutured together with a permanent suture, burying the mid portion underneath ('dorsal tucks'). These knots are buried beneath Buck's fascia.

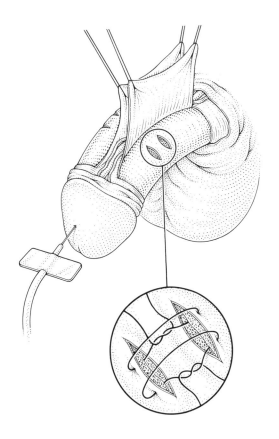

6

Skin cover

In all cases of hypospadias, the skin of the shaft of the penis is dissected to the penoscrotal junction or below. In the MAGPI procedure it is often possible to reapproximate the cylinder of penile skin back to the glans, in a manner similar to a circumcision, excising the redundant dorsal prepuce. It may be necessary to rotate the median raphe back to its ventral position in certain cases with torsion.

Alternatively, the dorsal preputial skin may be split down the midline permitting rotational flaps to be fashioned around each side, brought together in the midline in the ventrum and sutured up to the corona. The excess skin is excised obliquely.

Complications

Secondary surgery is required most commonly for fistulas. There should be a minimum interval of 6 months before closure is attempted. This can be done with a delicate excision of the epithelialized fistulous tract and reapproximation of the urethra and skin in two or three layers with fine sutures. No catheter is necessary. Stricture is the next most common complication and results from poor vascularization or, more commonly, overlap of the two suture lines with a kink. These require open revision. Internal optical urethrotomy is not very successful. Residual chordee may be corrected with dorsal tucks. Meatal stenosis may be revised with a meatoplasty. Urethral diverticula occur when urine leaks at the anastomosis, creating an epithelialized pocket which can be quite large. Tapering of the urethra may be required.

Outcome

The author favours the use of vascularized tissue. Free grafts of penile or preputial skin may do well for the early years but complications develop as the penis grows at puberty. It seems more logical to use vascularized skin, if possible, rather than to use the same skin as a graft. The buccal/bladder mucosal graft seems to be a better urethral substitute but long-term results are not yet available[11]. With delicate tissue handling, good plastic surgical principles and attention to the many details, a secondary surgery rate of less than 5% should be necessary in these patients.

References

1. Duckett JW. MAGPI (meatoplasty and glanuloplasty): a procedure for subcoronal hypospadias. *Urol Clin North Am.* 1981; 8: 513–19.

2. Arap S, Mitre AI, DeGoes GM. Modified meatal advancement and glanuloplasty repair of distal hypospadias. *J Urol* 1984; 131: 1140–1.

3. Firlit CF. The mucosal collar in hypospadias surgery. *J Urol* 1987; 137: 80–2.

4. King LR. One stage repair without skin graft based on a new principle: chordee is sometimes produced by skin alone. *J Urol* 1970; 103: 660–2.

5. Zaontz MR. The GAP (glans approximation procedure) for glanular/coronal hypospadias. *J Urol* 1989; 141: 359–61.

6. Duckett JW, Keating MA. Technical challenge of the megameatus intact prepuce hypospadias (MIP) variant: the pyramid procedure. *J Urol* 1989; 141: 1407–9.

7. Mathieu P. Traitement en un temps de l'hypospadias balanique et juxta-balanique. *J Chir (Paris)* 1932; 39: 481–4.

8. Duckett JW. Hypospadias repair. In: Frank JD, Johnston JH, eds. *Operative Paediatric Urology,* London: Churchill Livingstone, 1990: 203.

9. Duckett JW. Hypospadias. In: Gillenwater JY, Grayhack JT, Howards SS, Duckett JW, eds. *Adult and Pediatric Urology,* Vol 2. Chicago: Year Book Medical Publishers, 1991: 2125.

10. Keating MA, Duckett JW, Cartwright PC. Bladder mucosa in urethral reconstructions. *J Urol* 1990; 144: 827–34.

11. Duckett JW. Editorial comment. Dessanti A *et al.* Autologous buccal mucosa graft for hypospadias repair: an initial report. *J Urol* 1992; 147: 1081–4.

Further reading

Baskin LS, Duckett JW, Ueoka K, Seibald J, Snyder HM. Changing concepts of hypospadias curvature leads to more onlay island flap procedures. *J Urol* 1994; 151: 191–6.

Kinkead TM, Borzi PD, Duffy PG, Ransley PG. Long term follow up of bladder muscosa graft for male urethral reconstruction. *J Urol* 1994; 151: 1056–8.

Orchidopexy

John M. Hutson MD, FRACS

Professor of Paediatric Surgery, Department of Paediatrics, University of Melbourne and Director, Department of General Surgery, Royal Children's Hospital, Melbourne, Victoria, Australia

Principles and justification

Undescended testis is a common abnormality affecting 4–5% of male infants at birth. In preterm infants the incidence may be as high as 20% or more. A significant number of testes not in the scrotum at birth descend in the first 12 weeks after birth so that by 3 months of age the incidence of congenital undescended testes is approximately 1–2%. Some of those testes that descend late into the scrotum may reascend later in childhood, producing an acquired variant of undescended testes known as ascending testes.

Embryology

The urogenital ridge forms on the posterior abdominal wall and contains the mesonephros and its draining duct and the developing gonads. The primitive germ cells migrate from the yolk sac at about the sixth week of gestation, as the gonad in the male develops into a testis. By 7–8 weeks the testis is producing hormones that control its subsequent descent.

Descent of the testis

Descent of the testis occurs in two morphologically and hormonally distinct phases. The key structure in controlling the process is the gubernaculum, which is the embryonic ligament anchoring the testis and urogenital ridge to the inguinal region. The gubernaculum enlarges in the first phase to anchor the testis near the inguinal region as the embryo enlarges. This occurs between 10 and 15 weeks of gestation. In the second phase, which occurs between 28 and 35 weeks of gestation, the gubernaculum migrates out of the inguinal canal, across the pubic region and into the scrotum. The processus vaginalis develops as a peritoneal diverticulum within the elongating gubernaculum, creating an intraperitoneal space into which the testis can descend.

The hormone controlling the first phase of testicular descent is controversial, with conflicting evidence about whether müllerian inhibiting substance (MIS) is the active factor. In the second phase, testosterone acts apparently indirectly via the nervous system and the genitofemoral nerve which supplies the gubernaculum and scrotum. Calcitonin gene-related peptide (CGRP) has been identified recently within the genitofemoral nerve and has been postulated to act as a final common pathway for androgenic control of descent. Androgens probably cause masculinization of the genitofemoral nerve in the spinal cord between 15 and 25 weeks of gestation, and the masculinized nerve then controls the direction of gubernacular migration by the release of CGRP in the periphery.

Animal models of undescended testes, including the androgen-resistant mouse, the flutamide-treated rat, and the mutant TS rat, all show an absence or deficiency of gubernacular migration and an abnormality of CGRP physiology. This suggests that undescended testes in humans may be caused by physiologic or anatomic abnormalities of the genitofemoral nerve or its neuro-transmitter, CGRP. The most common cause of maldescent appears to be failure of gubernacular migration, leaving the testes in the groin or so-called 'superficial inguinal pouch'. Whether genitofemoral nerve anomalies are primarily anatomic or secondary to abnormal hormone development in mid-trimester is uncertain. In rare instances, undescended testes are caused by recognized anomalies in the hypothalamic–pituitary–gonadal axis or in the secretion or action of MIS. Recognizable hormonal syndromes, however, are rare causes of undescended testes in clinical practice.

Undescended testes

Congenital failure of gubernacular development or migration leads to arrest of gubernacular migration along the normal pathway or aberrant migration leading to an ectopic undescended testis in the perineal, prepubic or femoral regions. Many undescended testes are located in the superficial inguinal pouch, which is a subcutaneous space just above and lateral to the external inguinal ring and is just the processus vaginalis (with its contained testis) lying at the external ring or a little lateral to it. As this is the most common position for an undescended testis to occupy, it is not categorized as ectopic.

There is controversy about whether retractile testes are abnormal. These testes are located in the scrotum in infancy, but later in childhood tend to retract back out of the scrotum and often have an exaggerated cremaster reflex. It may produce an acquired variant of maldescent with the position of the testis becoming higher as the child gets older. Surgical intervention is not indicated unless the testis is no longer residing spontaneously in the scrotum. If the testis is near the top of the scrotum, regular follow-up is required to make sure that it does not ascend out of the scrotum with the passage of time.

A third variant of undescended testis is the ascending testis. This testis is commonly undescended on the day of delivery but reaches the scrotum within 12 weeks after birth. It may ascend back out of the scrotum later in childhood, probably because the spermatic cord is not elongating in proportion with the growth of the boy. It is controversial whether surgery is required, but many surgeons will elect to operate on such testes once they no longer reside within the scrotum. This often leads to orchidopexy being recommended in 8–11-year-old boys

Indications

Children are recommended for surgery for three common reasons: abnormal fertility in the undescended testis, a risk of testicular tumors in adult life, and the obvious cosmetic abnormalities. Although many undescended testes have an associated patent processus vaginalis, this is an uncommon presentation for an inguinal hernia. If an infant presents with an inguinal hernia in association with undescended testis, however, orchidopexy with associated herniotomy is performed immediately. Trauma and torsion to the undescended testis are alleged to be more common than when the testis is fully descended, although these are unlikely indications for surgery.

Germ cell development in the undescended testis is normal in the first 6–12 months, but then becomes abnormal subsequently due to secondary degeneration. This is caused by the undescended testes residing at a higher temperature (35–37°C) than when located in the scrotum (33°C).

The risk of malignancy in young adult men with undescended testes is approximately 5–10-fold that of the normally descended testis. These risk calculations are not based on current practice, however, but on results from children of a previous generation having orchidopexy at approximately 10 years of age. With the current practice of recommending surgery at a much younger age, it is hoped that the risk of cancer in the next generation will be lower, although this has not yet been proved. The risk of malignancy affects not only the unilateral undescended testis but also the contralateral descended testis in some patients.

Recommended age for orchidopexy

To prevent secondary degeneration of the testis with loss of germ cells and a progressively increasing risk of malignancy, orchidopexy is best performed in infancy. Although it is not proved conclusively for humans, it is clear in animal experiments that early surgery is better than a delayed operation. Operation can be performed at any time between 6 months and 2 years of age, depending on the experience of the surgeon. Those with less experience in pediatric surgery would be wise to delay surgery to the older end of this range, rather than to attempt orchidopexy in a young infant. For the inexperienced surgeon the risk of testicular atrophy secondary to surgery may be higher in younger infants.

Preoperative

Secondary preoperative preparation

In older boys with possible retractile testes, a course of gonadotrophins may be appropriate although this is controversial. In the rare circumstance of bilateral impalpable testes, a human chorionic gonadotrophin (hCG) stimulation test should be performed to determine whether testicular tissue is present at all. If the hCG stimulation test shows the presence of testicular tissue within the abdomen, the parents should be advised that laparoscopy is indicated at the beginning of the operation to determine the exact site and nature of the intra-abdominal testes.

Anesthesia

As orchidopexy is now a day-case procedure the type of anesthesia reflects the need for early mobilization. No premedication is usually required, although oral preparations such as chloral hydrate would be preferable to intramuscular injections. On admission to the day surgical unit, anesthetic cream containing lidocaine (lignocaine) and prilocaine is applied to the back of the hand so that intravenous access can be obtained without pain. An ilioinguinal nerve block, local anesthesia, or caudal anesthesia is provided to control pain for the first 4–6 h after operation.

Skin preparation and position of patient

The patient is placed supine on the operating table with the legs slightly apart. Povidone-iodine, or other appropriate antiseptic, is painted on the skin from the umbilicus to below the scrotum and perineum.

Operation

Standard orchidopexy for a palpable testis (which occurs in approximately 80–90% of cases) involves an inguinal incision, full exposure of the inguinal canal, separation of the processus vaginalis and mobilization of the testis and spermatic cord. The second part of the operation is the orchidopexy itself, or fixation of the testis in the scrotum.

Mobilization of the testis

1 A transverse skin crease incision is made over the inguinal canal. This incision is usually about one finger's breadth above the base of the penis in an infant. The medial end of the incision is level with the pubic tubercle, while the lateral end is at the mid-inguinal point.

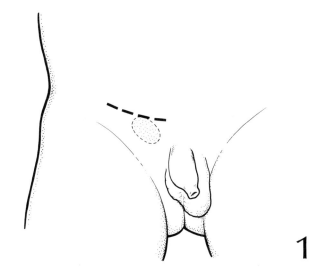

1

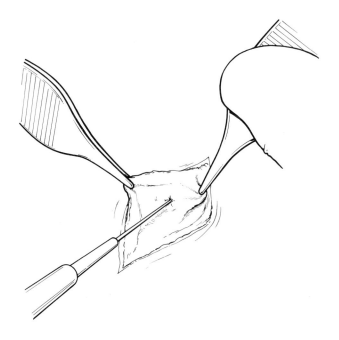

2

2 The incision is deepened through the subcutaneous fatty tissue with scissors or diathermy. The superficial fascia is in two layers: a more superficial fatty layer and a deeper, well developed fibrous layer known as Scarpa's fascia. The superficial inferior epigastric vein may be seen in the subcutaneous tissue running obliquely across the incision. Sometimes square-ended retractors can pull the vessel out of the way, and at other times it is best coagulated by diathermy and divided.

3 Once Scarpa's fascia has been divided, the external oblique aponeurosis can be distinguished deep to Scarpa's fascia by the oblique orientation of its fibers, which are absent in Scarpa's fascia. The surface of the external oblique muscle is cleared by placing square retractors under Scarpa's fascia to expose the lower border of the external oblique muscle where the inguinal ligament lies. A sweeping motion with closed scissors parallel to the external oblique fibers will expose the rolled edge of the inguinal ligament and the site of the external inguinal ring where the spermatic cord is seen bulging.

The inguinal canal is opened with a scalpel incision in the external oblique muscle with extension of the incision with scissors in line with the external ring. The incision can be extended with scissors by cutting the fibers towards the external ring, or by cutting laterally along the fibers from the external ring. The edges of the external oblique muscle are best stabilized with small artery forceps so that they can be identified easily later in the operation. The ilioinguinal nerve will run parallel to the incision, just under the fascia of the external

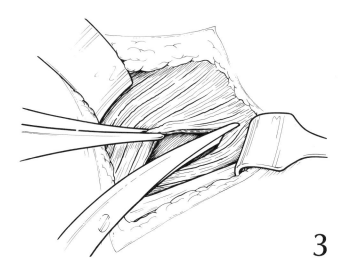

3

oblique muscle, and should be identified and carefully avoided. Accidental transection of the nerve will produce a sensory deficit in the region of the anterior scrotum. Blunt dissection is used to mobilize the inner layer of the external oblique aponeurosis off the surface of the spermatic cord, and the external ring is opened with scissors if this has not already been done.

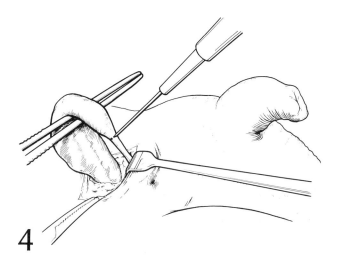

4

4 The testis and attached spermatic cord are mobilized with blunt dissection and delivered out of the wound. This should identify the abnormal attachment of the gubernaculum, which causes dimpling of the skin above and lateral to the neck of the scrotum. The gubernacular attachment is divided carefully with scissors or diathermy, taking care to avoid any structures within the processus vaginalis, such as the vas deferens, which may extend below the lower pole of the testis. The gubernaculum at this level is usually transparent with an occasional fine vessel and some fat and is easy to divide without risk to other structures.

5 A small artery forceps is placed on the gubernacular attachment to the testis and the tunica vaginalis and this is placed on tension. This enables the cremaster fibers surrounding the outside of the spermatic cord to be stripped off with blunt-ended forceps.

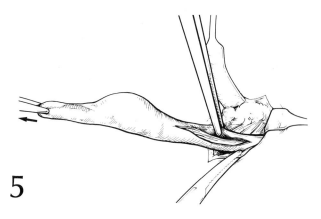

5

Dissection of the hernial sac

The processus vaginalis is commonly widely patent in the undescended testis. Careful separation of the patent processus vaginalis or obvious hernial sac from the vas deferens and the testicular vessels is an important part of the procedure, as this increases the effective length of the spermatic cord. The hernial sac may be stretched over the index finger while round-ended, non-toothed dissecting forceps gently sweep off the other cord structures, carefully avoiding direct application of the forceps on the vas deferens or vessels. Alternatively, the sac can be held with small artery forceps while the vas deferens and testicular vessels are isolated *en masse* off the sac. It is best to attempt to completely separate the hernial sac without opening it, as an unrecognized tear may extend through the internal ring into the peritoneum making closure of the hernial sac difficult. It is absolutely essential that the testicular vessels, and particularly the vas deferens, are visualized clearly before the sac is divided. It is important to note that the vas deferens is closely adherent to the posterior surface of the sac before dissection.

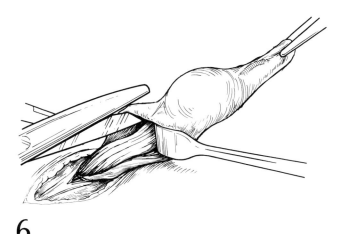

6 With the entire cord held on traction, the testicular vessels and vas deferens are separated from the hernial sac with a small retractor and adequately identified before clamping the hernial sac with artery forceps. The sac is then divided with scissors immediately distal to the artery forceps.

6

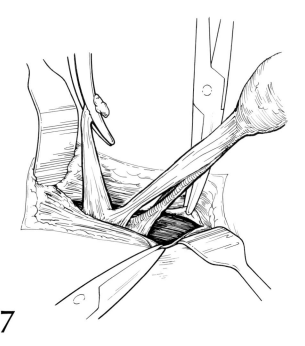

7 The divided processus vaginalis is pulled cranially to put the membrane under tension, and the testicular vessels and vas deferens are separated with blunt dissection from the posterior surface of the sac right up to the internal ring. At the junction between the processus vaginalis and the peritoneum proper, the translucent processus vaginalis becomes an opaque white membrane with a triangular widening of the base. At this level the vas deferens curves medially around the edge of the transversalis fascia, adjacent to the inferior epigastric vessels. By contrast, the testicular vessels pass cranially on the lateral side of the internal ring and disappear into the retroperitoneal space.

7

8 If the spermatic cord is not long enough for the testis to reach the scrotum, the retroperitoneal plane behind the processus vaginalis above the internal ring is developed, and a small Langenbeck's retractor is inserted to pull the peritoneal membrane anteriorly. This reveals the testicular vessels passing cranially in the retroperitoneum. The vessels tend to follow a gentle convex curve laterally, and there are a number of lateral fibrous bands attached to the vessels. These should be divided by sharp or blunt dissection once the testicular vessels themselves have been identified. Continuous traction on the testis allows the testicular vessels to be seen and preserved.

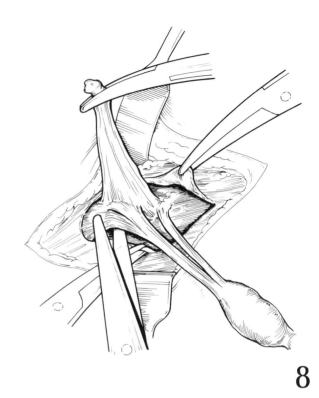

8

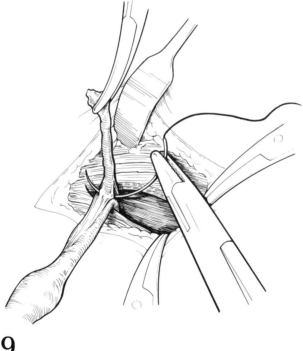

9

9 There should now be adequate length in the vas deferens and the vessels to allow the testis to reach the scrotum. The processus vaginalis is now twisted up to the internal ring to make sure that it contains no intraperitoneal contents, and it is transfixed and ligated at this level. At this point, if the length of the vas deferens is found to be a limiting factor in the position of the testis, the inferior epigastric vessels can be divided electively to gain an extra 0.5–1 cm.

10 Traction on the testis is now stopped and a finger is introduced through the incision and down to the scrotum, breaking down any fascial layers near the neck of the scrotum so that the tip of the index finger can reach the mid-scrotum. The scrotal skin is immobilized between the index finger internally and the thumb externally. A scrotal incision is then made, going just through the skin but not through the deeper tissues. This incision can be either horizontal (the author's preference) or midline in the scrotal septum. Horizontal incisions are associated with less bleeding.

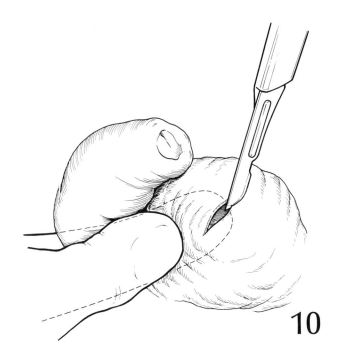

10

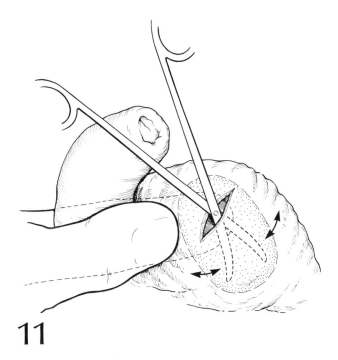

11

11 While the index finger is still inside the scrotum and the thumb is immobilizing the scrotal skin, a fine artery forceps or a pair of scissors is used to develop a subcutaneous pouch, which is usually just deep to the dartos muscle. This should be developed inferiorly more than superiorly, so that the external incision is placed near the cranial end of this subcutaneous pouch. Any troublesome bleeding is controlled by diathermy before proceeding further. This is an important step, as a scrotal hematoma around the testis will inevitably become infected and lead to wound breakdown.

12 A fine artery forceps is placed through the incision in the scrotum and pressed against the index finger internally. The index finger then guides the artery forceps back to the inguinal incision where the tip of the artery forceps is pushed bluntly through any residual fascial plane.

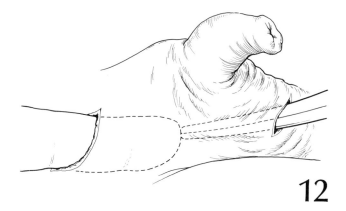

12

13 The artery forceps which has been pushed up through the scrotal incision to the inguinal incision then grasps the gubernacular attachments of the testis, making sure that the cord structures are not twisted. The testis and attached structures are then drawn gently down through the track made by blunt dissection and pulled through the 'button-hole' in the subdartos fascia and delivered through the scrotal incision.

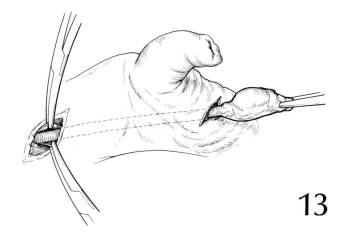

13

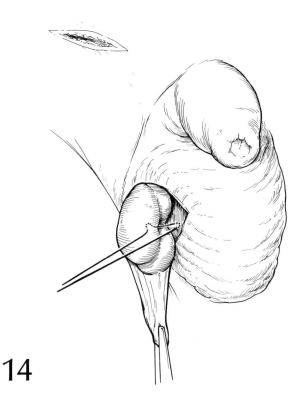

14

14 If the hole made by the artery forceps through the fascial planes between the two incisions is not too large, the testis will sit comfortably in the scrotal pouch like a button through a button-hole. If there is any concern that the testis may retract through a larger defect, it can be anchored to the midline scrotal septum with a 3/0 absorbable suture that passes through the tunica albuginea but does not need to pass right through the body of the testis. To enable this maneuver to be accomplished effectively, many surgeons will deliberately open the tunica vaginalis so that the anatomy of the testis can be defined precisely and recorded. In addition, any testicular appendages can be excised at this time. The testis, epididymis and adjacent coverings can then be placed in the subcutaneous scrotal pouch using blunt forceps.

15 The scrotal incision is closed with a 4/0 subcuticular absorbable suture.

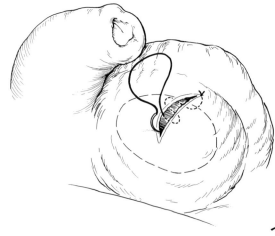

15

16 The surgeon now returns to the inguinal incision, where the external oblique aponeurosis is reconstituted with one to three interrupted sutures or a short continuous suture of 3/0 absorbable material.

The retractors are removed from the wound and the fibrous subcutaneous (Scarpa's) fascia is carefully identified and picked up with toothed forceps and closed with one or two interrupted sutures. The skin is approximated with a 4/0 subcuticular suture. The inguinal incision can be covered with a sterile semipermeable adhesive film dressing which provides a waterproof and childproof covering for the wound for the first 7–10 days. A similar dressing can be applied to the scrotal incision, or alternatively this can be sprayed with a plastic skin spray. Depending on the anesthesia used, local anesthetic infiltration to both the inguinal and/or scrotal wounds can be performed near the end of the procedure.

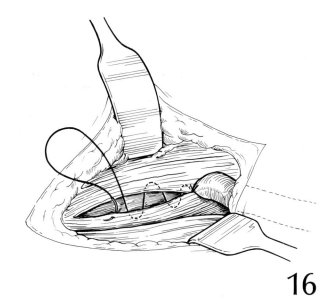

16

Postoperative care

The patient is discharged from the hospital the same day, unless an overnight stay is necessary, such as may be the case with bilateral impalpable testes. Most boys return to normal activities within 2–3 days, although they may need to refrain from active sport for 1–2 weeks.

The dressing is removed and the position of the testis checked after 1–2 weeks and again at 6 months after surgery.

Complications

Wound infection or hematoma are the two most common complications. Hematoma can be avoided by meticulous hemostasis with diathermy at the time of surgery. Wound sepsis can be avoided by placement of waterproof dressings on both incisions, which remain in place at least 1 week. The risk of testicular atrophy, which is determined at 6 months after surgery, should be less than 5%. In most series it is 1–2%. There is a small risk of retraction of the testis into the groin, particularly if there is significant sepsis or hematoma, or postoperative trauma.

Further reading

Bianchi A, Squire BR. Trans-scrotal orchidopexy: orchidopexy revised. *Pediatr Surg Int* 1989; 4: 189–92.

Bloom DA. Two-step orchiopexy with pelviscopic clip ligation of the spermatic vessels. *J Urol* 1991; 145: 1030–3.

Hutson JM, Beasley SW. *Descent of the Testis*. London: Edward Arnold, 1992.

Kogan SJ, Houman BZ, Reda EF, Levitt SB. Orchiopexy of the high undescended testis by division of the spermatic vessels: a critical review of 38 selected transections. *J Urol* 1989; 141: 1416–19.

Microvascular transfer of the testis

Adrian Bianchi MD, FRCS, FRCS(Ed)
Consultant Neonatal and Paediatric Surgeon, Royal Manchester Children's Hospital, Manchester, UK

History

Despite recent advances, the etiology of undescended testes remains unclear[1]. Ever since the days of John Hunter (1786) it has been postulated that a possible cause of undescended testes lay with the testes themselves. However, Mengel *et al.*[2] and Hadziselimovic[3] noted that most undescended testes show relatively normal histology at birth, but undergo a progressive and irreversible loss of spermatogonia and alteration in tubular structure if retained outside the scrotum beyond the second year of life. Disagreement still exists over the normality of the high inguinal and intra-abdominal testis. It is, however, accepted that these testes carry a greater degree of dysgenetic tissue which may account for the higher incidence of malignancy for these organs. Leydig cell function is usually preserved whatever the position of the testis, so that sufficient testosterone is produced to sustain virilization.

About 80% of undescended testes are palpable in the groin, lying along the normal pathway of descent or in an ectopic position. Most palpable testes are held up by a short processus vaginalis and have sufficient vascular and vasal length to allow transfer to the scrotum by conventional or trans-scrotal orchidopexy. It is the high inguinal and intra-abdominal testis with its short vascular pedicle that presents a major problem in achieving transfer to the scrotum with a full blood supply. Sudden division of the main testicular pedicle and reliance on the collateral circulation, as in the Fowler–Stephens technique, may cause a severe spermatogenic injury leading to virtual sterility.

The reliability of microvascular anastomosis of vessels of less than 1 mm diameter has made feasible the transfer of the high testis to the scrotum with a full blood supply[4].

Principles and justification

Indications and aims of orchidopexy

The indications are the same as for any position of the testis, namely to: (1) provide a normal genital appearance, avoiding psychologic distress to the child and the family and enhancing the development of a normal body image; (2) preserve and enhance spermatogenesis; (3) preserve endogenous hormone production; (4) avoid complications such as testicular torsion and inguinal hernia; and (5) possibly reduce the risk of malignancy directly and indirectly by allowing early detection of neoplasia by self-examination.

Indications for orchidectomy

Orchidectomy is indicated for those who demonstrate *in situ* or florid malignancy. Otherwise it should be reserved only for testes which have been proven to have no useful psychologic, spermatogenic or hormonal function.

Timing of orchidopexy

The incidence of undescended testes in the full-term normal child has risen from 1.8% in 1964 to about 4% in 1986. The incidence falls to 1.56% by the third month of life, after which spontaneous descent becomes less likely. Mengel *et al.*[5] and Hadžiselimovic *et al.*[3] have pointed out the progressive and irreversible loss of spermatogonia and the alteration in tubular architecture if the testis is retained outside the scrotum after the second year of life. Ludwig and Potempa[6] noted maximal fertility rates following orchidopexy before the second year of life, and Martin and Menck[7] and Pike[8] commented on the possibility of a reduced risk of malignancy following early orchidopexy. Furthermore, concomitant ligation of the processus vaginalis and testicular fixation removes the risk of testicular torsion and bowel strangulation in an inguinal hernia. By providing a normal genital appearance at an early stage, orchidopexy enhances the development of a normal body image in the growing child and relieves parental anxiety.

There is general agreement that orchidopexy should be undertaken after the first year of life when no further descent can be expected, and before the end of the second year when rapid progressive and irreversible damage occurs.

Operative options

Even after full retroperitoneal mobilization the vascular pedicle of the high inguinal and intra-abdominal testis is usually too short to allow tension-free transfer of the testis to the ipsilateral scrotum with a full blood supply. Several possible operative options have been proposed.

Multistage orchidopexy

Multistage orchidopexy with or without a Silastic wrap requires at least two operative interventions and is frequently unsuccessful.

Fowler–Stephens technique

Division of the main testicular pedicle and reliance on the collateral circulation from the flimsy vasal and cremasteric vessels (the Fowler–Stephens technique)[9] carries a high rate of atrophy (50–100%). Variations of this technique with preservation of a wide peritoneal band around the vasal vessels[10], or a two-stage technique with initial complete ligation or laparoscopic clipping of the testicular pedicle and subsequent scrotal transfer have recently been proposed, but still carry a significant rate of atrophy. Despite evidence of testicular circulation, these techniques expose the testis to a prolonged period of warm ischemia and inadequate venous drainage with consequent gross spermatogenic injury which renders surviving testes virtually sterile.

Microvascular orchidopexy

Microvascular orchidopexy immediately returns a full blood supply by anastomosis of the main testicular vessels to the inferior epigastric vessels. To date the procedure has been associated with a 92% testicular survival rate and testicular growth at puberty. The limited warm ischemia time of 45–90 min has not been followed by any noticeable morbidity.

'Refluo' technique

The 'Refluo' technique follows on the observation by Domini and Lima that testicular loss following the Fowler–Stephens approach was largely due to testicular congestion from inadequate venous drainage through the vasal collaterals[11,12]. The technique relies on the arterial inflow from the vasal vessels, but provides full venous drainage by microvascular anastomosis of the testicular to the inferior epigastric veins. This technique has acceptable testicular survival rates and limited spermatogenic injury. The authors are agreed that it is a useful 'fallback' position in the event of a failed arterial anastomosis.

The reliability of microvascular anastomosis, the high rate of testicular survival and the lack of injury to spermatogenic tissue suggest that microvascular orchidopexy is the preferred option for the management of the high testis on a short vascular pedicle.

Management of the child with impalpable testes

The management of the child with high or impalpable testes is essentially similar for unilateral or bilateral undescent. Management revolves around: (1) the presence, location and quality of testicular tissue; (2) the nature of the vascular pedicle and vas deferens; (3) the age of the child in relation to spermatogenesis; and (4) the risk of malignancy. The interrelation between these factors is outlined in the flow diagram (*Figure 1*).

Since the incidence of anorchia or monorchia is low, it is always important to attempt to locate an impalpable testis. Absence of response to a human chorionic gonadotropin stimulus does not exclude the presence of a hormonally non-functional severely dysgenetic gonad which carries the highest malignancy risk. Of the many possible means of investigation, laparoscopy remains the single most definitive means of locating and assessing an intra-abdominal testis. It is thus an essential investigation for all children with an impalpable testis. Diagnostic surgical exploration is contraindicated since it disrupts tissue planes and may jeopardize successful microvascular orchidopexy.

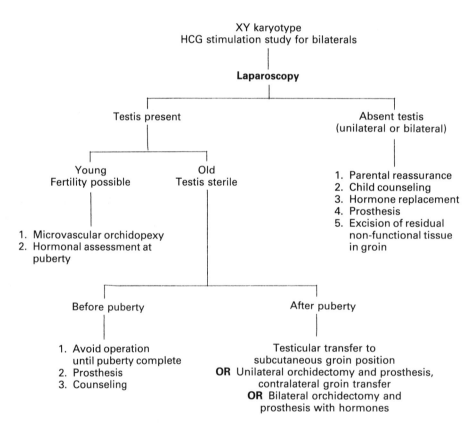

Figure 1   Flow diagram for management of the child with impalpable testes

Equipment

Operating microscope

Loupe magnification ($\times$ 3 to $\times$ 6) is only useful for preparatory vessel dissection and is insufficient for successful anastomosis of vessels of less than 1 mm diameter. Magnification of $\times$ 16 to $\times$ 25 or more can only be achieved with the operating microscope (e.g. Zeiss OPMI 6SDFC XY), which should be equipped with foot pedal control for focus, zoom magnification and XY coupling. Video attachments are helpful for record and teaching purposes and for maintaining interest in the operating room.

Instruments

Good quality microvascular instruments are essential to success and should include: (1) microvascular scissors with flat handles; (2) jeweller's forceps No. 5 or No. 3 (four should be available); (3) a vessel dilator with highly polished blunted ends; (4) microneedle holder with rounded handles and without ratchet; (5) micro-bipolar diathermy forceps and lead; (6) graded microvascular clamps. Individual clamps and 'clamps on bar or frame' suitable for arteries and veins of 0.3–1.5 mm diameter; (7) clamp applicator; (8) 10/0 monofilament nylon on a 3.75 mm 75 μm needle (W2870, Ethicon).

Preoperative

Anesthesia

There are no special requirements. Anesthesia consists of a routine safe general anesthetic with muscle relaxation.

Surgical technique

Successful microvascular anastomosis depends largely on the skill of the microvascular surgeon. This is acquired and maintained by regular application in the laboratory and clinically. It is wise to undertake only one testicular autotransplant at any one session. Microvascular orchidopexy for the contralateral testis is considered when the transferred testis is clearly established in the scrotum some 6 months after orchidopexy.

Anticoagulation

Only local wash of the vessel ends with a heparin–saline solution of 10 units per ml is required. No systemic anticoagulants or other antithrombotic agents are necessary.

Operation

Position and preparation

The child is placed supine on a heating blanket on the operating table in such a position as to allow the surgeon's knees to pass beneath the table. The surgeon and assistant position themselves and the operating microscope for maximum comfort and versatility. The microscope is adjusted for height and focus and the arm swung away from the operative field. A microscope cover is optional.

The child's bladder is emptied by suprapubic compression. Appropriate skin preparation (chlorhexidine in alcohol) and drapes are applied, allowing access to the groin and the scrotum.

Incision

1 An extended incision in the skin crease of the groin above the inguinal ligament is deepened through the external oblique aponeurosis which is split along the line of its fibers. The ilioinguinal nerve is safeguarded and the gubernaculum identified. Care is taken not to damage a long loop vas deferens passing down the inguinal canal. The gubernaculum is followed backwards to the internal inguinal ring where the inferior epigastric vessels become evident as they pass towards the lateral border of the rectus abdominis. At this point the testis may be visible, lying within the peritoneal cavity.

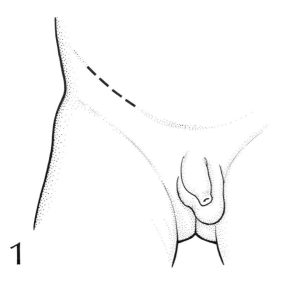

Testis, testicular vessels, vas deferens and vasal vessels

2 The peritoneal cavity is opened and the testis is delivered into the wound. All peritoneal attachments are carefully divided and the peritoneum is closed. All further dissection is undertaken retroperitoneally. Under direct vision the testicular vessels are mobilized by gentle blunt dissection while placing controlled traction on the testis. The vessels are followed high towards the origin of the testicular artery and beyond the confluence of the pampiniform plexus to form a single relatively large testicular vein. One or two venous branches passing to the perinephric tissues are consistent features and require division. These vessels could prove useful in the event of additional testicular venous drainage being required. The vas deferens is mobilized as far as is necessary, taking care to preserve its vascular supply. The mobilized testis could be passed beneath the lateral umbilical ligament to allow the vas deferens a straighter course towards the scrotum. The testis, with intact vessels and vas deferens, is placed aside and allowed to recover during preparation of the donor vessels.

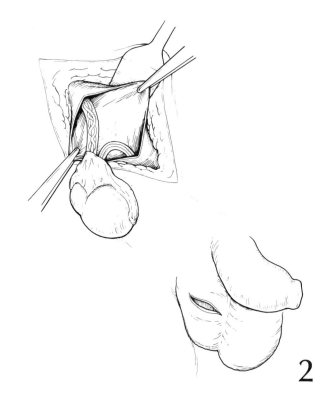

2

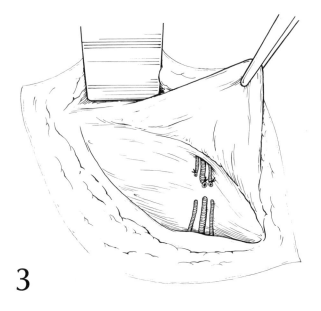

3

Inferior epigastric vessels

3 A donor vascular pedicle of sufficient length is prepared by following the inferior epigastric vessels to a high level beneath the rectus abdominis. This has the added advantage of reducing the diameter of the inferior epigastric artery, allowing for less discrepancy between it and the testicular artery. Several muscular branches are divided with bipolar diathermy. The inferior epigastric artery and one vein are clamped proximally with graded microvascular clamps. The proximal cut end of the second vena comitans is bipolar coagulated. The vein, however, is carefully preserved since it may serve as a vein graft should this be required. The vessels are divided high beneath the muscle and prepared for anastomosis. Under magnification with the operating microscope the vessel ends are cleared of all adventitia and resected back to ensure a clean undamaged intima. No instruments or cannulas, other than the vessel dilator, may be inserted into the lumen. The vessel ends are constantly washed with a heparin–saline solution (10 units/ml) and are never allowed to dry.

Subdartos pouch

As is routine for conventional orchidopexy, a pathway to the ipsilateral scrotum is developed by blunt finger dissection from the groin wound. A scrotal skin crease incision is made high on the scrotum and a pair of hemostat forceps is passed up towards the groin wound and left in position in preparation for testicular transfer.

Division of testicular vessels and scrotal transfer

4 The testicular vessels are divided high retroperitoneally only after all has been prepared for immediate anastomosis. The testis is passed through to the scrotum and exteriorized through the scrotal wound. Cold saline wraps may be applied but are unnecessary. Testicular perfusion is not performed since this is likely to cause catastrophic intimal injury. The testicular pedicle is of sufficient length to allow for comfortable microvascular anastomosis on the surface of the groin wound.

Vessel preparation and anastomosis

5a–d Under magnification with the operating microscope, the testicular artery and vein are cut back and cleaned of adventitia. One arterial and at least one venous anastomosis are required. In order to minimize possible testicular congestion because of inflow from the collaterals, the venous anastomosis is completed first and free venous flow established early. Venous anastomoses are usually end-to-end. A major discrepancy exists, however, between the testicular and inferior epigastric arteries such that an end-to-oblique or, better still, an oblique-to-oblique configuration is necessary to overcome this. End-to-side anastomosis or an interposition stepdown vein graft are also useful techniques.

All anastomoses are constructed with interrupted fine monofilament sutures on the smallest possible atraumatic needle (10/0 nylon on a 3.75 mm, 75 μm needle – Ethicon W2870). Accurate apposition of undamaged intima is essential for success. All vessel ends are washed constantly with heparin–saline (10 units/ml) and no other medication is given locally or systemically. Once the arterial anastomosis is completed the testis is revascularized. Anastomotic patency for more than 20 min is usually associated with long-term success. Evidence of developing venous congestion despite venous anastomotic patency is an indication for additional venous drainage. Thrombosis (usually within 5 min) at any of the anastomoses is an index of a faulty union for which the only treatment is resection and construction of a fresh anastomosis. In the event of repeated inability to establish arterial patency, the 'Refluo' principle (venous anastomosis only) of Domini and Lima[11, 12] can be used instead.

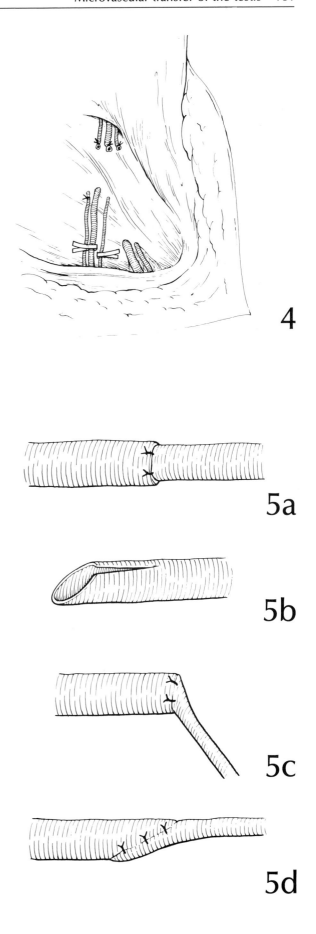

4

5a

5b

5c

5d

Testicular biopsy

Incision of the tunica albuginea on the body of the testicle and well away from the polar vascular network allows testicular tubular biopsy. Active arterial bleeding from the subcapsular plexus further confirms anastomotic patency. Following bipolar hemostasis the capsular wound is sutured with a 6/0 absorbable suture (Maxon).

Wound closure

The testis is placed in the prepared subdartos pouch where it must lie freely without any tension, thus requiring no fixation. All wounds are closed in layers, reconstructing the inguinal canal, with fine absorbable sutures (6/0 Maxon) ending with subcuticular skin sutures. No dressings are required.

Postoperative care

Since intraoperative anastomotic patency for more than 20 min has been associated with long-term success, no attempt is made at postoperative monitoring. Indeed, this is not a practical proposition, simply leading to additional discomfort for the child. Care is routine with early mobilization and discharge to all activities within 24–48 h.

Long-term follow-up

In view of the increased risk of malignancy all patients retaining previously high or intra-abdominal testes should receive appropriate counseling and must be taught testicular self-examination. Groin exploration and excision of any residual gonadal tissue gives added reassurance for those with a negative human chorionic gonadotropin stimulus after puberty when an intra-abdominal testis has been excluded at laparoscopy.

The role and value of early microvascular testicular transfer to the scrotum on a full blood supply can only be determined by long-term evaluation of its impact on the psychologic development of the child and his parents, on the child's eventual fertility, and on the incidence of testicular malignancy.

Outcome

A series of 51 testes in 42 boys, aged between 2 and 15 years, have been transferred to the scrotum with a full blood supply using microvascular techniques: nine children had bilateral transfer and 33 had a unilateral orchidopexy, some for a single testis after loss of the contralateral side. Total operating time was 2.5–3 h with a testicular ischemia time of 45–90 min. Hospital stay averaged 24–48 h. There has been no morbidity and no mortality. No testis was entirely normal histologically. Features were consistent with those expected in cryptorchidism with alteration in tubular architecture and varying degrees of interstitial fibrosis. Spermatogonia were present in 33 testes; the remainder showed Sertoli cells only. No testis showed carcinoma *in situ* or florid malignancy.

At follow-up 6 months to 12 years later, 47 testes are well placed in the scrotum providing excellent cosmesis, and four have atrophied. Testicular volume varies between normal and 75% of that expected for the child's age. All children going through puberty have shown an increase in testicular size, and none has required additional hormonal supplements. There have been no psychologic problems and parent satisfaction and relief of anxiety has been noticeable.

Conclusions

Autotransplantation of the high inguinal and intra-abdominal testis with a full blood supply is now a definite entity at any age. The testicular vessels in the 1–2-year-old infant are exceptionally well developed, possibly as a result of intrauterine hormonal stimulation, and do not constitute a problem. Vessel size is therefore not a bar to microvascular orchidopexy during the second year of life and before testicular damage becomes manifest.

Microvascular orchidopexy is accepted as a viable option. The value of early transfer (before 2 years of age) on a full blood supply, of the high inguinal and intra-abdominal testis to the scrotum still remains to be proven. Although satisfactory cosmetic and psychologic results are immediately apparent, the effect on spermatogenesis and on the incidence of malignancy must await considerable long-term follow-up, well into adulthood and middle age.

References

1. Hutson JM, Beasley SW. *Descent of the Testis*. London: Edward Arnold, 1992: 1–49.

2. Mengel W, Heinz HA, Sippe WG, Hecker WC. Studies on cryptorchidism: a comparison of histological findings in the germinative epithelium before and after the second year of life. *J Pediatr Surg* 1974; 9: 445–50.

3. Hadziselimovic F, Herzog B, Seguchi H. Surgical correction of cryptorchidism at 2 years: electron microscopic and morphologic investigations. *J Pediatr Surg* 1975; 10: 19–26.

4. Bianchi A. Management of the impalpable testis: the role of microvascular orchidopexy. *Pediatr Surg Int* 1990; 5: 48–53.

5. Mengel W, Zimmerman FA, Hecher WCH. *Timing of Repair for Undescended Testis*. Chicago: Year Book Medical Publishers, 1981.

6. Ludwig G, Potempa J. Der optimale zeitpunkt der behandlung des kryptorchismus. *Deutsch Med Wochenschr* 1975; 100: 680–3.

7. Martin DC, Menck HR. The undescended testis: management after puberty. *J Urol* 1975; 114: 77–9.

8. Pike MC, Chilvers C, Peckham MJ. Effect of age at orchidopexy on risk of testicular cancer. *Lancet* 1986; i: 1246–8.

9. Fowler R, Stephens FD. The role of testicular vascular anatomy in the salvage of high undescended testes. *Aust NZ J Surg* 1959; 29: 92–106.

10. Snyder HMcC, Duckett JW. Orchidopexy with division of spermatic vessels: a review of 10 year experience (abstract). *J Urol* 1984; 131 (Suppl.): 126A.

11. Domini R, Lima M. L'autotrapianto microvasculare 'Refluo' del testicolo: una nuova soluzione tecnica. *Rass Ital Chir Pediatr* 1989; 31: 213–23.

12. Lima M, Gentile C, Ruggieri G *et al*. Autotrapianto testicolare sperimentale: premessa all' autotrapianto testicolare 'Refluo' in eta pediatrica. *Rass Ital Chir Pediatr* 1989; 31: 243–6.

Testicular torsion

Su-Anna M. Boddy MS, FRCS
Consultant Paediatric Surgeon, St George's Hospital, London, UK

N. P. Madden MA, FRCS
Consultant Paediatric Surgeon, Chelsea and Westminster Hospital and St Mary's Hospital, London, UK

Torsion of the testis must be the first consideration in any child or young adult with acute scrotal pain. There are two peaks in the incidence: in the perinatal period and between the ages of 10 and 25 years.

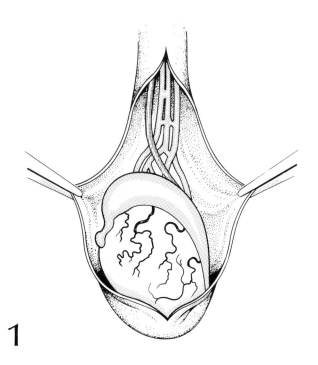

1

Diagnosis

Neonatal torsion

In the neonate the torsion is extravaginal. An intra-uterine or neonatal torsion may present as an impalpable testis. If a baby is born with a non-tender unilateral scrotal lump, surgical exploration is unnecessary. Exploration is indicated if the diagnosis is uncertain or the testis painful. Recent evidence[1] suggests that the contralateral testis should be fixed – probably electively at six months of age – to avoid subsequent torsion.

Intravaginal torsion of the testis

1 If the tunica vaginalis invests the whole of the epididymis and the distal part of the spermatic cord, the testis is in effect suspended in the scrotal cavity like a bell clapper and is free to rotate within the tunica vaginalis. This situation may be indicated by an abnormal horizontal lie of the testis. Testicular maldescent may also predispose to torsion. The torsion is usually towards the midline septum, that is, the right testis rotates in a clockwise direction and the left in an anticlockwise direction from the examiner's point of view.

Recurrent torsion

There is a history of episodic testicular pain, with or without swelling of the testis. The testis may lie more transversely in the scrotum, but may otherwise appear completely normal. However, the history alone indicates that both testes should be fixed by early surgery.

Differential diagnosis

Torsion of a testicular appendage

Torsion of a testicular appendage presents at 4–10 years of age. Careful palpation will reveal a tender nodule associated with the upper pole of the testis; the lower part of the testis is not tender. On transillumination this nodule may appear as a dark spot. If the diagnosis of torsion of a testicular appendage can be made on clinical assessment, neither hospital observation nor operation are mandatory.

Acute epididymo-orchitis

Unilateral epididymo-orchitis is common in adults but rare in children, in whom it is likely to be associated with infection or anomaly of the urinary tract.

Mumps orchitis

This rarely, if ever, occurs before puberty and appears within 3 days to 1 week after the onset of parotitis. It is usually bilateral.

Idiopathic scrotal edema

In this condition the erythema and swelling of the scrotal skin spread into the groin, perineum or base of the penis. Pain is not a major feature. The skin may be tender but the underlying testis and cord are normal. The peak incidence is at 4–6 years of age and the only treatment necessary is reassurance.

Incarcerated inguinal hernia

The symptoms and signs of torsion of an undescended testis closely resemble those of an incarcerated inguinal hernia – a painful tender swelling in the groin – but are associated with an empty scrotum. Since early surgical exploration is mandatory for both conditions differentiation is, perhaps, unnecessary.

Operation

Timing

In most cases the diagnosis of acute torsion of the testis must be made clinically unless techniques such as Doppler ultrasonography or radioisotope scanning are immediately available. Any delay in operation, once the diagnosis is suspected, will prejudice the survival of the testis.

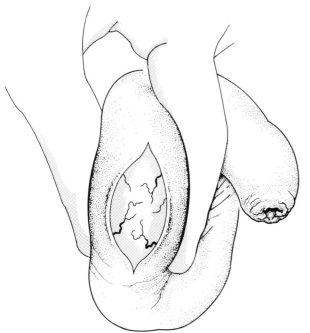

2 The testis is delivered from the scrotum through a vertical incision over its longitudinal axis. The skin, dartos fascia and tunica vaginalis are all incised. As the tunica vaginalis is incised the hemoserous fluid of the secondary hydrocele is released.

2

3 The testis is delivered from the tunica vaginalis and the cord untwisted.

The tunica albuginea is incised in order to release the pressure on the underlying tubules and to assess viability.

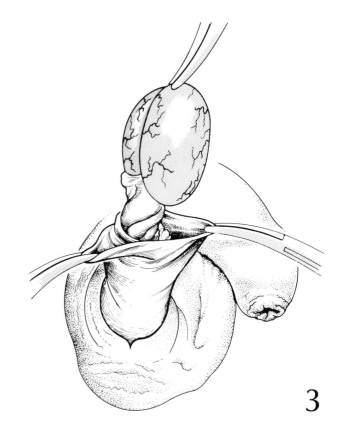

3

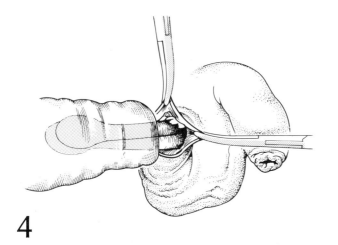

4

4 The untwisted testis is wrapped in moist, warm swabs and its colour carefully observed. While waiting to confirm whether perfusion has been re-established, the contralateral testis may be fixed.

Conservation or removal of the testis

If the testis is completely black and necrotic and is deemed non-viable then it should be removed. The spermatic cord is ligated within the scrotum with a strong absorbable suture and the testis removed. If there is any question that some perfusion might be re-established then the testis should be conserved. It is imperative to fix the contralateral viable testis.

Fixation of the testis

5   Testes should be fixed by three fine non-absorbable monofilament sutures such as 6/0 polypropylene. These should be placed between the tunica albuginea and the lateral wall of the scrotal cavity, at the upper and lower poles of the testis and at the equator.

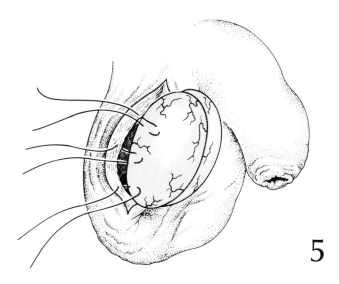

5

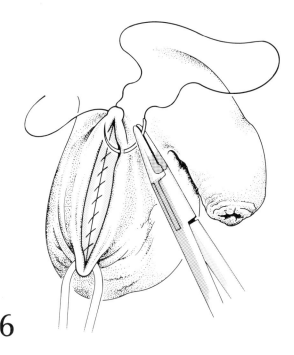

6

6   The wound is closed in layers using continuous 5/0 to 3/0 chromic catgut sutures, depending on the age of the patient. A scrotal support should be applied at the end of the operation.

Alternative method

Experimental evidence suggests that fixation of the testis in a scrotal pouch may cause less damage to the testis and, more importantly, offer better fixation preventing subsequent torsion[1,2].

7   The testis is delivered through a horizontal scrotal incision and the tunica vaginalis is everted. The testis is retracted superiorly onto the abdominal wall. A fine-toothed pair of forceps lifts the inferior margin of the scrotal skin incision. An adequate scrotal pouch can be made by blunt dissection. The testis – still everted from the tunica vaginalis – is placed in the scrotal pouch. The scrotal skin is closed with continuous or interrupted 4/0 chromic catgut (6/0 in infants).

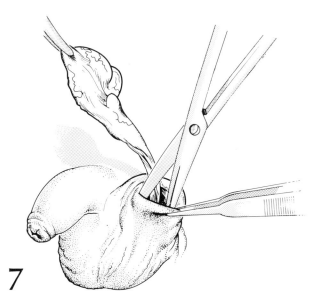

7

References

1. Mishriki SF, Winkle DC, Frank JD. Fixation of a single testis: always, sometimes or never. *Br J Urol* 1992; 69: 311–13.

2. Bellinger MF, Abromowitz H, Brantley S, Marshall G. Orchiopexy: an experimental study of the effect of surgical technique on testicular histology. *J Urol* 1989; 142: 553–5.

Circumcision, meatotomy and meatoplasty

J. D. Frank FRCS
Consultant Paediatric Surgeon and Urologist, Department of Paediatric Surgery, Bristol Royal Hospital for Sick Children, Bristol, Avon, UK

Principles and justification

Indications

1 A true phimosis is the *only* medical indication for circumcision. This is usually due to balanitis xerotica obliterans. Circumcision in the neonatal period should be avoided if possible because of the complications of meatal ulceration leading to meatal stenosis. Circumcision for social and religious reasons should therefore preferably be performed when the child is out of nappies.

The commonest causes of meatal stenosis are ulceration following an ammoniacal dermatitis in the circumcised child and previous hypospadias repair. The majority of these patients can be successfully treated by meatal dilatation, but a meatotomy may be required.

Stenosis may occasionally recur in children after a meatotomy. Meatoplasty is then required.

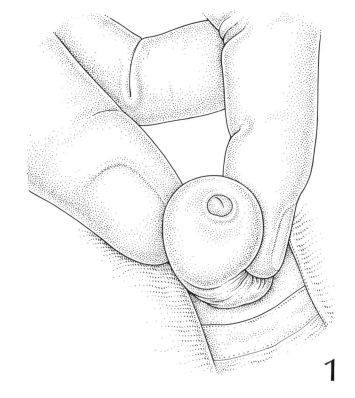

1

Preoperative

Anesthesia

General anesthesia is normally employed except in the neonatal period when a penile block may be used. The addition of caudal anesthesia to a full general anesthetic ensures a comfortable early postoperative period.

Operations

CIRCUMCISION

There are more ways of performing a circumcision than almost any other pediatric surgical operation apart from a hypospadias repair. The two most important considerations in planning the procedure are that it should have minimal complications and give a good cosmetic result. The following method appears to fulfill these criteria.

2a–c The scarred foreskin is dilated with artery forceps and completely retracted. Preputial adhesions are freed from the glans, and all smegma is removed and the glans cleaned completely.

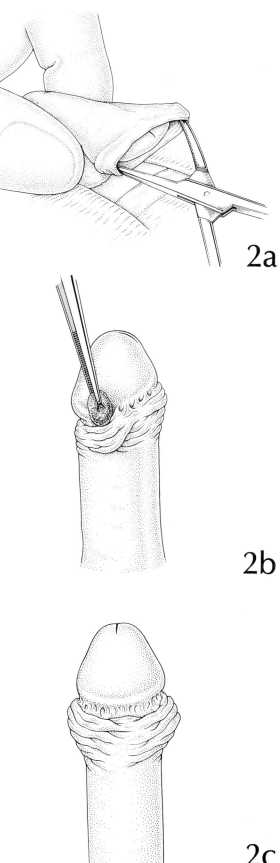

2a

2b

2c

3a–e

The foreskin is then elevated by placing one artery clip ventrally and one dorsally. A pair of sinus forceps is applied to the skin at the level of the coronal sulcus and closed gently. This movement will make it slide up and over the underlying glans, taking the skin with it. When the glans can be palpated inferior to the forceps, it can be safely closed and held tightly shut. Using long sharp scissors, a clean cut is then made just distal to the sinus forceps to remove the excess foreskin. If sufficient foreskin is not removed with the first cut, the procedure can be repeated and a little more skin excised. It is always better to leave a little too much rather than risk a deficiency of shaft skin.

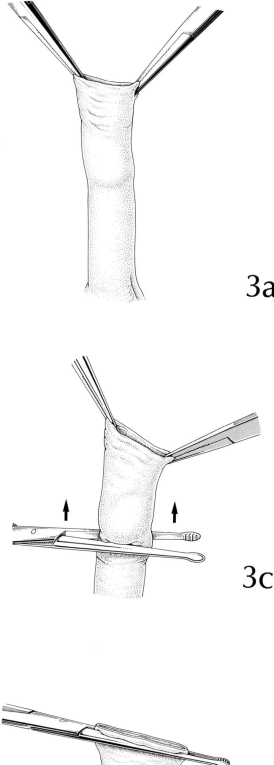

3a

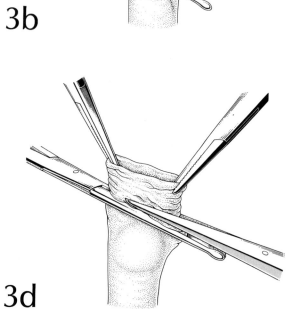

3b

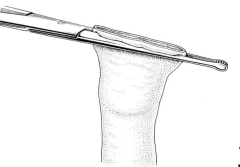

3c

3d

3e

4a–c The skin is then retracted and any bleeding points are grasped with artery forceps and ligated with fine catgut. The excess inner layer of the prepuce is trimmed, leaving a margin around the corona of approximately 3 mm. The wound is closed with interrupted 5/0 Dexon or plain catgut sutures.

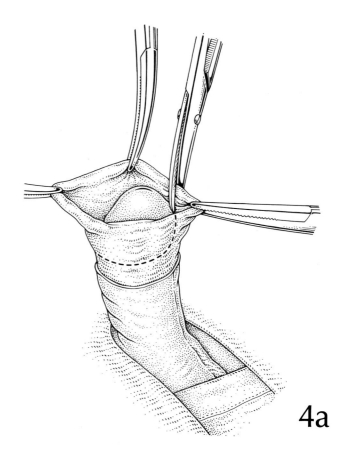

4a

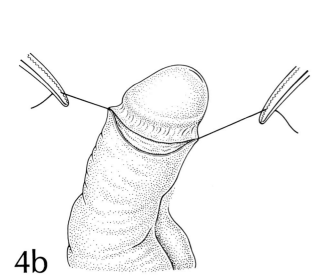

4b

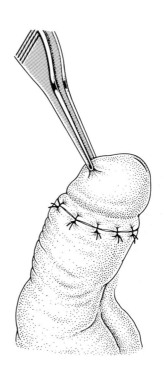

4c

Postoperative care

No postoperative dressing is necessary but some liquid paraffin may be poured over the penis to prevent the sheets adhering to it.

The child is allowed home on the same day and may start bathing the next day. No particular postoperative precautions are necessary.

Complications

Circumcision is often regarded as a minor surgical procedure, but there are probably more complications associated with this operation than with many other more complicated urological procedures. It should not be delegated to junior surgical staff without adequate training and supervision.

Hemorrhage

Careful hemostasis using bipolar diathermy at the time of surgery will prevent occurrence of a primary hemorrhage. Occasionally, however, a vessel will start bleeding after the patient has returned to the ward and in this situation ice cold saline dressings may stop the hemorrhage. If in doubt it is preferable to return the child to the operating theatre and deal with the bleeding point under anesthesia. Exclusion of a bleeding diathesis is obviously mandatory if the bleeding remains troublesome.

Sepsis

Infections after a circumcision are not infrequent, with a reported incidence of up to 10%. These infections normally settle after a few days with regular bathing but occasionally systemic antibiotics may be required. Deaths have been reported in the literature but should now be only of historical interest.

Fistulas

Urethrocutaneous fistulas following a circumcision are rare but are a difficult complication to treat as they usually occur at the level of the corona glandis. The two most common causes are excessive use of the diathermy or a suture placed too deeply in an attempt to stop bleeding of the frenulum. Surgical repair should be performed 6 months after the original circumcision.

Excision of too much or too little skin

If insufficient skin is excised the patient may suffer from a recurrence of the phimosis and require a further circumcision. Removal of excess skin will lead to a buried penis which will rarely require a skin graft.

Meatal stenosis

In younger children this complication occurs following a severe ammoniacal dermatitis, probably related to leaving the child in wet nappies. In the older child it is a complication of the balanitis xerotica obliterans that affects the glans and foreskin causing the original phimosis. It is not a complication of the circumcision *per se*. Treatment may necessitate a meatal dilatation, a meatotomy or, for recurrent stenosis, a meatoplasty.

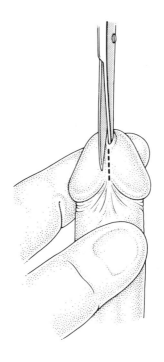

5a

MEATOTOMY

5a–c Once the meatus has been dilated, a pair of fine scissors is used to make a ventral incision through the meatus. A few fine 6/0 Dexon sutures are used to approximate the urethral mucosa to the skin.

The main complication of this procedure is that it creates a glandular hypospadias. This may affect the direction of the urinary stream but, providing the incision is not carried too far proximally, there should be no major problems.

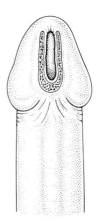

5b

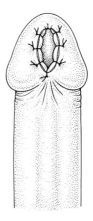

5c

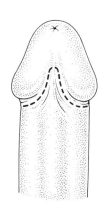

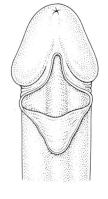

MEATOPLASTY

6a–f A tongue of ventral skin is first mobilized. An incision is then made proximally from the meatus until normal urethra is reached, and the tongue of skin is inlaid into the proximal part of the incision as shown. The wound is closed with 6/0 Dexon sutures.

This repair also creates a glandular hypospadias with occasional spraying.

6a

6b

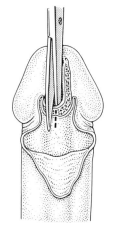

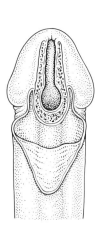

6c

6d

Further reading

Gairdner D. The fate of the foreskin. A study of circumcision. *BMJ* 1949; ii: 1433–7.

Griffiths DM, Atwell JD, Freeman NV. A prospective study of the indications and morbidity of circumcision in children. *Eur Urol* 1985; 11: 184–7.

Rickwood AMK, Walker J. Is phimosis overdiagnosed in boys and are too many circumcisions performed in consequence? *Ann R Coll Surg Engl* 1989; 71: 275–7.

Williams N, Kapila L. Complications of circumcision. *Br J Surg* 1993; 80: 1231–6.

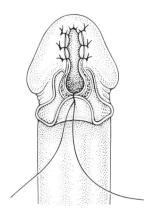

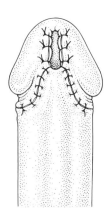

6e

6f

Bladder exstrophy closure and epispadias repair

Philip G. Ransley FRCS
Consultant Urological Surgeon, Great Ormond Street Hospital for Children, London, and Senior Lecturer in Paediatric Urology, Institute of Urology, University of London, UK

Patrick G. Duffy FRCSI
Consultant Paediatric Urologist, Great Ormond Street Hospital for Children, London, and Senior Lecturer in Paediatric Urology, Institute of Urology, University of London, UK

Principles and justification

The surgical treatment of the bladder exstrophy complex of anomalies is a highly specialized and difficult area of pediatric urology. Accordingly, it is most appropriate for exstrophy cases to be referred to a specialist center. The initial closure of the bladder is the beginning of a series of surgical steps aimed at achieving satisfactory cosmesis, urinary continence and a sexually adequate penis.

In boys (predominant in a ratio of three to one) the anomaly consists of an exposed everted bladder in continuity with an epispadiac penis. The pubic bones are widely separated and the external sphincter complex is represented only by a fibrous interpubic bar and has no recoverable muscle function. The penis itself is short and with upward chordee. In exceptional cases it can be very small and sex assignment as female may be appropriate.

The umbilicus is low set and there may be an accompanying umbilical hernia. Bilateral inguinal hernias are common. The perineum is foreshortened with an anteriorly placed anus, which may be abnormal.

In girls, the anomalies are similar with a bifid clitoris and a separate vaginal opening. The anus may be vestibular.

When isolated male epispadias occurs the penile defect ranges from a simple glanular anomaly to symphysial epispadias verging on complete exstrophy. In all but the most distal lesions the bladder neck and sphincter mechanisms are poorly formed and complete incontinence is usual. Isolated female epispadias is a very rare anomaly in which a bifid clitoris and a patulous urethral opening are obvious in a child with complete urinary incontinence.

The current surgical approach consists of early closure and later surgery for continence aiming, if possible, to achieve satisfactory urinary storage, continence and bladder emptying (by voiding or intermittent catheterization) by the time the child enters school. However, some patients will inevitably remain incontinent awaiting either an artificial sphincter or spontaneous improvement at puberty.

Epispadias repair is usually undertaken at 12–15 months of age following a short period of testosterone therapy. With late presenting exstrophy cases the repair may be performed as a single-stage procedure in conjunction with bladder closure, with or without osteotomy.

Surgical steps to closure

The surgical steps may be summarized as follows:

1. Closure of the bladder in the neonatal period within the first 24 h may proceed with approximation of the pubic bones without need for osteotomy. After 24 h osteotomy is advised and a modified Salter anterior osteotomy is currently recommended. Immobilization in a frog plaster is satisfactory and is recommended whether or not osteotomy is employed as it greatly facilitates postoperative nursing care.
2. Late closure may be combined with epispadias repair and osteotomy. External fixation may be required after the age of 3 years.
3. Carefully supervised testosterone therapy, usually 25 mg intramuscularly monthly for 3 months, is administered at the end of the first year of life.
4. Epispadias repair is undertaken at 12–15 months (single stage).
5. The upper tracts (ultrasound) and bladder capacity (cystogram under anesthesia) should be assessed annually.
6. Bladder neck reconstruction, with or without augmentation enterocystoplasty.
7. Bladder emptying is achieved by voiding or intermittent catheterization (urethral or suprapubic continent stoma).

In this chapter the basic techniques of bladder closure and epispadias repair are described but no attempt is made to give a detailed guide to the intricacies of the management of the patient with bladder exstrophy.

Preoperative

The neonate is transferred to the pediatric urology center from the maternity unit. It is appropriate that at least one parent should see the anomaly in order to appreciate its gravity and to understand the subsequent surgical procedures. However, neither parent is in a position to accept a detailed discussion at this stage. Surgery may be delayed for up to 24 h while avoiding the need for osteotomy but after 24 h pelvic ring closure without osteotomy is very difficult and poorly maintained. Cross-matched blood should be available. An ultrasound examination is recommended before surgical reconstruction in order to exclude an upper urinary tract abnormality.

Anesthesia

General anesthesia is required with the usual neonatal precautions. An additional caudal anesthetic is helpful, particularly for epispadias repair.

Operations

BLADDER EXSTROPHY CLOSURE

Position of patient

The patient is positioned flat and supine. Total lower body preparation with individual wrapping of the legs allows maximum maneuverability at the time of pelvic ring closure. A single intraoperative dose of gentamicin (2 mg/kg), metronidazole (7.5 mg/kg) and ampicillin (6 mg/kg) is administered intravenously as soon as venous access is established.

Skin incision

1 The umbilicus is ligated and trimmed but retained. Incisions are made beginning in the midline above the umbilicus, extending around the margins of the bladder and forwards on to the root of the penis as far as the distal limit of the verumontanum. The incisions are deepened with diathermy but the distal incisions may be left superficial at this stage.

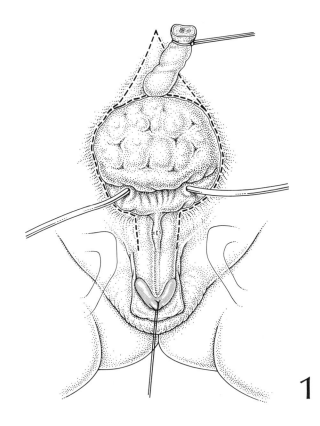

Bladder mobilization

2 The umbilical arteries serve as a guide to the extraperitoneal plane on each side. Careful blunt dissection opens up a plane behind the rectus muscles on each side, in front of the ureter (stent in position for palpation) and down to the pelvic floor at the bladder neck.

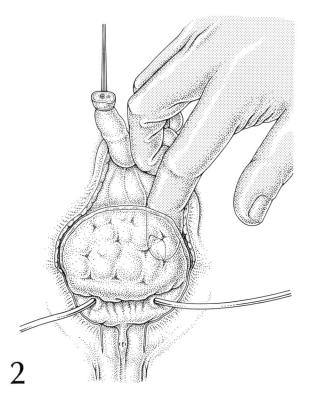

Completion of distal incisions

3 With a finger in position behind the abdominal wall, the distal incisions may be completed with diathermy. Superficial bleeding is encountered from erectile tissue and local infiltration with epinephrine (adrenaline) 1:200 000 into the prostate may be helpful. The interpubic bar tissue fusing with the bladder neck is now visible and is an important landmark.

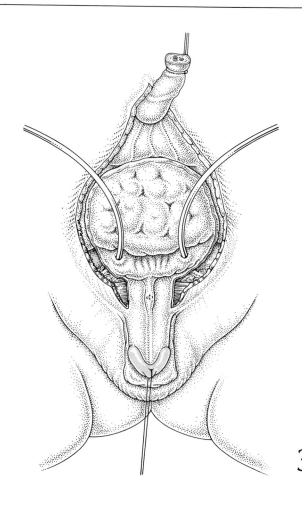

3

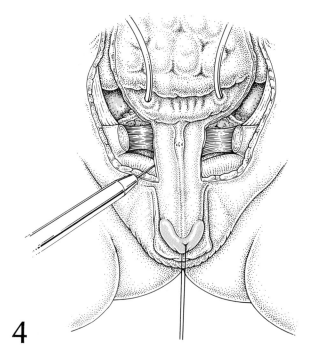

4

Dissection of posterior urethra

4 The verumontanum and the underlying prostate tissue are dissected free from the underlying interpubic bar tissue and corpora cavernosa in order to allow them to be recessed into the pelvis. The corpora are freed from the interpubic bar tissue and from the pubic bones but only for a sufficient distance to allow placement of the sutures that will hold the pubic bones together. Radical corporal mobilization is not performed.

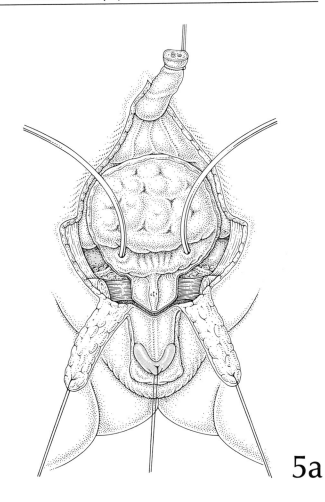

5a

Paraexstrophy skin flaps

5a, b Paraexstrophy skin flaps are no longer recommended on account of the long-term problems of stricture and stone formation with the incorporation of skin into the posterior urethra and bladder neck regions. In exceptional cases this procedure may be necessary because of an inadequate urethral plate.

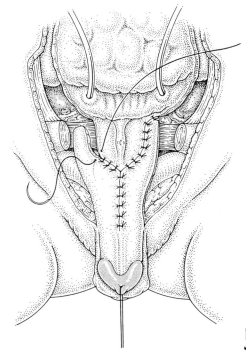

5b

Final urethral dissection

6 The bladder and prostate are now sufficiently free to drop back into the pelvis. The parallel urethral incisions may be extended a little further distally in order to create the segment of urethra that will come to lie behind the approximated symphysis.

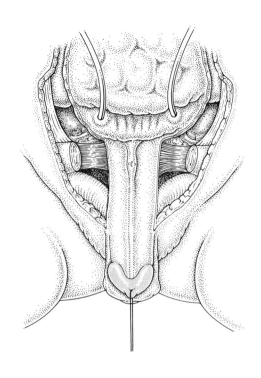

6

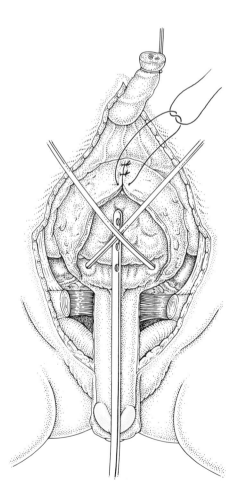

7

Bladder closure

7 A 10-Fr plastic Jacques catheter with opposed eyes is sutured to the bladder wall with 3/0 chromic catgut. Positioning of the catheter to ensure that all the eyes lie within the closed bladder lumen is important. The bladder edges are trimmed back to fresh muscle tissue, making sure that no marginal squamous epithelium is included in the bladder closure. Bladder closure begins from the apex using interrupted 3/0 polyglycolic acid sutures.

Closure of posterior urethra

8 The bladder closure continues through the bladder neck region to the base of the penis. A change to 5/0 polyglycolic acid is appropriate at this stage.

Incision of interpubic bar tissue and urethral wrap

9a, b The interpubic bar tissue is partially released from the posterior aspects of the pubic bones. This is an important step to provide support for the reconstructed posterior urethra and to define the boundaries between the abdominal cavity and the perineum. It may not be possible to achieve sufficient mobility for wrapping to be completed at this stage due to the wide separation of the pubic bones. In such circumstances the sutures are laid and closure completed as the pelvic ring is brought together in conjunction with abdominal closure.

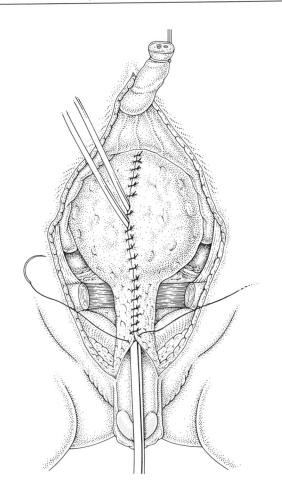

8

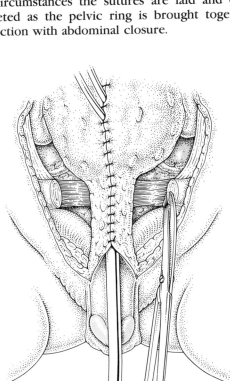

9a

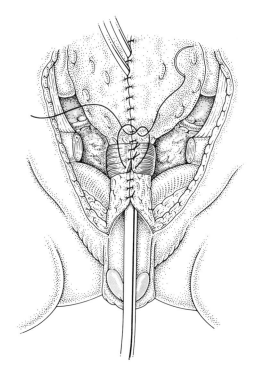

9b

Transpositional omphaloplasty and wound closure

10 The umbilicus is displaced to the apex of the abdominal incision.

Closure of the abdominal wound begins by bringing the rectus muscles together, starting from above and proceeding downwards. The aim is to even out the tension of closure throughout the whole length of the wound so that the strain of closure is not taken by the symphysial sutures alone. Vertical mattress sutures achieve this provided that the bites are placed at right angles to the oblique rectus margin and not horizontally, parallel to the transpyloric plane. A 2/0 polydioxanone suture is usually adequate but 0 may be advisable in the lower half of the wound.

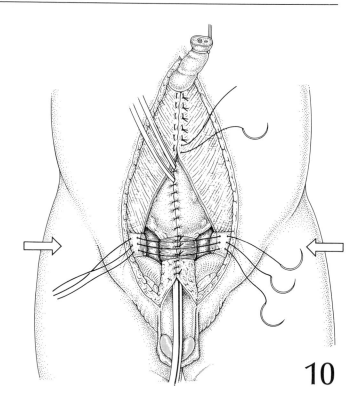

10

11a

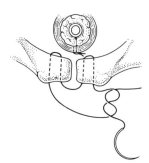

11b

Approximation of pubic bones

11a, b Three heavy (0 or 1) polydioxanone sutures are laid in position in the pubic bones before abdominal wall closure and are tied once rectus muscle approximation is complete. The precise placement is shown in *Illustration 11b* with the suture material traversing the gap between the pubic bones anteriorly. This helps to prevent a bowstring effect cutting back into the urethra if the bones separate a little postoperatively.

Final approximation of the pubic bones is completed last. Internal rotation of the hips and compression of the pelvis by an assistant is helpful.

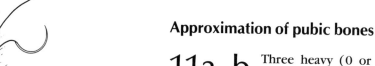

Skin closure

12 The skin is closed in two layers. The ureteric stent catheters come through the abdominal wound but the bladder is drained solely by the urethral catheter.

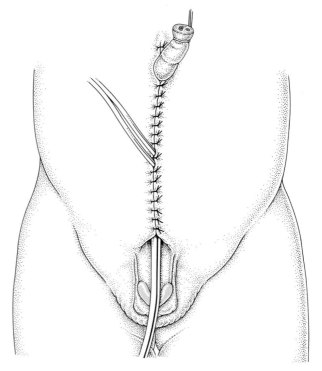

12

EPISPADIAS REPAIR

No special preparation is required. Cross-matched blood should be available.

Antibiotic cover is provided with a single intraoperative dose of gentamicin (2 mg/kg), metronidazole (7.5 mg/kg) and ampicillin (6 mg/kg).

Preoperative and perioperative infiltration with epinephrine (adrenaline) 1:200 000, especially around the base of the corpora and the prostate is required, but care should be taken to avoid intracorporeal injection.

Position of patient

The patient is positioned flat and supine.

Preliminary glansplasty

13 A longitudinal incision is made through the distal fusion of the lateral wings of the glans and the distal urethra. This is closed transversely using 6/0 polydioxanone sutures. This maneuver makes a great deal of difference to the final cosmetic appearance by displacing the terminal urethral meatus slightly ventrally.

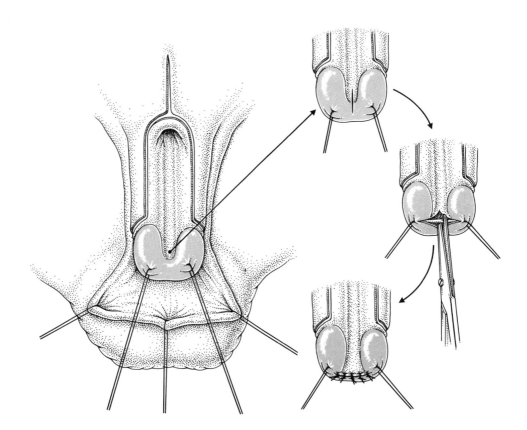

13

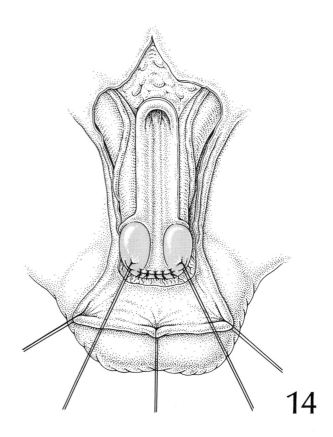

Skin incision

14 The incision begins in the midline above the urethral opening and is extended far enough upwards to provide good access to the proximal corpora for mobilization. It continues down on each side of the midline urethral strip (backed by corpus spongiosum) and sweeps ventrally around the coronal sulcus separating the prepuce and ventral skin from the corpora.

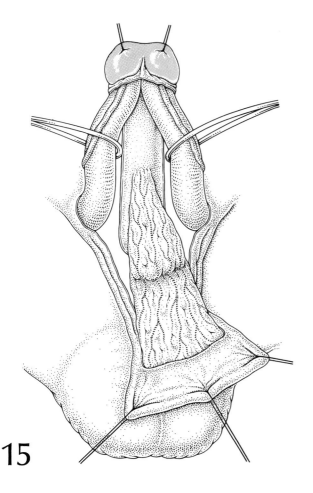

Mobilization of urethral plate

15 This step involves completely separating the urethral plate from the corpus cavernosum on each side so that the plate is free from the prostate proximally to the glans distally and can be transposed between the corpora on to the ventral surface of the penis. A vascular pedicle to the dartos muscle may be preserved.

Dissection commences proximally in the plane between the tough fibrous tissue of the corpora and the delicate spongy tissue of the urethral plate. By commencing the dissection proximally the process can move distally into a clear field if any bleeding is encountered. Alternate dorsal and ventral dissection is necessary until the urethral plate is completely free.

Dissection of neurovascular bundles and corporal bodies

16a, b The neurovascular bundles are well seen sweeping laterally and ventrally at the midpoint of the corpora. Artificial erection will show upward angulation of the corpora at the point where the neurovascular bundles move from the dorsal to the ventral surfaces of the corpora.

The neurovascular bundles are elevated and freed from the corpora. The corpora themselves are dissected free of adhesion to the pubic rami for 1–2 cm. Further dissection is not advantageous.

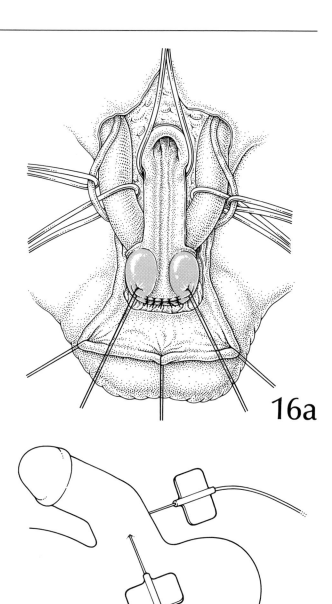

16a

16b

Tubularization of urethral plate

17 The urethral plate is now tubularized over a 10-Fr Silastic urethral stent or catheter. Interrupted 6/0 polydioxanone sutures are used. Urethral closure stops at the proximal end of the glans.

The urethra and dartos pedicle are displaced on to the ventral aspect of the penis.

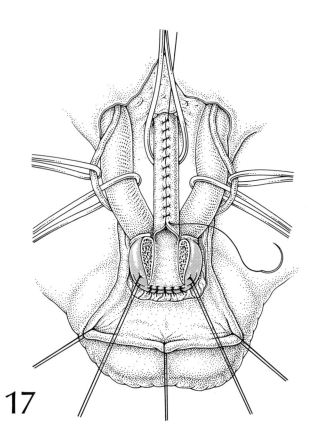

17

Chordee correction: cavernocavernostomy and corporal rotation

18 Cavernocavernostomy is performed in order to correct the distal corporal rotational abnormality and to secure the corpora in position. This corrects the upward chordee and serves to approximate the corpora on the dorsal aspect of the urethra.

An incision is made transversely in the dorsal aspect of each corpus at the site of maximum angulation. This incision opens as a diamond, elongating the dorsal surfaces of the corpora. The adjacent apices of each diamond are sutured together with double-ended 5/0 polypropylene (knots inside). Using a continuous stitch, the corpora are rotated through 90° as the two diamonds come face to face on the medial aspect of the corpora.

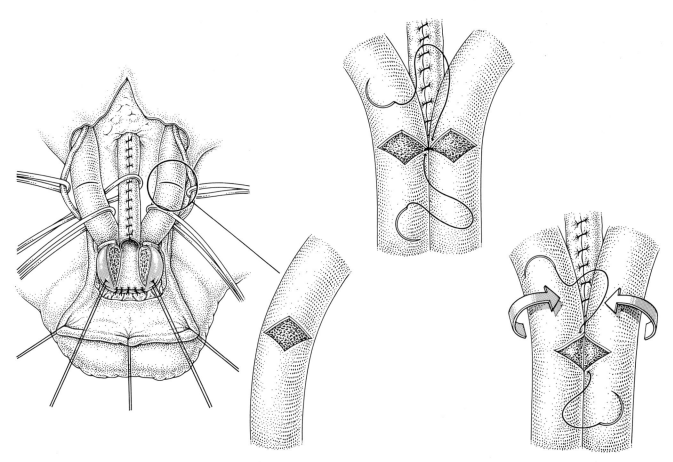

18

Glans closure

19 A broad strip of glans tissue is excised on each side and the glanular urethra closed. The flat raw surfaces of the glans are now brought together in two layers using vertical mattress sutures of 6/0 polydioxanone. The corporal rotation and approximation is reinforced between the site of the cavernocavernostomy and the glans using additional tacking sutures of 5/0 polydioxanone.

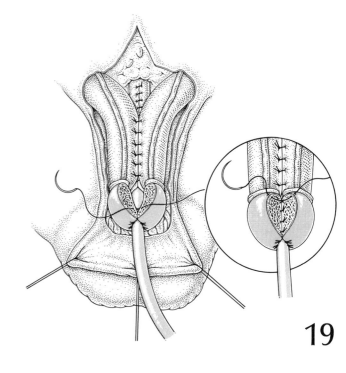

19

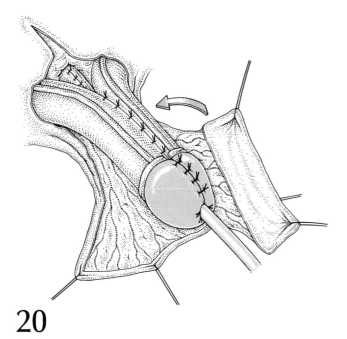

20

Mobilization of preputial skin

20 The inner layer of preputial skin is isolated on a vascular pedicle and brought on to the dorsal surface of the penis for skin cover. The ventral aspect is covered with the outer layer of preputial skin.

Skin closure

21 The transposed preputial skin may be deployed with its long axis lying either longitudinally or transversely on the dorsal aspect of the penis. Bilateral Z-plasty incisions at the base of the abdominal wall incision may be helpful in order to prevent scarring and retraction.

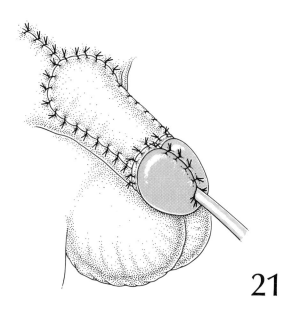

21

Postoperative care

Following bladder exstrophy repair a frog plaster with internal rotation of the hips, slight adduction and flexion of the knees provides effective immobilization and prevents troublesome hip flexion causing pooling of urine at the operation site. One of the most important factors for successful exstrophy closure is the maintenance of good stent and urethral catheter drainage. A high intravenous fluid intake is essential in the first few days after surgery to prevent crystalline deposits, to which the exstrophy patient seems very prone, from blocking these tubes. Ureteric stents are removed after 2 weeks, provided that wound healing is satisfactory. The plaster is maintained for 3–4 weeks. The neonate returns to theatre for an examination under anesthesia to ensure that there is a free urethral passage for urinary drainage before going home. Ultrasound review and repeat endoscopy is performed after 3 months.

After epispadias repair the penis is enclosed in a Silastic foam dressing for 1 week and the urethral catheter for 2 weeks. Bed rest for 1 week is advisable. Cystoscopy is performed 3 months after surgery.

Illustrations by Joanna Cameron

Ureterostomy

A. M. K. Rickwood MA, FRCS
Paediatric Urological Surgeon, Royal Liverpool Children's NHS Trust, Alder Hey, Liverpool, UK

History

During a period spanning the 1960s and 1970s, many infants and children – principally those with posterior urethral valves, neuropathic bladder and prune-belly syndrome – underwent urinary diversion by ureterostomy either as a temporary[1] or as a permanent[2] measure. Numbers of patients requiring a temporary ureterostomy have declined significantly because of the advent of percutaneous nephrostomy and cutaneous vesicostomy, and those requiring a permanent diversion have declined because of a better understanding of bladder dysfunction and its management.

Principles and justification

Cutaneous ureterostomy is advisable only with ureters that are substantially and chronically dilated. Mobilization of ureters of normal caliber to skin level risks ischemic necrosis, and this is also the case with acutely dilated ureters where vascularity tends to be attenuated. Ureterostomies should be fashioned proximally or distally; exteriorization of the mid ureter may cause problems with any subsequent reconstruction.

Proximal ureterostomies are for temporary diversion and aim to maximize free drainage of massively dilated and often atonic upper renal tracts. They are constructed as loop, Sober[3] or ring[4] formations; the advantage claimed for the last two is that when ureterostomies are formed bilaterally, as is usually the case, the bladder is not totally defunctioned. Distal

ureterostomies are for permanent, or at least long-term, diversion and are constructed as terminal stomas by detachment of the ureter from the bladder. As a rule both ureters are diverted to a single site, either by transureteroureterostomy or via a double-barrelled stoma.

Indications

Indications for ureterostomy are now few. Temporary proximal ureterostomy is preferred to percutaneous nephrostomy when drainage is likely to be necessary for an extended period. The principal indication is in the occasional male infant with posterior urethral valves in whom, after valve ablation, severe upper urinary tract dilatation persists and is compounded by compromised renal function, intractable urinary sepsis, or often both. As a rule, there is either ureteric atony or an element of ureterovesical obstruction, as can be demonstrated by antegrade pressure-perfusion studies; in the absence of these features, cutaneous vesicostomy is usually preferable. Exceptionally, similar considerations indicate proximal ureterostomy in infants with other forms of impaired bladder drainage, e.g. prune-belly syndrome or congenital neuropathic bladder.

The other indications for permanent or long-term distal ureterostomy include: (1) congenital neuropathic bladder, usually in patients with other major disabilities, where a more conservative approach has failed or is unrealistic. Those obliged to rely on a penile appliance or indwelling urethral catheter may consider an abdominal urinary stoma a preferable alternative; (2) vesical exstrophy, where further attempts to produce a continent bladder are unlikely to be rewarded; (3) miscellaneous conditions causing a combination of upper tract stasis and deteriorating renal function, when it is felt that diversion represents the best prospect of materially delaying the onset of end-stage renal failure.

In such cases, where there is chronic dilatation of one or both ureters, terminal ureterostomy has advantages over intestinal conduit diversion in being a lesser procedure and in avoiding the complications inherent in combined intestinal and urinary tract surgery.

Preoperative

Overall renal function should be ascertained and, where possible, individual renal function by radioisotope renography. Although the anatomy and degree of ureteric dilatation are usually adequately demonstrated by ultrasonography, it may be advantageous to assess ureteric peristalsis either by cystography, if there is vesicoureteric reflux, or by retrograde or antegrade contrast studies.

Better results can be anticipated in the presence of active ureteric peristalsis. Any electrolyte imbalance should be corrected as far as possible before the operation, and any urinary sepsis cleared or covered by appropriate antibiotic therapy. For distal terminal ureterostomy, a suitable stoma site must be selected; special care is necessary in patients with spinal deformities.

Anesthesia

General anesthesia is always employed.

Operations

PROXIMAL URETEROSTOMY

Incision

1 The exposure is common to all procedures. The patient is positioned obliquely, with the lumbar spine extended by a sandbag. The incision, about 5 cm long, extends downwards and forwards from the tip of the 11th or 12th rib, and for loop or ring ureterostomies, incorporates a shallow anterior or posterior V for formation of a skin bridge. The abdominal muscles are divided in the line of the skin incision.

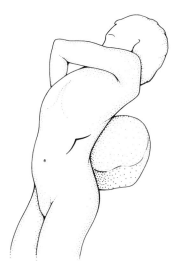

1

2 The peritoneum is retracted medially and the retroperitoneal space developed posteriorly to expose the proximal ureter, which is then freed from its bed to the level of the pelviureteric junction.

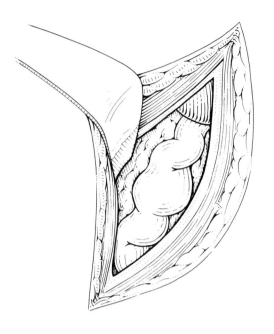

2

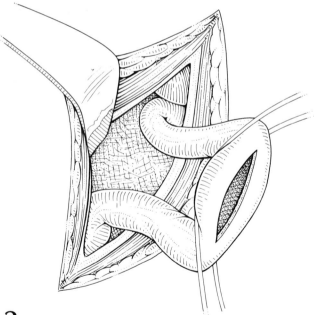

3

3 The ureter is usually tortuous, and division of the flimsy avascular adhesions uniting adjacent loops enables tension-free delivery to skin level without the need for dissection distally.

4 For a loop ureterostomy, the muscle layers are loosely approximated beneath the loop of the ureter.

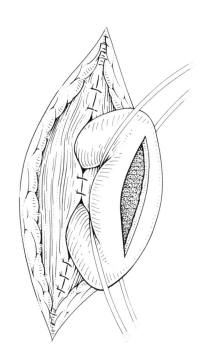

4

5 The skin bridge is anchored beneath the loop with non-absorbable sutures, e.g. 3/0 silk. The ureter at the apex of the loop is opened longitudinally and the ureteric wall sutured to the surrounding skin with 3/0 or 4/0 polyglactin (Vicryl) or coated polyglycolic acid (Dexon).

5

6 The ureteric and skin suture lines are completed. Although not routinely necessary, the proximal limb may be drained for a few days after operation via a fine (8–10-Fr) Foley catheter passed upwards to the renal pelvis.

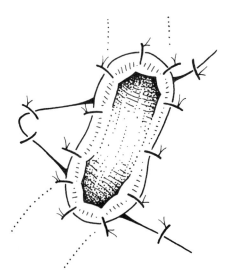

6

7 To construct a Sober ureterostomy[3] the ureteric loop is divided after mobilization at a level where the proximal limb lies comfortably at skin level. The distal limb is anastomosed to a corresponding aperture in the distal renal pelvis with interrupted 3/0 or 4/0 chromic catgut. The proximal limb is sutured to the skin as the stoma. External drainage of the anastomosis is provided via a 0.5-cm Penrose tube.

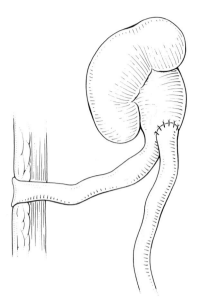

7

8 In the reversed Sober procedure, the distal limb of the ureteric loop forms the stoma while the proximal limb is anastomosed to it, en-Y, at a deeper level. This formation theoretically enhances onward urinary drainage, yet still adequately decompresses the upper urinary tract.

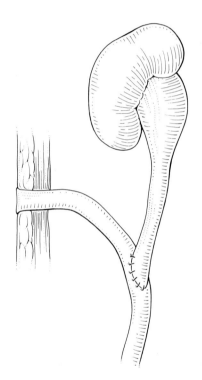

8

9 For a ring ureterostomy, both ureters are incised towards the base of the loop longitudinally for a distance corresponding to their diameter and are then anastomosed side-to-side by interrupted 3/0 or 4/0 chromic catgut sutures. If there is an element of secondary pelviureteric obstruction, the anastomosis can be constructed more proximally to the distal renal pelvis. The skin stoma is formed as for a loop ureterostomy, and the anastomosis is drained externally via a fine Penrose tube. With this formation the ureter is not divided, thus lessening the risk of ischemic necrosis.

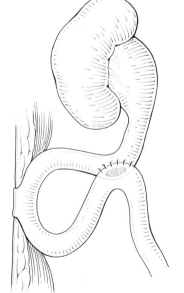

9

Closure of ureterostomy

10 With a Sober or ring ureterostomy, the stomal limb or limbs are mobilized to their confluence with the 'mainstream' of the urinary tract and are excised at this level. The ureteric defect is oversewn with a running 3/0 or 4/0 chromic catgut suture. Drainage can be external, via a Penrose tube, or internally via a percutaneous 6–8-gauge infant feeding tube entering the ureter distal to the suture line and running upwards to the renal pelvis.

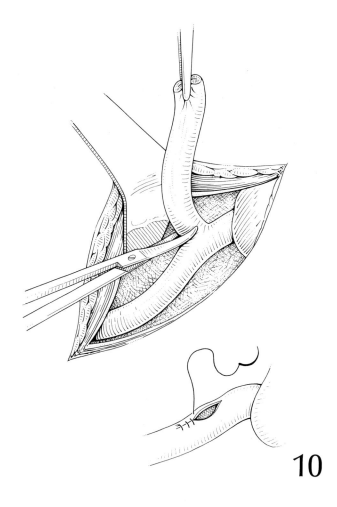

10

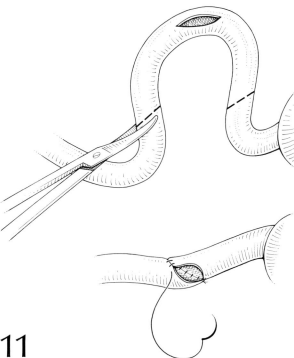

11 With a loop ureterostomy, both limbs are mobilized and then excised obliquely to enable a spatulated end-to-end anastomosis with 3/0 or 4/0 interrupted chromic catgut sutures. Drainage is as described above.

11

DISTAL URETEROSTOMY

Incision

12 The bladder is emptied with a urethral catheter. Access is transperitoneal, and in infants and most children adequate exposure is obtained through a high Pfannenstiel incision. A transverse, lower abdominal, muscle-cutting incision or midline subumbilical incision is preferable if difficulty is anticipated due to obesity or deformity.

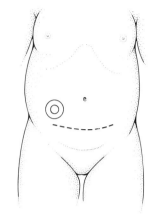

12

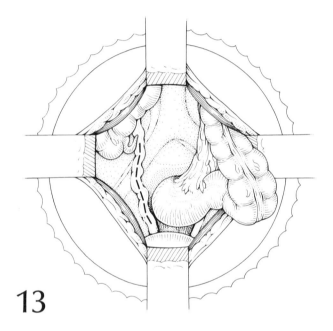

13

13 With the patient tilted slightly head downwards, the small intestine and cecum are packed upwards from the pelvis and a self-retaining (Denis Browne) ring retractor is inserted. Reflecting the sigmoid colon leftwards, the right ureter is identified as it crosses the iliac vessels, and an incision in the overlying peritoneum is carried downwards into the pelvis.

14 The pelvic ureter is mobilized with its surrounding adventitia, ligated close to the bladder with an absorbable suture and divided. Care should be taken to avoid excessive mobilization or damage to ureteric vasculature. The distal ureter is straightened, if necessary, by division of the flimsy adhesions uniting adjacent loops.

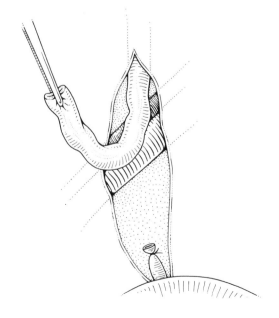

14

15 The sigmoid colon is reflected to the right, and the left ureter is similarly identified and mobilized.

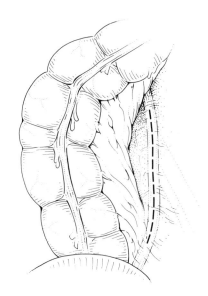

15

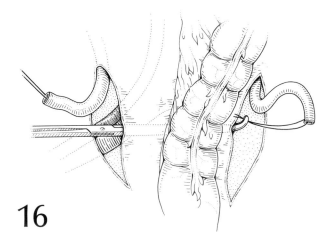

16

16 A tunnel is developed beneath the posterior peritoneum and sigmoid mesentery, commencing just above the pelvic brim and running slightly upwards away from the side of the stoma site. The chosen ureter is drawn through this tunnel and may be freed proximally along its lateral aspect for a few centimeters so that it follows a smooth curve medially.

17 If there is disparity between the diameter of the ureters, the larger is brought out ipsilaterally as the stoma and the smaller is anastomosed to it as a transureteroureterostomy. A V skin incision at the stoma site is deepened by cruciate division of the muscle layers to extraperitoneal level, from where a retroperitoneal tunnel of suitable caliber is developed by blunt dissection. The more dilated ureter is drawn through this tunnel, ensuring that it pursues a smooth path throughout.

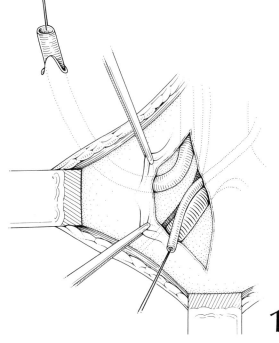

17

18 The smaller ureter is spatulated, and a corresponding incision is made in the larger ureter away from major ureteric vessels.

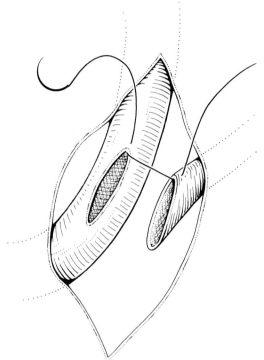

18

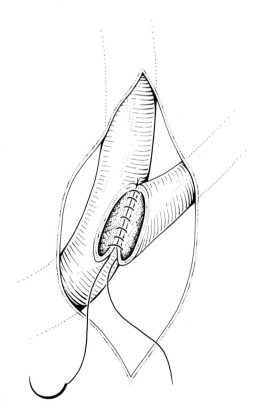

19

19 The posterior aspect of the anastomosis is constructed with a running all-layer suture of 3/0 or 4/0 chromic catgut. As a rule internal drainage is advisable, using 6–8-gauge infant feeding tubes, and these are most conveniently positioned at this stage, via the stomal limb and running up either ureter.

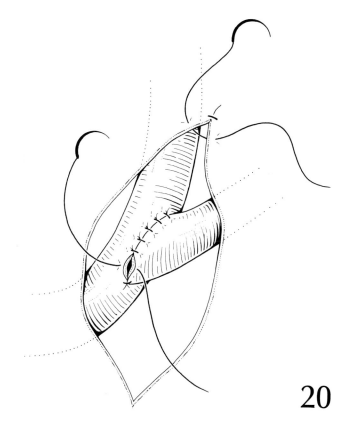

20 The anterior anastomosis is completed and then covered by closure of the retroperitoneum. External drainage of the anastomosis is unnecessary if internal ureteric drainage tubes are used.

20

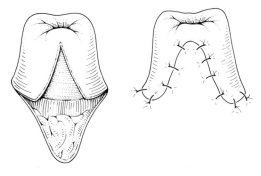

21

21 Where possible an everted stoma is formed, projecting about 1–1.5 cm. The risk of stomal stenosis is minimized by incorporating the V skin flap in the eversion. The stoma is sutured to the skin with 3/0 or 4/0 polyglactin or coated polyglycolic acid sutures.

22 When there is an insufficient length of ureter to form an everted stoma in the usual manner, skin flaps may be employed to achieve a similar effect.

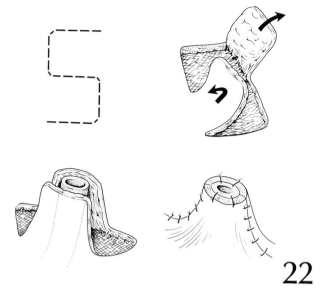

22

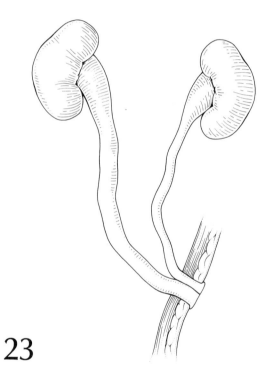

23

23 When both ureters are similarly dilated, a double-barrelled ureterostomy avoids the need for a transureteroureterostomy.

24 The two ureters are spatulated, conjoined distally, and then everted to form the stoma. It is usually unnecessary to drain this form of ureterostomy.

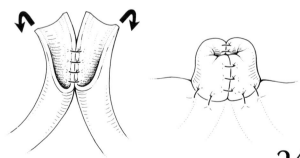

24

Postoperative care

Infants undergoing proximal ureterostomy tend to have precarious renal function, so that more than usual care is required with postoperative fluid and electrolyte balance. Severe natriuresis may follow relief of infantile obstructive uropathies. Antibiotic prophylaxis is advisable until free urinary drainage is established. Penrose tubes are removed once any urinary leakage has ceased.

Postoperative care of patients undergoing distal ureterostomy procedures follows the lines routinely adopted after any transperitoneal intervention. Nasogastric suction and intravenous fluids are usually advisable for 2–3 days after operation. Antibiotic prophylaxis is administered for as long as any internal drains remain *in situ*; with transureteroureterostomy, these are usually removed 5–7 days after operation.

Complications

Complications of loop and ring ureterostomies are rare except in the event of a major technical failure, e.g. a 180° twist on the ureteric loop. Ischemic necrosis of the stomal limb may complicate Sober procedures, and if extensive, necessitates abandonment of the ureterostomy and establishment of nephrostomy drainage.

Distal ureteric necrosis is the principal complication of distal ureterostomy. Minor degrees are manageable conservatively for 1–2 weeks, followed by mobilization of viable ureter to form a new stoma. More extensive necrosis necessitates conversion to a conduit diversion.

Outcome

Closure of proximal ureterostomies must be delayed until any bladder outflow obstruction, vesicoureteric reflux or ureterovesical obstruction has been corrected, and preferably until the distal ureter has acquired good peristalsis and more normal caliber. In many cases there has been appreciable permanent renal damage before initial treatment (and indeed often before birth), so that long-term prognosis must necessarily be cautious.

The short-term and medium-term results of terminal ureterostomies tend to be superior to those obtained with refluxing intestinal conduits[2], but in the long term this advantage may be lost[5], with recurrence of upper tract dilatation. Sometimes this has a remediable cause, e.g. stomal or substomal stenosis, or ureteroureteric stricture, but often the ureters lose effective peristaltic activity for no apparent reason. The resulting stasis may lead to stone formation, with a high rate of recurrence after removal or, less often, to end-stage renal failure.

References

1. Johnston JH. Temporary cutaneous ureterostomy in the management of advanced congenital urinary obstruction. *Arch Dis Child* 1963; 38: 161–6.

2. Shapiro SR, Peckler MS, Johnston JH. Transureteroureterostomy for urinary diversion in children. *Urology* 1976; 8: 35–8.

3. Sober I. Pelviureterostomy. *J Urol* 1972; 103: 473–5.

4. Williams DI, Cromie WJ. Ring ureteroureterostomy. *Br J Urol* 1975; 47: 789–92.

5. Rickwood AMK. Urinary diversion in children. In: Ashken MH, ed. *Urinary Diversion*. Berlin: Springer-Verlag, 1982: 22–58.

Surgical reconstruction of intersex abnormalities

Michael L. Gustafson MD
Surgical Research Fellow, Pediatric Research Laboratories, Massachusetts General Hospital, Boston, Massachusetts, USA

Patricia K. Donahoe MD
Marshall K. Bartlett Professor of Surgery, Massachusetts General Hospital, Boston, Massachusetts, USA

Principles and justification

For an infant to develop as an 'anatomically correct' male or female, a complex cascade of molecular and morphological events must occur during ontogeny. An embryo's *genetic sex* is determined by its chromosomal constituents, in particular genes on the X and Y chromosomes. The *gonadal sex*, or formation of an ovary or testis, is guided by these genes and other secondary pathways. The gonads, in turn, produce hormones that regulate differentiation of the internal and external genitalia, thus determining *phenotypic sex*. When an abnormality exists in one or more of the above steps, an intersex infant with incongruent genetic, gonadal and phenotypic sex results. The etiology of such ambiguous genitalia formation can be divided into four main categories: male pseudohermaphroditism, female pseudohermaphroditism, mixed gonadal dysgenesis and true hermaphroditism. Clinically, these intersex patients represent one of the great challenges in pediatric surgery. Their management demands accurate gender assignment, active participation in family support and counseling, and creative surgical interventions.

Male pseudohermaphrodites

By definition male pseudohermaphrodites have a 46XY karyotype but deficient masculinization of their external genitalia. This phenotype may result from abnormal testicular development, impaired testosterone biosynthesis or conversion to dihydrotestosterone (DHT), or decreased androgenic response of genital target tissues[1]. Males with the persistent müllerian duct syndrome are also included under this category as rare variants.

Deficiencies in several different enzymes of the steroid metabolism and androgen synthesis pathway, which are inherited as autosomal recessive traits, can result in deficient testosterone production. Deficiencies in 20–22 desmolase, 3β-hydroxysteroid dehydrogenase, and 17α-hydroxylase interfere with normal cortisol production as well, while 17–20 desmolase and 17-ketosteroid reductase defects result in isolated testosterone deficiency. Placental human chorionic gonadotrophin (hCG) is required for androgen production by the fetal testis, so placental insufficiency may also be associated with deficient masculinization. The inability to convert testosterone to DHT because of a steroid 5α-reductase deficiency results in a form of male pseudohermaphroditism referred to as pseudovaginal perineoscrotal hypospadias[2–4]. This autosomal recessive defect is characterized by normally differentiated testes but deficient external genitalia, with a clitoris-like phallus, severe perineoscrotal hypospadias and an undifferentiated prostatic utricle into which drain the Wolffian ducts.

The testicular feminization syndrome results from complete expression of a defect in androgen receptor function. This X-linked recessive trait leads to the formation of normal female external genitalia in an individual with a 46XY karyotype. Testes are often found in the labioscrotal folds, and therefore diagnosis is suspected in girls with bilateral inguinal hernias containing palpable gonads. Patients with the persistent müllerian duct syndrome are phenotypically normal 46XY males who typically present in later childhood with uterus inguinale (retained uterus and fallopian tubes in an inguinal hernia sac) and unilateral or bilateral cryptorchidism.

Female pseudohermaphrodites

Almost all cases of female pseudohermaphrodites are secondary to congenital adrenal hyperplasia, an autosomal disorder caused by one of several adrenal steroid synthetic enzyme deficiencies, of which 21-hydroxylase is the most common[5]. Overproduction of adrenal androgens secondary to adrenocorticotrophic hormone stimulation produces a virilized female phenotype, with prostatic enlargement and masculinization of the external genitalia. Müllerian duct structures form normally in the absence of müllerian inhibiting substance (MIS) but the distal vagina fails to reach the perineum. In the most severe anomaly, referred to as high vaginal atresia, the proximal urethra is conjoined to a highly shortened vagina.

Mixed gonadal dysgenesis

Patients with mixed gonadal dysgenesis are characterized by disordered formation, early senescence and neoplastic transformation of their gonadal tissue[6,7]. Many of these 45X/46XY, 46XY or 45XO patients have a dysgenetic testis on one side and a streak ovary on the other, although considerable gonadal variability can occur, such as unilateral gonadal agenesis, bilateral streak gonads and unilateral gonadal tumors[7,8]. In the absence of appropriate gonadal induction as a testis, seminiferous tubular differentiation does not occur and MIS is produced only poorly or too late, leading to retention of müllerian ducts. Leydig cell differentiation may be deficient or delayed, resulting in subnormal or late production of testosterone and incomplete masculinization. Ovarian tissue is also poorly differentiated, probably due to the absence of a second X chromosome.

True hermaphrodites

True hermaphrodites have both testicular and ovarian tissue that is well developed and non-dysgenetic[9]. Such patients usually have a 46XX karyotype, although 46XY karyotypes and complex mosaicisms have been reported. The two gonadal tissue types may be present in a wide variety of combinations; they often occur together to form ovotestes or appear separately as a testis on one side and an ovary on the other. Müllerian duct structures are often present on the side of the ovary but regress on the side of the testicular gonad.

Assignment of gender

The primary consideration during the assignment of gender in intersex patients is the potential for future sexual and reproductive function, which is largely dependent on the size of the phallus and the ability of the external genitalia to respond to androgenic stimulation. It is only when patients present during early infancy with a sex assignment that would not permit sexual function despite aggressive medical and surgical treatment that reassignment is warranted. In intersex children presenting later, the authors generally support the previously assigned sex, because gender identity has often been established and a change could have devastating consequences.

The mean stretched phallic length in the term infant is 3.5 cm (3rd to 97th percentile 2.8–4.2 cm); in premature infants, mean length at 34 and 28 weeks is 2.8 and 2.2 cm respectively[10]. The mean width at term is 1.1 cm (3rd to 97th percentile 0.9–1.3 cm), at 34 weeks 0.9 cm and at 28 weeks 0.8 cm. If the phallus in a term infant is less than 1.5×0.7 cm, insufficient phallic growth is likely and female gender assignment is recommended; this is particularly true for the syndrome of complete androgen resistance. In contrast, phallic growth in patients with 5α-reductase deficiency, hypopituitarism or true hermaphroditism is adequate in response to early testosterone therapy. This confirms androgenic response of the genital structures, often results in an adequate phallic size before toilet training, and avoids gender uncertainty by caretakers. The response in the severely affected patient with chordee and a hypospadiac penis at the penoscrotal junction can be striking. Reconstruction involves release of chordee, staged hypospadias repair and correction of the prepenile bifid scrotum; removal of retained müllerian duct structures and/or orchiopexy may also be indicated[1,11].

In patients with male pseudohermaphroditism, mixed gonadal dysgenesis, true hermaphroditism to whom female gender is assigned and all patients with female pseudohermaphroditism, surgical reconstruction consists of clitoral recession, labioscrotal reduction and exteriorization or construction of a vagina[12,13]. An abnormal communication between the reproductive and urinary tracts at the verumontanum of the urethra is usually present in these patients, creating a urogenital sinus defect. The vast majority of such patients have a vagina which enters the urethra distal to the external urethral sphincter but in a small percentage a high short vagina enters the urogenital sinus proximal to this sphincter, creating a phenotype known as high vaginal atresia. These patients almost always have severely masculinizing congenital adrenal hyperplasia[14].

Early one-stage repair of patients in the first group is generally undertaken at 3–6 months of age, but may also be performed in the neonatal period if the social situation dictates. Staged repair of the second group of children has traditionally consisted of early clitoral recession and labioscrotal reduction, followed by vaginal pull-through at 2–4 years of age[11–15], but this requires two operations and has a high incidence of vaginal stenosis. Early one-stage surgical reconstruction has been shown to be favorable in these patients[16]. Bilateral rotated buttock flaps may be used to augment the vaginal introitus, as a secondary procedure in patients in whom stenosis has occurred after primary pull-through, or in those in whom vaginal exteriorization has been delayed until after infancy, when very little perineal tissue remains to augment the introitus and the pelvis has elongated[17]. If no vaginal remnant is present, as is the case in male pseudohermaphrodites with no retained müllerian ducts, vaginal replacement is performed in late adolescence.

Operations

PERINEAL RECONSTRUCTION IN INFANTS RAISED AS MALES

Severe penoscrotal deformities encountered in male pseudohermaphrodites are often more safely repaired in multiple stages. The smaller the phallus, the later the institution of reconstructive procedures to correct the chordee. During the first operation, all ventral fibrous tissue is removed down to and proximal to the bifurcation of the corpora cavernosa to allow straightening of the penile shaft. A second operation is then performed 6 months later to create a neourethra from the distal end of the native urethra (exiting at the penile midshaft, penoscrotal junction or perineum) to the tip of the glans. This is accomplished using a composite graft constructed from adjacent tubularized midscrotal tissue, dorsal perineal flaps and/or a free mucosal bladder graft. A third, much delayed, procedure involves correction of prepenile and bifid scrotal deformities. Placement of a testicular prosthesis may need to be considered at a later stage.

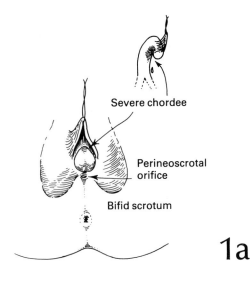

1a

First stage of hypospadias repair

1a–c A circumferential incision is made 2 mm below the corona of the glans. The chordee is released by excising ventral scar from Buck's fascia outward, carrying the excision well beyond the bifurcation of the corpora. The remainder of the penis is degloved on its dorsal and lateral aspect and the dorsal hooded foreskin unfolded to form one layer; this tissue is then transferred to the ventral surface by creating either bilateral Byars' flaps or a midline button hole.

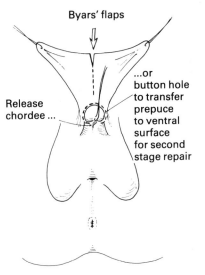

1b

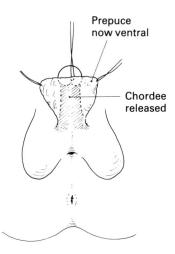

1c

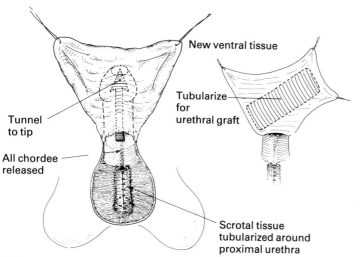

New ventral tissue

Tunnel to tip

All chordee released

Tubularize for urethral graft

Scrotal tissue tubularized around proximal urethra

2a

Second stage of hypospadias repair

2a–c Midscrotal tissue is tubularized around the meatal opening and a Jackson–Pratt stent to create the proximal neourethra. A tunnel for the remainder of the neourethra is then created flat against the corpora cavernosa from this point to the tip of the glans. A rectangular graft of skin is harvested from the now ventral foreskin flap, defatted, tubularized around the Jackson–Pratt stent, and joined to the proximal neourethral tissue. Multiple layers are used to close the ventral penile shaft, particularly over the proximal anastomosis; excess foreskin is used for exterior reconstruction. Occasionally the glans must be split to complete second-stage repair. In this case, closure of the glans around the distal graft and stent can be augmented by advancing ventral subcoronal skin.

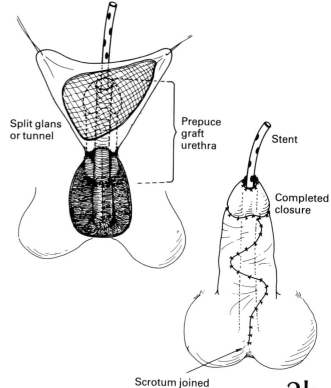

Split glans or tunnel

Prepuce graft urethra

Stent

Completed closure

Scrotum joined

2b

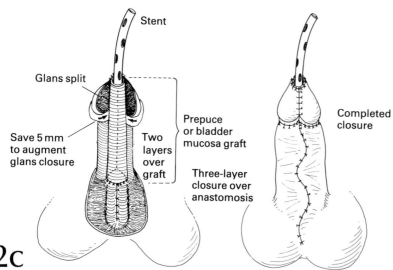

Stent

Glans split

Save 5 mm to augment glans closure

Two layers over graft

Prepuce or bladder mucosa graft

Three-layer closure over anastomosis

Completed closure

2c

Bladder graft to form neourethra

3a–d If local tissue is insufficient for creation of a neourethra, bladder mucosa may be used for neourethral extension. The bladder is opened in the midline through the serosa and muscularis, leaving the mucosa intact. The bladder mucosal graft is then carefully measured, harvested, tubularized over a fenestrated stent, anastomosed to the proximal neourethra in a beveled fashion, tunneled to the meatus, and sutured to the tip. These grafts may stenose at the meatus, and should be dilated with a metal sound 2 weeks after surgery for another 2–3 weeks. Longitudinal trim may be required later, because these fragile grafts tend to stretch.

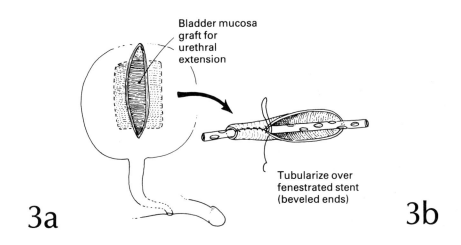

Bladder mucosa graft for urethral extension

Tubularize over fenestrated stent (beveled ends)

3a   3b

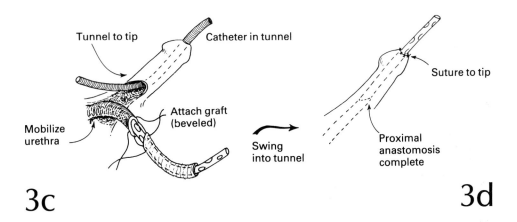

Tunnel to tip   Catheter in tunnel

Mobilize urethra

Attach graft (beveled)

Swing into tunnel

Suture to tip

Proximal anastomosis complete

3c   3d

Repair of the prepenile scrotum

4a–f Intersex children often have a bifid shortened scrotum associated with scrotal tissue anterior to the dorsal base of the penis. This anomaly is repaired by displacing scrotal skin posteriorly and the penis anteriorly. The base of the penis is advanced forward onto the anterior abdominal wall by creating a square, distally based flap which circumscribes the base of the penis. This is dropped distally to restore normal scrotal length. The abdominal wall is then undermined and swung around the base of the penis to join ventrally in the midline. It is important to mobilize the anterior abdominal wall flaps sufficiently so that midline separation does not occur. The scrotum is then closed in the midline and laterally.

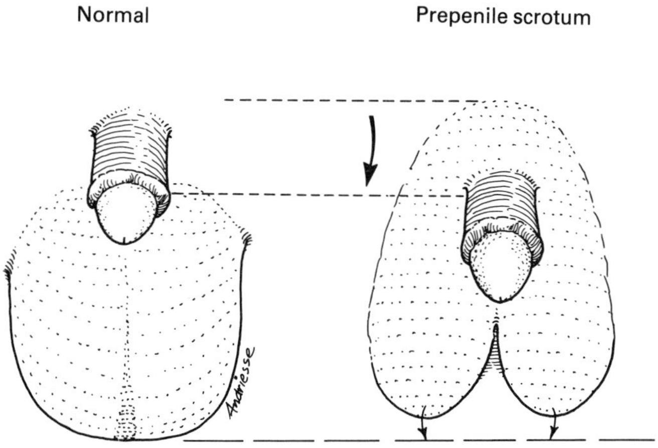

4a

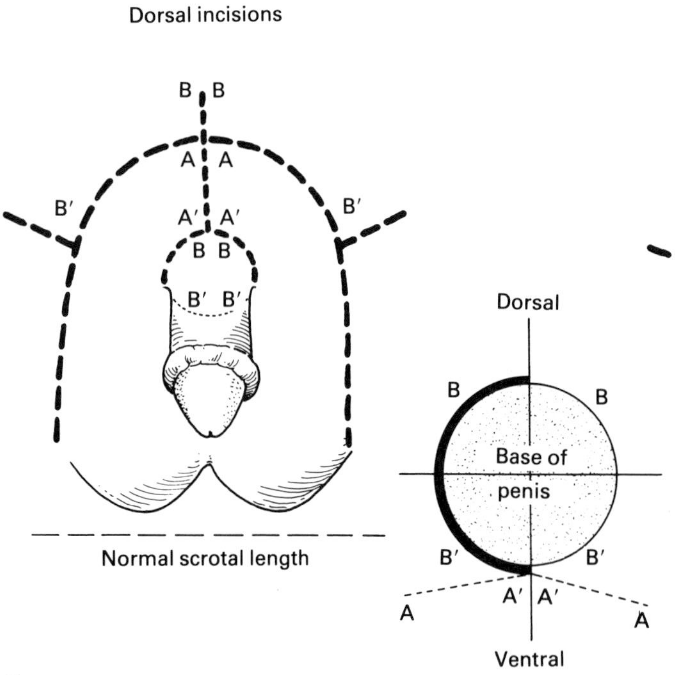

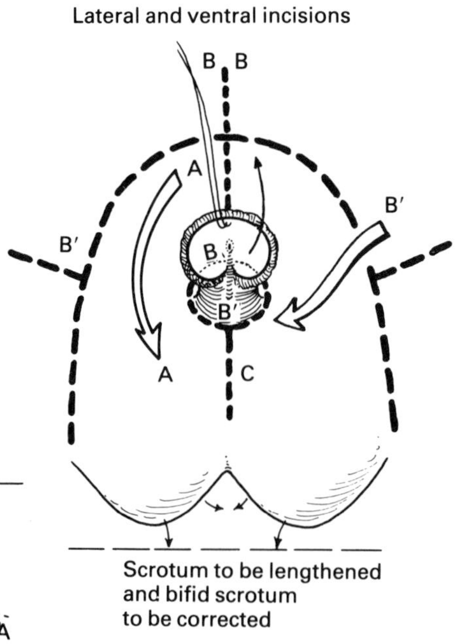

4b

4c

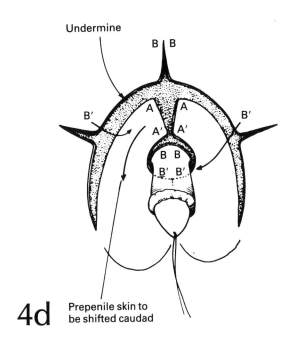

4d

Undermine

Prepenile skin to
be shifted caudad

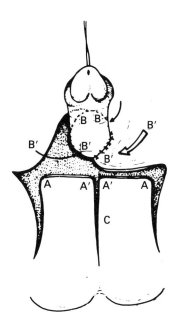

4e

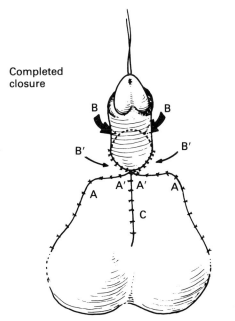

Completed
closure

4f

Removal of retained müllerian ducts and creation of a neoseminal vesicle

5a–c In males with retained müllerian ducts the vas deferens often lies within the side wall of the dilated vagina; its course, however, cannot usually be palpated in the thickened vaginal wall. Therefore a strip of vagina surrounding the predicted course of the vas is preserved when the uterus and vagina are resected. The vaginal strip is then turned in and tubularized from the proximal vas to the point of union with the urethra using interrupted sutures.

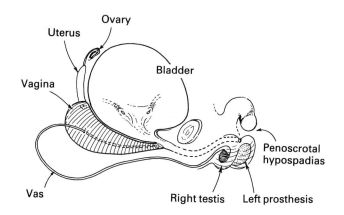

5a

PERINEAL RECONSTRUCTION IN INFANTS RAISED AS FEMALES

The first step in the surgical evaluation of intersex children assigned the female gender should be cystoscopy to determine whether the vagina enters the urogenital sinus distal or proximal to the external urethral sphincter. The former anatomy is found in 95% of these cases, including infants with mixed gonadal dysgenesis, true hermaphroditism and less severely masculinizing forms of the adrenogenital syndrome. Their management calls for combined clitoral recession, labioscrotal reduction, and flap vaginoplasty at 1–6 months of age. The remaining 5% of children represent the most severely masculinizing forms of congenital adrenal hyperplasia.

Although the genital and vaginal tissues are certainly more fragile during infancy, early combined repair of clitoromegaly, labial scrotal hypertrophy and high vaginal atresia is no more difficult than delayed vaginal exteriorization at age 2–4 years[16], the age at which reconstruction has been recommended. In fact, the tissues are more mobile at this early stage. In addition, labia minora flaps can be used to fill in below the recessed clitoris and labia majora flaps used to augment the lateral vaginal introitus. Advancing the anterior island of perineal skin inferiorly also has the advantage of displacing the abnormally high urethral meatus toward a more normal posterior position. Paradoxically, bilateral rotated buttock flaps are more often required to complete vaginal exteriorization if the repair is delayed[17], most probably due to the vagina being pulled further back up into the pelvis with growth. The authors have also used these flaps to augment the introitus in patients referred with vaginal stenosis following previous vaginal exteriorization procedures.

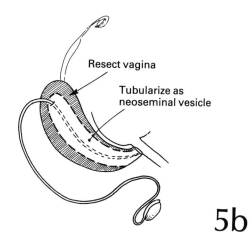

5b

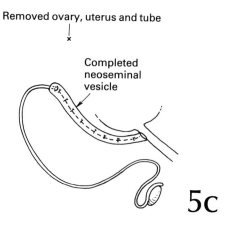

5c

Clitoral recession, labioscrotal reduction and flap vaginoplasty for high vaginal atresia

6 In a lateral view of the pelvis of a patient with high vaginal atresia the urethrovaginal fistula is seen proximal to the external urethral sphincter. A Fogarty balloon catheter inserted into the vagina provides orientation during dissection from below, while a Foley catheter drains the urinary bladder.

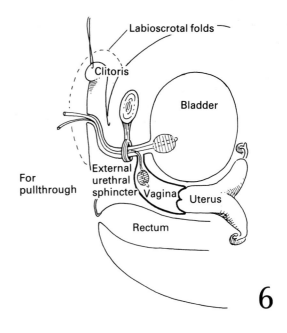

7 Dissection begins by creating an inverted U flap based posteriorly on the rectum. The Fogarty and Foley catheters exit from the anteriorly displaced urethral meatus.

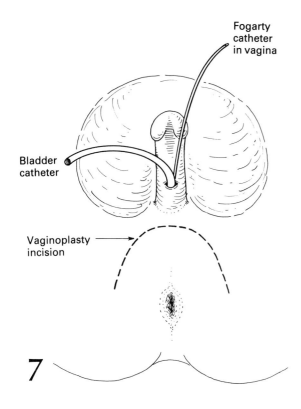

8 Careful dissection and full mobilization of the posterior vaginal wall from the anterior rectal wall are essential. This is performed with the operator's finger in the rectum.

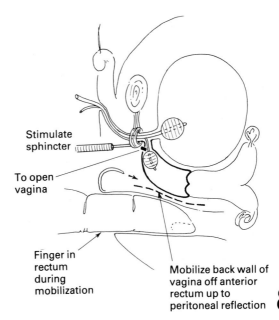

9 The external urethral sphincter should be identified with the nerve stimulator and the distal vagina
opened just below its confluence with the proximal
urethra.

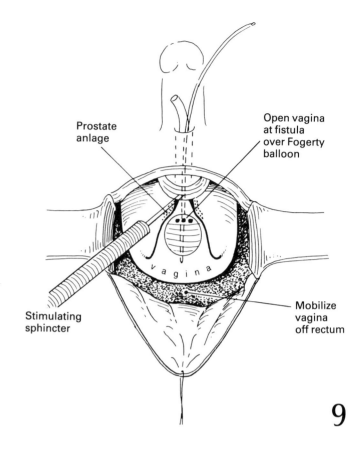

Prostate
anlage

Open vagina
at fistula
over Fogerty
balloon

Stimulating
sphincter

Mobilize
vagina
off rectum

v a g i n a

9

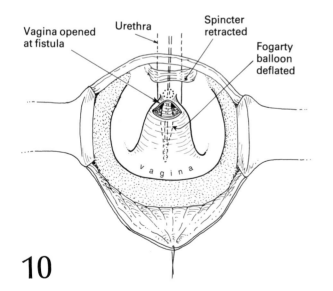

Vagina opened
at fistula

Urethra

Spincter
retracted

Fogarty
balloon
deflated

v a g i n a

10

10 With the external sphincter retracted, the
posterior wall of the vagina is opened and the
Fogarty balloon deflated.

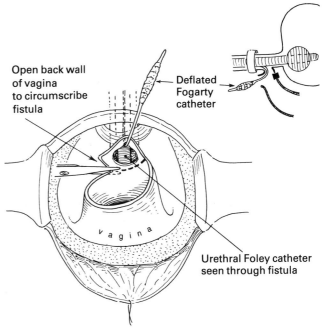

11 The Fogarty catheter is then passed out of the vaginal opening and retracted superiorly. This allows the Foley catheter to be seen in the proximal urethra through the urethrovaginal opening. The posterior wall of the fistula is circumscribed sharply under direct vision.

11

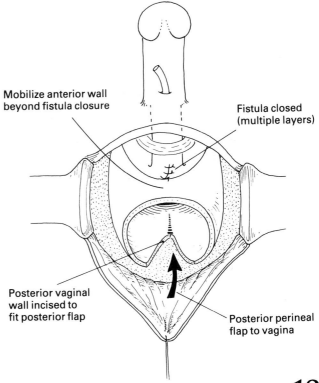

12 The urethra is closed longitudinally with interrupted sutures and the anterior vaginal wall mobilized forward by dissection from the bladder neck. The posterior vaginal wall is opened in the midline to widen the introitus before turning in the posterior inverted U flap.

12

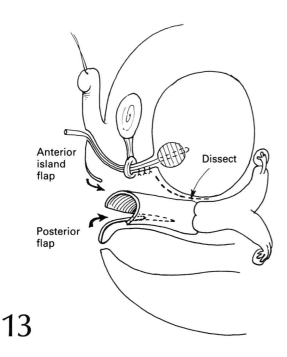

13

13 Mobilization of the vagina from the bladder neck is essential to avoid apposition of suture lines at the urethrovaginal fistula closure site. Following clitoral recession, the vagina is ready for anastomosis to the anterior island and posterior U flaps.

14 The skin of the clitoris is circumscribed just below the glans. Ventral dissection releases an anterior island of skin on the perineum. Dorsal shaft skin is dissected to the corporal bifurcation and then divided in the midline to create bilateral Byars' flaps. The dorsal neurovascular bundle is carefully dissected and retracted upward to allow resection of the mid body of the clitoral shaft to this same level.

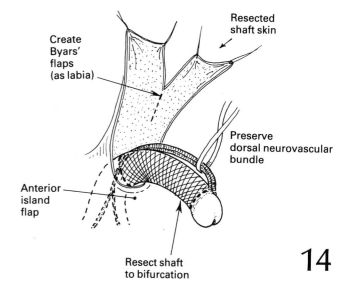

14

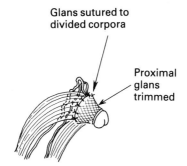

15

15 Following resection of the mid body of the clitoris, the glans is trimmed to a normal size and sutured to the base of the transected corpora cavernosa.

16 The posterior inverted U flap has been turned into the divided posterior vaginal wall to augment the introitus. Byars' and labioscrotal flaps are advanced posteriorly to create labia minora and majora, respectively. The Byars' flaps are also used to fill in the defect below the recessed clitoris and to allow the anterior perineal island flap to be advanced inferiorly and inward to augment the introitus anteriorly.

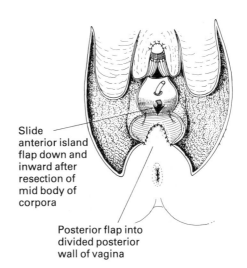

Slide anterior island flap down and inward after resection of mid body of corpora

Posterior flap into divided posterior wall of vagina

16

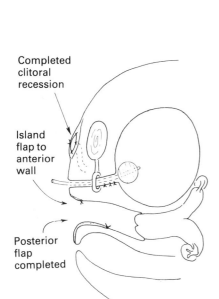

Completed clitoral recession

Island flap to anterior wall

Posterior flap completed

17

17 The urethral meatus in the anterior island flap should be displaced to a more normal position. Aggressive mobilization of the vagina both anteriorly and posteriorly brings it to the perineum without tension.

18 The introitus of the mobilized vagina is augmented by the posterior U flap, the anterior perineal island and labioscrotal folds. Byars' flaps and labioscrotal folds are advanced posteriorly to create labia minora and majora with a normal appearance.

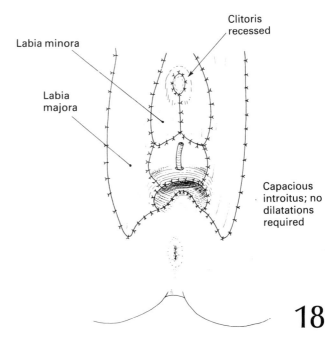

Clitoris recessed

Labia minora

Labia majora

Capacious introitus; no dilatations required

18

Acknowledgments

Illustrations 1–4 have been modified from ref 11, *Illustration 5* from ref 18 and *Illustrations 6–18* from ref 16 with permission of the publishers.

References

1. Donahoe PK, Crawford JD, Hendren WH. Management of neonates and children with male pseudohermaphroditism. *J Pediatr Surg* 1977; 12: 1045–57.

2. Opitz JM, Simpson JL, Sarto GE *et al*. Pseudovaginal perineoscrotal hypospadias. *Clin Genet* 1972; 3: 1–26.

3. Walsh PC, Madden JD, Harrod MJ, Goldstein JL, MacDonald PC, Wilson JD. Familial incomplete male pseudohermaphroditism, type 2: Decreased dihydrotestosterone formation in pseudovaginal perineoscrotal hypospadias. *N Engl J Med* 1974; 291: 944–9.

4. Peterson RE, Imperato-McGinley J, Gautier T *et al*. Male pseudohermaphroditism due to steroid 5-α-reductase deficiency. *Am J Med* 1977; 62: 170–91.

5. Miller WT, Levine LS. Molecular and clinical advances in congenital adrenal hyperplasia. *J Pediatr* 1987; 111: 1–17.

6. Federman DD. *Abnormal Sexual Development: A Genetic and Endocrine Approach to Differential Diagnosis*. Philadelphia: WB Saunders, 1967.

7. Donahoe PK, Crawford JD, Hendren WH. Mixed gonadal dysgenesis, pathogenesis and management. *J Pediatr Surg* 1979; 14: 287–300.

8. Robboy SJ, Miller T, Donahoe PK *et al*. Dysgenesis of testicular and streak gonads in the syndrome of mixed gonadal dysgenesis. *Hum Pathol* 1982; 13: 700–16.

9. Donahoe PK, Crawford JD, Hendren WH. True hermaphroditism: A clinical description and a proposed function for the long arm of the Y chromosome. *J Pediatr Surg* 1978; 13: 293.

10. Feldman KW, Smith DW. Fetal phallic growth and penile standards for newborn male infants. *J Pediatr* 1975; 86: 395–8.

11. Donahoe PK, Powell DM, Lee MM. Clinical management of intersex abnormalities. In: Wells SA, ed. *Current Problems in Surgery*. St. Louis: Mosby-Year Book, 1991: 515–79.

12. Hendren WH, Donahoe PK. Correction of congenital abnormalities of the vagina and perineum. *J Pediatr Surg* 1980; 15: 751–63.

13. Donahoe PK, Hendren WH III. Perineal reconstruction in ambiguous genitalia infants raised as females. *Ann Surg* 1984; 200: 363–71.

14. Donahoe PK, Crawford JD. Ambiguous genitalia in the newborn. In: Welch KJ, Randolph JG, Ravitch MM *et al*., eds. *Pediatric Surgery*. Chicago: Year Book Medical Publishers, 1986: 1374–5.

15. Hendren WH, Crawford JD. Adrenogenital syndrome: The anatomy of the anomaly and its repair: some new concepts. *J Pediatr Surg* 1969; 4: 49–58.

16. Donahoe PK, Gustafson ML. Early one-stage surgical reconstruction of the extremely high vagina in patients with congenital adrenal hyperplasia. *J Pediatr Surg* 1994; 29: 352–8.

17. Dumanian GA, Donahoe PK. Bilateral rotated buttock flaps for vaginal atresia in severely masculinized females with adrenogenital syndrome. *J Plast Reconstr Surg* 1992; 90: 487–91.

18. Donahoe PK. Neoseminal vesicle created from retained Müllerian duct to preserve the vas in male infants. *J Pediatr Surg* 1988; 23: 272–4.

Illustrations by Peter Cox

Myelomeningocele

Karin M. Muraszko MD
Assistant Professor of Pediatric Neurosurgery, C.S. Mott Children's Hospital, University of Michigan, Ann Arbor, Michigan, USA

Principles and justification

Myelomeningocele is the most severe of the spinal dysraphic states and still the most common, though its incidence is decreasing with improved prenatal maternal nutrition and through the availability of prenatal screening mechanisms[1,2]. Myelomeningocele is a central nervous system fusion defect. Neural tube defects affect females more frequently than males and there have been clusters of increased incidence of myelomeningoceles in certain populations such as the Irish, British, Sikhs, and the Egyptians of Alexandria. Siblings of an affected child show an increased risk for neural tube defects when compared with the general population. The rate of recurrence ranges from about 1% to nearly 10% in different series. A clear correlation between maternal diet and neural tube defects has been determined. A seven-fold reduction in neural tube defects has been achieved with folate and vitamin supplementation during pregnancy.

Embryology

The central nervous system begins as a focal proliferation of ectoderm. The central groove develops and forms two folds of neural tissue. At approximately gestational day 20–28, the lips of this fold touch and the tube fuses. The fusion of this fold starts at the center to eventually become the craniovertebral junction. This fusion proceeds in a caudal and cephalic direction. The caudal section is the last to close. A plane develops between the neural ectoderm which has fused and the overlying superficial ectoderm. Between these layers migrate mesenchymal cells which give rise to the arch of the vertebrae and the paraspinal muscles. Myelomeningocele represents a failure of fusion of the neural fold, leaving the vertebral arches open and the unfused spinal cord or neural placode either exposed or covered by a thin membrane. It is important to distinguish a myelomeningocele from less severe defects such as meningoceles which consist only of a spinal fluid-filled sac with meningeal and cutaneous coverings. Meningoceles contain no spinal elements but can occasionally contain some nerve roots. True meningoceles are rare. Lipomyelomeningoceles are usually covered by well developed dermal elements and fat and consist of spina bifida with associated abnormalities of the spinal cord and extension of fat into the spinal canal.

Associated problems

Like most congenital anomalies, spina bifida is a spectrum of disorders. Myelomeningocele represents the most severe of these spinal dysraphic states and includes anomalies of the brain such as the Chiari II malformation and hydrocephalus, and has implications for other organ systems such as the genitourinary and musculoskeletal systems. Most children with myelomeningocele have some degree of weakness of their lower extremities and many have significant orthopedic problems. As a result of denervation, muscle imbalance ensues and can result in abnormalities at the hip, knee and foot. Anesthesia of various portions of the skin can lead to pressure sores, particularly later in life. Anorectal neuropathy may cause a variety of defecatory dysfunctions.

Urologic abnormalities are common in children with myelomeningocele and are best managed with intermittent catheterization. Careful follow-up with evaluation of kidney and bladder function is extremely important.

The cornerstone of management of children with myelomeningocele is a multidisciplinary team that treats and assesses the various needs of both the child and the family. The development of cerebrospinal fluid diversionary devices (shunts) in the 1950s has allowed these children to be successfully managed and has dramatically changed the outlook for them.

Selection criteria

The controversial discussion about the selection of children for myelomeningocele repair has largely subsided as more effective means of diagnosis and treatment have been developed. Before the development of successful methods of treating hydrocephalus, selection of candidates for non-treatment was commonly practiced[3]. With shunting devices available the cognitive outcome for these children has significantly improved and, in most centers, children with myelomeningocele receive early repair. Although discussion among various groups including ethicists, clerics, jurists, administrators, legislators and physicians still continues, most children now receive repair of their myelomeningocele and are treated by a team with a variety of specialists. At best, selection criteria as to which children should not be repaired are inconsistent. Studies which discuss the outcome of such unrepaired children must be viewed cautiously, as many who were not initially treated received later repair, and not all who were left unrepaired died as had been anticipated[4]. The ease of care of children with myelomeningocele is greatly improved following repair, and thus even chronic care facilities often will not accept children with open defects. Unless associated additional central nervous system defects or other congenital anomalies are of such a magnitude as to suggest that meaningful survival is unlikely, repair of the child with myelomeningocele is now standard.

Preoperative

Assessment

The principles involved in the repair of children with myelomeningocele consist initially of a complete evaluation of the child including detailed physical and neurologic examination. Ultrasonographic imaging of the head, spine above and below the area of defect, and kidneys can be an important adjuvant to constructing a surgical plan for an individual child. If there are any associated intracranial or spinal abnormalities on ultrasonographic examination, computed tomographic scanning or magnetic resonance imaging should be performed to evaluate these abnormalities more carefully. Radiographs of the spine can identify additional anomalies (e.g. diastematomyelia) which may require

repair at the time of initial surgery. Blood should be cross-matched and available.

Preparation

Infants born with myelomeningocele require the skilled services of a multidisciplinary team. After initial determination of cardiorespiratory stability the child may be transferred to an appropriate institution. The lesion itself should be covered with moist sterile gauze dressings surrounded by a protective plastic sheet. The use of sponges impregnated with bacitracin ointment covered by a thin plastic layer is recommended to prevent additional skin breakdown.

Emergency operative intervention is seldom necessary in neonates with myelomeningocele. The repair can be safely carried out within the first 48–72 h after delivery. Delaying closure for more prolonged periods may increase the risk of central nervous system infection and may decrease motor function by increasing the trauma to the exposed neural placode. Deterioration of motor function occurred in children left untreated and a 37% incidence of ventriculitis was found in children in whom repair was delayed[5,6].

Most myelomeningoceles are in the lumbosacral region, although they can occur anywhere along the spinal cord. Assessment with good spinal ultrasonography can help to alert the surgeon to associated anomalies such as diastematomyelia, arachnoid cysts and intradural masses such as dermoids which may complicate the repair of the myelomeningocele. If significant hydrocephalus is found on preoperative ultrasonography, concurrent shunting of the child should be considered. If ventriculomegaly is mild to moderate, shunting need not be performed at the same operation as the myelomeningocele repair. Most children will, however, require shunting in the first days to months of life. It should also be borne in mind that unshunted children are more likely to leak from their repair site and thus to experience more problems with breakdown of the repair site and associated infections.

Anesthesia

General endotracheal anesthesia with overhead warming lights is appropriate. Occasionally, intraoperative use of a nerve stimulator is necessary to distinguish functioning nerve roots so paralytic agents must be used appropriately and no longer be present when stimulation is planned. Intravenous lines must be of sufficient size to accommodate blood transfusion. Careful assessment of blood loss is necessary as blood loss can be significant, particularly when rotational flaps are employed. A Foley catheter is generally used for bladder drainage and proves a useful adjunct in keeping the repair site clean and dry during the postoperative period.

Operation

Position of patient

1 Repair of the myelomeningocele is performed with the child in the prone position. Careful attention to the position of the neck is important, as almost all children with myelomeningocele have Chiari II malformations and most will also have hydrocephalus. Positioning of the head, which is often large, must therefore be done to avoid undue kinking of the internal jugular veins and undue extension or flexion of the cervical spine. The abdomen must be hanging free so that intra-abdominal pressure is not increased. Increases in intra-abdominal pressure lead to compression of Batson's venous plexus and result in increased engorgement and bleeding by epidural veins. The author has found that the use of a foam rubber donut which has been cut out at the top and bottom acts as an excellent bolster. Various bolsters and rolls have been employed with the goal always to allow the abdomen to be hanging free. Careful attention to positioning of the upper extremities to avoid brachial plexus stretching is necessary. The lower extremities also require careful positioning and padding as congenital dislocation of the hips and multiple orthopedic anomalies are often present.

The central neural placode and membranous areas are cleansed with sterile saline and the surrounding areas of skin are cleansed with an iodinated solution. Iodinated solutions should not be applied directly to the neural placode. Most surgeons find magnifying loupes useful. Occasionally the operating microscope can also be of benefit. Bipolar electrocoagulation should be available as it is employed throughout the procedure to control bleeding.

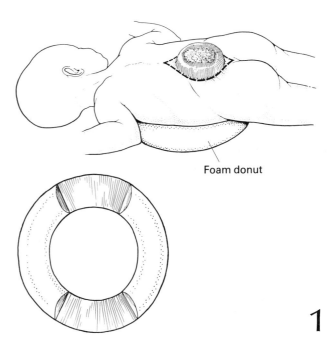

Foam donut

1

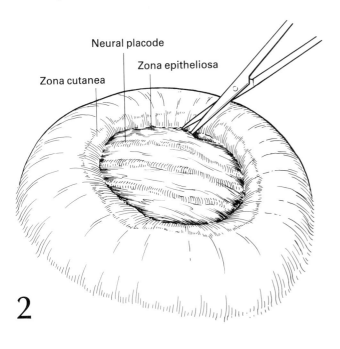

Neural placode

Zona epitheliosa

Zona cutanea

Freeing the neural placode

2 Dissection of the neural placode begins at the lateral aspect of the placode at the junction of the zona epitheliosa and the edge of the hemangiomatous skin (zona cutanea). This can be done with sharp iris scissors or tenotomy scissors. A significant amount of yellowish cerebrospinal fluid will egress when the sac is opened which deflates the cystic portion of the myelomeningocele sac. At this point careful inspection of the interior of the sac is necessary.

2

3 Examination of the contents of the sac demonstrates that the floor of the sac is formed by the glistening white dura which is adherent to the surrounding fat and mesodermal elements. Medially, nerve roots can be seen passing from the neural placode down into the spinal canal which is often flattened relative to a normal canal.

The sharp dissection is carried out on either side and then completed at the cephalic and caudal end. It should be noted that at the upper end the placode is nearly a normal spinal cord and is invested by normal arachnoid and has the typical cylindrical shape of the spinal cord.

At the upper end of the neural placode filamentous adhesions may bind the cord/placode to the dura. These should be carefully divided. Dissection of the placode from the zona epitheliosa and the hemangiomatous skin edges is important and it is here that magnification proves to be particularly helpful. Dissection is most difficult at the cephalic and caudal portions of the placode as there are usually multiple adhesions both to the dura and surrounding skin. Occasionally, additional laminectomies and dural opening are necessary to achieve adequate exposure of the spinal cord to free adhesions. An important goal of myelomeningocele closure is the untethering of the neural placode as well as repair of the skin/dural defect. Freeing of these adhesions allows the cord to slide more gently within the dural sac.

Inspection of the internal contents should include a check for fibrocartilaginous or bony spurs near the level of the first intact lamina. Such spurs, often seen on preoperative radiographs, suggest a narrowed intervertebral space, if a vertebral body anomaly is seen, or if a midline septum is seen on ultrasonographic examination. A laminectomy at one or two levels above the lesion may be necessary to adequately visualize such septae.

The adhesions of the terminal portion of the placode can be quite dense. Where there are significant fibrous bands, use of a nerve stimulator can often help to distinguish these bands from functioning neural tissue.

Placement of the neural placode back into spinal canal

4 The edges of the neural placode should be carefully inspected to be certain that no dermal elements are included in the placode. Pieces of the membranous tissue of the zona epitheliosa and thin parchment skin from the zona cutanea should be sharply debrided from the edges of the placode. The placode, if completely freed of adhesions, should rest within the spinal canal.

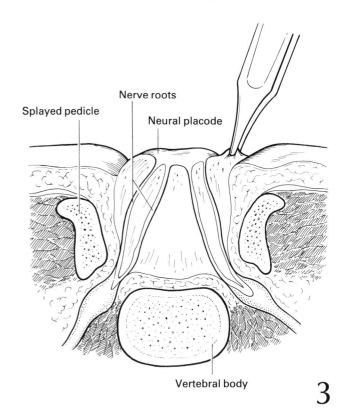

Splayed pedicle — Nerve roots — Neural placode — Vertebral body

3

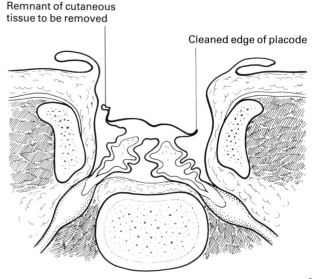

Remnant of cutaneous tissue to be removed — Cleaned edge of placode

4

Reconstitution of the neural tube

5   Controversy exists as to whether reconstitution of the neural tube is beneficial. If the neural placode is very thin, the edges may be brought together to reconstitute the neural tube. A few sutures of 6/0 polypropylene (Prolene) can be placed into the arachnoid elements at the edge of the placode to reconstitute the tube. It is hoped that this maneuver will decrease tethering and prevent adherence to the surrounding dura. Care must be taken not to place these sutures through neural elements and reconstitution of the tube should not be performed if the edges of the placode do not easily come together or if the placode is thick.

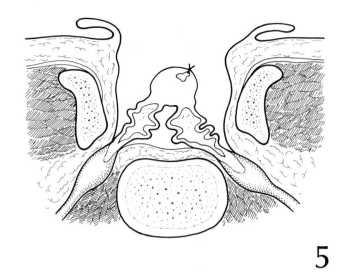

5

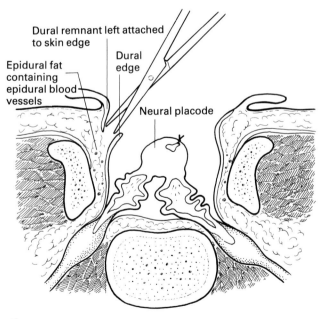

6

Identification of the dural edges

6   One of the most important aspects of repair of a child with myelomeningocele is achievement of a water-tight dural closure. The dura is a glistening white structure which is adherent to the edges of the myelomeningocele sac. It is most easily identified by carefully examining the upper end of the sac near where the neural placode is reconstituted into a normal spinal cord. It may not be reconstituted at the lower end, depending on the level and extent of the myelomeningocele defect. The dura is dissected initially at the upper end off the paraspinous fascia. Care must be taken to go high enough up along the walls of the sac to provide sufficient dura to close over the placode and to obtain a water-tight closure. It is important that the dural closure is sufficiently capacious to prevent strangulation of the neural placode.

Dissecting of the dural edges

7 A cuff of residual dura is left along the skin edges and can be used to anchor subcutaneous stitches to assist in the closure of the skin edges. An important landmark in identifying the plane of dissection to free the dura from the surrounding tissue is the identification of epidural fat. This epidural fat is more loosely developed than subcutaneous fat and has within it a rich blood supply including epidural veins. These epidural veins can be quite large and should be coagulated where necessary.

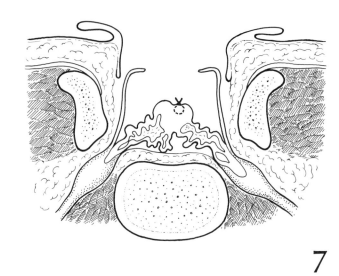

7

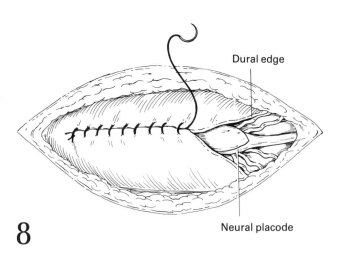

Dural edge

Neural placode

8

Closing the dura

8 The dural edges should be brought together using a running stitch. A 4/0 or 5/0 polypropylene running stitch works well to close the dura in a water-tight fashion. If insufficient dura is available, a piece of paraspinous fascia may be used as a patch to complete the repair. If insufficient fascia is available, cadaveric dura or fascia can also be used as a patch.

Closing the fascia

9 Where possible the fascia should be closed over the dura. This is usually not possible across the entire area, as there is probably insufficient fascia. In addition, as the pedicles of the spine are widely bifid, the fascia usually ends quite laterally from the dura. Splitting of the fascia into a superficial and deep layer laterally can provide a sufficient amount of fascia so that it can then be closed over the midline. Here again, closure of the fascia should not cause strangulation of the placode. A complete fascial closure, although useful, should not be attempted if it results in pressure on the placode.

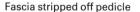
Fascia stripped off pedicle

Dural closure

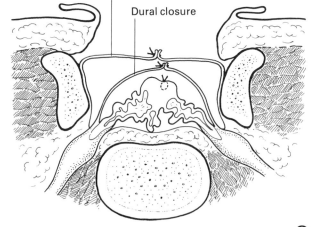

9

Skin closure

The closure of the skin defect in a myelomeningocele repair is the single most difficult element of the repair. Serious consideration must be given to employing the talents of a pediatric plastic surgeon when dealing with a large defect. Important factors which contribute to the breakdown of the skin repair are use of poor quality skin, placing the skin under tension at the suture line, and inadequate dural closure or hydrocephalus resulting in leakage of cerebrospinal fluid.

10 All of the skin surrounding the area should be employed. Parchment skin cannot be used as it will break down. If the defect in the skin is less than half the width of the back a primary closure can be achieved by careful undermining of the skin. The direction of the closure is not important but avoidance of pressure and stretching of the skin edges is important. Undermining the skin edges using blunt finger dissection is useful. Division of the tight fibrous band tethering the subcutaneous tissue and skin near the iliac crest can be particularly helpful in mobilizing skin in the lower lumbar area. Occasionally, especially if there is significant kyphotic deformity, resecting part of the pedicles may be helpful in closing the skin. In more severe cases kyphectomy may have to be performed to achieve skin closure. This should be done in conjunction with an orthopedic surgeon.

The skin should be closed in two layers making use of the residual dural cuff that is still attached to the skin edges. Interrupted 3/0 absorbable suture works well in the subcutaneous tissues. Vertical mattress sutures using 4/0 or 5/0 nylon can be used along the skin edges. Intravenous fluorescein can demonstrate the blood supply to the skin and may be helpful in identifying places where there are non-viable areas.

11 Adequate closure may not be possible in large defects and the use of various flaps must be considered. Relaxing flank incisions may allow closure of the undermined skin.

12 The use of S-shaped rotational flaps allows mobilization of adequate skin in some large defects.

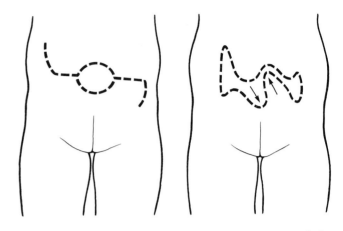

12

Postoperative care

The mortality rates from repair of myelomeningoceles range from 2% to 19% but intraoperative deaths are exceedingly rare. Early postoperative deaths are also exceedingly rare (about 2%) and are usually associated with respiratory failure or severe infection, particularly meningitis.

The repair site is covered with a light non-compressive dressing. Use of plastic drapes to keep stool from contaminating the wound should also be employed. Maintenance of a clean dressing is crucial. The child should be kept off the repair site and can be nursed in a lateral position. Use of a Foley catheter or intermittent catheterization is necessary to prevent stasis and avoid urinary tract infections. Because neonatal ureteric peristalsis may be weak, hydronephrosis may develop. Ultrasonographic examination of the kidneys can be helpful in identifying such problems.

Wound care must be meticulous and the wound must be inspected regularly to look for areas of breakdown. Bacitracin ointment or silvadene are useful in keeping the wound moist and clean. Small areas of wound breakdown will usually respond to local management and will eventually granulate. Wound care is particularly important when lateral releasing incisions have been employed.

Leakage of cerebrospinal fluid is probably the result of progressive hydrocephalus and 85–95% of children

with myelomeningocele will require shunting during the first days to weeks of life. Repeated cranial ultrasonography and careful head measurements can identify progressive hydrocephalus. A ventriculo-peritoneal shunt is most commonly employed to relieve hydrocephalus. Recent studies do not suggest an increased risk of infection if the shunt is placed at the same time as the repair. However, children with myelomeningoceles are still at increased risk of shunt infections and physicians must always be on the alert for shunt infections in the first few weeks after repair.

Occasionally the Chiari II malformation may become symptomatic during the first few months of life. It is characterized by downward displacement of the vermis into the cervical spinal canal, causing compression of the underlying brainstem and spinal cord. Symptoms include apnea, stridor, high-pitched cry and lower cranial nerve paresis. Initial evaluation must always be directed toward evaluation of the shunt, but if this proves negative consideration must be given to early decompression of the Chiari II malformation. It must be remembered that a small percentage of children, despite adequate decompression of their Chiari II malformations, still have intrinsic developmental anomalies of their brainstem which result in brainstem dysfunction, necessitating tracheostomy and insertion of feeding tubes.

Outcome

Counseling and education of the parents and caregivers of children with myelomeningocele must be considered a vital part of postoperative care. Multidisciplinary management of these children permits most to lead productive and fulfilling lives. As the technical ability to treat these children and the radiographic capacity to image their associated abnormalities is improved, and most importantly, as we learn from long term follow-up of these children, it is clear that the outcome for most is good.

Survival for children with myelomeningocele is improving. Most tertiary care centers find that 95–98% of these children will survive with aggressive medical management. Associated abnormalities of the central nervous system, particularly complications related to the Chiari II malformation and other systemic anomalies, account for mortality in many of the present day non-survivors. Antibiotic therapy has greatly decreased the mortality associated with ventriculitis. Ventriculoperitoneal shunting has successfully managed progressive hydrocephalus. McLone has shown that intellectual function is significantly lower in children in whom meningitis has developed in the postoperative period. Some form of learning disability will be present in 70–80% of cases and special education or special programs will be required while in school. Routine evaluation with computed tomographic scans of the head in the first few years of life can be helpful in identifying indolent shunt malfunction. As the children grow older, school performance can be used to follow intellectual function.

Some 80–90% of children with myelomeningocele have neurogenic bladder dysfunction. Among the lifelong risks associated with this dysfunction are urinary stasis and infection, trabeculation and diverticula of the bladder, ureteric reflux, hydronephrosis and renal failure. The use of intermittent catheterization has reduced the incidence of hydronephrosis and urinary tract infections. It has also improved continence so that, with regular catheterization, more than 90% can now achieve continence. Improvement in urologic management means that urine diversionary procedures are now infrequently employed. Control of defecation can be achieved in 50–75% of patients with the assistance of careful dietary management, use of dietary supplements such as bran, and use of enemas and suppositories.

Multiple orthopedic problems can occur. Scoliosis occurs in 65–75% of patients and may require surgical correction. Significant kyphosis is seen in 5–10% of patients and may require surgical correction if respiratory function is impeded. Many lower extremity deformities may occur and often require surgical correction or bracing. Use of orthotics in these children requires the specialized attention of a pediatric orthotist and will improve the functional outcome.

Careful neurologic monitoring is necessary. Delayed neurologic complications in these children can occur because of several problems. Recognition or consideration of indolent shunt malfunction must always be considered when there is clinical deterioration of any type in a child with myelomeningocele. Chiari II malformation may cause bulbar compression and result in lower cranial nerve dysfunction. It may also result in syringomyelia or cervical cord dysfunction which may manifest itself with upper extremity weakness or numbness. Magnetic resonance imaging has greatly improved our understanding of the Chiari II malformation by allowing an excellent view of the malformation.

Changes in segmental motor or sensory deficits, evidence of increasing spasticity, change in bladder or bowel function, progressive neuromusculoskeletal deformity at the ankle or leg and progressive scoliosis may occur secondary to tethering of the spinal cord. Because all children with myelomeningocele have evidence of a tethered cord on magnetic resonance imaging, careful clinical evaluation must still be employed to determine if such tethering is clinically significant and warrants further surgery to untether the spinal cord. In addition, less common causes of progressive deficit may include dermoid cyst formation, diastematomyelia with septum, and arachnoid cyst formation.

It cannot be overemphasized that shunt malfunction is the most common cause of clinical deterioration in children with myelomeningocele. It must always be considered, and shunt function must be carefully evaluated before such deterioration is attributed to other causes such as Chiari II malformation or tethered cord.

References

1. Reigel DH. Spina bifida. In: McLaurin RL, Schut L, Venes JL, Epstein F, eds. *Pediatric Neurosurgery – Surgery of the Developing Nervous System.* 2nd edn. Philadephia: WB Saunders, 1989: 35–52.

2. Brock DJ, Sutcliffe RG. Alpha-fetoprotein in the antenatal diagnosis of anencephaly and spina bifida. *Lancet* 1972; 197–9.

3. Charney E, Weller SC, Sutton LN, Bruce DA, Schut LB. Management of the newborn with myelomeningocele: time for a decision making process. *Pediatrics* 1985; 75: 58–64.

4. McCullough DC. Surgical treatment of meningomyelocele. In: Raimondi AJ, Choux M, DiRocco C, eds. *The Pediatric Spine vol. 1. Development and the Dysraphic State.* New York: Springer-Verlag, 1989: 160–78.

5. McLone DG. Results of treatment of children born with a myelomeningocele. *Clin Neurosurg* 1983; 30: 407–12.

6. McLone DG, Naidich TP. Myelomeningocele: outcome and late complications. In: McLaurin RL, Schut L, Venes JL, Epstein F, eds. *Pediatric Neurosurgery – Surgery of the Developing Nervous System.* 2nd edn. Philadephia: WB Saunders, 1989: 53–70.

Ventricular shunting procedure

Robert C. Dauser MD
Assistant Professor of Neurosurgery, Texas Children's Hospital, Houston, Texas, USA

Principles and justification

Hydrocephalus results from a buildup of cerebrospinal fluid (CSF) within the intracranial compartment. This fluid is continuously produced by the choroid plexus tissue located in each of the four cerebral ventricles. Flow then proceeds out of the brain through the small openings in the fourth ventricle, the foramina of Luschka and Magendie. Circulation through the subarachnoid spaces of the basilar cisterns and up over the cerebral hemispheres then leads to the arachnoid granulations of the venous sinuses, where reabsorption into the bloodstream occurs.

Occasionally, over-production of CSF due to an imbalance between production and absorption, such as with a choroid plexus papilloma, produces hydrocephalus; more commonly, however, a blockage to the normal circulatory flow of CSF at some point along the path prevents the fluid from re-entering the bloodstream, despite a steady rate of secretion. The result is an accumulation of fluid within the ventricles, or hydrocephalus. The disorder is classified as *obstructive* if the blockage prevents fluid from escaping the ventricular system within the brain, or *communicating* if the CSF is able to flow out of the fourth ventricle but reabsorption is prevented by a blockage somewhere more peripherally along the pathway.

Early treatment of hydrocephalus was largely unsatisfactory. Lumbar or ventricular punctures gave only temporary relief at best, while surgical removal of the choroid plexus aimed at removing the source of CSF production failed to control the pathologic process. In addition, trials of various medications to slow CSF production have not yielded lasting disease control. The modern era of the surgical treatment of hydrocephalus began with the development of valve mechanisms for shunting systems in the late 1950s.

Etiologies of hydrocephalus

Congenital anomalies are common causes of hydrocephalus. The narrow aqueduct is often blocked, leading to dilatation of the lateral and third ventricles. An X-linked form of such aqueductal stenosis may be seen as an inherited trait. Children born with myelomeningoceles almost always have an associated Chiari II malformation with downward herniation of the posterior fossa tissue into the cervical canal. The flow of CSF is impeded in these children, usually by obstruction at the incisura or aqueduct. Occlusion of the outlets of the fourth ventricle produces hydrocephalus in another congenital disorder, the Dandy Walker malformation.

Certain acquired disorders may also lead to hydrocephalus. Neoplasms growing along the CSF circulatory pathways may block flow. Children are especially prone to tumors growing within the fourth ventricle or elsewhere in the posterior fossa, with hydrocephalus resulting from occlusion of the CSF spaces within this crowded region. Masses near the third ventricle or aqueduct can produce similar results. Finally, diffuse spread of neoplasm throughout the subarachnoid spaces may block flow and absorption of CSF at multiple sites.

Inflammatory blockage of the subarachnoid spaces may reduce fluid flow and absorption, resulting in hydrocephalus. Infections, such as meningitis from bacteria, fungi or mycobacteria, are common causes. Hemorrhage can lead to similar pathology. Preterm infants are prone to intraventricular bleeds, which are seen in 40% of children born before 35 weeks' gestation or weighing less than 1500 g. Other causes of hemorrhage that can lead to hydrocephalus include bleeding from aneurysms or arteriovenous malformations or head trauma.

Clinical features

Infants may present to the physician after the disease has progressed considerably. The infant skull is composed of separate bones with open suture lines and fontanels, allowing the head to expand and pressure to release as the ventricles dilate. For this reason, an increase in the head circumference percentile detected by the pediatrician on routine examination may be the only clue to the diagnosis. Fontanel tension may increase as pressure rises, and scalp veins may dilate. Non-specific signs of pressure, such as irritability, lethargy, vomiting, poor feeding and developmental delay may also be seen.

Pressure from the dilated third ventricle on the collicular plate of the brainstem can produce paralysis of upward gaze and downward deviation of the eyes, resulting in the whites of the eyes being visible above the irises, or 'sunsetting'. Inward deviation of one or both eyes occurs with sixth cranial nerve palsies as a result of increased intracranial pressure. Papilledema may be seen on fundoscopic examination in some patients.

In older children and adults the skull no longer expands, and the pressure release mechanism is lost. As pressure from hydrocephalus rises, headache and vomiting are frequently seen, especially in the morning. Papilledema and sixth nerve palsy can be noted, and as the disease progresses frank coma and brainstem compression occur.

Diagnostic examination

1a–d
Non-invasive studies such as computed tomography (CT) and magnetic resonance imaging (MRI) make the diagnosis of hydrocephalus straightforward. In addition, contrast enhancement may detect an underlying cause such as a neoplasm. Ultrasonography can be used to detect ventriculomegaly in a young infant with an open fontanel. Lumbar puncture carries with it some risk in these patients until pressure within the cranium has been relieved, because acute herniation may result from pressure release below.

Choice of procedure

Once the diagnosis of hydrocephalus has been made in a patient with clinical signs and symptoms, treatment must be initiated. Medical treatment has no long-term benefit, and punctures of the ventricle or lumbar space afford no lasting relief, because the production of CSF continues steadily. The only effective treatment is therefore to implant a mechanical shunting device which continuously drains fluid from the ventricle into an extracranial compartment. The peritoneal cavity is by far the most desirable site of drainage because enough extra tubing can be inserted to allow for future growth, the insertion technique is simple, and no foreign body is placed directly into the bloodstream, which would increase the risk of infection.

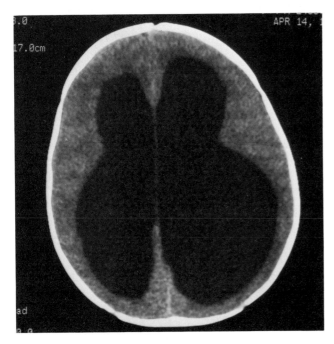

1a

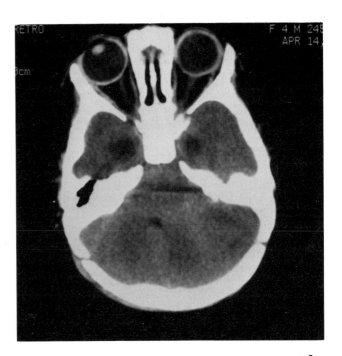

1b

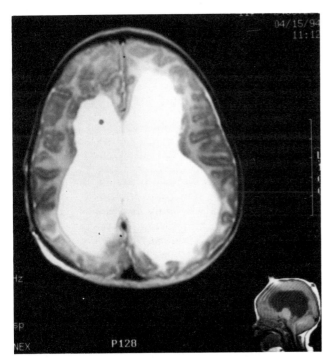

1c

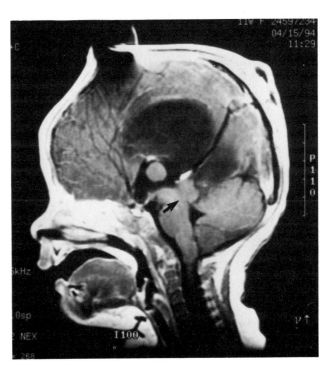

1d

(a) CT scan through the mid portion of the lateral ventricles in an 11-week-old infant presenting with a large head, lethargy, vomiting and a firm fontanel; ventricles are extremely large. (b) CT scan of the same patient through the posterior fossa, demonstrating normal fourth ventricle, suggesting blockage at aqueduct of Sylvius. (c) MRI scan of the same patient showing large lateral ventricles. (d) Sagittal MRI scan; the aqueduct of Sylvius (arrow) is occluded.

Preoperative

Assessment and preparation

When a child or adult is seen with the clinical picture described above, the examination usually proceeds with some combination of ultrasonography, CT scanning or MRI scanning. This both confirms the diagnosis and searches for a cause for the hydrocephalus (*Illustration 1*).

If the patient is acutely ill, shunting is often done on an emergency basis. Medical measures such as intubation with hyperventilation, or the administration of an osmotic diuretic such as mannitol may provide a lifesaving reduction in intracranial pressure until definitive surgical treatment can be instituted. Rarely, an emergency ventricular puncture is required in the acutely decompensating patient. The timing of surgery is based on the severity of the illness.

Anesthesia

Shunts are always placed under general anesthesia. The anesthetist must take measures such as hyperventilation to reduce intracranial pressure during the induction and until pressure is surgically relieved to avoid a surgical catastrophe. Mannitol may also be given if the patient is in severe difficulty with intracranial pressure. Antibiotics should be given before the skin incision is made, as evidence suggests that the infection rate is lower if this practice is maintained[1].

Operation

Selection of shunt material

Many different types of shunt devices exist, none being clearly superior to the rest. The catheters that enter the ventricle and the peritoneal cavity are made of Silastic, which is extremely non-reactive. Some type of valve is placed within the shunt system to reduce the rate of flow and to prohibit backflow. As most shunt occlusions are caused by the holes in the ventricular catheter becoming blocked by tissue from the ependymal lining of the ventricle, and because collapse of the ventricular wall from overdrainage seems to enhance this process, many surgeons feel that a high-pressure valve may prevent this complication. However, a small infant may not tolerate a high-pressure valve. Although slit valves placed on the distal end of the peritoneal catheter are available, there is evidence that these valves are more prone to problems than valves placed more proximally near the cranial end of the shunt[2]. Each surgeon should become very familiar with one type of shunt and use it regularly, which should reduce the likelihood of complications.

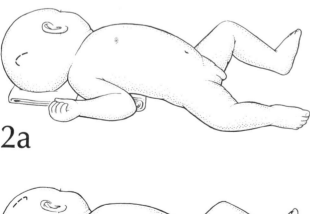

2a

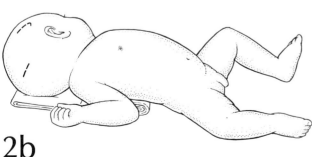

2b

Positioning and preparation

2a, b One of the most serious complications seen with ventricular shunt placement is infection and for this reason it is vital that meticulous attention is paid to preparation of the operative field. Scrubbing and then painting with iodine solution is recommended, followed by placement of an iodine-impregnated adhesive plastic drape over the entire field. Hair should be carefully excluded from the incision sites, but with careful draping technique, shaving can be limited to small patches directly surrounding the areas of interest. In children, infiltration of the sites of incision with lidocaine–epinephrine (lignocaine–adrenaline) solution reduces blood loss from the skin edges. The head is generally turned full lateral to keep anatomical landmarks consistent; placing a lift under the shoulder reduces cervical stress with this maneuver.

PLACEMENT OF THE VENTRICULAR CATHETER

The proximal portion of the shunt consists of the ventricular catheter and usually the lateral ventricle is the site of placement. The holes in the distal end of the tube should reside in the frontal horn anterior to the foramen of Monroe, away from the choroid plexus tissue posterior to the foramen which commonly occludes the small holes in the catheter. There are two acceptable methods of placing this portion of the shunt[3].

Frontal approach

3 Placing the ventricular catheter by way of a frontal burr hole has several theoretical advantages: less brain is traversed than with the posterior approach, and the distance to the ventricle is shorter, making cannulation of very small ventricles easier. In addition, none of the holes in the tubing lie along side the choroid plexus if the catheter has been placed correctly in the ipsilateral frontal horn, making occlusion less likely. The disadvantage to the anterior approach is that a longer subgaleal tunnel is required, and an extra incision behind the ear is necessary to tunnel to the abdominal wound.

The burr hole is placed 3 cm lateral to the midline just in front of the coronal suture. It is important to place the curvilinear incision well anterior to the skull opening so that the shunt material itself does not lie directly under the wound, which would predispose to breakdown and infection. The burr hole can be made with either a power drill or a simple hand twist drill. In small infants the opening can be created by biting away a small portion of the frontal bone anterior to the coronal suture with a rongeur. The dura is then coagulated with bipolar cautery and opened carefully with a scalpel. The pia is coagulated and opened, avoiding cortical vessels.

Correct placement of the ventricular catheter is most important in avoiding future shunt malfunction. The catheter is passed through the brain essentially perpendicular to the skull, aimed at the inner canthus of the ipsilateral eye. Palpation of the nose and orbit through the drapes can aid in this maneuver. Aiming too medially will result in the catheter crossing to the opposite side, and aiming too far posteriorly will result in placement behind the foramen of Monroe adjacent to the choroid plexus. The catheter should be 6 cm long in an adult, and somewhat shorter in an infant. The length can be adjusted slightly if necessary to achieve more optimal flow.

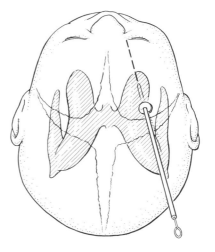

3

Parieto-occipital approach

4 A more posteriorly placed burr hole allows one fewer incisions and a shorter subgaleal tunnel. However, it may be more difficult to cannulate small ventricles with this approach, and more critical brain tissue must be traversed. In addition, even if the tip of the catheter enters the ipsilateral frontal horn, some of the more proximal holes in the catheter may lie alongside the choroid plexus, predisposing to occlusion.

The burr hold is made 3 cm above and 3 cm behind the ear, with dural and pial openings proceeding as with the frontal approach. The catheter is passed parallel to the sagittal suture, aimed at the midpoint of the forehead. The body of the lateral ventricle lies approximately half way between the top of the ear and the top of the skull, and travels parallel to the sagittal sinus. The length of the catheter should allow the tip to extend 1 cm anterior to the coronal suture to place the tube within the frontal horn. Care must be taken to avoid aiming too low, as this may injure the internal capsule fibers or place the catheter erroneously into the temporal horn, leading to almost certain malfunction. A lateral skull radiograph taken in the operating room should detect such a problem.

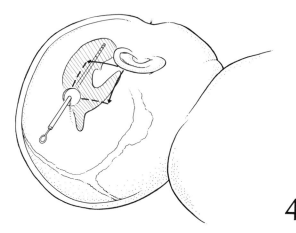

4

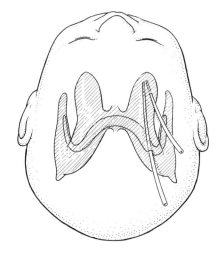

5

5 With either approach, adequate CSF flow must be demonstrated before the catheter position is accepted. Sluggish flow may mean that the interhemispheric fissure has been cannulated. If the ventricles are large, pulsatile flow should be seen with successful catheter placement, although with very small ventricles this may be more confusing.

DISTAL CATHETER PLACEMENT

Peritoneal cavity

6 A small incision is made just off the midline over the rectus abdominis muscle. The anterior rectus fascia is opened vertically and the muscle fibers split longitudinally. The posterior rectus sheath and peritoneum are picked up with straight hemostats and opened until the peritoneal cavity is visualized as a large open space. Care must be taken to open both the final layers and avoid entering the preperitoneal space. On occasion, adherent omentum may make this distinction difficult and dissection must continue until the issue is resolved, which sometimes requires opening in a different location. When the distal catheter is finally placed, it must pass easily and freely without obstruction or coiling within a confined area.

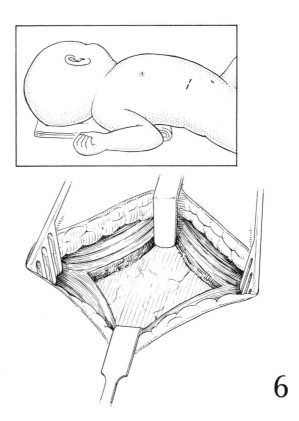

6

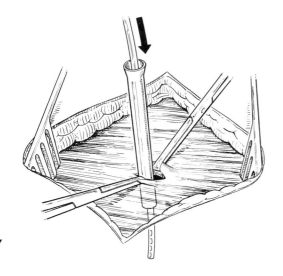

7

7 Some surgeons place the distal catheter using a very small incision and a trochar. Although this is simple and fast, it has been known to cause bowel perforation and a small laparotomy is the preferred method of placement.

Venous system

Although the peritoneal cavity is the preferred site of distal catheter placement, this may not be possible because of peritonitis, dense adhesions, or failure of the peritoneal cavity to absorb sufficient CSF. The right atrium of the heart is the next best site for placement.

8 With the head turned full laterally, a transverse incision is made 2–3 cm below the angle of the mandible just anterior to the sternocleidomastoid muscle. The platysma is split and the common facial vein is isolated if visible. Vessel loops are placed around this vein and a venotomy allows passage of the Silastic atrial catheter towards the internal jugular vein and into the right atrium. If this approach is unsuccessful the internal jugular vein may be isolated directly with vessel loops, a venotomy created inside a purse-string suture in the vessel wall and the atrial catheter passed directly towards the heart. The catheter should be irrigated with heparinized saline to avoid thrombus formation.

Multiple methods have been used to achieve correct catheter length, the simplest of which seems to involve holding the catheter over the chest wall to estimate the appropriate length to the right atrium, and then placement of the catheter followed by chest radiography to adjust the final length. The tip of the catheter should lie within the right atrium proximal to the tricuspid valve, usually at the level of the fourth thoracic vertebra. A short catheter will be outgrown quickly and may thrombose, while a catheter that is too long may cause cardiac irritation and arrhythmia.

Difficulty may be encountered in obtaining venous access. If the technique described above is unsuccessful, the external jugular route of entry, often with the help of curved guidewires, may be effective. The cephalic vein (found by dissection in the deltopectoral groove) or the subclavian vein (by direct puncture) can also be tried. These more unusual approaches will not be discussed further in this chapter.

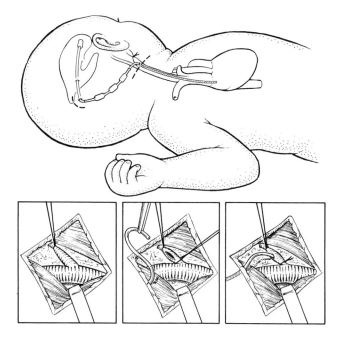

8

Tunneling and connections

9 Following placement of the ventricular catheter and exposure of the site of distal shunt placement, the shunt device itself is tunneled between the incisions. The tunneling device supplied usually consists of a steel rod, curved at the end, which is passed within the subcutaneous space. The rod carries with it a sheath through which the shunt tubing is passed, followed by removal of the sheath.

Alternatively, a heavy suture can be passed via the shunt tunneller and tied to the shunt tubing, which is then pulled through the tunnel. Connections are made and tied securely with non-absorbable sutures. Fewer connections make disconnection less likely, and the present trend seems to be towards one- or two-piece shunt systems. The final step with the peritoneal shunt is to pass all slack into the peritoneal cavity, making sure that the tubing is not kinked. Generally the entire length of peritoneal catheter should be inserted, which avoids the problem of the catheter becoming too short.

Wound closure

Wounds are closed in layers with absorbable sutures.

Postoperative care

Antibiotics do not need to be continued in the immediate postoperative period. The neurologic condition of the patient is closely monitored; the preoperative symptoms of increased intracranial pressure should resolve quite rapidly. If no improvement is seen, shunt malfunction must be suspected and appropriate measures taken to correct the problem. Diagnosis is made by CT scanning and, if necessary, by shunt tap. The site over the reservoir is carefully prepared with iodine and a 23-gauge butterfly needle inserted with sterile technique. This allows measurement of the opening pressure, removal of CSF for temporary relief, and examination of the fluid. A high opening pressure with good flow suggests obstruction of the distal system, such as the valve or distal catheter. Inability to obtain CSF implies a blocked or improperly placed ventricular catheter. Plain radiography of the shunt system may diagnose a poorly placed catheter or a kink in the tubing.

One of the most serious and common problems following shunt insertion is infection. This occurs in at least 5% of cases, usually within the first few weeks following surgery. Leakage of CSF from a wound in the immediate postoperative period makes this complication far more probable. Symptoms include fever, pain and redness along the shunt, drainage of pus from an incision, meningeal signs or peritonitis. Abdominal pain is often noted as the infected CSF becomes walled off

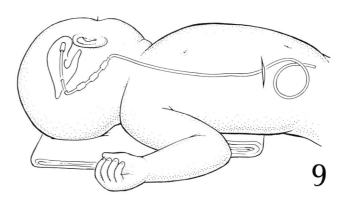

9

into a pseudocyst. Drainage into this structure is poor, leading to elevated intracranial pressure and symptoms such as headache, lethargy and vomiting. CT scanning may show recurrent enlargement of the ventricles. Diagnosis is confirmed by shunt tap, which may show elevated pressure, pleocytosis with a predominence of neutrophils, and a positive Gram stain and culture. Abdominal ultrasonography may show a pseudocyst containing the end of the peritoneal catheter.

Treatment of the infected shunt requires that the CSF is drained into an external container while antibiotics are administered, either by removing the entire shunt and replacing it with a ventriculostomy, or by cutting down over the distal catheter over the chest wall and connecting to an external drainage system. Antibiotics that penetrate the CSF well are given intravenously and adjusted according to Gram stain, culture and sensitivity results. If initial results are inconclusive, both Gram-negative and Gram-positive antibiotic coverage should be given until further results are obtained. After the CSF has been sterile for 1 week the shunt may be reinserted, usually at the same site, after the entire old shunt has been removed.

In patients with extremely large ventricles before shunt placement, rapid decompression of these ventricles may lead to subdural hematoma or fluid collection. This may be avoided by placing a higher resistance shunt, and by keeping the patient horizontal for an adjustment period. Treatment of this problem can be troublesome, and involves draining the collections while increasing the resistance of the shunt. In some patients with chronically elevated pressure from hydrocephalus, shunting can lead to headaches from low pressure, as seen following lumbar puncture. These headaches are often worse when the patient is upright, and are relieved by lying down. A waiting period (sometimes of several weeks) allows adjustment to the new pressure and relief of the headache, but persistence occasionally requires an increase in the resistance of the valve or placement of an antisiphon device.

Outcome

If shunt infection occurs, it is usually within the first few weeks following surgery; however, any infection seen within 6 months is assumed to be a result of intraoperative contamination. Diagnosis and treatment is as described previously.

Shunt malfunction is usually due to obstruction of the ventricular catheter, and may occur at any time. A recent study noted a 73% rate of ventricular catheter obstruction 7 years following shunt placement[4]. Symptoms of malfunction include headache, irritability, confusion, decline in school performance or developmental milestones, vomiting or papilledema, sometimes with visual loss. The infant may experience rapid head growth, bulging of the fontanel, or splitting of the cranial sutures. Diagnosis is made by CT scan, in general, but in perhaps as many as 15% of cases the CT scan may show no evidence of ventricular enlargement despite shunt malfunction. Shunt tap with assessment of flow and pressure is helpful in these equivocal situations. Radiographs of the shunt system may show disconnection of the tubing or a short distal catheter. Once the diagnosis has been made, operative exploration is carried out, replacing any non-functional component.

Patients should be followed on a long-term basis for shunt malfunction. A baseline CT scan, taken at a time when the shunt is known to be working, is helpful for future comparisons. Most surgeons feel that it is unlikely for a patient to outgrow the need for the shunt, and follow the rule 'once a shunt, always a shunt'. If the peritoneal catheter becomes too short, it should be electively lengthened in most instances. With good medical care, and if there are no severe underlying brain disorders that affect intelligence, patients with hydrocephalus can expect to live productive and relatively normal lives with an adequately functioning shunt.

References

1. Haines SJ, Walters BC. Antibiotic prophylaxis for cerebrospinal fluid shunts: a metanalysis. *Neurosurgery* 1994; **34**: 87–93.

2. Sainte-Rose C, Piatt JH, Renier D, Pierre-Kahn A, Hirsch JF, Hoffman HJ *et al*. Mechanical complications in shunts. *Pediatr Neurosurg* 1991; **17**: 2–9.

3. Rekate HL. Treatment of hydrocephalus. In: McLaurin RL, Schut L, Venes JL, Epstein F, eds. *Pediatric Neurosurgery*, 2nd edn. Philadelphia: WB Saunders, 1989: 200–18.

4. Serlo W, Fernell E, Heikkinen E, Anderson H, von Wendt L. Functions and complications of shunts in different etiologies of childhood hydrocephalus. *Child Nerv Syst* 1990; **6**: 92–4.

Syndactyly

David M. Evans FRCS
Consultant Hand Surgeon, Royal National Orthopaedic Hospital, Stanmore, Middlesex, UK

Principles and justification

During embryonic development a process of programmed cell death is required to establish the separate digits by absorption of the intervening cells. If this fails, varying degrees of syndactyly occur. Some forms of syndactyly are inherited, including Apert's syndrome (acrocephalosyndactyly), which is an autosomal dominant condition, and orofacial–digital syndrome, which is dominant X-linked. Syndactyly occurs in about 7/10 000 live births, and is twice as common in boys as in girls. Syndactyly and polydactyly may occur in the same hand.

Simple syndactyly involves a skin connection between otherwise normal digits and is the most common form. The more complicated forms of syndactyly are much more difficult to treat and involve sharing other tissues (bone, joints, tendons and neurovascular structures) or syndactyly between abnormal digits, which may be short, lacking joints or other structures, or abnormal in number, either reduced or increased. The patterns are infinitely variable, but fall into the following groups.

Symbrachydactyly

The digits are short and may be reduced in number, and there is a basic failure of skeletal development at the extreme of which there are only nubbins of soft tissue, usually with a nail remnant.

Acrosyndactyly

The syndactyly is fenestrated proximally, usually in association with ring constriction syndrome.

Acrocephalosyndactyly (Apert's syndrome)

This is usually complete syndactyly of all four limbs and three broad nails and a jumble of bones, associated with a severe craniofacial abnormality.

Poland's syndrome

This form of symbrachydactyly is associated with a small arm, hypoplasia of the ipsilateral breast and absence of the sternocostal head of the pectoralis major muscle.

Typical cleft hand

If the third ray is absent there is usually associated syndactyly of the first web space.

'Superdigit'

This is a form of syndactyly in which the digits merge completely at either the proximal or distal end, but are more or less separate at the other end. It is not possible to make two digits out of this complex, and treatment is designed to make a more acceptable single digit or to leave it alone entirely.

Indications for separation

A child with a congenital malformation of the hand will not perceive a functional deficit and will only become aware of the abnormal appearance when it is pointed out by others. The request for surgical correction usually comes from the parents and is often based on esthetic considerations. Syndactyly in the hand should usually be separated unless there is a definite contra-indication, e.g. a sharing of structures without which one of the digits would not remain a viable functioning unit. Each digit needs a neurovascular bundle, stable joints and a full set of flexor and extensor tendons. This is never a problem with simple syndactyly, but difficulties are more likely to occur when the digits are joined more closely or are otherwise abnormal. Each pair of digits has to be evaluated carefully, including study of the surface anatomy, the presence or absence of flexion creases (a useful guide to the presence of flexor tendons), assessment of independent movement if possible and radiographic examination. If there is doubt about any of the above-mentioned structures, a plan should be made to reconstruct them or the digits should be left joined together.

The first web space should always be separated to provide an independently functioning thumb, and digits of unequal length or with joints in different positions will develop secondary deformities if left connected. For the same reasons these categories of syndactyly merit separation early, at around the age of 6 months, while digits presenting none of these problems can be separated later if preferred, although 6 months is a good age for surgery if a child is generally fit.

Neighboring clefts may be best separated in stages to avoid a shortage of skin for flaps, although the risk to the circulation has been overemphasized, except in digits with deficient neurovascular bundles. The hand with syndactyly in all the webs can be treated by separation of the first and third cleft at one sitting and the others at another. Simple syndactyly of the smaller toes is of no functional importance and should not be divided in childhood, as a graft failure could lead to scar contracture with difficulties in growth, gait or footwear. Separation in adolescence or adulthood is a matter of choice for the patient. As in the hand, separation of unequal toes may be indicated, particularly when the big toe is involved, and when there is associated polydactyly.

Principles of surgical technique

In many cases surgery is undertaken for esthetic reasons, and it is vital in addition that no deterioration in function is produced through subsequent scar contracture or through loss of use in digits that cannot exist independently. Where there was a functional indication for surgery this must be met in all respects; it is usually found that functional and esthetic considerations are closely linked and where one is satisfied, the other will also be.

The factor most likely to lead to contracture and impaired growth is the presence of a longitudinal scar, particularly on the volar aspect of the finger. To avoid this, steep zigzag incisions must be used. There is always a skin deficiency and the best use must be made of local flap skin to line the base of a new cleft and to provide continuity of flap skin around each finger at strategic points to break the line of skin grafts. This should be done only with oblique or transverse scars. Alternatively, the incisions can be designed to provide enough skin to clothe one finger completely or with only a small graft proximally, leaving a larger skin defect on the other finger into which is placed a single full-thickness skin graft, still with zigzag margins. This is the technique which will be described in this chapter. It has the advantage of leaving one finger with a single zigzag scar and the other with a single graft, and therefore with fewer scars. It also makes it possible to cover exposed joints or tendons, including reconstructed pulleys on one finger in more complicated cases, in which soft tissue can be preserved on the other finger to provide a graft bed. For example, with a shared flexor tendon sheath, all the sheath can cover the tendons on one finger, allowing skin grafting, while skin is available for cover of the tendon and reconstructed pulleys on the other. Skin expansion has not been of value for syndactyly, and although some cases have more skin available than others, the possibility of complete closure without tension is rare.

Skin replacement should be accurate, using full-thickness free skin grafts by choice, as these have less tendency to contract and a greater capacity for growth than split skin. A high rate of graft success and skin flap survival should be ensured by accurate planning, delicate tissue handling, hemostasis and effective postoperative splinting.

Operation

1 Separation is carried out under general anesthesia with tourniquet control. The incisions are planned to leave no straight longitudinal scars, and no scars crossing the web from finger to finger. It is standard practice to share available skin equally between the two digits, filling remaining defects with skin grafts, but cover of one digit as completely as possible with flap skin and the other with a single large graft will be described here. To achieve this the zigzag incisions are moved away from the interdigital line on palmar and dorsal surfaces just enough to allow the zigzag flaps to interdigitate accurately on the favored finger, which is a matter of choice. The ring finger is usually favored to allow comfortable wearing of a ring. More skin needs to be available proximally than distally. Flap skin is needed to line the web which should shelve from dorsal to distal, and should be positioned to match the neighboring clefts. A dorsal flap is preferred for this purpose.

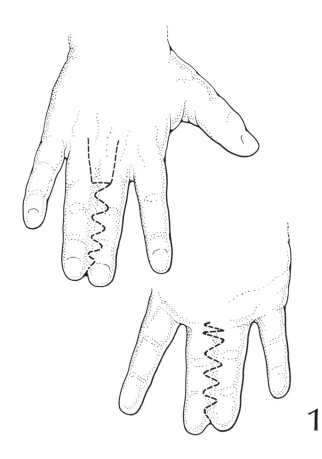

2 The small triangular flaps are raised only as far as the line of separation of the fingers, and there is no need to raise flaps that are going to stay where they are. All flaps should be raised close to the subdermal plane to disturb the veins and lymphatics in the subcutaneous tissue as little as possible.

The two long narrow flaps at the proximal end of the palmar incision are designed to sit on either side of the dorsal web flap, breaking the line of scar tissue extending into each digit[1]. This is a most important step to prevent 'web creep'.

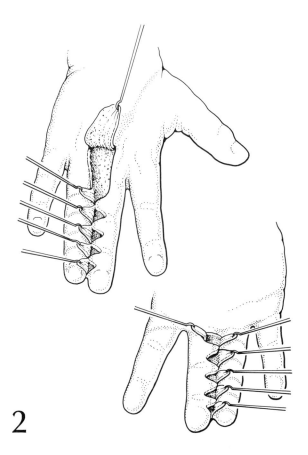

3 Separation of the soft tissues in the web is completed under direct vision preserving the neurovascular bundle to each finger. If there is a common digital nerve it should be split into components for each finger, using magnification. If a common digital artery extends into the web, one branch has to be sacrificed, selecting the branch to the finger which is most likely to have an arterial supply.

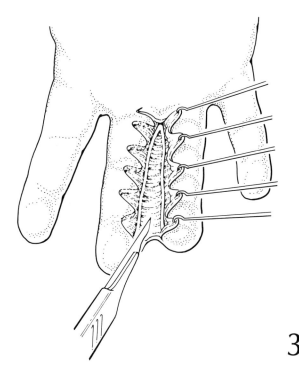

3

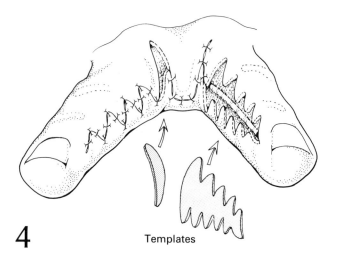

4

Templates

4 The proximal dorsal flap is sutured through the base of the web to the transverse proximal palmar incision, and the two narrow 'Moss' flaps[1] are placed alongside its tip, using one suture for each; 6/0 catgut is used throughout for skin closure in the hand. The zigzag flaps are then interdigitated to produce complete closure on the favored finger, sometimes leaving a crescent-shaped defect proximally needing a graft. On the finger with less skin, distal flaps can usually be closed, and the proximal defect presents an ideal surface for a single full-thickness skin graft, with no straight longitudinal edges. A template of this defect is carefully prepared using either a suture packet or thin rubber from a Martin's bandage. At this stage the tourniquet is released.

5 The patterns are placed in the groin crease, taking care to stay lateral to the likely line of future pubic hair growth which should be marked beforehand. The most accurate way to transfer the shape of the pattern to the groin is with a scalpel, lightly marking the detailed edges.

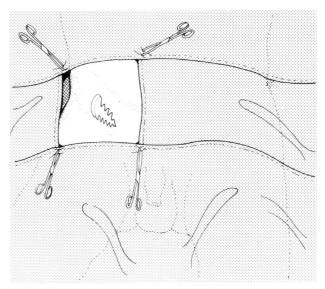

5

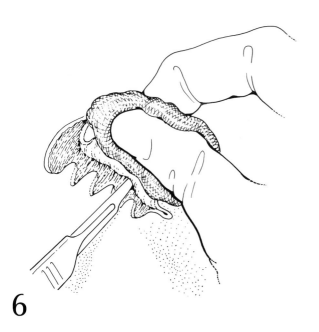

6

6 The graft is then raised immediately beneath the dermis. Using a dry swab the graft is folded back as it is cut and this allows elevation of the graft by sharp dissection without the need for further thinning. The groin wound is slightly undermined and closed with a subcuticular suture (5/0 polydioxanone (PDS) or Maxon are useful for this); the irregular edges can usually be interdigitated.

7 After checking for hemostasis, the skin graft is accurately sutured into the defect and, if the pattern was carefully made, should fit perfectly. The convexity of the defect and slight tension on the graft make the use of a tie-over dressing unnecessary in this situation.

The postoperative dressing is of great importance. One layer of tulle gras against the wounds reduces adhesion; dressing gauze is then loosely wrapped around the fingers and packed in each cleft. Plaster wool and plaster of Paris or synthetic slabs are used, always above-elbow and never constricting. It is best to place a slab on the palm and a slab on the dorsum with the hand flat, and the splint extending beyond the fingers. The elbow should be at 90°. It is difficult to keep small limbs in dressings and they should be carefully applied. A sling of elasticated surgical tubular stockinette is made (as described in the chapter on pp. 827–829). The plaster and dressing can be removed after 1 week without any need for anesthesia or sedation.

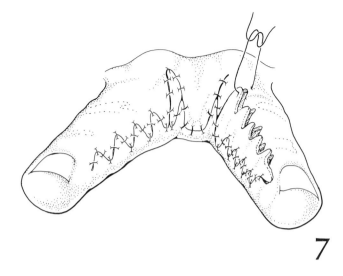

7

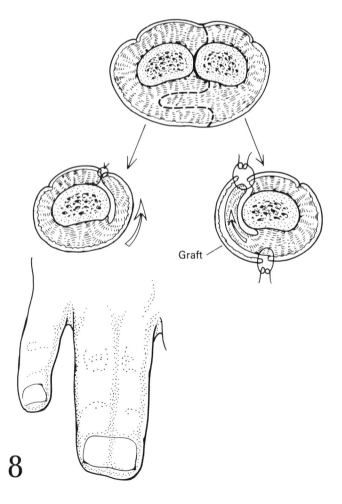

Graft

8

8 Closely syndactylized fingertips may have a broad, single nail, and separation leaves both fingers without a nailfold and often with exposed bone. Long narrow transverse flaps can be kept to make each nailfold, and a subcutaneous flap taken from the pulp of one fingertip can be used to cover the bone, leaving extra skin to cover the other. Alternatively, composite toe pulp grafts have been described[2], or a thenar flap can be used.

9 Additional procedures may be needed in complicated cases. A common flexor tendon sheath needs careful reconstruction, making use of all available sheath for the finger with less skin, covering the sheath with the skin graft, and reconstructing annular pulleys in the finger that has full skin cover. Similar maneuvers may be needed to cover exposed bone or reconstructed ligaments and osteotomy sites. In Apert's syndrome this is a common problem, but it is always possible when raising the skin flap to cover one finger and to leave a subcutaneous tissue flap borrowed from that finger to provide soft tissue cover for the finger with less skin, so that a graft can be applied.

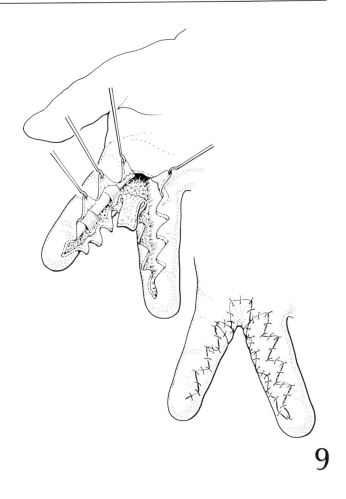

9

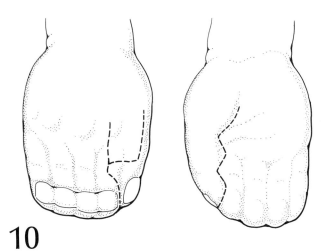

10

10 Syndactyly of the first web space is usually associated with short fingers. A large dorsal skin flap is needed to fill the base of the defect and is best taken from the dorsum of the thumb. Zigzag margins are left when possible.

11 A full web space release may be necessary and may need to be supplemented by an osteotomy of the base of the first metacarpal bone to bring the thumb into the correct relationship with the other digits. In cases associated with thumb hypoplasia an opponensplasty may also be required, using either a spare tendon of flexor digitorum superficialis or abductor digiti minimi if it is present. The gaps between the flaps are grafted in the usual way.

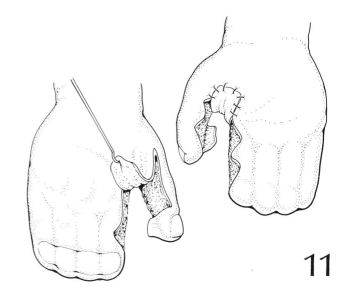

11

Postoperative care

The dressings need not be disturbed for 7–10 days provided there are no signs of infection or bleeding, but if the child is troubled by the hand or develops pyrexia the hand should be inspected. Full-thickness grafts often blister and require further dressings until they heal.

As soon as the wounds are dry and healed the hand may be left uncovered and the child can start to use it. Children regain function well without help in most cases, but any tendency for a finger or web space to contract should be immediately overcome by splinting, and refusal to use a finger or hand requires careful re-education, preferably by the child's mother. A therapist can help by encouraging play involving the reconstructed hand showing the parents how to continue this between therapy sessions.

Complications

Loss of grafts may be due to hematoma or infection and should be avoidable. If this is recognized frequent dressings should start and the defect should be regrafted with a split-skin graft at the earliest opportunity. If healing by secondary intention is allowed a contracted scar is inevitable.

If a scar contracture does develop it should be released early to avoid secondary joint changes. A Z-plasty release is indicated, but the Z flaps may need to be supplemented with further skin grafts.

Correction of secondary web contracture

12 If a secondary web contracture does occur, it can be corrected using a double Z-plasty, e.g. the 'jumping man' procedure described by Mustardé[3] for correction of epicanthic folds. The tight scar is split in an anteroposterior direction, with a triangular palmar flap which advances dorsally. Elongation on either side is provided with a Z-plasty which is three-dimensional around the curve of the web.

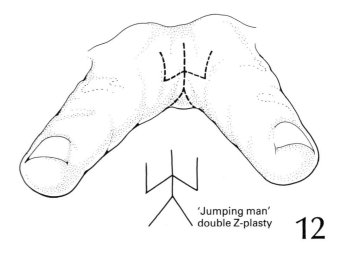

'Jumping man'
double Z-plasty

12

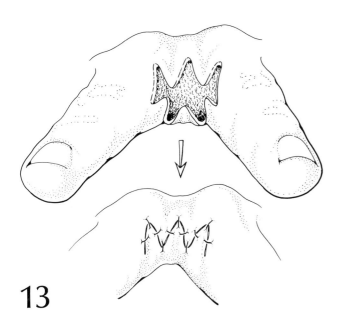

13

13 Release of underlying scar tissue allows the flaps to interdigitate in such a way that contracture should not recur.

References

1. Moss ALH, Foucher G. Syndactyly: can web creep be avoided? *J Hand Surg [Br]* 1990; 15: 193–200.

2. Sommerkamp TG, Ezaki M, Carter PR, Hentz VR. The pulp plasty: a composite graft for complete syndactyly fingertip separations. *J Hand Surg [Am]* 1992; 17A: 15–20.

3. Mustardé JC. Epicanthus and telecanthus. *Br J Plast Surg* 1963; 16: 346–56.

Polydactyly

David M. Evans FRCS
Consultant Hand Surgeon, Royal National Orthopaedic Hospital, Stanmore, Middlesex, UK

Principles and justification

Polydactyly, or duplication of the fingers, occurs in approximately eight per 10 000 live births. Its incidence relative to other congenital anomalies of the hand varies in different ethnic groups, however, from 15% reported by Flatt[1] in the USA to 40% in Hong Kong[2]. Any of the digits may be involved, but the thumb is the most common digit, radial (or preaxial) polydactyly forming between 70%[3] and 95%[2]. Central polydactyly, less common than postaxial polydactyly (affecting the ulnar side of the hand) is more often associated with a reduction malformation, e.g. cleft hand, and with syndactyly. Syndromes featuring polydactyly include Ellis–van Creveld syndrome (short limbs and cardiac abnormalities; autosomal recessive); trisomy 13 (midline facial cleft); and Laurence–Moon–Biedl syndrome (retinitis pigmentosa, obesity and mental retardation; autosomal recessive). Mirror hand is an extremely rare form of polydactyly in which the ulnar half of the limb is duplicated as a mirror image, with absence of the radial half. The double ulna causes problems with elbow movement. The profusion of digits provides ample material for separation, but this is an extremely complex procedure.

In its mildest form, polydactyly consists of a small rudiment attached by a narrow stalk of skin and blood vessels. Better developed supernumerary digits are connected either at a joint or the shaft of the bone, and the digit to which they are attached is likely to be abnormal, particularly in the case of the thumb. More than one extra digit may be present, and complex forms occur in which conflicting distal and proximal relationships make a supernumerary digit appear to arise skeletally from one digital ray, yet be syndactylized to another.

Indications

The purpose of removal of extra digits is to restore the hand to a normal configuration. Few cases of polydactyly have any functional problem before treatment, and it is therefore vital that function and growth are not disturbed by the effects of ill-conceived surgery. Careful distinction should be made during preoperative evaluation between those cases in which deformity may result from inadequate surgery (particularly those involving the thumb) and extra digits which can be simply removed leaving a normal hand. The feature most likely to be associated with subsequent deformity is connection of the two digits at a joint, but simple soft tissue or bone connection can be associated with problems also. Because these problems are most commonly encountered in polydactyly of the thumb, this will be given prominence in this chapter.

Operations

1 A floppy supernumerary digit with a stalk should be accurately removed under sterile conditions. The traditional ligature around the stalk leaves a bump in the scar which requires revision later. It is possible to excise the digit including the whole stalk under local anesthesia in neonates, as the needle prick is quickly forgotten and the baby easy to hold, particularly if it can be given a feed. One 6/0 catgut suture is required. This method is unsuitable for older babies, for whom general anesthesia should be used.

More completely formed preaxial or postaxial digits are removed under general anesthesia with a tourniquet. There is no strong reason to do this early, but any age from 6 months to 4 years is suitable. After that any deformity that does exist may become more firmly established.

2 A zigzag incision borrowing some spare skin from the extra digit will avoid a straight scar. The feeding vessels are ligated and the digital nerves cut short and touched with a diathermy, taking special care to avoid damage to the neurovascular bundles running to the neighboring digit. The skin can be trimmed to leave a flat scar without tension.

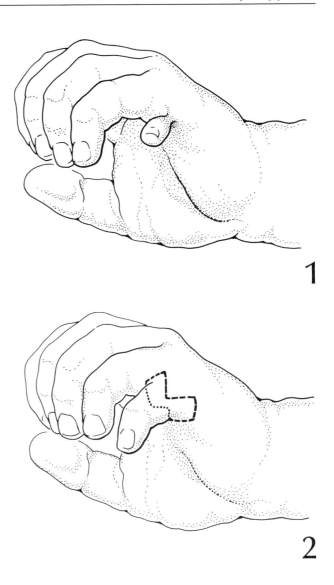

1

2

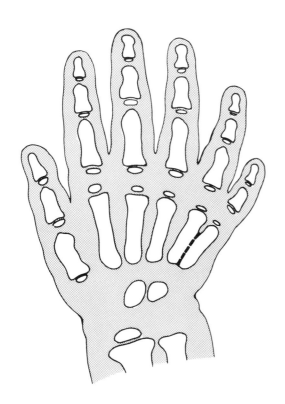

3 When the accessory digit arises from the shaft of the neighboring metacarpal bone or phalanx, the bone should be trimmed to leave a smooth shaft. A small bump left behind may grow into a prominent swelling. If an epiphysis is close it must not be damaged.

3

POLYDACTYLY OF THE THUMB

4 Wassel[3] provided the generally accepted classification of thumb polydactyly. This serves reasonably well, although the various forms are more variable than his schemes suggest and form a spectrum. Furthermore, this classification is based on the skeletal arrangement only, but there are other variations to consider, including the longitudinal alignment of the digital segments and the soft tissues, particularly tendons.

The principle underlying surgical management is one of making the best use of material from both digits to construct a thumb that is correctly aligned longitudinally, with the joints and epiphyseal plates at right angles to its long axis, and with normally aligned long tendons and stable collateral ligaments. This should be accomplished in one stage and should leave the thumb able to move as near normally as possible and relate properly to the remaining digits. To achieve this in some of the more complicated cases is extremely demanding technically, yet if the opportunity is lost, later correction of the residual deformity is even more difficult.

There are two ways in which tissue from the thumbs can be shared, and each has its place. For Wassel types I, II and sometimes III, the Bilhaut–Cloquet method of sharing equal contributions from the two digits after excising a central wedge is appropriate, provided the two halves are fairly equal in size. For more proximal or very unequal cases, the lesser digit should be excised, making use of components as necessary when performing maneuvers to rectify any deformity in the remaining digit.

5 The Bilhaut–Cloquet procedure was described by Bilhaut in 1889[4]. It is applicable to types I–III duplication when the two halves are equal, although slight irregularities can be accommodated. The central portion of each digit is excised to allow the outer portions to be approximated, and if designed correctly this procedure can leave a thumb close to normal in size and appearance.

The original description recommends a straight split down each digit in a wedge shape, splitting the two nails. This inevitably leaves a ridge or a gap down the nail, and the incision shown here, by which one nail (the larger if there is a difference) is moved across to the center of the new thumb, usually keeping just the nailfold on the side where the nail is removed, gives a small but perfectly formed nail. On the pulp the incision should be convex inwards to provide a little extra prominence, with a small proximal zigzag.

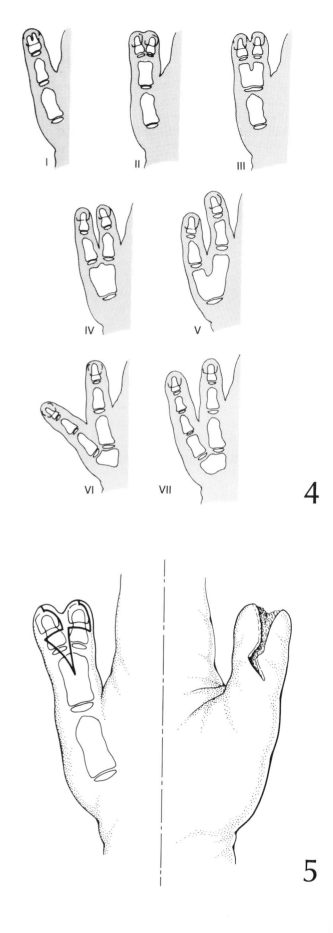

4

5

6   The nail is dissected off the distal phalanx keeping the germinal and sterile matrix intact, and the two distal phalanges are exposed down to the joint. The technique is illustrated for a Wassel type II duplication, and the procedure for Wassel types I and III has to be adapted appropriately. The inner part of each distal phalanx is excised with a fine oscillating saw. It is advisable to take a little over half the width of each, so that the slight inevitable gap leaves a phalanx of appropriate width, otherwise the thumb is too wide. The two halves are wired together with fine interosseous wire, making sure that both the epiphyseal lines and the joint surfaces match exactly. This is technically difficult. If the phalanges are of slightly different length, it is possible to excise a central segment of one, but the procedure is even more difficult.

The excision can be extended into the middle phalanx in exactly the same way, but again the technical problems are compounded by the need to exactly match the joints and growth plates. It is most important to preserve the insertion of the extensor and flexor tendons on both remaining hemiphalanges.

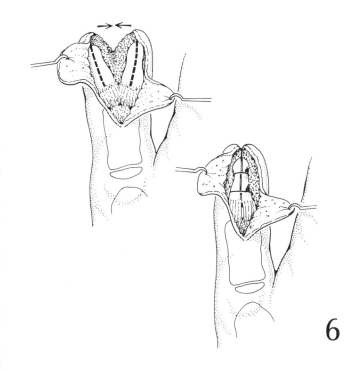

6

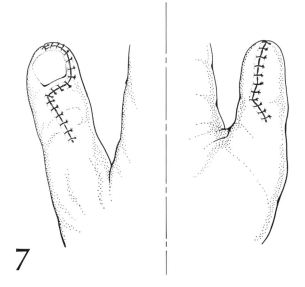

7

7   The nail is laid across the reconstructed distal phalanx and the skin closed with 6/0 catgut. The advantage of this method over the alternative of removing one half and realigning the other is that the reconstructed thumb is symmetric and internally stable.

The thumb and hand should be rested in a splint and elevated, and movement encouraged under supervision after about 10 days. It is not uncommon for there to be some limitation of interphalangeal flexion, but the intact carpometacarpal and metaphalangeal joints should allow normal function to develop.

8 Wassel types V, VI and VII polydactyly require careful amputation of the lesser (usually radial) digit, and interference with the remaining one is only necessary if it is not normally aligned. This requires careful preoperative assessment. If the carpometacarpal joint is entered, a bony prominence may need to be trimmed and the capsule should be carefully closed.

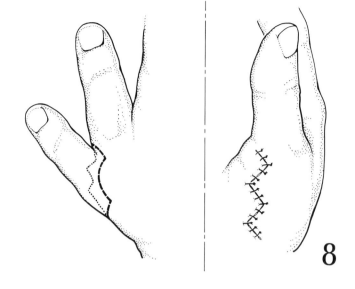

8

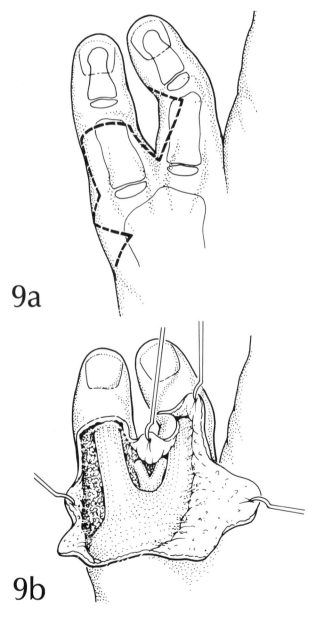

9a

9b

9a, b The most challenging thumbs fall into the Wassel type IV group, which comprises about half of all thumb polydactylies. Similar principles are applied to Wassel types III, V, VI and VII when there is a zigzag deformity in the preserved thumb. In order to leave a straight, stable, growing thumb, the joints and epiphyseal lines must be at right angles to its axis, and the extensor tendons must have a direct line of action in the axis of the thumb.

This requires careful preoperative assessment by examination and radiography. It is wise to keep skin from the thumb to be removed so that there is ample available for zigzag closure, and proximal and distal extension should be in a zigzag form. Wide dissection is needed to expose the tendinous anatomy and gain access to the metaphalangeal and interphalangeal joints.

Elevation of the flaps reveals the extensor mechanism, which splits as a Y, so that the line of approach is deviated inwards. The same arrangement is often found in the flexor pollicis longus muscle, which can just be seen in the illustration, pulled inwards.

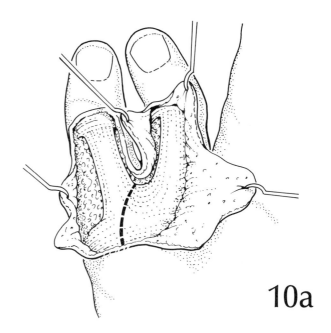

10a, b

The extensor mechanism is split, taking care to maintain continuity to the remaining thumb, and spare tendon from the discarded thumb can be used to reconstruct retinacular bands to hold the tendon in the midline of the thumb. Dissection proximally reveals the tendons of the abductor and flexor pollicis brevis muscles, and these are detached from the discarded thumb. A ligamentoperiosteal flap is constructed on the radial side of the broadened metaphalangeal joint[5] with the proximal attachment kept intact. The redundant thumb is then disarticulated from the metaphalangeal joint.

10a

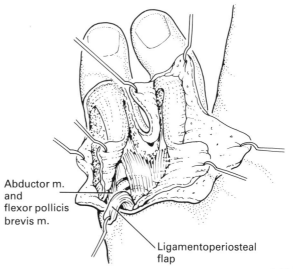

Abductor m. and flexor pollicis brevis m.

Ligamentoperiosteal flap

10b

11 Exposure of the whole flexor pollicis longus muscle is now possible. The tendon running towards the discarded thumb is divided, and this leaves most of the flexor pollicis longus muscle without a pulley system. Once the redundant thumb has been removed, ligating the vessels and dividing the nerves with preservation of those to the remaining thumb, it is possible to restore the smoothed-off flexor pollicis longus muscle to its correct line of pull, if necessary dissecting a pocket and using preserved retinacular tissues to construct a pulley. Very occasionally the insertion of this muscle is so radial that part of it has to be detached and rolled over in an ulnar direction for reattachment. It is better not to detach the whole insertion.

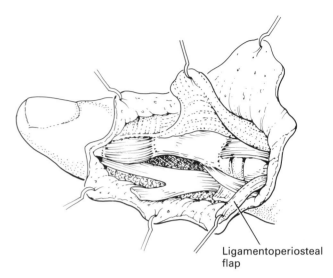

Ligamentoperiosteal flap

11

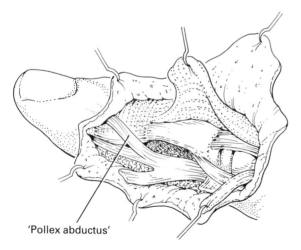

'Pollex abductus'

12

12 Occasionally an oblique connection is found between the flexor pollicis longus and the extensor mechanism, giving rise to a condition referred to by Lister[6] as 'pollex abductus'. The tendinous band is instrumental in producing and perpetuating a vicious lateral angulation and must be excised as part of the primary procedure.

13, 14 Having prepared the tendons of the new thumb, the skeleton should be realigned. The usual pattern in a retained ulnar thumb is ulnar deviation at the metacarpophalangeal joint and radial deviation at the interphalangeal joint. If mild, an osteotomy of the metacarpal head is all that is needed, but the author usually prefers a double osteotomy – a closing wedge osteotomy at the metacarpal head and an opening wedge osteotomy of the neck of the proximal phalanx, using the wedge of bone from the metacarpal to maintain the position of the distal osteotomy. The metacarpal wedge excision is distal to the origin of the retained ligamentoperiosteal flap, and includes the prominent boss where the discarded thumb was previously articulated.

A wedge is cut accurately from the metacarpal just below the head, using a fine saw. The proximal surface of the wedge is perpendicular to the long axis of the metacarpal, and the distal surface is parallel to the joint surface articulating with the retained thumb. The osteotomy need not penetrate the opposite cortex, but the gap should close easily and is held with a K-wire running down the length of the thumb or obliquely across the metaphalangeal joint only. It is more secure if a small interosseous wire is inserted in the outer cortex. The wedge of bone is held in place in the proximal phalangeal osteotomy with the same longitudinal wire after opening the osteotomy wide enough to correct the alignment of the distal phalanx. The slight laxity of the distal interphalangeal joint means that the position of the distal phalanx has to be slightly overcorrected, as it will settle back slightly when released. Preserved periosteum sutured over the graft where possible helps to keep it in place.

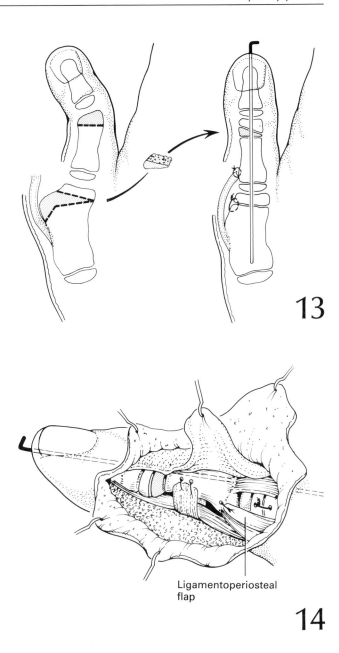

13

Ligamentoperiosteal flap

14

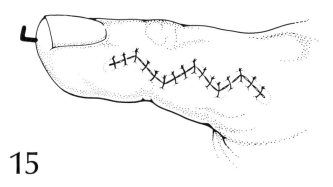

15

15 The tourniquet is released and hemostasis is secured. The skin is sutured leaving a neat, flat, zigzag suture line without tension.

CENTRAL POLYDACTYLY

16 In central polydactyly the extra digit is often syndactylized to another central digit, and the skin is redistributed to leave a smooth web with zigzag scars. Often the skeletal components of the extra digit do not extend into the metacarpal area, but if they do, all skeletal components must be excised.

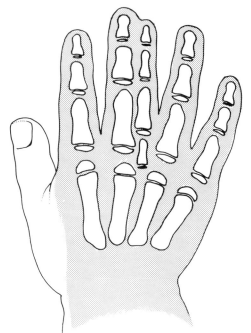

16

Postoperative management

A well-padded, non-constricting dressing is applied, over which is placed a plaster or synthetic splint supporting the whole hand with the wrist in extension and the thumb web maintained. In small children the splint should extend above the elbow and should not be circumferential. Splinting of osteotomies and ligament repairs should be retained for 4 weeks, after which wires can be removed. Some support is advisable for a further 2 weeks, but can be removed intermittently.

References

1. Flatt AE. *The Care of Congenital Hand Anomalies*. St Louis: Mosby, 1977.

2. Leung PC, Chan KM, Cheng JC. Congenital anomalies of the upper limb among the Chinese population in Hong Kong. *J Hand Surg* 1982; 7: 563–5.

3. Wassel HD, The results of surgery for polydactyly of the thumb. *Clin Orthop Rel Res* 1969; 64: 175–93.

4. Bilhaut. Guérison d'un pouce bifide par un nouveau procédé opératoire. *Congrès Français Chirurg* 1889; 4: 576–80.

5. Manske P. Treatment of duplicated thumb using a ligamentous periosteal flap. *J Hand Surg [Am]* 1989; 14: 728–33.

6. Lister G. Pollex abductus in hypoplasia and duplication of the thumb. *J Hand Surg [Am]* 1991; 16: 626–33.

Illustrations by Marks Creative Consultants

Popliteal cysts

J. A. Fixsen MChir, FRCS
Consultant Orthopaedic Surgeon, Great Ormond Street Hospital for Children, London, UK

Principles and justification

Popliteal cysts in children are common in the first decade, with a maximal incidence around the age of 6 years. They present as a cystic swelling which transilluminates and arises between the medial head of the gastrocnemius muscle and the semitendinosus and semimembranosus tendons[1]. They are more common in boys and a traumatic origin has been suggested[2].

Unlike such cysts in adults, they are very rarely associated with intra-articular pathology. There is a rapid fall in incidence after the first decade, suggesting a high spontaneous recovery rate, and this is supported by Dinham[3], who showed a 73% spontaneous disappearance rate over a mean period of 20 months. Surgery is indicated only if there is serious doubt about the nature of the lesion, if it persists and causes pressure symptoms, or if the parents are unduly anxious about it. It is important to remember that there is a considerable risk of recurrence after surgery (42% in the series reported by Dinham[3]).

Preoperative

Anesthesia

For accurate dissection and removal of the cyst it is essential to carry out the operation under general anesthesia with a tourniquet.

Operation

Position of patient and incision

The patient lies prone. A curving longitudinal incision centered over the cyst is made. A transverse incision with vertical extensions at each end is preferred by some surgeons.

Exposure and removal of cyst

1, 2 The deep fascia is divided and the cyst is exposed and carefully dissected out from the surrounding structures. It lies between the semitendinosus and semimembranosus tendons medially and the medial head of the gastrocnemius muscle laterally. The wall of the cyst is intimately attached to these structures and sharp dissection is necessary to remove it adequately. If possible, the cyst should be kept intact during the procedure.

The majority of cysts communicate with the cavity of the knee joint through an opening in the posterior capsule which remains after removal of the cyst. As intra-articular pathology is so rare in children, it is not necessary to enlarge this opening to inspect the intra-articular structures unless pathology is suspected. The opening is sutured with chromic catgut. The tourniquet is removed and hemostasis obtained. The wound is closed in layers suturing the deep fascia and skin. Care should be taken with the skin sutures to avoid an ugly scar. A subcuticular polyglycolic acid suture can be used, as this is self-absorbing and gives a good cosmetic result.

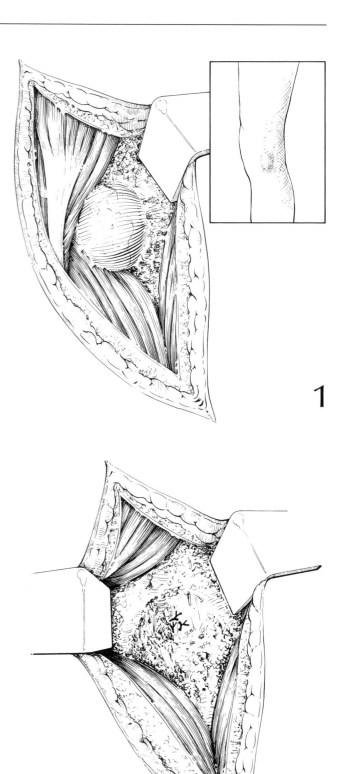

1

2

Postoperative care

A firm cotton wool and crepe bandage is applied. The patient is mobilized with crutches and allowed home as soon as he is comfortable. The procedure is commonly carried out as a day case. Skin sutures are removed at 10–14 days when the wound is healed and full use of the knee is then encouraged.

References

1. Wilson, PD, Eyre-Brook AL, Francis JD. A clinical and anatomical study of the semimembranosus bursa in relation to popliteal cysts. *J Bone Joint Surg* 1938; 20: 963–84.

2. Gristina AG, Wilson PD. Popliteal cysts in adults and children. A review of 90 cases. *Arch Surg* 1964; 88: 357–63.

3. Dinham JM. Popliteal cysts in children: the case against surgery. *J Bone Joint Surg* 1975; 57B: 69–71.

Trigger thumb

David M. Evans FRCS
Consultant Hand Surgeon, Royal National Orthopaedic Hospital, Stanmore, Middlesex, UK

Principles and justification

Trigger thumb affects two quite distinct age groups. It occurs in small children, probably as a congenital abnormality, although it is often not noticed until some months after birth. It also occurs as a degenerative condition usually after the age of 40 years, and often associated with trigger finger. It may present as part of an inflammatory condition, e.g. rheumatoid arthritis.

In congenital trigger thumb a nodule forms in the tendon of flexor pollicis longus and becomes trapped proximal to the A1 pulley, producing a 20–30° flexion deformity of the interphalangeal joint of the thumb. The phenomenon of triggering backwards and forwards through the stenosed sheath is not usually observed in this age group, and the presentation as a flexion deformity of the interphalangeal joint may give rise to diagnostic confusion. There is sometimes compensatory hyperextension of the metacarpophalangeal joint, and a hard nodule is always palpable in the tendon, thrown into greater prominence by the hyperextension. The presentation of the swelling over the flexor tendon combined with interphalangeal flexion deformity is pathognomonic.

Dinham and Meggitt[1] found that 12% of cases resolved spontaneously, but this finding was not confirmed by Ger et al.[2] who recommended surgical release without delay. Surgical release is indicated by the age of 2.5 years to avoid any risk of loss of full hyperextension at the interphalangeal joint.

Congenital trigger thumb occasionally runs in families, but it is usually an isolated lesion on one side only; congenital trigger finger is rare but does occur.

Operation

Release of trigger thumb in children requires full operating theater facilities, general anesthesia and tourniquet control. The principal hazard of the operation is digital nerve damage.

Incision

1 A 1.5–2-cm incision is made in the proximal crease of the thumb, where it meets the thenar skin. The incision should not reach the loose skin fold of the first web.

Surgical access to the base of the thumb is awkward, but is made easier if an assistant holds the hand with the wrist flexed and the thumb gently extended and abducted so that its palmar surface faces the surgeon. Another assistant provides retraction. This position is preferable to a flat hand because it relaxes tension on the digital nerves and the skin, making nerve injury less likely.

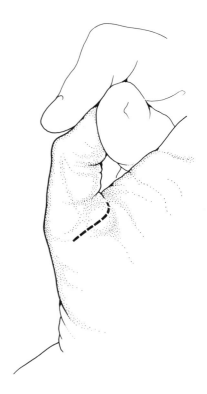

1

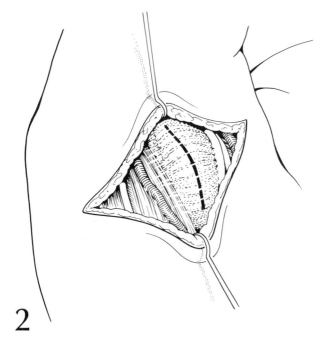

2

2 Using gentle dissection the incision is opened and the radial digital nerve identified. Usually it lies to the radial side of the flexor apparatus, but it may be sited between the tendon and the skin, and the two digital nerves may be side by side in this position. If so, they are carefully retracted to expose the A1 pulley on its radial side, with a tendon nodule bulging below it.

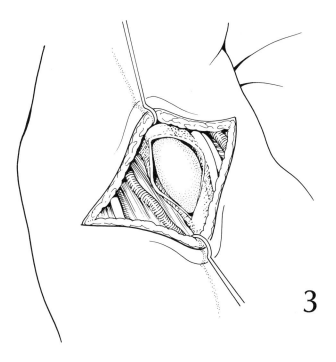

3

3 The A1 pulley is divided with a scalpel at its radial edge; if it is divided in the midline the tendon can bowstring out of the sheath. The glistening white tendon is exposed and the nodule can be easily palpated. The interphalangeal joint should now extend freely and the full excursion of the tendon can be checked. If the nodule is still held distally the sheath should be divided further, but no more of the sheath should be opened than is necessary. There is no indication for interfering with the nodule itself as it will gradually resolve.

The tourniquet is released to allow hemostasis to be checked, the integrity of the digital nerves is confirmed and the wound is closed with 6/0 chromic catgut.

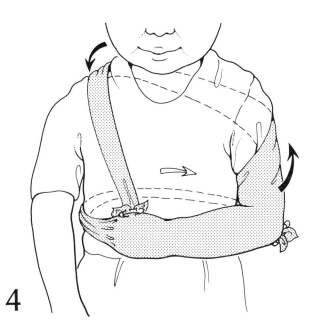

4

4 A well-padded bandage is held on with adhesive tape, and a sling is made out of elastic net tubular stockinette to rest the limb. There is no need to splint the thumb at this stage.

Postoperative care

The child's parents should make sure that the thumb moves freely. Usually the child will extend it spontaneously, but if necessary gentle passive extension should be done daily starting on the third day after operation. The dressing can be removed after 1 week.

References

1. Dinham JM, Meggitt BF. Trigger thumbs in children: a review of the natural history and indications for treatment in 105 patients. *J Bone Joint Surg [Br]* 1974; 56: 153–5.

2. Ger E, Kupcha P, Ger D. The management of trigger thumb in children. *J Hand Surg [Am]* 1991; 16: 994–7.

Surgical treatment of thermal injuries

Heinz Rode MMed(Surg), FCS(SA), FRCS(Ed)
Associate Professor, Department of Paediatric Surgery, Red Cross Children's Hospital, Rondebosch, South Africa

D. M. Heimbach MD
Professor of Surgery, University of Washington Burn Center, Harbor View Medical Center, Seattle, Washington, USA

History

A burn is one of the most serious injuries that can be inflicted and, although many problems are still unresolved, substantial progress has been made since Neanderthal man treated burns with plant extract or when ancient Romans used a mixture of bran and honey, cork and ashes or vinegar. The modern treatment of burns is a logical exercise in resuscitation, infection control, surgical wound care, nutrition and psychologic and physical rehabilitation.

The Indian Tilemaker caste is credited with the earliest recorded method of skin grafting and Reverdin performed the first epidermic graft. Thiersch, in 1874, used more extensive pieces of skin, Wolfe utilized a free full-thickness graft to repair a defect on the lower eyelid, and Lustgarten described in 1891 the technique of early excision and grafting of small burns. Although allografts have also been used for centuries, Brown of St Louis established the practical aspects of biological skin dressings as life-saving procedures in extensively burnt patients.

In modern times a combination of early eschar excision and auto- or allografting (cadaver skin), biological and synthetic skin substitutes have transformed burn care management substantially with a 50% predicted survival for a burn of 98% total body surface area (TBSA).

Principles and justification

Superficial thermal injuries which will heal spontaneously within 3 weeks can be clinically identified.

Hot water scald burns in children are best left for 2 weeks to assess the need for operative intervention, thereby reducing the area for excision by 66%.

Early excision and grafting should be considered the treatment of choice for all burns that will not heal by primary intention within 3 weeks and it is crucial to diminish burn size and to graft essential functional areas.

Surgery should be delayed in burns which are more than 24 h old on admission. These wounds are potentially infected and should be swabbed or a quantitative biopsy performed (one biopsy per $24 \, cm^2$ of burnt tissue). Debridement should be carried out, topical therapy applied and surgical excision postponed for 24 h or longer.

Surgical excision may safely be undertaken in the presence of inhalational injury, although operative time and blood loss must be kept to a minimum.

Beta-hemolytic *Streptococcus* infection is a contraindication to surgical excision and grafting and routine burn wound cultures should be performed on alternate days until the burns are excised.

Burn severity

The severity of the burn is determined by the age of the patient, the depth and size of the burn, the anatomic site, concomitant disease or injury and the physiologic status of the patient. Skin does not reach adult thickness until puberty; hence, the younger the child the deeper the burn.

Burn depth

1 No objective clinical methods are available to determine the depth of thermal injury and a standardized method has been adopted. Most burns are a combination of superficial and deeper burns and the best assessment can be made 2–3 days after the injury when wound evolution is completed.

Superficial partial thickness: destruction of only superficial layers of the skin

These wounds will epithelialize spontaneously within 3 weeks; excision is contraindicated and the wounds rarely cause functional or cosmetic defects or hypertrophic scars. They may never completely match the color of the unburned surrounding skin. These wounds characteristically have an erythematous, moist, homogeneous surface with blister formation, are painful and hypersensitive to touch, blanch readily and have a normal to firm texture on palpation.

Indeterminate depth (deep dermal burn): destruction of epidermis and varying amounts of dermis

These wounds are difficult to assess during the first 3 days after injury due to the ongoing evolution within the burn wound which can be modulated by infection and dehydration. These wounds present with a reticulated red, white dry surface and may blister. Capillary circulation may be sluggish or absent when pressure is applied to the wound. Pain is perceived as discomfort and the wound is often less sensitive to pinprick than the surrounding normal skin. The burn is depressed in comparison with the surrounding skin and the healing time for these wounds may be variable. Hypertrophic scar formation is commonly encountered in the long term.

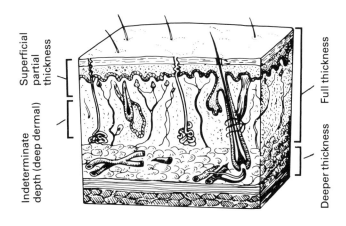

1

Unequivocally full thickness: total irreversible destruction of all elements of the skin with or without extension into the deeper tissues and structures

These wounds will not heal spontaneously within 3 weeks and have unsatisfactory functional and cosmetic results. There is general consensus that the best treatment entails early eschar excision and immediate grafting. These wounds may mimic the appearance of an indeterminate burn and are usually mottled, white, red or charred and dry in appearance, insensitive to pain and leathery to palpation. Blisters are unusual and if present are thin walled and do not enlarge. Clotted superficial vessels may be visible. The surface of the burn is usually depressed relative to adjacent unburned skin and the appearance of the burn remains static with little change over the ensuing days.

Estimating the extent of the burn

2   The extent of the burn is expressed as a percentage of the TBSA involved. Two methods of assessment are used. (1) The open hand of a child amounts to approximately 1% of the TBSA. (2) Different age-related values are used to calculate the percentage area burned, because the body proportions change with age. These are shown in *Table 1*.

Table 1

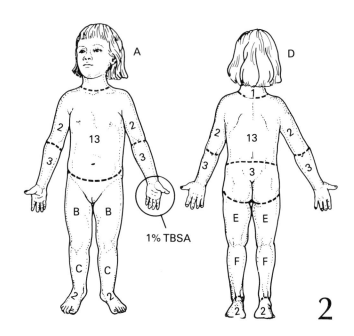

1% TBSA

2

	Age (years)				
	<1	1	5	10	15
A/D Head	10	9	7	6	5
B/E Thigh	3	3	4	5	5
C/F Leg	2	3	3	3	3

Management

Emergency management

At the scene of the injury smouldering or hot clothing should be removed immediately and the adequacy and patency of the airway ensured. Small burns are immersed in cold water or covered with cold, wet compresses for at least 30 min to reduce the depth of injury and relieve pain and discomfort. Larger burns (> 25% TBSA) should not be treated with cold water, as this may result in hypothermia, and should be covered with dry, clean dressings. Copious irrigation of the wound with water is indicated for chemical burns; neutralizing agents should not be used. In electrical burns the patient's circulation and ventilation must be evaluated. For suspected inhalation injury, 100% oxygen is given by face mask or endotracheal tube as soon as possible and a patent airway is maintained. Oral fluids should be withheld initially.

Definitive treatment

Minor burns

Initial therapy of minor burns should include administration of analgesics, cleaning the wound with bland soap and water or detergent, removal of topically applied agents and shaving hair where necessary. Dead tissue should be debrided and any tar removed with soft paraffin in a water base. Topical antibacterial agents and occlusive dressings (gauze and elastoform) or an adhesive polyurethane sheet should be used to dress the wound and tetanus toxoid administered.

Follow-up therapy: the patient should be encouraged to move the affected area. Local topical therapy is applied every 2–3 days until the wound is healed. Prophylactic antibiotics are not usually necessary. The wounds should be examined regularly (daily/once a week) as necessary.

Major burns

Initial therapy should include ensuring patency of the airways and checking the fluid requirement. For resuscitation, colloids should be given at a dose of 3.5 ml/kg/percentage burn for the first 24 h, reduced to 1.5 ml/kg/percentage burn during the second 24 h, and 60–120 ml/kg/day for fluid maintenance. The wound should be carefully cleaned and debrided and surface pus swabs taken for bacteriological culture. Topical therapy, analgesics and other medications (such as antacids, antibiotics and tetanus toxoid) are given as needed. Escharotomy is performed if necessary. A nasoduodenal tube may be needed in large burns and, if the burn is greater than 20% TBSA, a bladder catheter should be inserted.

Ongoing therapy involves preventing and correcting hypovolemia and management of the wound. Nutritional support (enteral feeding within 6–12 h) may be necessary. Function should be restored if possible by early grafting and care must be taken to prevent and treat any complications that arise. The patient may need rehabilitation and psychologic support.

Surgical management

The depth and extent of the burn wound will determine the surgical approach.

Anesthesia

Pediatric burns represent a unique challenge due to the nature of the operation and the concomitant physiologic responses to injury. Important components of anesthetic management are maintenance of an adequate airway especially in the presence of inhalation injury, choice of anesthetic agent, maintenance of hemodynamic stability and temperature, the use of pharmacologic agents, the position of the patient during surgery and continual monitoring.

Premedication in the form of trimeprazine (2 mg/kg) and droperidol (0.1 mg/kg) is administered. Anesthesia is induced by ketamine 2 mg/kg intramuscularly on arrival in the operating room, complemented with nasal oxygen (30–50%) and nitrous oxide. Intramuscular midazolam 0.5 mg/kg may be added for major burns. Anesthesia is maintained with a continuous infusion of ketamine (16–32 µg/kg/min). Inhalational agents are occasionally used.

Inhalational injury is not a prerequisite for intubation and bronchoscopy should be performed in all children with suspected or diagnosed pulmonary burns.

The ambient temperature should be 28–32°C and all anesthetic gases and fluids are heated to 37°C. Vascular access is critical. A large-bore cannula is usually placed subclavicularly or into the internal jugular vein. Concomitant arterial access is established in large burns or if the estimated blood loss will exceed 40 ml/kg. Maintenance fluid is given as isotonic crystalloids at 4 ml/kg/h and blood loss is replaced volume/volume to maintain the hematocrit above 30%. The child is thoroughly showered and washed with 3% PVP iodine soap at 37°C and intraoperative antibiotics given for all excisional procedures and for 5 days postoperatively. A urinary catheter with a temperature probe is inserted and surgery usually limited to 2 h. Postoperatively the child is kept in a recovery area and constantly monitored until fully awake with satisfactory vital signs.

Releasing escharotomy

3 Releasing escharotomy must be performed where a circumferential deep burn is impeding circulation to more distal parts, especially around the arms, legs or over the chest where respiration may be impaired.

The releasing escharotomy must traverse the dead tissue as far into the subcutaneous layer as necessary to encounter viable tissue and must extend from normal skin proximal to normal skin distally to prevent deep tissue death. Excessive bleeding can be problematic if the escharotomy is performed incorrectly or too deeply into the adjacent tissue.

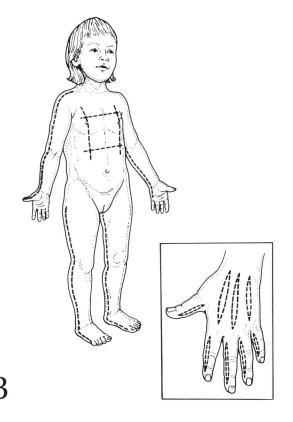

3

Timing and extent of excision

In general terms, excision is carried out as soon after injury as possible (i.e. as soon as the cardiovascular system is stable and resuscitation is completed, metabolic and physiologic balance restored and vital signs, urine output, hematocrit and albumin levels are satisfactory). This time may vary from a few hours to several days. Excision is therefore an elective procedure in a stable patient. The order of priority of areas of major excision (every alternate day) are the posterior trunk, anterior trunk and clavicular area, one lower extremity, second lower extremity, both upper extremities and hands, and all unhealed areas on the face, neck and head.

The amount to be excised at each procedure depends on the stability of the patient, the burn size, availability of auto- and allografts, the volume of blood loss incurred during the procedure and the adequacy of anesthesia. Most deep burns of less than 40% TBSA should be excised and grafted within the first few days as adequate donor sites are usually available. In large burns the principle is to reduce the burn surface area expeditiously.

4 The excised wound is covered with a widely meshed 3:1 autograft which in turn is overlaid with a 2:1 meshed allograft.

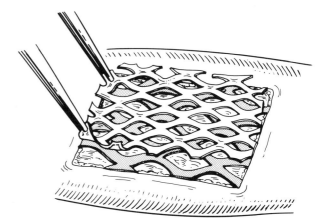

4

SURGICAL EXCISION

Burns < 10% TBSA

Excision and autografting are performed using meshed 1.5:1 or 2:1 or sheet grafts. Sheet grafts are placed on all vital and visual areas (face, neck, chest, hands) and all small grafted areas.

Burns 10–30% TBSA

Excision and autografting are performed with meshed 1.5:1 or 2:1 or sheet grafts. Sheet grafts are placed on all vital and visual areas (face, neck, chest, hands).

Burns 30–40% TBSA

Sufficient donor sites are usually available to graft the excised bed despite the fact that about 30% TBSA is unavailable for donation (face, neck, hands, feet). The grafts should be meshed at 1.5:1 or 2:1, or temporary allografts used.

Burns > 40% TBSA

Donor sites are limited and it is impossible to cover all the excised wounds with autografts primarily. The method preferred is to perform total or sequential (20% TBSA every alternate day) excision. Skin cover should then be applied (autograft 1.5:1, 2:1 or 3:1 and/or autograft 3:1 with allograft 2:1 overlay and/or synthetic skin substitutes).

Skin substitutes

Allografts are used only as a temporary biological cover and should be removed before rejection becomes evident. In practice this means removal every 10–12 days and replacement with pool allografts or permanent replacement with autograft when available. If this procedure is followed the likelihood of rejection and poor donor bed is reduced. If allografts are left for more than 14 days removal can only be achieved by excision. Alternative methods (xenografts, cultured keratinocytes and other biological skin substitutes) are not reliable for routine use and at best function only as temporary skin cover.

In general terms three anatomically different methods of removing eschar are used: (1) tangential or sequential excision; (2) fascial excision; and (3) delayed escharectomy.

TANGENTIAL OR SEQUENTIAL EXCISION

This method entails the sequential excision of thin layers of burn eschar until a viable bed is encountered. If done adequately the minimum amount of living tissue is sacrificed with satisfactory functional and cosmetic results.

5 Excision is best performed using a hand-held dermatome, held at a tangent to the wound surface and using guards of variable thickness to control the level of excision (± 0.02 cm (0.008 inch)). Excision over uneven surfaces or bony prominences can be aided by subeschar injection of saline. The appropriate level of excision or end point is characterized by a shiny white surface with brisk arteriolar or punctate bleeding or viable yellow non-hemorrhagic subcutaneous fat globules with briskly bleeding vessels in all areas. Dark pink-brown hemorrhagic fat is non-viable and must be removed; residual necrotic areas will jeopardize graft take. Dissection may become difficult once the level of excision has gone beyond the dermis. It may be very important to preserve subdermal fat over bony prominences for esthetic reasons but grafting onto subdermal fat results in a lower success rate. Blood loss may be substantial and effective control of hemorrhage must be established. It is advisable to limit excision to 25–100 cm^2, control hemorrhage and then to proceed with further excision. Tangential excision is best done within the first 1–5 days before hypervascularity and wound infection become established. A maximum of $\pm 20\%$ TBSA should be excised at any one time.

Once excised to the appropriate level and hemostasis is secured, an immediate split-thickness skin graft is performed. Sheet grafts are placed on important cosmetic and functional areas. To prevent desiccation of exposed and viable tissue, mesh grafts should not be expanded more than 1.5:1–2:1. If greater expansion is needed, temporary skin substitutes (cadaver or biobrane) should overlay the autograft. The latter method is also used for all excised and non-grafted areas.

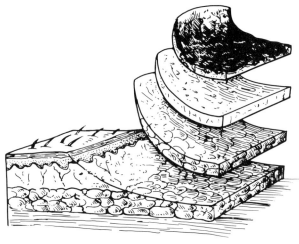

5

FASCIAL EXCISION

6 This method is generally reserved for very large life-threatening or deep full-thickness burns. The excision is performed using a combination of sharp dissection, traction and hemorrhage control. The amount excised at each procedure is determined by the stability of the child, blood loss and the availability of autografts or skin substitutes. The excision is preferably limited to approximately 20% TBSA at any one time. Fascial excision assures a viable bed for skin grafting with moderate blood loss, especially if done under tourniquet control; an excellent graft take may be expected if done within the first few days after injury. By incising at the periphery of the eschar vertically downward to the level of the deep investing fascia, a flap of eschar is raised and the dissection extended until all the dead tissue down to fascia level has been excised. It is preferable to leave a thin layer of fat over the subcutaneous bony prominences and tendon sheaths. Complete hemostasis with electrocoagulation should minimize blood loss substantially but bleeding often occurs from the skin edges. Topical vasoconstrictive agents could be applied to the fascia as the dissection proceeds. At completion the extremity is wrapped with a pressure bandage and elevated for 10 minutes. The excised area is covered with an expanded split-thickness skin graft. If the ratio exceeds 2:1 the autograft should be covered with a 2:1 meshed cadaveric allograft. The major disadvantage of this method is that it causes damage to lymphatics and cutaneous nerves, loss of subcutaneous fat, long-term cosmetic deformity and distal edema.

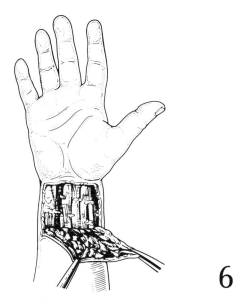

6

DELAYED ESCHARECTOMY

Delayed escharectomy after 1 week or spontaneous eschar separation allows for the formulation of a bed of granulation tissue. Daily debridement by means of hydrotherapy (showering or bathing), or coarse mesh gauze dressings will hasten eschar separation. The burn wound is ready for split skin grafting when there is a shiny slightly granular pinkish/red uniform bed of granulation tissue with no debris or evidence of infection.

Donor skin procurement

7 All unburned areas can serve as donor sites although 30% of the TBSA is unsuitable for donor skin. The preferred donor sites are the legs, buttocks and back and best color match between donor and recipient can be obtained from the 'blushing' area of the body for facial and neck burns. Donor skin thickness should be between 0.02 cm (0.008 inch) (thin) and 0.025 cm (0.010 inch) (thicker). Thicker grafts are more pliable and cause less scarring. Skin grafts are best procured with an electric dermatome or a Goulian or Watson dermatome.

Grafts are usually meshed with a Tanner mesher at a ratio of 1.5:1, 2:1 or 3:1, or used as sheet grafts on vital or cosmetically important areas.

Bleeding can be brisk and substantial and is best controlled with pressure, topical epinephrine (adrenaline) and early application of pressure dressings.

Subcutaneous injection of saline and vasopressin will greatly facilitate graft procurement over bony or uneven prominences. Donor sites are usually ready for reuse after 14 days.

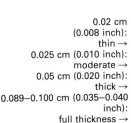

0.02 cm (0.008 inch): thin →
0.025 cm (0.010 inch): moderate →
0.05 cm (0.020 inch): thick →
0.089–0.100 cm (0.035–0.040 inch): full thickness →

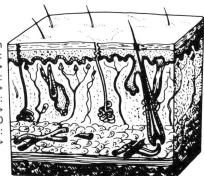

7

Hemostatic control

Bleeding from excised areas should be minimized by limiting excisional procedures to 25–100 cm² at any one time until hemostasis is ensured. Other methods employed are local pressure for 10 min, diathermy coagulation, suture ligation and the topical application of sponges soaked in 1:10 000/1:30 000 epinephrine (adrenaline) solution to the excised bed for 10 min. The latter should not be used in patients with cardiac disease or arrhythmias.

Skin graft placement

The procured skin is grafted onto the recipient area at the time of eschar excision, directly from the mesh board. Grafts are placed with the shiny or cut surface facing the prepared bed, either longitudinally or transversely over joints. The edges should be approximated or slightly overlapping and secured with surgical clips, sutures, or fine mesh gauze.

Wound dressings

Recipient area

In general terms the recipient area is covered with an occlusive dressing to prevent infection, avulsion and desiccation of the graft, and to allow for graft vascularization (3–4 days if grafts are placed on dermis or fascia and 5–7 days if placed on fat). Both sheet and mesh grafts are covered with a layer of fine mesh gauze, impregnated with topical antibiotics, followed by an absorbable dressing and an elastic dressing and splinting in a functional position where indicated. Sheet grafts may be left exposed, especially on the face and neck areas. The outer dressings, down to the layer of fine gauze, are taken off the following day to remove any blood clots or wound exudate. These dressing changes are repeated every day. The innermost dressing in contact with the graft is removed on day 5 with the aid of hydrotherapy.

Donor site

The area is covered with a topical agent; an adhesive polyurethane sheet may be used for limited areas. Discomfort is minimal, a rapid healing is experienced and the dressing is either left intact until healing has occurred or removed after a few days.

Early reconstruction

Early reconstructive principles form an integral part of all surgical procedures and long-term problems can be circumvented or minimized by proper positioning, supportive splints and pressure devices, judicious use of skeletal traction and suspension through maintaining joint excursions and mobility. Pressure garments are required if the burn wound has taken more than 3 weeks to heal and in those which were grafted.

Further reading

Alexander JW, MacMillan BG, Law E, Kittur DS. Treatment of severe burns with widely meshed skin autograft and meshed skin allograft overlay. *J Trauma* 1981; 21: 433–8.

Artz CP. Historical aspects of burn management. *Surg Clin North Am* 1970; 50: 1193–200.

Desai MH, Herndon DN, Broemeling L, Barrow RE, Nichols RJ Jr, Rutan RL. Early burn wound excision significantly reduces blood loss. *Ann Surg* 1990; 211: 753–62.

Desai MH, Rutan RL, Herndon DN. Conservative treatment of scald burns is superior to early excision. *J Burn Care Rehabil* 1991; 12: 482–4.

Heimbach DM, Engrav LH. *Surgical Management of the Burn Wound.* New York: Raven Press, 1984.

Heimbach DM. Early burn excision and grafting. *Surg Clin North Am* 1987; 67: 93–107.

Heimbach DM, Herndon D, Luterman A *et al.* Early excision of thermal burns – an international round table discussion. Geneva June 22, 1987. *J Burn Care Rehabil* 1988; 9: 549–61.

Heimbach D, Luterman A, Burke J *et al.* M. Artificial dermis for major burns. A multi-center randomized clinical trial. *Ann Surg* 1988; 208: 313–20.

Herndon DN, Parks DH. Comparison of serial debridement and autografting and early massive excision with cadaver skin overlay in the treatment of large burns in children. *J Trauma* 1986; 26: 149–52.

Herndon DN, Barrow RE, Rutan RL, Rutan TC, Desai MH, Abston S. A comparison of conservative versus early excision. Therapies in severely burned patients. *Ann Surg* 1989; 209: 547–53.

Janzekovic Z. A new concept in the early excision and immediate grafting of burns. *J Trauma* 1970; 10: 1103–8.

Janzekovic Z. The burn wound from the surgical point of view. *J Trauma* 1975; 15: 42–62.

Muller MJ, Herndon DN. The challenge of burns. *Lancet* 1994; 343: 216–20.

Tompkins RG, Remensnyder JP, Burke JF *et al.* Significant reductions in mortality for children with burn injuries through the use of prompt eschar excision. *Ann Surg* 1988; 208: 577–85.

Management of major trauma

Steven Stylianos MD
Assistant Professor of Surgery, Columbia University College of Physicians and Surgeons, and Attending Pediatric Surgeon, Babies' Hospital, New York, USA

Burton H. Harris MD
Professor of Pediatric Surgery, Tufts University School of Medicine, Chief of Pediatric Surgery, New England Medical Center, and Director of the Kiwanis Pediatric Trauma Institute, Boston, USA

'If a disease were killing our children in the proportions that accidents are, people would be outraged and demand that this killer be stopped.'

C. Everett Koop MD, ScD

Injury is the most important threat to the health of children in the USA and the leading cause of death after the first year of life in developed countries. Each year nearly 13 million children aged up to 14 years attend emergency rooms in the USA; 360 000 are hospitalized, 8000 die, and a significant number are left with a permanent disability.

The energy and interest of pediatric surgeons in the care of injured children is as old as the specialty of pediatric surgery itself. William E. Ladd became the father of pediatric surgery because of his interest in the special needs of injured children. In 1917 a collision between a French munitions ship and a Norwegian freighter caused an enormous explosion in the harbor in Nova Scotia, leaving 2000 killed, 9000 injured, and 31 000 homeless. Pleas for medical help were issued throughout the USA and Canada, and the Boston team was led by Dr Ladd. He was so moved by the medical differences of the children that he decided upon his return to devote himself exclusively to the surgical care of infants and children.

As a result of the advances in resuscitation and transport of victims of pediatric trauma, pediatric surgeons treat increasing numbers of children who survive severe multiple injuries. Most seriously injured children sustain the common triad of closed head trauma, abdominal injuries and long bone fractures, and diagnostic and treatment strategies for pediatric trauma patients should be planned for the multiply injured child.

Resuscitation

A child with multiple injuries admitted to a medical facility should be treated by an organized team of surgeons, physicians and nurses. The composition of the team will vary, but the senior surgeon should be the team leader. Preparation is mandatory, and includes equipment appropriate to children of varying ages and the establishment of a resuscitation protocol (*Table 1*). The 'check-list approach' is the surest way to accomplish the essential steps of diagnosis and treatment while individualizing care for each patient[1].

Airway control, vascular access, spinal precautions and temperature regulation must be assured throughout the initial evaluation and treatment of injured children. Specific details of airway management, pharmacologic therapy and central venous access in injured children are published elsewhere[2, 3].

Delay in establishing venous access may be life-threatening in the critically injured child. Percutaneous access to the subclavian, internal jugular or femoral veins can be hazardous in small, hypovolemic patients.

Table 1 Trauma receiving unit checklist: Kiwanis Pediatric Trauma Institute, Boston, USA

1. Immobilize neck
2. Remove clothing
3. Perform 60 s examination
4. Apply ECG leads
5. Draw blood for complete blood count, type and crossmatch
6. Nasal oxygen
7. Establish intravenous access
8. Venous cutdown
9. Lateral radiography of cervical spine
10. Foley catheter and temperature probe
11. Endotracheal intubation
12. Insert nasogastric tube
13. Peritoneal lavage
14. Insert arterial line
15. Dress open wounds
16. Complete physical examination
17. Take history
18. Chest radiography
19. Check laboratory results
20. List positive findings

Each of these steps should be considered by the trauma team leader as a do/don't-do decision

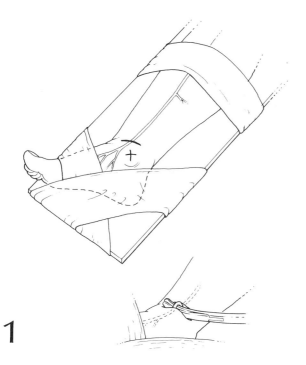

1 Venous cutdown requires surgical training, equipment and lighting often unavailable before reaching hospital.

2 Intraosseous infusion is an efficient alternative for achieving rapid vascular access during resuscitation. The device should be removed as soon as intravenous access is obtained. Infusions of crystalloid, blood, epinephrine (adrenaline), atropine, sodium bicarbonate, calcium chloride, succinylcholine (suxamethonium), mannitol, morphine, phenytoin, and glucocorticoid all can be successfully administered by intraosseous infusion. Training programs for intraosseous infusions are included in the curriculum of paramedics in the USA.

The indications for emergency department thoracotomy in children are the same as those currently accepted for adult trauma victims. Children *in extremis* with penetrating injuries have a survival rate of 5–36% following emergency department thoracotomy. Loss of vital signs and cardiac electrical activity before reaching the emergency department following blunt trauma defines the group least likely to benefit from emergency department thoracotomy.

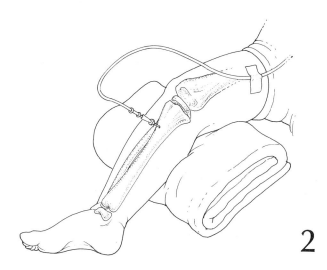

2

Diagnosis of blunt abdominal injuries

Recognition of significant abdominal injuries in children with blunt multisystem trauma can be difficult. Physical examination is inaccurate in more than 30% of cases, particularly in those patients seen soon after injury, or with central nervous system injuries and an abnormal neurologic examination. Evaluation may be further confounded by rib fractures, pelvic fractures, abdominal wall contusions and gastric dilation, all of which may contribute to the inaccuracy of the abdominal examination in children. It is no surprise that advances in diagnosis have paralleled the development of new imaging technology. Prompt and accurate recognition of abdominal injuries, now possible with computed tomographic (CT) scanning, allows for focused treatment plans[4]. In many centers CT scanning has become the single, global non-invasive test most commonly used to evaluate pediatric trauma patients, replacing sonography, radioisotope scans and diagnostic peritoneal lavage as the diagnostic test of choice. Double-contrast abdominal CT is recommended in all hemodynamically stable children with altered mental states after blunt trauma, in those with specific abdominal findings on physical examination, and in children with hematuria. For the hemodynamically unstable patient for whom a decision about laparotomy must be made in the first 20 min after admission, diagnostic peritoneal lavage performed in the emergency department is the procedure of choice.

Treatment of specific abdominal injuries

Diaphragm

Rupture of the diaphragm following blunt trauma is caused by cephalad transmission of a sudden increase in abdominal pressure. Herniation of abdominal viscera usually occurs through the posterolateral aspect of the diaphragm. The pathologic anatomy is a central circular defect, and the left hemidiaphragm is affected in over 70% of cases. The stomach is the most frequently displaced abdominal organ followed by the colon, small bowel, spleen and liver.

Goals in treatment are diagnosis at or before the first celiotomy, safe return of the herniated viscera into the abdomen, and a tension-free closure. The abdominal approach allows inspection of the viscera. Primary repair of the diaphragm is possible in most cases, and the use of prosthetic material or paracostal fixation is reserved for cases in which the muscle is avulsed from the chest wall. Interrupted non-absorbable sutures over pledgets are preferred for the repair. Repair of asymptomatic diaphragm injuries by a thoracic approach may be advisable because of the possible formation of pleural adhesions.

Spleen

The spleen is the organ most frequently injured in blunt abdominal trauma and the one surgeons work hardest to preserve. The findings of left upper quadrant tenderness with evidence of blood loss should prompt imaging of the spleen in the hemodynamically stable child. Abdominal CT scanning is useful because it produces anatomic images defining the presence and extent of splenic injury and identifies associated injuries and the degree of hemoperitoneum.

Non-operative treatment of isolated splenic injuries in stable patients is now standard practice in pediatric surgery[5]. This departure from the traditional practice of splenectomy for trauma is a response to increasing evidence of the important role of the spleen in cellular and humoral immunity. The evolution of non-operative therapy is seen in *Table 2*. The finding of non-bleeding splenic injuries at celiotomy led many to question the need and safety of exploration of stable patients with these injuries, but pediatric surgeons at The Hospital for Sick Children in Toronto were the pioneers of the expectant treatment of children with splenic laceration[5].

Children with hemodynamic compromise unresponsive to fluid resuscitation, and those with continued abdominal hemorrhage from splenic injuries, require celiotomy to stop blood loss.

Table 2   Treatment of children with splenic injuries

Author	Study period	No. of patients	Splenectomy	Repair	Non-operative treatment	Splenic salvage
Wesson	1974–79	63	15 (24)	4 (6)	44 (70)	48 (76)
King	1977–80	49	6 (12)	15 (31)	28 (57)	43 (88)
Pearl	1981–86	75	3 (4)	7 (9)	65 (87)	72 (96)

Figures in parentheses are percentages.

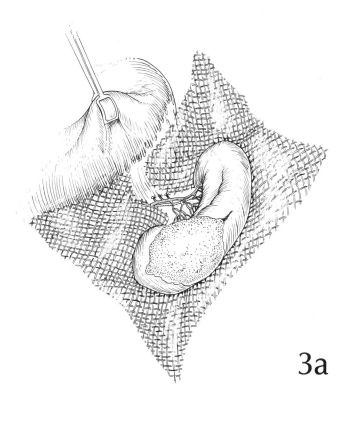

3a

3a, b Several surgical options are available which share as a goal the preservation of as much parenchyma as possible. The segmental anatomy of the spleen lends itself to partial splenectomy, splenorrhaphy, mesh wrapping (*Illustrations 3a, b*) using woven polyglycolic acid mesh, branch splenic artery ligation, and autotransplantation of splenic fragments. Each of these procedures has been successful in preserving filtering and synthetic funtions.

The importance of arterial inflow for pneumococcal clearance has been shown in experimental conditions, suggesting that splenic artery ligation and autotransplantation are unattractive alternatives.

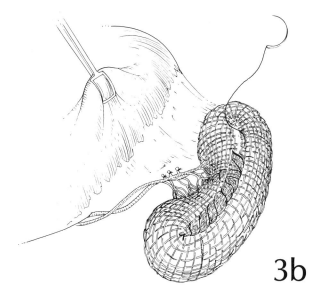

3b

Liver

Liver injuries are more often solitary in children than in adults, and are the second most common abdominal injury. Double-contrast truncal CT scanning has allowed rapid, non-invasive anatomic diagnosis, and an anatomic classification of hepatic injuries has been proposed[6]. CT scanning has replaced blood tests, sonography and isotope scans as the diagnostic method of choice in stable patients.

Operative repair is no longer considered mandatory for treatment of blunt liver injuries in hemodynamically stable children, duplicating the saga of the spleen. The amount of hemoperitoneum seen on the CT scan is not an indication for exploration if peripheral perfusion is normal. Abdominal exploration for liver injury in children is reserved for patients with a falling blood pressure, continuing transfusion requirements greater than 40 ml/kg, evidence of retrohepatic caval or hepatic vein injury, or suspicion of associated bowel injury. In a recent review of 342 children with blunt liver injuries from five institutions, 89% were successfully managed without operation[7].

Surgical management of life-threatening liver injuries begins with evacuation of abdominal blood and manual compression of the hepatic parenchyma while restoration of an adequate circulating blood volume is accomplished. When bleeding is active, temporary occlusion of the portal triad (the Pringle maneuver) should be performed. This allows hemostasis and debridement of the damaged parenchyma to be accomplished under direct vision. All devitalized tissue must be removed to decrease the risk of abscess formation. Use of a viable omental pack to cover the debrided hepatic surface and fill dead space may decrease the need for external drains and help prevent postoperative infection. Debridement need not follow anatomic planes and formal lobectomy with hepatic artery ligation is rarely indicated for blunt injury.

Continued hemorrhage despite occlusion of the portal triad suggests hepatic vein or retrohepatic vena caval injury. Many children with such injuries can present without initial hemodynamic compromise, only to experience acute hypotension when the liver is mobilized and its tamponade effect released. Availability of an autotransfusion device can assist in rapid restoration of blood volume in this setting, but requires skilled personnel and strict attention to replacement of coagulation factors. Extending the midline abdominal incision as a median sternotomy while compressing the liver against the diaphragm and retroperitoneum can aid exposure and control of such injuries. Initial enthusiasm

for atriocaval shunts has decreased with reports of 60–90% mortality from major trauma centers. Others advocate direct finger fracture of the hepatic parenchyma to expose the vascular injury after portal triad occlusion with atriocaval shunts.

The early morbidity and mortality of severe hepatic injuries are related to the effects of massive blood loss and replacement of large volumes of cold blood products. If evidence of coagulopathy, hypothermia, and acidosis exist before control of hemorrhage has been obtained, abdominal packing with planned re-exploration may be life-saving. In less urgent circumstances, percutaneous angiographic embolization of hepatic arterial branches can be a valuable adjunct in treating postoperative hemorrhage and hemobilia after liver injury.

Kidney

Renal injuries in children are often caused by high energy impact associated with motor vehicle accidents or other serious abdominal trauma. Hematuria is present in 41–68% of children following blunt abdominal trauma. Most authors report direct correlation between the amount of hematuria and the severity of genitourinary injury, but renovascular injuries may result in no hematuria and bladder contusion or disruption often causes large amounts of blood in the urine. The magnitude of hematuria requiring diagnostic evaluation following blunt abdominal trauma continues to be a subject of debate, as does the otpimal imaging study for detection of renal injuries.

The majority of blunt renal injuries are treated without operation when uncontrolled hemorrhage or other indications for abdominal exploration are absent. This approach is safe and effective in 80% of children. Successful renal salvage at operation by partial nephrectomy or nephrorrhaphy depends on the severity of both the renal injury and associated injuries. Collecting system injuries should be repaired with absorbable sutures after evacuation of pelvic clots and debridement of devascularized parenchyma. Intravenous infusion of indigo-carmine (a vital dye excreted in the urine) at operation may help to identify sites of extravasation, and proximal control of the renal artery and vein before opening Gerota's fascia may facilitate retroperitoneal exploration. Nephrectomy is recommended for major renal injuries in hemodynamically unstable patients with multiple injuries, and in those patients with avulsion injuries. Vascular repair can be attempted within 12 h of injury and in the absence of multiple injuries.

The 'seatbelt syndrome'

A decrease in motor vehicle-related fatalities has occurred in association with mandatory seatbelt legislation. Concurrently, a pattern of injuries caused by lap-belt restraints has emerged[8].

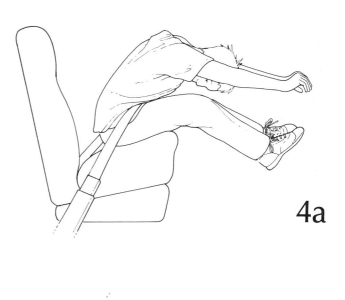

4a, b

This 'seatbelt syndrome' includes abdominal wall contusion, injury to a hollow viscus and vertebral fracture. The mechanism of injury is hyperflexion of the torso caused by deceleration forces with the lap-belt as a fulcrum. Children are at a particular risk of these injuries owing to their higher center of gravity, thin abdominal wall, non-prominent iliac crest, and immature supporting structures of the vertebral bodies.

Bowel injuries associated with lap-belt use can occur by several mechanisms: compression against the vertebral column with a crush injury and delayed necrosis and perforation, shearing of the bowel and mesentery at fixed points in the retroperitoneum with subsequent ischemia, and immediate closed-loop burst injuries on the antimesenteric border when fluid-filled loops are subjected to sudden increases in intraluminal pressure (*Illustration 4b*). This injury is often associated with a Chance fracture of the lumbar spine.

Children who present with a linear band of ecchymosis across the lower abdominal wall should be evaluated for these injuries. Other lap-belt injuries include abdominal wall contusions, major vascular injuries, and vertebral fractures. The vertebral injuries associated with hyperflexion (Chance fractures) may escape detection on plain abdominal radiographs and abdominal CT scans. Lateral lumbosacral plain films are indicated in all children with lap-belt injuries before immobilization is removed.

Repair of blunt intestinal injuries requires debridement or resection of all devascularized tissue. Peritoneal irrigation and systemic antibiotics allow most small bowel perforations to be managed with primary repair or anastomosis even if diagnosis and operation are delayed and peritoneal contamination has occurred.

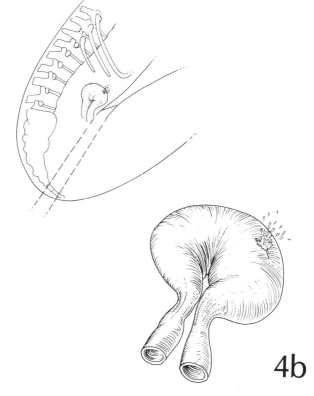

Conclusions

Recent advances in the delivery of trauma and critical care in children have resulted in improved outcome following major injuries. Continuous evaluation in a monitored setting with repeated abdominal examinations, serial hematocrit determinations, careful attention to fluid requirements, and immediate availability of anesthesia, operating theater and blood products are essential components of successful management. Although the last decade has seen increasing emphasis on non-operative treatment, the pediatric surgeon should remain the principal physician in multidisciplinary care of these critically injured children; the decision not to operate is always a surgical decision.

Pediatric trauma care has become an art form practiced by many pediatric surgeons who regard it as their field of special interest. The emotional and physiologic differences of young patients and the need to cope with pediatric trauma as a syndrome are now acknowledged to require special techniques and organization best provided by pediatric trauma centers. Improved outcome has been documented beyond doubt, and the trauma center movement in the USA has matured to the point where legislative and regulatory bodies and insurance carriers are directing seriously injured patients to specialized facilities.

We hear so much about the rare diseases that it is possible to forget that trauma kills more children than all other diseases combined. Seventy years after Dr Ladd's vision, the day may finally be at hand in which every pediatric hospital and children's service makes a special effort to provide advanced pediatric trauma care.

The essential ingredient of pediatric trauma care is commitment to the special needs of injured children: personal, institutional and community commitment.

References

1. Harris BH, Latchaw LA, Murphy RE, Schwaitzberg SD. A protocol for pediatric trauma receiving units. *J Pediatr Surg* 1989; 24: 419–22.

2. American Academy of Pediatrics and American Heart Association. *Textbook of Pediatric Advanced Life Support.* Dallas, USA, 1990.

3. American College of Surgeons Committee on Trauma. *Textbook of Advanced Trauma Life Support.* Chicago, USA, 1989.

4. Taylor GA, Fallat ME, Potter BM, Eichelberger MR. The role of computed tomography in blunt abdominal trauma in children. *J Trauma* 1988; 28: 1660–4.

5. Pearl RH, Wesson DE, Spence LJ *et al.* Splenic injury: a five year update with improved results and changing criteria for conservative management. *J Pediatr Surg* 1989; 24: 428–31.

6. Moore EE, Shackford SR, Pachter HL *et al.* Organ injury scaling: spleen, liver, and kidney. *J Trauma* 1989; 29: 1664–6.

7. Oldham KT. Liver and spleen trauma in children. In: Harris BH, Coran AG, eds. *Progress in Pediatric Trauma* 3rd edn. Boston: Nobb Hill, 1989: 95–101.

8. Taylor GA, Eggli KD. Lap-belt injuries of the lumbar spine in children: a pitfall in CT diagnosis. *Am J Roentgenol* 1988; 150: 1355–8. Published erratum appears in *Am J Roentgenol* 1988; 151: preceding 641.

Illustrations by Angela Christie

Principles of fetal surgery

Thomas M. Krummel MD
John W. Oswald Professor and Chair, Department of Surgery, Chief, Division of Pediatric Surgery,
Pennsylvania State University, College of Medicine, Hershey, Pennsylvania, USA

History

Without a clear understanding of the natural history of a fetal anomaly, rational fetal therapy is impossible. The fetus could not be considered a patient until after the development of prenatal ultrasonography. Based on the accumulated experience of the last 20 years, serial high-resolution sonograms by skilled sonographers permit accurate prenatal diagnosis and identify prognostic features upon which treatment can be considered.

Over the last 20 years, the surgical treatment of a number of congenital anomalies has been pioneered and refined by Harrison, Adzick and their colleagues[1,2]; the techniques depicted in this chapter are based on their experience.

A significant impediment to the surgical treatment of the fetus (who might benefit from the operation) is the risk to the mother (who will not directly benefit from the operation). Extensive experience in the rigorous non-human primate model is mandatory to minimize risks of morbidity or late reproductive loss. It would be reckless for a surgeon who does not have such experience to offer open fetal operation to a woman.

Fetal obstructive uropathy

Since the early 1980s the natural history of fetal obstructive uropathy has been deciphered. Animal models have been developed which mimic the human condition with renal dysplasia and pulmonary hypoplasia, and treatment algorithms have been developed[1].

Fetus with space-occupying lung lesion

These were not originally throught to be problematic prior to birth but prenatal ultrasonography has identified a small group of fetuses who present with distress. A number of infants with congenital cystic adenomatoid malformation (CCAM) of the lung will demonstrate polyhydramnios and fetal hydrops, and a high risk of death.

Fetus with sacrococcygeal teratoma

Prenatal diagnosis of a sacrococcygeal teratoma has several implications. Under most circumstances, a large teratoma will preclude vaginal delivery; elective cesarian section at term is recommended. Serial sonograms have also identified a small group of fetuses with severe, potentially life-threatening, physiologic perturbations. The presence of polyhydramnios, fetal hydrops, and placentomegaly is highly predictive of mortality.

Fetus with congenital diaphragmatic hernia

No other fetal lesion has engendered more heated discussion regarding prenatal treatment than congenital diaphragmatic hernia. Most of this controversy has centered on the actual fetal mortality resulting from this lesion; when diagnosed prenatally, the mortality has been clearly documented at 60%[2]. Such prenatal experience has delineated the 'hidden mortality' associated with a prenatal diagnosis.

Principles and justification

It is important to emphasize that the vast majority of correctable malformations are well handled with established surgical techniques after delivery. Some defects may require preterm delivery (urinary obstruction, fetal hydrops) or cesarian section delivery at term (conjoined twins, giant omphalocele, meningomyelocele or sacrococcygeal teratoma).

In a few cases an easily correctable anatomic malformation leads to life-threatening damage or developmental delay of a key organ, jeopardizing the life of the infant. Such anomalies, if reliably detected early, amenable to prenatal correction and if repaired, permit resumption of normal organ development; these patients may be considered for prenatal operation. Maternal safety must always be safeguarded.

Indications

Open fetal surgical intervention poses unique technical, ethical and legal challenges. The International Fetal Medicine and Surgery Society has suggested general criteria for undertaking fetal therapy.

The fetus should be a singleton, in whom a detailed sonographic examination and genetic studies show no concomitant abnormalities. The family must be fully counseled about risks and benefits and should agree to treatment, including long-term follow-up to determine efficacy. A multidisciplinary team that includes a perinatologist experienced in fetal diagnosis and fetal sampling or intrauterine transfusion, a geneticist, a sonographer experienced in the diagnosis of fetal anomalies and the pediatric surgeon and neonatologist who will manage the infant after birth should concur in the plan for innovative treatment. Committed anesthetists and other support staff are also essential. The institutional review board must approve. There should be access to a level III high-risk obstetric unit and neonatal intensive care unit, as well as bioethical and psychologic consultation.

In general, an organized fetal treatment program is required, where state-of-the-art clinical care is interdigitated with ongoing research. Because the efficacy of fetal surgery is not yet clear, all clinical cases must be subjected to the scrutiny of uninvolved colleagues.

Fetal obstructive uropathy

High-grade bilateral obstruction (or unilateral in a solitary kidney) will adversely affect renal development; the diminished fetal urine excretion results in oligohydramnios and may result in fetal pulmonary hypoplasia. Either problem exists as a spectrum, depending on the lesion and its duration.

Fetus with space-occupying lung lesions

An expanding thoracic mass may produce ipsilateral pulmonary compression, mediastinal shift with vena caval obstruction and consequent fetal hydrops. The development of hydrops is an ominous sign. Although some such lesions disappear, if they are persistent and profoundly symptomatic, prenatal treatment may be warranted. Microcystic lesions seem to have a worse prognosis with more frequently associated hydrops and pulmonary hypoplasia leading to death before or after birth.

Fetus with sacrococcygeal teratoma

A large teratoma will acquire considerable blood flow; such a 'vascular steal' will invariably siphon off an ever-increasing output from the distal aorta, away from the placenta. The resultant high-output cardiac failure may kill the fetus.

Fetus with congenital diaphragmatic hernia

As with all considerations for prenatal treatment, selection criteria strive to identify the fetus at greatest risk of dying with conventional postnatal care. Current inclusion criteria include an otherwise well single fetus of less than 30 weeks' gestation with a distended intrathoracic stomach and a left-sided congenital diaphragmatic hernia. Exclusion criteria, importantly, include the presence of an intrathoracic herniated left lobe of the liver with an umbilical vein/ductus venosus above the diaphragm. This specific contraindication results from the technical inability to reduce such a liver lobe without compromising umbilical vein blood flow and risking fetal death[1,2].

Preoperative

For the mother, routine preoperative studies are indicated. Preoperative tocolysis begins with administration of an indomethacin suppository (100 mg); perioperative antibiotics are indicated to minimize the risk of chorioamniitis.

Assessment necessary for the fetus depends on the procedure to be undertaken, and will be included under each specific anomaly.

Anesthesia

1 The mother is placed supine with a roll under her right side to displace the uterus medially off the inferior vena cava. Inhalational halothane is administered for maternal and fetal anaesthesia and uterine relaxation. Intraoperative maternal care and monitoring include electrocardiography, pulse oximetry, central venous pressure and arterial catheters, large-bore intravenous cannulas and a bladder catheter.

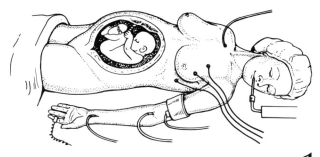

1

Operations

Maternal incision

2 A low transverse skin incision is made in the mother's abdomen. A vertical midline fascial incision is made if the placenta is posterior (anterior hysterotomy); the transverse incision is deepened through the muscle layers if the placenta is anterior (posterior hysterotomy). A fixed ring retractor facilitates uterine exposure. Intraoperative ultrasonography is used to confirm the placental and fetal positions, and to direct intramuscular injection of narcotics and paralytic agents if necessary.

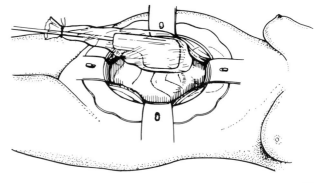

2

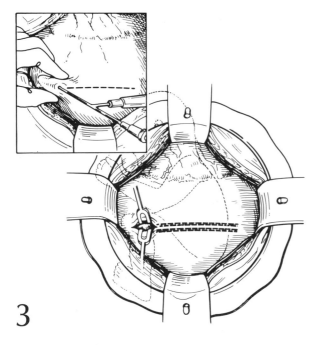

3

Hysterotomy

3 The hysterotomy is located parallel to and at least 6 cm away from the edge of the placenta and yet should provide appropriate fetal exposure. Amniotic fluid is aspirated via a trocar and the hysterotomy incision begins with the electrocautery, then is opened with a Lactomer stapling device which places parallel lines of absorbable staples in the uterine wall and membranes. This device fuses the membranes to the uterine wall and provides hemostasis. Specially designed reverse-biting clamps are placed at the apices and on either edge[2]. Throughout the operation, warm saline should be used to bathe the uterus and fetus.

Fetal incision

4 The fetal operative site is exposed and the specific procedure begun. Throughout the procedure, the condition of the fetus must be monitored with pulse oximetry and a radiotelemetry implant[3], which maintains fetal ECG and temperature during the operation and until delivery. Fetal intravenous access, if needed, is best accomplished via an interosseous route[3].

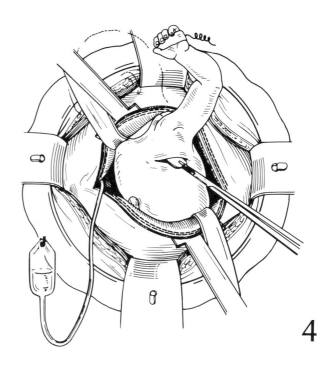

4

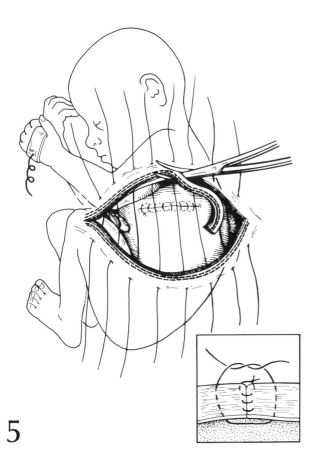

5

Wound closures

5 Once the fetal operation is complete, the fetus is returned to the uterus. Long-term absorbable monofilament sutures are placed as stays, the staple line excised and the hysterotomy closed in a continuous fashion for a watertight repair; fibrin glue may be helpful. Warmed saline with antibiotics is used to replace amniotic fluid volume. The maternal laparotomy incision is closed in layers.

FETAL VENTRICULOMEGALY[1]

Treatment is technically feasible, but currently the fetus with ventriculomegaly is not treated. Initial attempts at treatment used sequential needle aspiration; a percutaneously placed, valved shunt was subsequently developed to be deployed with ultrasound guidance. Although this has increased the chances of survival there is a concomitant increase in the number of moderately or severely handicapped infants.

FETAL OBSTRUCTIVE UROPATHY[1, 2]

Selection criteria for prenatal decompression attempt to identify the fetus with significant yet reversible renal impairment; in the vast majority of patients obstruction is due to posterior urethral valves. Harrison and Adzick[1, 2] have developed an algorithm based on the sonogram and bladder aspiration. Renal function outcome is predicted by sonographically normal renal parenchyma, and fetal urine with sodium concentration <100 mg/l, chloride <90 mg/l, osmolarity <210 mosmol/l and β_2-microglobulin <2 mg/l.

6, 7 Beyond 28 weeks' gestation, percutaneous ultrasound-guided placement of a vesico-amniotic Harrison catheter is the first option. The catheter is loaded into a hollow stylet, the uterus and fetal bladder are punctured and the catheter discharged. Maintenance of catheter position and function is difficult; a bulbed catheter has recently been developed to circumvent this difficulty.

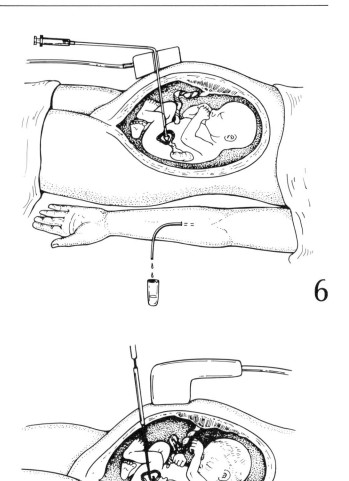

6

7

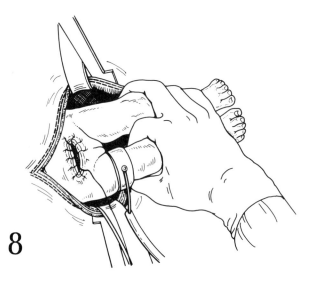

8

8 Before 28 weeks' gestation, or if vesicoamniotic shunting fails, open surgical decompression is warranted. Less than 3% of over 300 cases of bilateral hydronephrosis have come to open fetal operation. The operation of choice is marsupialization of the bladder to the abdominal wall. Following hysterotomy, the lower fetal abdomen is exposed. A suprapubic incision is carried down to and into the dilated bladder. An open vesicotomy is constructed with long-term absorbable sutures.

The hysterotomy and maternal incisions are then closed; preterm labor is treated as described previously. Once urinary drainage is established, amniotic fluid volume can be restored, with a chance to ameliorate pulmonary hypoplasia.

FETUS WITH SPACE-OCCUPYING LUNG LESION1[1,2]

An isolated CCAM producing hydrops between 24–32 weeks of gestation (*Illustration 9a*) may be considered for treatment. Before 24 weeks the outlook is dismal, and after 32 weeks induced labor and postnatal operation are more appropriate.

A thoracoamniotic shunt may occasionally be placed for a macrocystic lesion with a dominant cyst, though it may dislodge or fail. This technique is similar to that described for catheter drainage of the obstructed bladder.

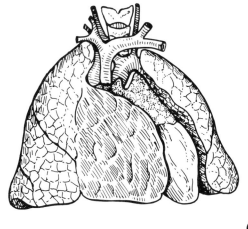

9a

9a, b The maternal laparotomy and hysterotomy are performed as described earlier, as are fetal monitoring and exposure. A thoracotomy incision is opened and the CCAM allowed to decompress itself through the incision. An anatomic resection is performed based on the lobe(s) of origin with a stapler, and the fetal chest is then closed. The uterus and mother's abdomen are closed as previously described and tocolysis begun.

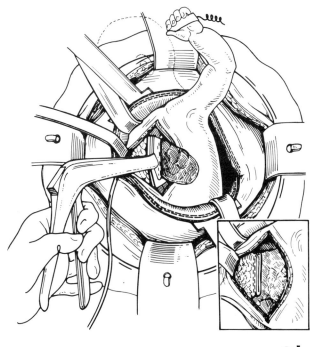

9b

FETUS WITH SACROCOCCYGEAL TERATOMA

The size-for-dates discrepancy associated with poly-hydramnios will prompt the first ultrasound examination, and concurrent Doppler studies demonstrating high distal aortic blood flow with a 'steal' suggest a lower chance of the pregnancy going to term. The subsequent development of fetal hydrops indicates a very poor prognosis. There may also be profound maternal consequences as a result of fetal distress; the maternal 'mirror' syndrome of severe pre-eclampsia is well documented, and may further justify fetal operation.

Maternal pre-eclampsia is treated in the standard fashion. Maternal and fetal care, monitoring and operative exposure are accomplished in the usual fashion.

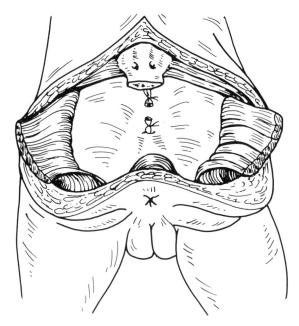

10a

10a, b Excision is performed in a manner similar to that used in the neonate. A chevron incision, coccygectomy and control of the middle sacral arterial supply to the tumor are performed. The tumor is then resected and the wound closed.

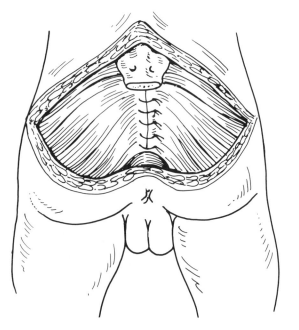

10b

FETUS WITH CONGENITAL DIAPHRAGMATIC HERNIA[1,2]

Polyhydramnios as a consequence of a functional gastric outlet obstruction at the diaphragm should indicate sonographic study for diagnosis. The inclusion and exclusion criteria detailed above must be met. The parents should always be counseled extensively before the procedure is carried out.

11a–c
Harrison and colleagues have evolved the operative technique currently used[1,2]. The lateral aspect of the fetus is exposed. Simultaneous thoracic and subcostal incisions are made. A Goretex silo is then sutured along the lower edge of the subcostal incision. The herniated viscera are reduced into the silo, the diaphragmatic defect closed with a patch and the silo then completed. The maternal operation is completed as described earlier; tocolytic management is crucial as always.

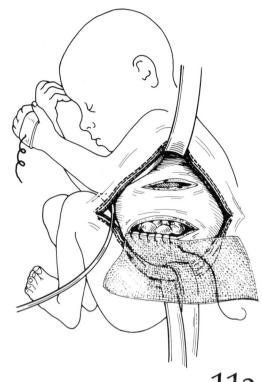

11a

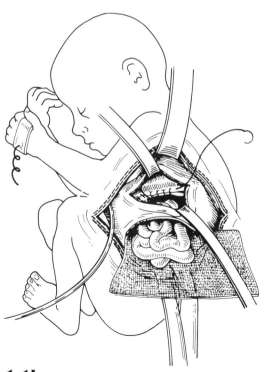

11b

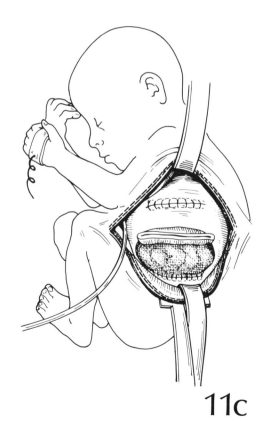

11c

The future – fetoscopy

Despite extraordinary work and phenomenal progress, open fetal surgery remains a daunting challenge. Not only are the operative difficulties formidable, the tocolytic management is also extremely complex and continues to be the rate-limiting step.

Management of preterm labor has made a quantum leap with the use of the radiotelemeter[3] and the advent of nitric oxide therapy in one of several modes[2]. The recent application of minimally invasive surgical techniques to fetoscopy[4] will no doubt further reduce the morbidity/mortality of fetal manipulations.

12 Transuterine placement of endoscopic lens systems and instruments may permit a variety of operative manipulations and reduce the high risk of mortality of the open operations.

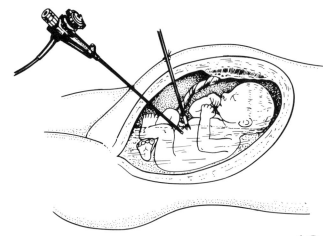

12

Postoperative care

Tocolytic therapy begins as anesthesia is completed and includes patient-controlled analgesia, continued indomethacin and an evolving regimen of nitric oxide compounds. The maintenance of a quiet relaxed uterus continues to be a formidable challenge. Monitoring continues during inpatient recovery and then as an outpatient using telemetry monitoring and serial fetal ultrasonographic scans. Delivery is always by cesarian section.

Outcome

Fetal obstructive uropathy

Eight fetuses have undergone open urinary decompression[2]. One was removed because of a cloacal anomaly and one was delivered 2 weeks after surgery (maternal cessation of tocolytics) and died of pulmonary hypoplasia. Six fetuses were delivered at 32–36 weeks; two died at birth of pulmonary hypoplasia. Neither had normal amniotic fluid volumes restored. Four survivors resulted from restoration of normal amniotic fluid volumes and no significant neonatal respiratory distress was seen. One child died of unrelated causes and two have normal renal function. One child required a renal transplant at 3 years of age.

Fetus with space-occupying lung lesion

To date, eight patients have undergone surgical resection of CCAM lesions producing life-threatening hydrops. There have been five survivors with good long-term development[2].

Fetus with sacrococcygeal teratoma

Two infants with large sacrococcygeal teratomas, high output failure and hydrops have been operated upon in the prenatal period (24–26 weeks' gestation)[2]. Resection and closure were accomplished but both subsequently died. Maternal pre-eclampsia led to delivery at 26 weeks and death from pulmonary causes in one fetus; the second was also delivered at 26 weeks with minimal pulmonary problems but because of immature histology of the teratoma, re-resection was attempted when the neonate was 2 weeks old. During this procedure the neonate died of an air embolus.

Fetus with congenital diaphragmatic hernia

Harrison's early experience was frustrating; with the current techniques developed, 14 fetuses have been operated upon[2]. Repair was successful in nine patients and four survived.

Conclusion

Surgical care of the human fetus is currently at a stage similar to that of orthotopic liver transplantation before the availability of cyclosporin. The evolution of fetal techniques to include telemetry, control of preterm labor and minimal yet effective manipulation may well provide an equivalent of 'cyclosporin' for fetal surgery.

References

1. Harrison MR, Golbus MS, Filly RA, eds. *The Unborn Patient: Prenatal Diagnosis and Treatment*, 2nd edn, Philadelphia: WB Saunders, 1990.

2. Adzick NS, Harrison MR. The unborn surgical patient. *Curr Probl Surg* 1994; 31: 1–68.

3. Jennings RW, Adzick NS, Longaker MT, Lorenz HP, Estes JM, Harrison MR. New techniques in fetal surgery. *J Pediatr Surg* 1992; 27: 1329–33.

4. Estes JM, MacGillivray TE, Hedrick MH, Adzick NS, Harrison MR. Fetoscopic surgery for the treatment of congenital anomalies. *J Pediatr Surg* 1992; 27: 950–4.

Principles of transplantation: kidney

Robert M. Merion MD, FACS
Associate Professor of Surgery and Chief, Division of Transplantation, University of Michigan Medical School, and Director, University of Michigan Kidney Transplantation Program, Ann Arbor, Michigan, USA

History

Successful renal transplantation in human identical twins was first achieved by Joseph Murray and his colleagues at the Peter Bent Brigham Hospital in Boston in the 1950s. This accomplishment was recognized by the award of a Nobel Prize to Murray in 1990, by which time living-related and cadaveric renal transplantation in infants and children were routinely performed as the optimum therapy for end-stage renal disease. The development of effective methods of chemical immuno-suppression, including cyclosporine (cyclosporin) has greatly improved success rates in recent years.

Principles and justification

Any pediatric patient with end-stage renal disease should be actively considered for renal transplantation. Even infants and neonates, previously thought to have a poor outcome, have been found recently to do well from medical as well as developmental perspectives[1]. Adequate recipient size is one of the few absolute physiologic prerequisites for operation. In order to permit an adult donor kidney to fit comfortably in the recipient's abdominal cavity, an arbitrary weight of 7 kg is sought. Absolute contraindications to renal transplantation include pre-existing malignancy, systemic infection that cannot be eradicated (including human immunodeficiency virus), and absence of patent major abdominal vasculature for anastomosis.

Preoperative

Assessment and preparation

A team approach including the transplant surgeon, pediatric nephrologist, social worker, nurse specialist and transplant coordinator facilitates a good outcome.

Aggressive nutrition and dialysis, usually by a peritoneal method such as nocturnal cycling or intermittent ambulatory peritoneal dialysis, is required to allow growth of small infants with renal failure. If possible, childhood immunizations should be administered before transplantation and previous exposure to chicken-pox (or immunization if this is available) is desirable. The child must be free of acute infectious illness at the time of transplantation.

Unlike adult recipients, children are much more likely to have an inadequate lower urinary tract due to obstructive uropathy or congenital genitourinary abnor-malities. An evaluation of the lower urinary system should be complete and inadequacies must be identified and corrected before transplantation. Strategies for achieving a satisfactory lower urinary tract may include training for intermittent self-catheterization, bilateral native nephroureterectomy, bladder augmentation (usually with colon), or construction of an intestinal conduit.

Adequate social support must be in place. Postopera-tive outpatient visits and occasional readmissions to hospital are the rule rather than the exception. Transportation arrangements must be secure. The child's caregivers must have a thorough understanding of the warning signs of post-transplant infection and organ dysfunction.

Anesthesia

General anesthesia for renal transplantation follows the usual principles for major abdominal procedures in children. Attention to intraoperative fluid management and maintenance of temperature are particularly critic-al. The child should be given warmed intravenous fluids and a ventilator with a temperature-regulated humidi-fier should be used. Monitoring of arterial blood pressure is mandatory for infants and children weighing less than 15 kg and central venous pressure should be monitored for all renal transplant recipients regardless of age or size.

Operation

Position of patient

Renal transplantation is performed with the patient in the supine position. A urinary catheter is placed into the bladder or urinary reservoir and connected to a three-way system to allow for instillation of povidone-iodine (Betadine) solution at the time of urinary reconstruction. The head should be extended and turned to one side for placement of a central venous catheter at the beginning of the procedure. If a peritoneal dialysis catheter is in place, any residual fluid should be drained using a sterile technique and the clamped catheter should be secured on the patient's left side. The neck, anterior chest wall and abdomen are prepared with an iodinated solution.

Central venous catheter placement

1 At the beginning of the procedure an indwelling central venous catheter of the Hickman type should be inserted via an incision over the external jugular vein or via the percutaneous approach to the internal jugular vein in larger children. The tip of the catheter should be positioned at the junction of the superior vena cava and the right atrium and confirmed by fluoroscopy. The catheter should follow a gently curved course and exit on the anterior chest wall. Following insertion, the catheter is passed to the anesthetic team to be connected to an in-line pressure monitoring system.

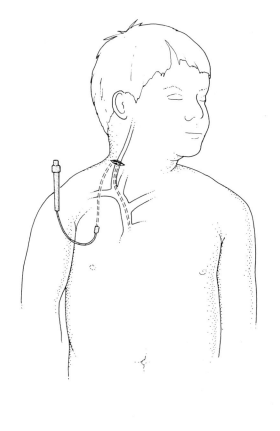

1

Incision

2 A curvilinear incision on the right abdomen, which will allow access to the retroperitoneum, major vessels (iliac vessels, vena cava and aorta) and the bladder is used. The incision starts at the midline about one finger-breadth superior to the pubic symphysis, extends lateral to the rectus abdominis muscle and then curves superiorly to about the level of the umbilicus. In small children and infants the incision must be carried nearly to the costal margin to permit adequate exposure.

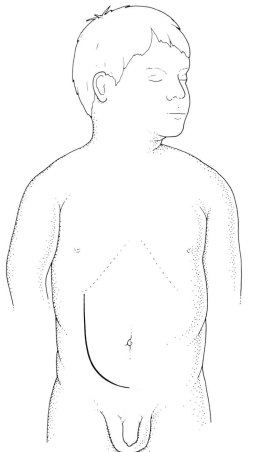

2

Exposure

3 The external oblique, internal oblique and transverse abdominis muscles are divided, as is the rectus abdominis medially. Extreme care should be taken to avoid entry into the peritoneal cavity. Damage to the peritoneal cavity is most likely at the most superior and inferior aspects of the dissection, particularly if there have been previous episodes of peritonitis. Inadvertent tears should be closed with absorbable sutures to prevent leakage of residual dialysis fluid into the operative field. The peritoneum is swept medially and superiorly to expose the iliac vessels, inferior vena cava and distal aorta. The inferior epigastric vessels are ligated and divided medially. The spermatic cord should be conserved by careful dissection and medial retraction. In girls the round ligament should be divided. At this point a self-retaining Bookwalter rectractor system should be assembled to maintain exposure for the remainder of the procedure.

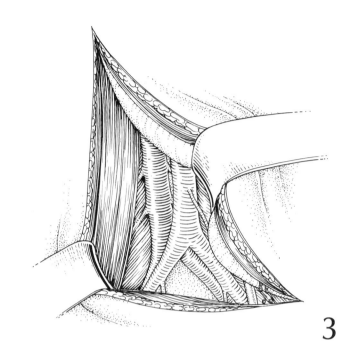

3

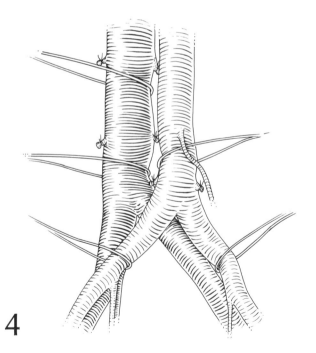

4

Vascular dissection

4 The inferior vena cava and distal aorta should be used for vascular reconstruction in children weighing less than 15 kg. Circumferential dissection of the distal vena cava is accomplished first. Lumbar veins are divided between fine silk ligatures to free a segment of vena cava approximately 2–3 cm in length. The distal aorta and proximal common iliac arteries are controlled with rubber vessel loops. The inferior mesenteric artery does not usually need to be divided. At least one set of lumbar arteries is generally encountered. Care should be exercised during dissection of the aorta to avoid disruption of the abdominal lymphatic trunk.

Preparation of donor kidney

Before administration of heparin and clamping the vessels, the donor kidney is brought to the operative field in a bath of sterile iced saline solution. The renal artery and vein are cleaned of surrounding tissues and side branches are secured. The renal vein should be kept relatively short, usually not longer than 1.5 cm, to prevent kinking. If the donor kidney is of cadaveric origin, a decision must be made whether or not to utilize the entire length of the renal artery with a Carrel patch of donor aorta. Usually this will result in a renal artery that is too long unless the recipient weighs more than 30 kg. The renal artery from a living-related donor kidney should be spatulated. The kidney may be wrapped in a moistened laparotomy pad with a 'keyhole' fashioned for the vessels. This facilitates handling of the kidney in the wound.

Vascular anastomoses

The recipient is given heparin, 50–70 units/kg body weight. Full-dose heparinization is unnecessary. Vascular clamps should be carefully chosen to avoid obscuring the field. In infants, tension on double-looped rubber vessel slings is all that is required. This technique has the advantage of elevating the vessels in the field. During construction of the vascular anastomoses, the anesthetic team should volume load the recipient to a central venous pressure of 15–18 cmH$_2$O and administer mannitol, 1 g/kg. These maneuvers will counteract the effects of revascularization and its attendant destabilizing effect due to volume shift. A transplanted adult kidney may account for 20% of the circulating blood volume of a 7-kg infant.

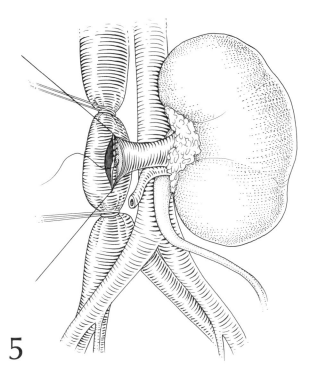

5

5 A longitudinal incision is made in the vena cava and 6/0 or 7/0 polypropylene sutures are placed at the apices. The assistant positions the kidney medially in the wound. The medial side of the anastomosis is performed first from within the lumen of the vein followed by the lateral side from the outside. Following completion of the venous anastomosis the kidney is rotated toward the operator's side.

6 The aorta is occluded and incised. A 4-mm aortic punch is used to fashion an orifice on the anterior surface of the aorta. This anastomosis is started with a running 6/0 polypropylene suture at the superior aspect. The 'back wall' of the anastomosis is performed from the inside and the 'front wall' from the outside.

Revascularization ensues at the completion of the vascular anastomoses. Heparin need not be reversed with protamine sulfate unless troublesome bleeding occurs. Following establishment of hemostasis, attention is turned to the urinary reconstruction.

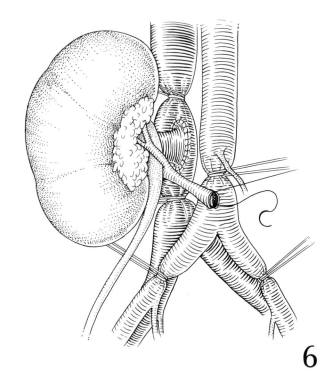

6

External ureteroneocystostomy

If the bladder is to be used for urinary reconstruction, the urinary catheter is clamped and povidone-iodine solution is instilled to distend the bladder and sterilize its contents. The author's preferred technique is an external ureteroneocystostomy, and the results with this method have been previously reported[2]. The principles of this technique include direct anastomosis of the ureter to bladder mucosa and construction of a submuscular tunnel to prevent reflux into the transplanted kidney.

A site is chosen anteriorly near the dome of the distended bladder. The choice of site should take into account the course of the transplanted ureter. An appropriate balance must be struck between the need for an adequate ureteric length to reach the anastomotic site when the bladder is empty and the requirement of avoiding excessive redundancy and the attendant risk of ureteric obstruction. Keeping in mind that the blood supply to the transplanted ureter is completely dependent on small branches from the lower pole renal artery, the tendency should be to err on the side of a shorter ureter.

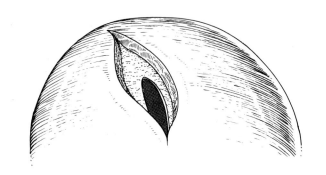

7 The muscular coat of the bladder is divided sharply and small vessels are carefully electrocoagulated. The bladder mucosa is exposed over an area of about 4 cm². An ellipse of mucosa is excised at the distal side of the mucosal dissection. The presence of the bladder catheter should be confirmed visually at this time, as in children a thickened peritoneum adjacent to the bladder can fool even the most experienced surgeon.

7

8a, b After sizing and spatulation of the transplant ureter, the anastomosis is completed with running 5/0 monofilament absorbable sutures. Traction sutures are placed at the 'heel' and 'toe' of the anastomosis. Careful placement of sutures and avoidance of excessive ureteric handling are critically important to avoid stenosis or obstruction. Only the smallest of bites should be taken on the ureter. Construction of the anastomosis should proceed from 'toe' to 'heel' and then back to the 'toe' on the opposite side.

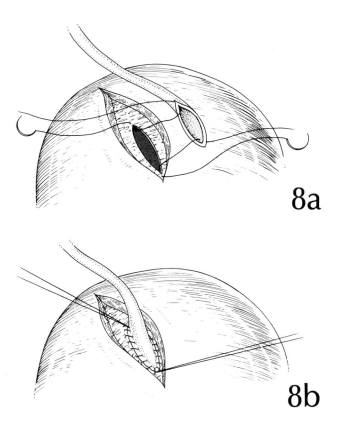

8a

8b

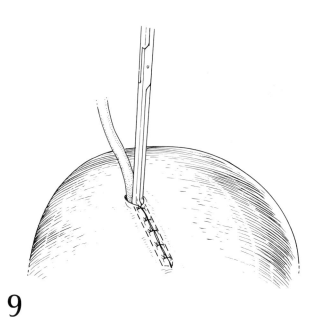

9

9 On completion of the anastomosis the ureter is laid in the submuscular space and the bladder muscle is closed over it using interrupted 4/0 monofilament absorbable sutures over a distance of 1–2 cm. When completed, the tunnel should still admit the end of a right-angled clamp, thus ensuring that the ureter will not be obstructed within the tunnel.

Wound closure

The transplanted kidney should lie comfortably within the iliac fossa. In extremely small infants (<7 kg) it may be necessary to open the peritoneum and convert the transplant to an intraperitoneal allograft, but this is required in fewer than 10% of cases. No fixation of the kidney allograft is needed. On removal of the self-retaining retractor, the peritoneal contents will hold the kidney against the iliopsoas and false pelvic side wall. No drains are used. The wound is irrigated and a two-layer fascial closure is completed with interrupted non-absorbable sutures. Absorbable suture material should be avoided for the fascial closure because of the deleterious effects of immunosuppressive agents on wound healing. No sutures are placed in the subcutaneous tissues and the skin is closed with a running, absorbable, subcuticular suture.

Postoperative care

General care and infection prophylaxis

Infants and small children are managed in a pediatric intensive care unit. Although most recipients are extubated in the operating room, small infants with an adult-sized kidney may require mechanical ventilation for 1–2 days. The urinary catheter is left in place for 3–5 days. Satisfactory bladder emptying may be assured if necessary with occasional post-micturitional catheterization. Prophylaxis against bacterial infection should be given for 3 days and then discontinued if donor renal vein cultures are negative. Prophylaxis is given for 1 month against opportunistic infection. This includes trimethoprim and sulfamethoxazole for *Pneumocystis carinii*, acyclovir for herpes virus and nystatin for candidiasis. Patients at high risk of cytomegalovirus infection (donor serology positive or recipient serology negative) are given a course of human immunoglobulin. The mean hospital stay is 10–14 days for uncomplicated cases.

Immunosuppression

Immunosuppressive therapy is commenced immediately before operation with corticosteroids and azathioprine. After operation induction immunotherapy is given with antithymocyte globulin administered for 10 days. Cyclosporin is withheld until renal allograft function is satisfactorily recovered in order to avoid the nephrotoxic effects of this agent. A deliberate steroid taper is pursued over several months and many pediatric patients can eventually be transferred to alternate-day steroids. Long-term maintenance immunosuppression consists of cyclosporin, azathioprine and steroids.

Outcome

The overall results of renal transplantation in children have improved steadily in recent years. The most important advances have included aggressive pretransplant dialysis and nutritional management, meticulous surgical technique and cyclosporin-based immunosuppression. The author's group has had a special interest in transplantation in very young patients with end-stage renal failure, and the transplant and developmental outcomes have been excellent even among recipients less than 1 year of age with renal failure[3]. Results with parental living-related donors, the preferred donor source, have been even more gratifying, with a 1-year actuarial patient survival rate of 100% and a 1-year actuarial graft survival rate of 95%[4].

References

1. Yuge J, Cecka JM. Pediatric recipients and donors. *Clin Transplant* 1990; 425–36.

2. Ohl DA, Konnak JW, Campbell DA, Dafoe DC, Merion RM, Turcotte JG. Extravesical ureteroneocystostomy in renal transplantation. *J Urol* 1988; 139: 499–502.

3. Tagge EP, Campbell DA, Dafoe DC *et al.* Pediatric renal transplantation with an emphasis on the prognosis of patients with chronic renal insufficiency since infancy. *Surgery* 1987; 102: 692–8.

4. Bunchman TE, Ham JM, Sedman AB *et al.* Superior allograft survival in pediatric renal transplant recipients. *Transplant Proc* 1994; 26: 24–5.

Principles of transplantation: liver

Kai-Chah Tan FRCS(Ed)
Consultant Surgeon, Liver Transplant Surgical Service, King's College Hospital, London, UK

The clinical introduction of cyclosporin as an immuno-suppressant has resulted in a dramatic improvement in survival after liver transplantation. Currently, the 1-year survival in children approximates 80%. Most surviving recipients enjoy an excellent quality of life, with normal growth patterns and often with complete relief of the stigmata of chronic liver disease.

The number of pediatric liver transplants performed has increased substantially over the last decade resulting in a universal shortage of size-matched donor organs, particularly for smaller children. Although organ availability has improved with increased public awareness and a better system of sharing and distribution, the waiting-list mortality remains around 25%. In addition, the clinical deterioration of many of these children during the long waiting period compromises their eventual outcome. Operative techniques have been devised to help overcome this problem, including size reduction of adult livers, split liver grafts and the use of the left lateral segment from living donors. These technical innovations will be illustrated.

Principles and justification

Indications

The indications for which pediatric liver transplantation has been performed are listed in *Table 1*.

The most common indication for liver transplantation in children is biliary atresia. Portoenterostomy has cured some of these patients, but for those in whom portoenterostomy has failed and who remain jaundiced there is a progressive fibrosis of the liver with repeated attacks of cholangitis. Most of these patients will die before reaching 5 years of age.

Inborn errors of metabolism, as a result of partial or complete deficiencies of specific liver enzymes or abnormal products of hepatic synthesis, constitute the second most common indication. Since the metabolic specificity of the donor is retained, such patients can be treated by transplanting a normal liver. In the majority, the disease process has damaged the liver and it is the hepatic decompensation or the development of malignant tumors that prompts its replacement. Alpha$_1$-antitrypsin deficiency is the most common inborn error of metabolism for which liver transplantation is

Table 1 Indications for pediatric liver transplantation

Cholestatic diseases
  Biliary atresia
  Sclerosing cholangitis
  Ductular paucity (Alagille's syndrome)
  Familial cholestasis
Metabolic diseases
  Byler disease
  Wilson's disease
  α_1-antitrypsin deficiency
  Crigler–Najjar
  Glycogenosis (type 1)
  Tyrosinemia
Miscellaneous
  Chronic active hepatitis
  Acute hepatic failure
  Neonatal hepatitis
  Tumors
  Budd–Chiari syndrome
  Congenital hepatic fibrosis

performed. Cirrhosis develops in 15% of patients with the homozygous phenotype PIZZ. Following liver transplantation the phenotype of the recipient becomes that of the donor, and the α_1-antitrypsin level is restored to normal.

Wilson's disease is an autosomal recessive disorder of copper metabolism with excessive copper deposition in the liver, basal ganglia, kidney and other organs. The hepatic disease may be acute and self-limiting or may progress rapidly to fulminant failure and death. Liver transplantation is the only treatment for these patients.

Other rare disease conditions for which transplantation has been carried out are listed in *Table 1*.

The decision to perform a liver transplant in a child with fulminant liver failure from viral or toxic hepatitis is more difficult, since about 20% of such cases may recover from the initial insult. Features predicting poor prognosis include progressive encephalopathy, worsening prothrombin time, metabolic acidosis, cardiovascular instability and rapid shrinkage of the liver. In patients with these indicators liver transplantation is the only treatment.

Evaluation of potential recipients

Potential pediatric liver transplant recipients must be carefully evaluated after referral from their primary physician. The purpose of the evaluation is to: (1) confirm the diagnosis and assess the status and progression of the disease; (2) determine the technical feasibility of the procedures; (3) identify occult infection and malignancy; and (4) assess metabolic and nutritional deficiencies. It should be a multidisciplinary approach involving the surgeon, hepatologist, anesthetist and radiologist. Further advice is often sought from the nutritionist, psychologist, social worker and transplant nurse specialist or coordinator. The various tests are outlined in *Table 2*.

A complete history and physical examination should be undertaken. Blood type is determined so that an ABO-compatible donor liver can be accepted and the blood bank informed. A coagulation profile allows for appropriate correction either with vitamin K, clotting factor replacement or exchange transfusion. Screening for hepatitis is mandatory, and serum α-fetoprotein levels should be measured and ultrasonography and computed tomographic (CT) scanning should be performed if malignancy is suspected. A chest radiograph is routinely performed, arterial blood gases should be measured and, if possible, lung function tests should be carried out. These children often have renal dysfunction and blood urea and serum creatinine levels should be obtained. If necessary amino acid excretion and 24-h creatinine clearance should be evaluated.

Anemia is common and may be secondary to poor nutrition and bleeding varices. Upper gastrointestinal endoscopy should be performed and bleeding varices injected before transplantation.

Table 2   Investigations in pediatric liver transplant patients

General
 Chest radiography
 Serum electrolytes, blood gas, magnesium, uric acid, cholesterol, triglycerides, ammonia, amino acids, transferrin
Hematology
 Full blood count, clotting profile
 Blood group, tissue typing and cytotoxic antibodies, immunoglobulins, complements
Hepatic
 Liver function tests, α-fetoprotein
 Ultrasonography, ^{99m}Tc-liver scan, portal/hepatic venography, CT scan of chest and abdomen
Renal
 Urinalysis
 Blood urea and serum creatinine (24-h creatinine clearance)
Pulmonary and cardiovascular
 (Pulmonary function tests)
 ECG (echocardiography)
Infectious screen
 Cultures: urine, sputum, blood, ascitic fluid, stools, nasal and throat swabs
 Hepatitis screen
 Antibodies: cytomegalovirus, Epstein–Barr virus, herpes simplex virus, HIV, measles, varicella
Specific tests related to primary liver disease
Social and psychiatric assessment

Malnutrition is common. These patients are often anorexic and hypercatabolic in addition to suffering significant steatorrhea from poor biliary drainage. An assessment of nutritional status is important and an aggressive regimen to correct deficiencies should be implemented. Liver transplantation should ideally be timed to coincide with a positive nitrogen balance.

Bacterial infection is common in children with end-stage liver disease. Any infection should be considered a contraindication to transplantation and aggressively treated. Bacterial, fungal and viral cultures are obtained of urine, sputum, blood and perhaps ascitic fluid. Baseline titer to cytomegalovirus, herpes simplex virus and Epstein–Barr virus are determined. These children should be immunized; however, live vaccinations should be given at least 1 month before liver transplantation.

Anatomic evaluation is important since vascular and visceral anomalies are not uncommon, particularly in children with biliary atresia. Ultrasonography is useful in determining the patency and size of the portal vein. Failure to visualize the portal vein is an indication for celiac angiography or splenoportography. Transplantation has been successful in the presence of visceral anomalies such as abdominal situs inversus and the polysplenia syndrome.

The psychologic assessment and emotional preparation of the child and family is important. Once the child is accepted into the program, priority on the waiting list is assigned according to the immediacy of the need. Since the wait can be long, continued outpatient monitoring of the child is necessary.

Operations

DONOR OPERATION

The liver is obtained from a heart-beating donor diagnosed by stringent criteria as brain-stem dead. Most donors die either from severe head injury, spontaneous intracranial bleed, anoxia or primary brain tumor. Both donor and recipient should be ABO blood group compatible but tissue typing is not required. They should have normal or near normal liver function tests and virology screening, which should include hepatitis A, B, C, HIV and cytomegalovirus, must be negative. Nowadays most donor livers are removed as part of a multiorgan procedure in which various combinations of kidneys, liver, pancreas, heart or heart/lungs are procured.

Incision

1 A midline incision is made from the suprasternal notch to the pubic symphysis. The sternum is opened in the midline with a Gigli saw, giving access to the intrathoracic organs and liver. A careful examination of the abdominal viscera is performed to exclude unsuspected injury or disease. Any abdominal sepsis or gross hepatic injury would preclude its use. The liver is mobilized by incising the falciform and left triangular ligaments. With the gastrohepatic ligament exposed, a search should be made for the presence of a hepatic arterial branch from the left gastric artery. If present, it must be preserved in continuity with the celiac axis.

Dissection

2 The porta hepatis is dissected next. A search is made for an anomalous hepatic artery arising from the superior mesenteric artery; it may be the only artery to the liver. If present, it lies posteriorly to the portal vein for a short distance from its origin before crossing it from left to right and must be preserved in continuity with the superior mesenteric artery.

If the hepatic arterial supply is 'normal', the gastroduodenal and right gastric arteries are divided between ligatures followed by that of the left gastric and splenic arteries. The common bile duct is divided close to the upper border of the duodenum. The portal vein and hepatic artery are skeletonized and isolated.

The right peritoneal attachments of the liver to the diaphragm are carefully dissected to identify the retrohepatic and infrahepatic vena cava. The right adrenal vein is divided between fine ligatures and the entry of the renal vessels identified. Finally, the vena cava is fully mobilized leaving the liver attached only by its vascular pedicles.

The superior mesenteric vein is identified at the base of the mesentery of the transverse colon, dissected and encircled. The cecum and ascending colon together

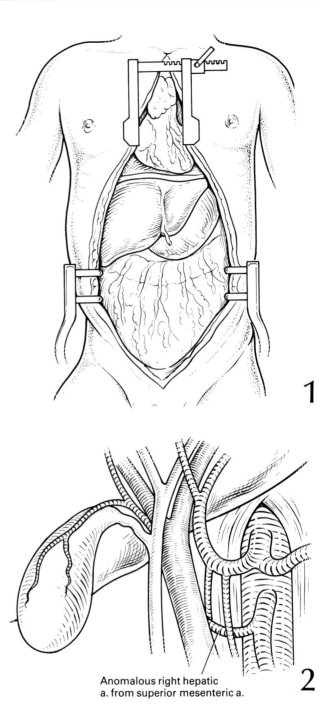

Anomalous right hepatic a. from superior mesenteric a.

2

with the mesentery of the small intestine are mobilized. Once the infrarenal vena cava and aorta are identified they are dissected and encircled below the renal vessels. The inferior mesenteric artery is ligated in continuity to prevent loss of the cold perfusate into its vascular bed. The other abdominal organs to be retrieved are similarly dissected.

At this stage the cardiac team should commence mobilizing the heart or heart–lung; the latter may involve the use of cardiopulmonary bypass and hypothermia. The donor is then heparinized.

Perfusion

3   A large-bore cannula is inserted into the distal aorta and connected to 1 litre of Marshall's solution from a drip stand at a height of about 1 m above the organ. A smaller cannula is inserted into the superior mesenteric vein and threaded into the portal vein to lie just before the confluence. This is connected to 1 litre of University of Wisconsin (UW) solution about 0.5 m above the organ. A large cannula may be inserted into the infrarenal vena cava for eventual bleeding off into a bag but, if the heart is not retrieved, the donor can be bled into the chest.

The aorta above the diaphragm is encircled with tape. When all surgical dissection is completed the supra-diaphragmatic aorta is clamped and the infrarenal vena cava is incised to drain blood from the donor before infusion of cold perfusion solutions to minimize organ congestion. The cold solutions are infused slowly initially and once the flow is satisfactory this is followed by rapid infusion. The ventilation and circulation are now stopped.

Normally 1−2 litres of Marshall's solution and 1−2 litres of UW solution (50 ml/kg) have to be infused into the aorta and portal vein, respectively. With this technique both the liver and kidneys should be cooled together. Iced saline slush is poured over the liver and the abdominal viscera to provide additional surface cooling. When the organs are cold and have become blanched they are removed. The celiac axis is removed with a short portion of the aorta. The portal vein is freed and transected beyond the confluence of the splenic and superior mesenteric veins. The vena cava above and below the liver is transected. The liver is removed with a suprahepatic cuff of diaphragm.

The gallbladder is incised to wash out the bile with cold saline. Failure to remove the bile will lead to autolysis of the ducts during the cold ischemia period with subsequent sludge formation. On the bench the liver is perfused with 500 ml of UW solution. The liver is

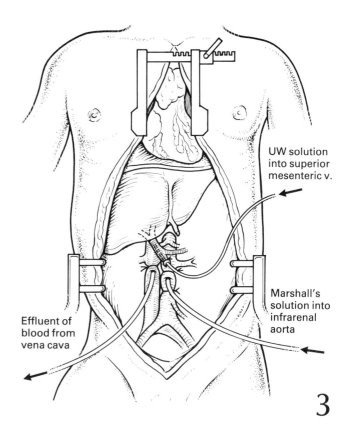

UW solution into superior mesenteric v.

Marshall's solution into infrarenal aorta

Effluent of blood from vena cava

3

packed in sterile plastic bags and stored in ice for transportation.

When the kidneys are removed the iliac arteries and veins are retrieved in case subsequent vascular reconstructions become necessary. It is important that the arteries are dissected to below the inguinal ligaments.

Once the liver is brought back to the recipient hospital it is cleaned and prepared. This 'bench work' normally takes about 30 min and entails trimming the suprahepatic diaphragmatic cuff and closing the origins of the phrenic vessels. The infrahepatic vena cava is checked for the origin of the right adrenal vein and other small veins and closed with 4/0 polypropylene (Prolene) sutures. Both the hepatic artery and portal vein are now examined.

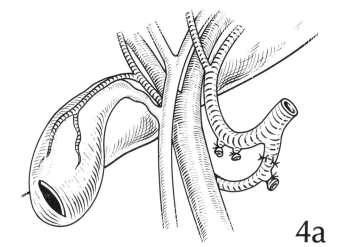

Arterial reconstruction

4a, b

In the presence of an anomalous hepatic arterial supply, various vascular reconstructions have been described which bring them together as a single trunk for anastomosis in the recipient. Usually the superior mesenteric artery is anastomosed to the splenic stump of the celiac trunk. The common hepatic artery can also be anastomosed to the superior mesenteric artery.

Rapid cooling technique

In an unstable donor the meticulous dissection before perfusion of the preservation solutions should be avoided. A rapid core cooling technique should be used. The ice-cold UW solution is infused directly into the abdominal aorta once the abdomen has been opened and the donor heparinized. In this instance the blanched structures and the absence of arterial pulsation make dissection more difficult and considerable surgical expertise and experience are needed to avoid damage.

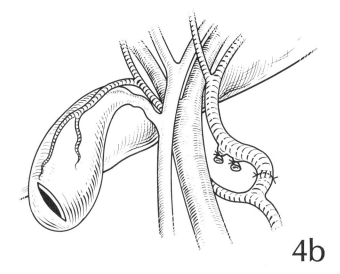

RECIPIENT OPERATION

Anesthesia

These children often suffer from multisystem disorders, either related to or coexistent with their liver disease. Preoperative presentations vary from a child with fulminant hepatic failure complicated by coagulopathy, cerebral edema and acute renal failure to that of a small undernourished child with biliary atresia and multiple previous upper abdominal operations. Great emphasis is placed on prediction and prevention of problems and a team approach with liaison between surgeons, pediatricians and anesthetists is essential. The procedure may involve massive transfusion (perhaps up to five estimated blood volumes) and adequate supplies of blood and components are essential.

The anesthesia is based on opiate analgesia supplemented with isoflurane supplied in an oxygen air mixture. Atracurium is used for muscle relaxation. Nitrous oxide is avoided because of the potential for distention of the bowels during the long surgical procedure. Nasal intubation is preferred (in the absence of a severe coagulopathy).

Invasive hemodynamic monitoring and vascular access for rapid infusion is initiated at induction and is supplemented by nasopharyngeal and rectal temperature probes, oximetry, capnography and monitoring of neuromuscular transmission. Blood is analyzed at least hourly for hemoglobin, platelet count, prothrombin time and electrolytes (including ionized calcium and blood glucose). Thromboelastography has been found to be an invaluable adjunct to the monitoring of coagulation. Fluid replacement can thus be rapidly adjusted to meet changing situations. Temperature hemostasis is aided by high ambient temperatures, the use of radiant heaters during induction of anesthesia, an efficient warming mattress and the warming and humidification of anesthetic gases. All intravenous fluids must be warmed to normal body temperature. Wrapping the extremities of the patient in impervious reflective sheeting is also important. Venovenous bypass is seldom required in pediatric liver transplantation.

Surgical procedure

The recipient procedure can be classified into three components: (1) hepatectomy; (2) engraftment of organ; and (3) hemostasis and closure of abdomen.

The recipient hepatectomy may be exceedingly difficult in children with biliary atresia where dense adhesions from previous surgery may bind the portal structures, duodenum, Roux limb and transverse colon into a mass of unrecognizable structures. The presence of portal hypertension with massive thin-walled varices and coagulopathy may further complicate this dissection.

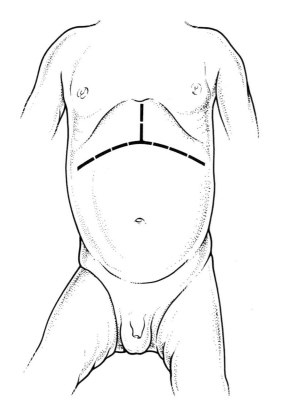

Incision

5 The abdomen is entered using cautery through a bilateral subcostal incision, and this may occasionally be extended vertically in the midline to the xiphoid process for extra exposure. The upper abdomen is held open with a Thompson retractor with its adjustable blades.

5

Hepatectomy

6 If the porta hepatis is dense and unrecognizable, unscarred tissue planes such as the posterolateral aspect of the liver may be dissected first. The hepatic flexure of the transverse colon and the duodenum are reflected from the right lobe of the liver and the Roux limb is identified and traced to the hilum. Once the portoenterostomy is detached, the portal structures lying below are easily identified.

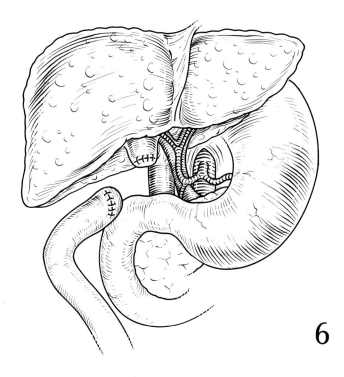

6

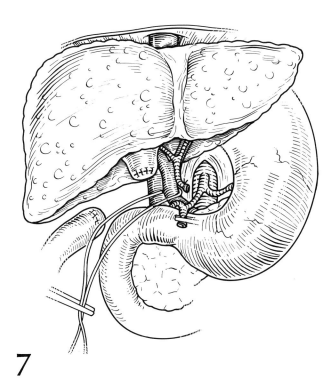

7

7 When the porta hepatis is dissected first, the common bile duct is identified and divided between ligatures. In children with biliary atresia the portoenterostomy is taken down and the Roux-en-Y limb preserved for later anastomosis. The hepatic artery is dissected and divided between two bulldog vascular clamps. The portal vein is dissected and isolated. If the portal vein is small the dissection should be taken to its confluence. The gastrohepatic ligament is then divided between ligatures.

8 The falciform and triangular ligaments together with the right peritoneal reflection are incised.

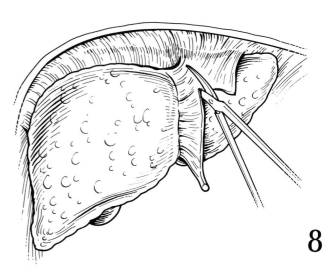

8

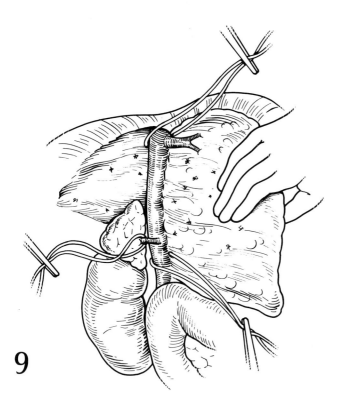

9

9 The liver is retracted medially into the wound and the right lobe is dissected from the retroperitoneum. The right adrenal vein should be identified and divided between fine ligatures. The retrohepatic space should be carefully dissected until both the suprahepatic and infrahepatic vena cava are encircled.

10 In children venovenous bypass is not necessary. The portal vein is divided between two Cooley vascular clamps. Both the suprahepatic and infrahepatic vena cava are clamped with Satinsky clamps, the former with a cuff of diaphragm and the latter above the renal veins.

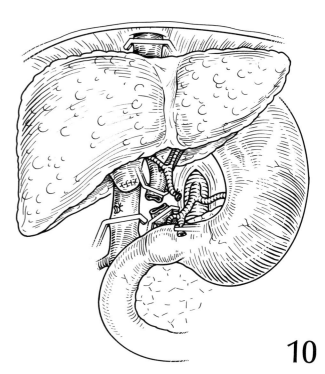

10

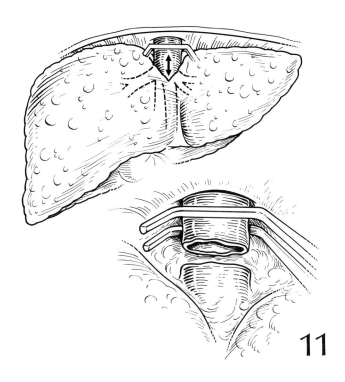

11 The suprahepatic vena cava is divided; extra length can be obtained by transecting into the substance of the liver at the confluence of the hepatic veins.

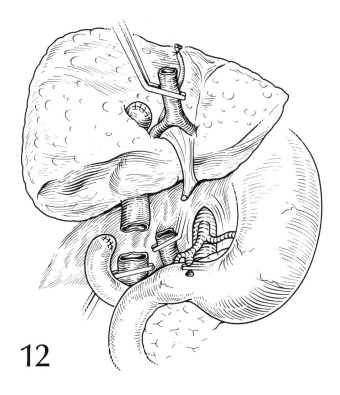

12 The infrahepatic vena cava is next divided and the liver is removed.

13 With the removal of the liver, meticulous hemostasis of the retroperitoneum should be obtained with a combination of cautery and suture ligation. This is important because hemostasis is much more difficult to secure behind the implanted donor liver.

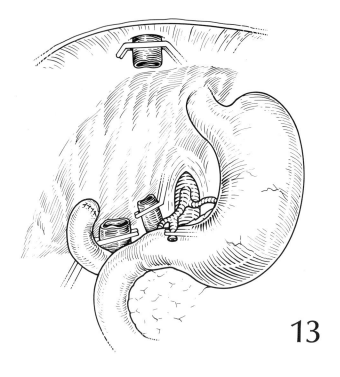

13

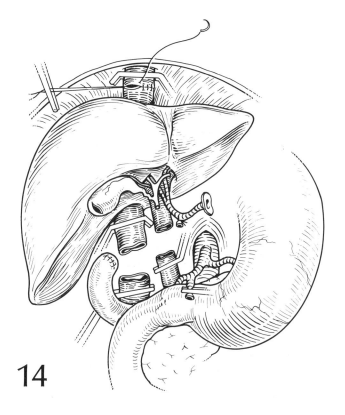

14

Engraftment

14 The engraftment should begin with the suprahepatic vena cava anastomosis. This is performed with a continuous 3/0 or 4/0 polypropylene suture. In an infant where the inferior vena cava is narrow, the anterior wall should be closed with interrupted sutures.

15 The infrahepatic vena cava anastomosis is performed next; the anterior wall is left incomplete. The liver is then flushed with 500 ml of normal saline via the portal vein to wash out the hyperkalemic preservation solution. The effluent is allowed to flush out of the incompletely anastomosed infrahepatic vena cava. The infrahepatic vena cava anastomosis is completed at the end of the flush.

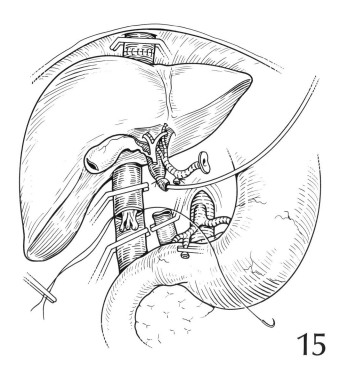

15

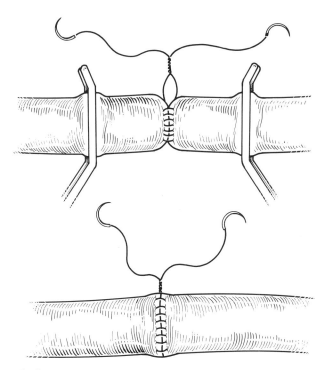

16

16 The portal anastomosis is performed next, care being taken to ensure that there is no redundancy in length otherwise there will be resultant kinking. The anastomosis should be performed with a continuous 5/0 or 6/0 polypropylene suture with a growth factor of about one-quarter to one-third the diameter of the vessel. This technique is important in preventing stenosis when these small vessels are anastomosed.

The patient is checked for stability and it is useful to anticipate that reperfusion of the graft may result in acidosis and hyperkalemia, both of which are deleterious to the heart. The vascular clamps are removed in succession. The suprahepatic clamp is removed first followed by that of the infrahepatic. A search is made for major bleeding points and, if the patient is stable, the portal clamp is then removed and the liver is perfused with portal blood. An effort is made to identify and secure major bleeding points before rearterialization. Care should be taken to see that the 'growth factor' of the portal venous anastomosis is taken up as the vessels expand with the restoration of blood flow. An additional suture may be needed at the end of the suture line to prevent bleeding. The gallbladder is removed at this stage by a retrograde dissection. The cystic duct is tied with a 3/0 polyglactin (Vicryl) ligature.

17a–c The donor hepatic artery is flushed with heparin–saline to remove air and blood clots and a bulldog clamp is applied to prevent retrograde flow of blood from the donor liver which may interfere with the anastomosis. The hepatic artery is anastomosed end-to-end and an effort is made to anastomose it using branch patches. The anastomosis is performed with either interrupted or a continuous 6/0 polypropylene suture with 'growth factor'.

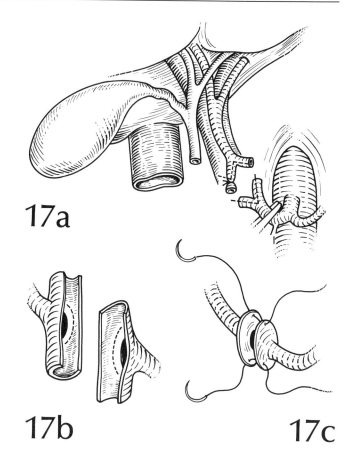

17a

17b   17c

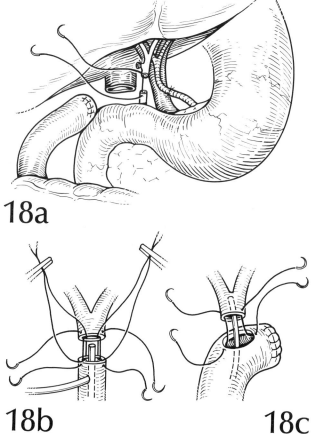

18a

18b   18c

18a–c A duct-to-duct anastomosis is preferred using interrupted 6/0 polydioxanone (PDS). An 8-Fr T tube is inserted via the recipient duct. The posterior row of sutures is placed before the ends of the ducts are 'rail-roaded' together and the sutures tied. The upper end of the T tube is inserted into the donor duct and the anterior layer of the anastomosis is then completed (*Illustration 18b*). An operative cholangiogram can be carried out.

A Roux-en-Y choledochojejunostomy is performed in cases of biliary atresia and sclerosing cholangitis. In addition, a choledochojejunostomy is preferred if the caliber of the duct is small or if there is gross disparity between donor and recipient ducts such as occurs with a reduced liver. A 40–45-cm loop of jejunum is prepared and brought up to the porta hepatis in a retrocolic fashion. A small opening is made in the antimesenteric side and the anastomosis is performed with interrupted 6/0 polydioxanone. A 4-Fr or 5-Fr feeding tube is used either as an internal stent or brought out through the jejunal loop (*Illustration 18c*).

Hemostasis and closure

19 Complete hemostasis should be secured before closure. All the vascular anastomoses are checked and often a few additional sutures are needed at the corners to secure hemostasis. Bleeding at this juncture is often secondary to a coagulopathy and thromboelastography is particularly useful in monitoring and guiding the correction of coagulation defects. The abdomen is closed with absorbable sutures after two closed sump drains are placed on either side of the liver.

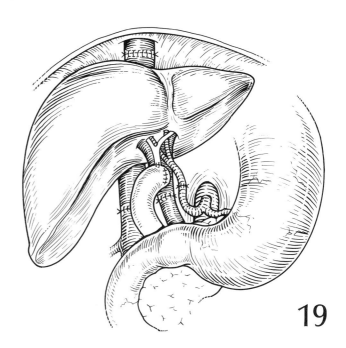

19

MODIFICATIONS OF TECHNIQUE

Liver reduction techniques

The major technical modification of the standard transplant procedure concerns the use of reduced size livers in children. Reduced liver graft techniques have been greatly facilitated by the prolonged preservation time associated with the use of the UW solution.

The principal reason for the use of reduced size liver grafts in children is the lack of size-matched cadaveric organ donors. About 30% of children with end-stage liver disease die while on the waiting list for a transplant. The 1-year survival rate for children transplanted with a reduced size liver is more than 65%, and there is no functional difference between the reduced size grafts and those transplanted whole.

The reduction technique is based on the segmental anatomy of the liver. In practice three types of liver graft are possible: the right lobe (segments V, VI, VII, VIII), the left lobe (segments II, III, IV) and the left lateral segment (segments II, III).

The liver reduction should be performed as a bench procedure in the recipient operating room. The liver must be totally immersed in cold (4°C) UW solution throughout the procedure. The extent of reduction is determined by visual comparison between the donor liver and the recipient hepatic fossa. In using the right or left lobe of the liver, the parenchyma transection is carried along the principal plane slightly to the left or right of the middle hepatic vein, respectively. The biliary and vascular radicles of the lobe to be used are carefully ligated with fine ties. The structures of the portal triad can be transected within the parenchyma. The donor vena cava is left with the lobe to be used and the other lobe is discarded. With the completion of transection the surface is tested for further biliary or vascular leakages by perfusing the vessels and common bile duct. The leakage points identified are oversewn. The surface is dried and sprayed with a layer of fibrin glue. The inplantation of the lobe is performed as for a whole graft.

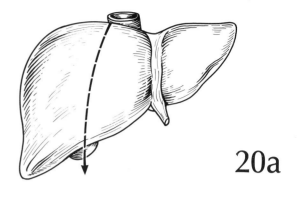

20a

20a–c Both the right and left lobes can be used with an intact donor inferior vena cava. With this technique, however, it is unsafe to transplant across a donor:recipient weight disparity of greater than 3:1. In order to increase the pool of pediatric donor organs, particularly for smaller children, the left lateral segment is used.

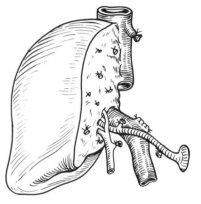

20b

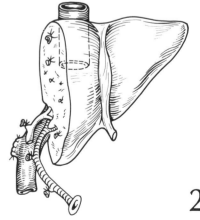

20c

21a–c With this technique the left hepatic vein or the common trunk of the middle and left hepatic veins is used for venous outflow and the retrohepatic vena cava of the recipient is retained. With this technique, a donor:recipient weight ratio of greater than 10:1 has been crossed successfully. This technique of transplanting the left lateral segment involves transecting the parenchyma just to the right of the falciform ligament. The right extrahepatic portal structures are divided, the stump of the right hepatic duct and artery are suture ligated, and the right branch of the portal vein is closed with a continuous 6/0 polypropylene suture. A cuff of the left hepatic vein or the common trunk is obtained for anastomosis to the recipient vena cava. It is important to ensure a wide anastomosis to prevent outflow obstruction and the triangulation technique is useful using a continuous 5/0 polypropylene suture (*Illustration 21c*). Although the common hepatic artery and main portal trunk can be used for the implantation, only the left hepatic duct is used as the blood supply of the common bile duct is often compromised here.

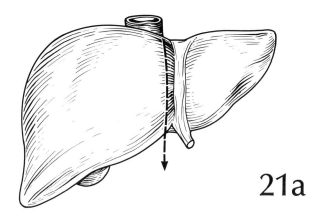

21a

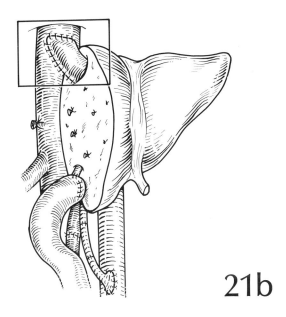

21b

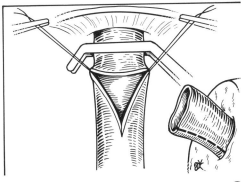

21c

Split liver technique

22 In order to increase the pool of donor liver grafts further the 'split liver' technique was developed. In this technique the donor liver is 'split' along the principal plane into two grafts for transplantation into two patients.

In most cases the inferior vena cava remains with the right graft (segments V, VI, VII, VIII) which should also carry the right portal vein, common hepatic duct and the right or common hepatic artery. The left graft (segments II and III) should be left with the main portal trunk, the left hepatic duct and the left or common hepatic artery. The venous outflow of this graft should be the left hepatic vein. Segments I and IV should be discarded. Interpositional vascular grafts are often required.

It is important to note that the bench procedure for a 'split' may take 3–4h and the recipient procedures should be timed accordingly. A bench cholangiogram should be obtained to minimize the dissection of the extrahepatic bile ducts; an angiogram is optional.

The hepatectomy for the right graft recipient is the same as for the standard transplant procedure. The inferior vena cava should, however, be preserved in the recipient of the left graft by 'filleting' off the native liver.

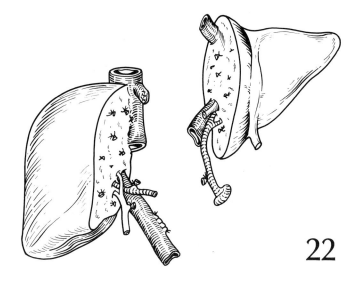

22

Living-related technique

An increasing number of living-related liver transplants have recently been performed. In this technique the left lateral segment of the liver of a suitable parent is retrieved and transplanted into the child. In addition to having a compatible blood group, the volume ratio of the donor segment and the hepatic fossa of the child should be suitable. A preoperative hepatic angiogram is performed to ensure suitability of the arterial supply and a CT scan to estimate the volume of the left lateral segment.

The operation is performed electively. The abdomen of the donor is opened through a bilateral subcostal incision. Once the left side of the liver is mobilized the left hepatic vein and left portal triad structures are dissected and isolated by slings. The parenchyma is transected just to the right of the falciform ligament. Great care is taken to ligate the vascular and biliary radicles individually on both sides of the transection.

The bile duct and blood vessels are transected at the last moment and the liver segment is then perfused with ice-cold UW solution as a bench procedure. A suitable length of the donor saphenous vein should be retrieved for use as an interpositional graft.

The recipient procedure should have been commenced once the donor liver segment is judged suitable. The hepatectomy is as described on pp. 579–589. The implantation is similar to that for a left lateral segmental graft except that the vascular interposition conduit will be the saphenous vein of the donor.

The patient and graft survival with this technique is superior to that of cadaveric grafting. Compared with cadaveric transplants, the living-related grafts have better early function and immunorejection is not only less common, but tends to be less severe. Patients are likely to stay in hospital for a shorter period.

Postoperative care

The patient is nursed in the intensive care unit and ventilated for 24–48 h. The arterial blood pressure, pulmonary wedge pressure, temperature, blood loss and urine output are continuously monitored. Blood loss should be carefully replaced either by whole blood or blood products. Any signs of hepatic dysfunction would necessitate Doppler ultrasonographic examination of the hepatic artery and portal vein and, if indicated, angiographic studies.

Nasogastric suction is continued for 4–5 days or until bowel function returns. Chest radiographs are performed daily for the first week and evidence of atelectasis, pleural effusion and pneumonia will need immediate attention. The blood urea, serum creatinine, electrolytes, calcium, phosphate, full blood count and liver function tests are determined daily for the first week. An ultrasonographic study is made on the fifth postoperative day and at weekly intervals. A good 'picture' of the liver parenchyma and biliary tree can be obtained, together with the flow of the hepatic artery and portal vein.

Immunosuppression consists of: (1) intravenous methylprednisolone, 2 mg/kg/day for 5 days, then oral prednisolone tapered progressively to 0.2 mg/kg/day within 4 weeks; (2) intravenous azathioprine, 1–2 mg/kg/day; and (3) intravenous cyclosporin 1–5 mg/kg/day.

Prednisolone and azathioprine are given intraoperatively, but cyclosporin is commenced on the first or second postoperative day depending on renal function. The dose of cyclosporin is adjusted to maintain a whole blood level of 100–300 ng/ml. Once gastrointestinal function returns the patient is started on oral cyclosporin, 10–30 mg/kg/day. Encouraging results have recently been reported with the new immunosuppressive agent FK506.

Complications

Bleeding

Postoperative bleeding is diagnosed when increasing transfusion requirements are needed to maintain systemic blood pressure and hemoglobin levels. The drain loss and degree of abdominal distension may also be a good guide. Increasing intra-abdominal pressure associated with a drop in urine output is an indication for early re-exploration.

Acute cellular rejection

A sudden increase in the plasma levels of liver synthetic enzymes together with a low-grade fever should lead to a suspicion of acute cellular rejection. If possible a liver biopsy should be performed. Acute rejection is treated with methylprednisolone, 20 mg/kg/day, for 3 days and may be repeated. A response is usually seen within 48 h. For intractable acute rejection antilymphocyte globulins, particularly the monoclonal antibody OKT3, have been used. An alternative is to switch the immunosuppression to FK506.

Vascular occlusions

Thrombosis of the hepatic artery following liver transplantation is a devastating event. It is more common in pediatric recipients, particularly in the younger and smaller patients. It presents as an acute deterioration of hepatic function leading to hepatic gangrene and death unless the patient is urgently retransplanted. It may present insidiously with delayed bile leakage or intermittent sepsis of unknown origin. If hepatic artery thrombosis is suspected it should be investigated with Doppler ultrasonography, angiography or both.

Portal venous occlusion is uncommon and acute occlusion presents with variceal hemorrhage, ascites, abdominal pain or deteriorating hepatic function and will necessitate surgical correction. Late portal venous stenosis presents with complications associated with portal hypertension and may be amenable to balloon angioplasty.

Vena caval occlusion is rare and presents with ascites and lower trunk edema. The suprahepatic anastomosis is more commonly involved and balloon angioplasty is possible.

Biliary complications

Although these may occur in isolation, often they are associated with arterial pathology since the biliary tree is solely dependent upon the hepatic artery for its blood supply. These include anastomotic dehiscence and bile leak, and necrosis of the duct resulting in strictures and obstruction. They may present with fever, right hypochondrial pain and jaundice. Diagnosis is made by ultrasonography and cholangiography. Anastomotic strictures and bile leaks may be treated with balloon dilatation and stent placement. Reconstructive surgery may be required and it is important to perform angiography before this.

Renal complications

Many of the patients have preoperative renal dysfunction as a result of hepatorenal syndrome, ascites and variceal hemorrhage. The majority should rapidly improve following liver transplantation provided care has been taken to avoid hypotension, venous compression from a tense abdomen and nephrotoxic drugs, particularly cyclosporin.

Infections

Infectious complications remain the major cause of mortality and morbidity after liver transplantation. Many of these children suffer from severe malnutrition associated with their chronic liver disease. A broad-spectrum preoperative antibiotic regimen is used. Fluconazole or amphotericin is given to children transplanted for fulminant liver failure and retransplantation.

Most severe infectious complications occur within the first 2 months after transplantation and these include most of the viral and fungal infections. Bacterial infections are usually due to biliary or vascular line problems. Fungal infections are usually caused by the *Candida* and *Aspergillus* species.

Viral infections are still the major cause of post-transplant morbidity and mortality. Cytomegalovirus is the most common and presents with low-grade fever, malaise and muscle ache. Diarrhea, gastrointestinal ulceration and pulmonary symptoms are also common presentations. Children develop the disease either as a primary infection when graft from a cytomegalovirus-positive donor is used or as a reactivation infection. Symptomatic patients should be treated with a course of gancyclovir and, if appropriate, the level of immunosuppression should be decreased.

Other opportunistic viral infections include herpes simplex (HSV-1 and -2), varicella zoster, Epstein–Barr and adenovirus. All are capable of infecting the allograft. Treatment consists of a reduction in the level of immunosuppression and a course of intravenous acyclovir.

Outcome

The results of pediatric liver transplantation have improved dramatically in the last decade with the clinical introduction of cyclosporin. A 1-year survival rate of more than 75% is now regularly reported and, in those patients transplanted electively, a survival rate of 85–90% is expected.

The indications for pediatric liver transplantation are widening each year and sicker and smaller children are increasingly being transplanted. This has led to a mushrooming of pediatric liver transplant centers in North America and Western Europe. The last few years have seen a universal shortage of pediatric donor organs and, as described above, various technical innovations have been devised by transplant surgeons to alleviate this problem. The earlier technique of reducing an adult liver is now being criticized because of the increasing dearth of adult livers. Techniques such as split liver and living-related liver grafting will be increasingly popular in the foreseeable future.

Further reading

Broelsch CE, Emond JC, Whitington PF, Thistlethwaite JR, Baker AL, Lichtor JL. Application of reduced-size liver transplants as split grafts, auxiliary orthotopic grafts and living related segmental transplants. *Ann Surg* 1990; 212: 368–77.

Calne RY, Rolles K, White DJ *et al.* Cyclosporin A initially as the only immunosuppressant in 34 recipients of cadaveric organs: 32 kidneys, two pancreases, and two livers. *Lancet* 1979; ii: 1033–6.

Emond JC, Heffron TG, Whitington PF, Broelsch CE. Reconstruction of the hepatic vein in reduced size hepatic tranplantation. *Surg Gynecol Obstet* 1993; 176: 11–17.

Shaw BW, Iwatsuki S, Starzl TE. Alternative methods of arterialization of the hepatic graft. *Surg Gynecol Obstet* 1984; 159: 490–3.

Starzl TE, Iwatsuki S, Shaw BW. A growth factor in fine vascular anastomoses. *Surg Gynecol Obstet* 1984; 159: 164–5.

Tan KC. Liver transplantation. In: Howard ER, ed. *Surgery of Liver Disease in Children*. Oxford: Butterworth-Heinemann, 1991: 224–38.

Illustrations by Mark Iley

Small bowel transplantation

Daniel H. Teitelbaum MD
Assistant Professor of Pediatric Surgery, University of Michigan Medical School, C.S. Mott Children's Hospital, Ann Arbor, Michigan, USA

Principles and justification

Indications

Candidates for small bowel transplantation have irreversible intestinal failure as a consequence of one of several bowel dysfunction syndromes. These include short bowel syndrome, absorptive abnormalities (e.g. microvillous atrophy) and dysmotility problems (e.g. total intestinal aganglionosis, extensive and severe neuronal intestinal dysplasia and visceral myopathies). Most infants with short bowel syndrome, even those with inordinately short lengths of remaining intestine, can eventually be weaned off parenteral nutrition. At least 1–2 years of intensive nutritional support should be tried before considering bowel transplantation for an infant with short bowel syndrome. This approach applies equally for patients with other forms of malabsorption and dysmotility disorders.

Preoperative

Prolonged total parenteral nutrition may lead to cholestasis and eventually to liver cirrhosis. All candidates for bowel transplantation must be screened for signs of liver failure using both functional tests (i.e. protein C and S levels) and histopathologic examination of liver biopsies. In the presence of significant liver dysfunction, a combined small bowel and liver transplant is indicated. Intravenous line sepsis is also common in patients requiring prolonged parenteral nutrition. These infective episodes often recur and can lead to the development of an infective thrombus in the central venous system. A white cell nuclear scan may help to identify such sequestered areas of infection, which must be eliminated before transplantation. Bacterial overgrowth of the dilated and poorly motile intestine requires attention before transplantation. Selective decontamination of the intestine should be considered.

Operations

HARVEST OF INTESTINE

The bowel is neither irradiated nor irrigated, as the incidence of graft-versus-host disease and the amount of bacterial contamination are fairly low. If time permits, both donor and recipient should receive oral antibiotics (amphotericin B, mycostatin, tobramycin and polymyxin B) for selective bacterial decontamination.

1 A standard mobilization of the intra-abdominal organs is performed. The bowel is perfused with chilled University of Wisconsin solution through an aortic cannula. The entire length of the small intestine is harvested on a pedicle of the superior mesenteric artery. Alternatively a Carrel patch of aorta is used.

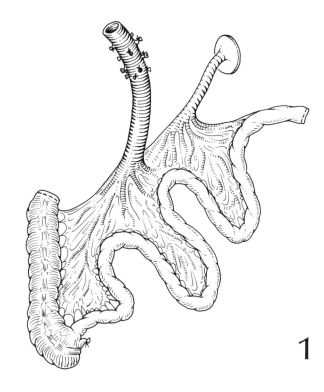

1

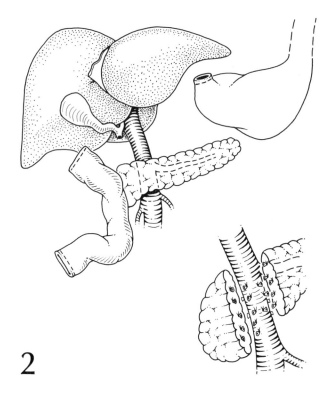

2

2 The duodenum is divided with an automatic stapler. The pancreas is also divided with cautery and multiple sutures, using the index finger as a guide to protect the portal vein. In this fashion a long segment of portal vein is harvested for venous drainage. The intestine is kept moist and on ice until transplantation. Ischemia times of up to 10 h after harvest are acceptable.

ISOLATED SMALL INTESTINE TRANSPLANT

Although commonly only the small intestine is used, additional segments of the colon may reduce high enteral losses which are characteristically seen after operation in these patients. If the colon is used, it should be irrigated with a neomycin solution on a separate table in the operating room before transplantation. An appendectomy is performed.

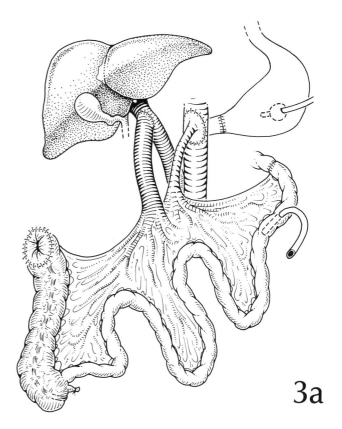

3a

3a, b The arterial supply is anastomosed to the aorta and the venous drainage placed into the native portal vein in piggy-back fashion. Alternatively, the venous drainage can be placed directly into the inferior vena cava if access to the portal vein is not possible.

The proximal bowel is anastomosed to the proximal remnant of the recipient's intestine. The distal bowel is brought out as an end stoma. This stoma allows accurate assessment of enteral output and access for frequent endoscopic inspection of the transplanted bowel.

Depending on the anatomy of the residual intestine of the recipient, it may be an advantage to construct an end-to-side anastomosis between the recipient colon to the side of the donor intestine just proximal to where the stoma exits the abdominal cavity.

A feeding jejunostomy is placed through the most proximal portion of the transplanted bowel so that slow enteral feeds may be administered in the early postoperative period. A gastrostomy tube should be placed to facilitate drainage due to gastric atony, as well as for enteral feeds.

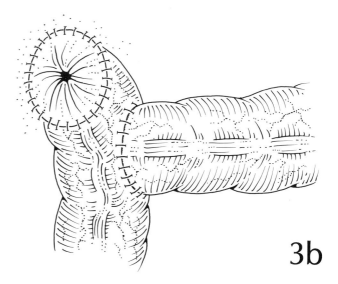

3b

COMBINED LIVER AND SMALL INTESTINE TRANSPLANT

4 For a combined liver and small bowel transplant, a Carrel patch comprising the hepatic artery and superior mesenteric artery is used. The donor portal vein is harvested in the same way as for the isolated small intestinal transplant. The Carrel patch is then anastomosed to the aorta. The recipient's portal vein can be anastomosed to the donor's portal vein in an end-to-side fashion.

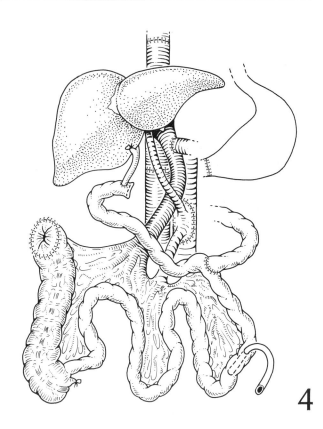

4

Postoperative care

Nasogastric decompression is maintained until gastro-intestinal activity is restored. Gastric output is often high because many of the patients have persistent gastric atony. To avoid this problem, a pyloroplasty is often performed, as shown in *Illustration 4*. Jejunal feeding is started with a slow continuous pump, using an elemental diet. Endoscopic surveillance of the mucosa should be performed at least twice weekly and several biopsies should be taken with each endoscopy.

Complications

The predominant complications are rejection and infection. A flattened mucosa with ulceration is consistent with rejection. Infections are mostly enteric in origin, with bacterial and fungal organisms predominating[1]. Patients are maintained on selective bacterial decontamination for at least 1 month after transplantation. High enteral losses can be a problem, even if no rejection is indicated at biopsy. These can be corrected with dietary supplements and medication, but may be easier to control with the addition of a colonic segment.

Acknowledgment

Illustration 2 has been adapted with permission from Starzl *et al.*, *Surg Gynecol Obstet* 1991; 172: 335–44.

Reference

1. Reyes J, Abu-Elmagd K, Tzakis A, *et al*. Infectious complications after human small bowel transplantation. *Trans Proc* 1992; 24: 1249–50.

Further reading

Starzl TE, Todo S, Tzakis A, *et al*. The many faces of multivisceral transplantation. *Surg Gynecol Obstet* 1991; 172: 335–44.

Todo S, Tzakis AG, Abu-Elmagd K, *et al*. Intestinal transplantation in composite visceral grafts or alone. *Ann Surg* 1992; 216: 223–34.

Pediatric interventional radiology: an overview

M. Victoria Marx MD
Assistant Professor of Radiology, University of Michigan Medical Center, Ann Arbor, Michigan, USA

Ramiro J. Hernandez MD
Professor of Pediatric Radiology, University of Michigan Medical Center, Ann Arbor, Michigan, USA

Interventional radiology is the branch of medicine that specializes in a wide variety of vascular and non-vascular, invasive, diagnostic and therapeutic procedures using imaging guidance. Examples of vascular interventional radiologic procedures include diagnostic angiography, percutaneous transluminal angioplasty, percutaneous vessel embolization, placement of venous access devices and inferior vena cava filter placement. Non-vascular interventional radiologic procedures include percutaneous gastrostomy or gastrojejunostomy, nephrostomy tube placement, biliary drainage tube placement and a variety of interventions in the biliary tree and upper urinary tract such as stone removal and stricture dilatation. Other interventional radiologic procedures include percutaneous biopsy as well as drainage of abscesses and other types of fluid collections.

Imaging modalities used for guidance of these procedures include fluoroscopy, computed tomographic (CT) scanning and ultrasonography. Although non-ferrous instruments do exist, the use of magnetic resonance imaging (MRI) for guidance of interventional procedures is limited by the configuration of the equipment. MRI units designed with easy access for interventions are under development.

Modern interventional radiology began with Seldinger and his technique for placing a guidewire and catheter safely into an artery. Almost all of the procedures listed above came into being because of innovation with guidewires and catheters placed through a tiny hole in the skin. Concurrent developments in imaging and catheter technology were also crucial to the development of safe and effective interventional procedures. Although most percutaneous interventions were first developed for and in adults, almost all are now available for children because tools of appropriate size have been developed[1].

The goal of this chapter is to provide an overview of the types of interventional procedures available for pediatric patients, the typical indications for use of interventional radiology in children and special considerations about pediatric interventional procedures.

Background

In the 18 months between July 1992 and December 1993, the Vascular/Interventional Division at the University of Michigan had 362 pediatric patient visits (a pediatric patient was defined as anyone under 20 years of age). Case breakdown is given in *Table 1*. The information in this chapter, including indications for procedures, preferred tools and techniques, and peri-procedural decision-making, is taken from experience at the Univeristy of Michigan. Practices will vary from one institution to another.

Table 1 Types of procedures performed on pediatric patients (age < 20 years) by the Interventional Radiology Division at the University of Michigan from July 1992 to December 1993. These do not include esophageal foreign body retrievals, intussusception reduction, biopsies or abscess drainages

Procedure	Number of visits	Mean age (years)
Vascular		
Diagnostic	110	14
Interventional	35	
Gastrointestinal		
Initial feeding access	38	7
Tube maintenance	95	
Biliary		
New intervention	17	3
Tube maintenance	25	
Genitourinary		
New intervention	21	5
Tube maintenance	21	
Total	362	10

Patient preparation

Physical evaluation of a patient includes history taking, physical examination, appropriate imaging tests, laboratory tests and pre-procedure orders. These steps, along with close communication between the interventionalist and the referring surgeon, ensure that the right procedure is performed with the best procedural plan and that patient safety will be optimized.

Important points to note in the history are previous surgery, allergy history, contrast history and social history (*see below*). Important points in the physical examination are weight, body habitus, pulse, location of scars and of subcutaneous tubing such as ventriculoperitoneal shunt tubing. Knowledge of the patient's weight and peripheral pulses is necessary before angiography or vascular intervention to gauge permissible contrast load and to detect possible arterial injury related to catheter insertion. Knowledge of the patient's body habitus and locations of subcutaneous tubing is particularly important if percutaneous access to an abdominal organ is planned. If the torso is particularly twisted, CT scanning may be helpful in planning the approach.

Laboratory testing before interventional procedures should include blood urea nitrogen and creatinine, as well as platelets, prothrombin time and partial thromboplastin time. Baseline renal function should be known before carrying out vascular procedures to detect possible contrast nephropathy after the procedure. Coagulation status should be normal or near normal. The relative urgency of the intervention will dictate how aggressively correction of abnormal coagulation parameters is pursued. In unusual circumstances (such as coagulopathy due to ongoing hemorrhage or sepsis) the procedure may be necessary despite coagulopathy. In these cases, appropriate blood products must be available. Hematocrit should be followed before and after embolization for hemorrhage. Complete blood count should be followed before and after manipulation in an infected or potentially infected organ or cavity.

Pre-procedure orders should include 'nil by mouth except medications' for 1–8 h before the procedure (length of time will vary with patient age and weight). It is best not to discontinue enteric medications which may include anticonvulsants, antispasmodics or immunosuppressive drugs. Antibiotics should be administered before any procedure in patients with a vascular graft, in those undergoing vessel embolization, and before accessing any organ or cavity that could be infected.

Preparation must also include careful explanation of the procedure to the patient (if possible) and the family. This is not difficult if a 'one-time' procedure such as an angiogram is planned. However, if the initial procedure is placement of a long-term tube such as a gastrostomy tube, nephrostomy tube or biliary drainage tube, careful explanation of long-term care issues is necessary. Placement of such a device represents a major change in lifestyle. The tubes require care, development of trouble-shooting skills and many follow-up visits to the interventional radiology suite. It is vital that the person who will actually take care of the child should be included in the discussion — that person may not be the legal guardian. The complexity of the child's social situation should never be underestimated. It can be very helpful to show the tube to the child and family before insertion, to let them handle it and get used to it.

Anesthesia

The choices of anesthesia are: none, enteric sedation, intravenous sedation and general anesthesia. If sedation is used it can be administered and monitored by either a member of the surgical team who accompanies the patient, a member of the interventional team, or by anesthesia personnel.

The choice of the most appropriate method of anesthesia depends on many variables including type of procedure (expected pain level, need for patient immobility), patient age and personality, training, experience and number of interventional personnel, physical location of the interventional suite, and availability of anesthesia support. In addition, standards of care regarding pediatric sedation and monitoring have been published within the disciplines of pediatrics[2] and anesthesia, and they are uniform in at least one regard: a patient who has been sedated must be monitored by a person whose *only* job is to monitor the patient[2].

There is no single correct anesthesia protocol. The approach used in the Interventional Radiology Division at the University of Michigan is as follows: when sedation is necessary for normally functioning patients over 36 kg in weight and over 14 years of age, intravenous sedation monitored by interventional radiology personnel is used. For smaller and younger children, and for teenagers who are functionally much younger than their age, the type of anesthesia used is left to the discretion of the anesthesia department staff. With this approach no anesthesia-related complications in pediatric patients have been experienced.

The authors' experience has been that sedation with chloral hydrate is rarely adequate for interventional procedures in which the child is being repeatedly stimulated. Outpatient procedures are possible with proper preparation, recovery facilities and personnel.

Tools and techniques

Miniaturization of tools has been the key to increasing the likelihood of success and the safety of pediatric intervention[1]. All interventions available to adults are now possible even for very small children. Micropuncture needle kits have increased the safety of arterial puncture and have decreased the risk of hemorrhagic complications following puncture of intra-abdominal organs. Atraumatic guidewires that are 0.012–0.018 inches in diameter are used. Catheters in sizes as small as 2.2 Fr are available for vascular diagnostic and interventional procedures. For drainage procedures, small self-retaining catheters have been developed for placement into the kidney, liver, stomach and fluid collections.

During vascular procedures the risk of fluid and contrast overload can be minimized by using small syringes (1–3 ml) and non-ionic contrast in low concentration.

A variety of technical advances in angiographic equipment design make it possible to minimize the radiation exposure of the child during these procedures. Attention on the part of the interventionalist to lead shielding and fluoroscopy time can further ensure that radiation exposure is kept as low as possible.

Procedures and complications

DIAGNOSTIC ANGIOGRAPHY

Most vascular anatomic information necessary to surgeons is available via non-invasive imaging studies. The use of diagnostic angiography is limited. Indications include penetrating and non-penetrating trauma, renal vascular hypertension, aortic dissection or coarctation, evaluation for major aortic branch stenosis caused by systemic vascular disease such as neurofibromatosis or Takayasu's arteritis, peripheral vascular insufficiency caused by embolus, thoracic outlet syndrome or popliteal artery entrapment (*Figure 1a, b*), follow-up of surgical or percutaneous vascular intervention, vascular malformation evaluation (*Figure 2a, b*), evaluation for possible acute deep venous thrombosis or pulmonary embolism, and questions related to organ transplantation. Typical indications before organ transplantation include evaluation of renal donor anatomy and recipient portal vein patency when ultrasonography is equivocal. Indications after transplantation include evaluation of arterial and venous anastomoses.

With two major additions, the complications of angiography in children are the same as those seen in adults: contrast allergy, contrast nephropathy, vascular injury, hematoma and hemorrhage, stroke (for procedures involving catheterization of the brachiocephalic arterial tree), and death. The two significant additions (*Figure 3a, b*) are acute femoral arterial spasm resulting in thrombosis, and leg length discrepancy resulting from chronic femoral arterial thrombosis[3]. The former is manifested by acute signs of peripheral ischemia and may require emergency treatment. The mechanism of the latter is poorly understood but well documented, particularly in children who undergo catheterization under the age of 5 years. Close monitoring of the peripheral pulses in the extremity being accessed is necessary. Heparinization and intra-arterial administration of glyceryl trinitrate during the procedure are recommended.

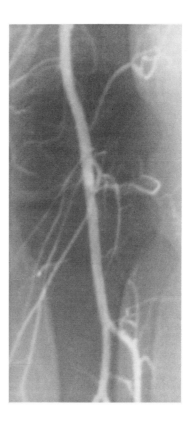

1a

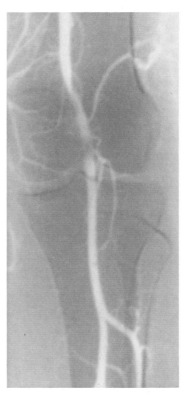

1b

Figure 1   Arteriographic evaluation of a 17-year-old tennis player with claudication. The popliteal artery is normal in appearance at rest (a), but narrows with the foot in dorsiflexion (b), indicating popliteal artery entrapment

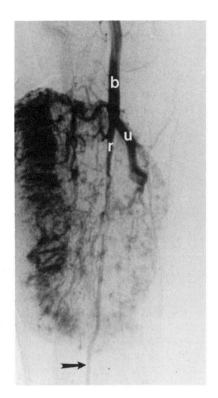

2a

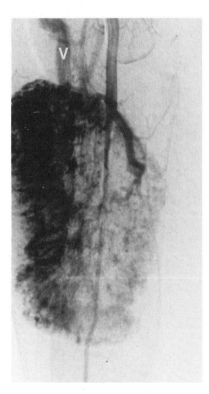

2b

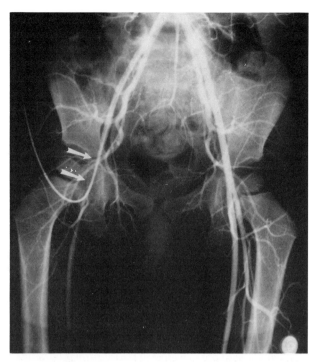

3a

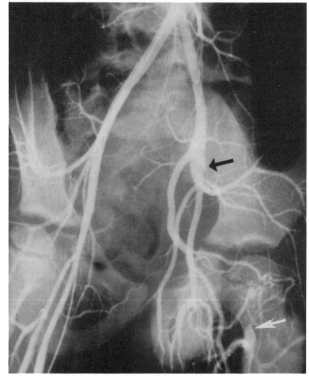

3b

Figure 2   Arteriogram of a large arteriovenous malformation of the forearm of an infant associated with hemorrhage and skin breakdown. (a) Arteriography demonstrates multiple arterial feeders from the brachial (b), ulnar (u) and radial (r) arteries. Flow to the hand is minimal (arrow). (b) Later phase film shows marked capillary staining of the malformation and shunting to the venous system (v)

Figure 3   Acute and chronic complications of arterial catheterization. (a) The right common femoral artery is in spasm (arrows) around the percutaneously placed catheter. Note the normal sized left common femoral artery. (b) Angiographic evaluation of leg length discrepancy which in this child is due to chronic occlusion of the left external iliac and common femoral arteries, the sequelae of a cardiac catheterization performed as an infant. The black arrow indicates the point of occlusion and the white arrow the point of reconstitution. Note the large collaterals provided by the left internal iliac artery

VASCULAR INTERVENTIONS

Over the past 10 years, percutaneous vascular interventions have gained increased acceptance for pediatric patients, particularly for those children who are critically ill and are not good candidates for surgery, who do not have a long life expectancy, or who have problems for which there is no good definitive operation (i.e. complex arteriovenous malformations infiltrating major muscle groups). Principles, tools and techniques are the same as those used in the adult.

Percutaneous embolization

Typical indications for vascular embolization include arterial gastrointestinal hemorrhage, post-traumatic hemorrhage, hemoptysis due to chronic inflammatory lung disease such as cystic fibrosis, spontaneous or iatrogenic (i.e. post-biopsy) hemorrhage from a solid organ, control of symptoms of a vascular malformation, control of hypersplenism, control of hypertension and varicocele occlusion (*Figure 4a–c*). The embolic agents typically used are surgical gelatin sponge (Gelfoam), polyvinyl alcohol particles (Ivalon), absolute alcohol,

sodium tetradecyl sulfate (Sotradecol), and metallic occlusion coils. Detachable balloons and glue have application in the management of vascular malformations but are available in only a few centers.

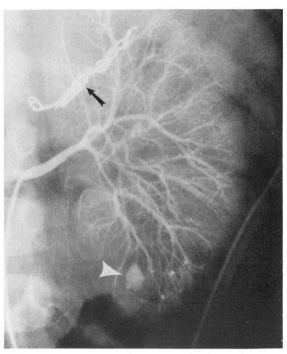

4b

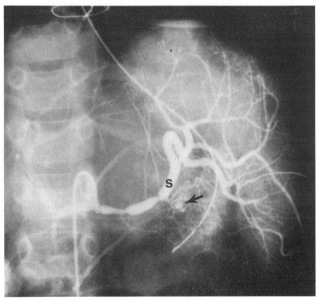

4a

Figure 4   Two arterial embolization procedures in one patient with multiple medical problems. (a) Acute pancreatitis complicated by hemorrhage from the pancreatica magna artery (arrow) was treated with coil embolization of the splenic artery (s). Note catheter-induced spasm of the proximal splenic artery. (b) Two years later the same patient developed gross hematuria after a left renal biopsy requiring transfusion. Left renal arteriogram demonstrates a lower pole pseudoaneurysm (arrowhead). The arrow indicates coils in the previously embolized splenic artery. (c) Following Gelfoam embolization of the branch supplying the pseudoaneurysm, the left nephrogram is partially preserved

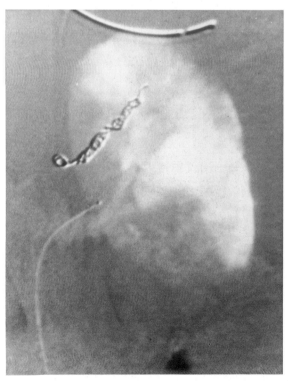

4c

The choice of embolic agent depends on the nature of the lesion to be occluded as well as operator preference and the catheter system being used. Hemorrhage from a point source that is likely to heal with time such as a duodenal ulcer, a renal biopsy site, or a point of post-traumatic hemorrhage can be stopped reliably with Gelfoam. Hemoptysis due to inflammatory hypertrophy of bronchial artery branches is best treated with Ivalon, as is palliation of hypersplenism. Occlusion of a large vessel such as the gonadal vein or a traumatically transected artery greater than 2 mm in diameter is best achieved with occlusion coils.

The choice of embolic agent can be particularly critical for occlusion of an arteriovenous malformation. A large simple arteriovenous fistula with no intervening capillary bed can be occluded with metallic coils or, where available, detachable balloons. A complex arteriovenous malformation with multiple feeders and a capillary nidus is best approached with Ivalon. A venous malformation can be sclerosed with a liquid agent.

Complications of embolization include those listed for diagnostic angiography as well as tissue necrosis and inadvertent placement or spontaneous migration of the embolic agent to an unintended site[4, 5]. Tissue necrosis is most likely to occur with the use of small Ivalon particles (150–250 μm) or a liquid sclerosing agent in the arterial tree. Tissue necrosis is typically accompanied by pain, fever, nausea and elevated white blood cell count. Supportive care and antibiotic medication is recommended. If tissue necrosis is not an intended result of the embolization procedure, development of symptoms suggesting tissue necrosis must be investigated thoroughly to ensure that a complication such as bowel infarction after occlusion of a colonic bleeding site is not overlooked.

Liquid sclerosants must be used with extreme caution even in the venous system. Perivascular inflammation can lead to scarring and clinically significant neuropathy if a nerve is in close proximity to the vein being sclerosed. Severe inflammation after treatment of an arteriovenous malformation may be treated with steroids.

Coil migration can occur if the coil is the wrong size. Paradoxical embolization to the lungs can occur with any agent if there is a significant degree of arteriovenous shunting in the lesion being occluded. Care must be taken to choose the size of the embolic agent carefully in this setting. Fatal pulmonary insufficiency has been reported in infants following Ivalon embolization of an arteriovenous malformation[5].

Lytic therapy

Lytic therapy is an alternative to surgical thrombectomy for acute vascular occlusion. Use of catheter-directed local lytic therapy in children is, however, limited. Indications can include aortic thrombosis due to umbilical artery catheter placement, peripheral arterial embolus, dialysis graft thrombosis and thrombosis of a vascular anastomosis (i.e. after liver transplantation). In the latter two instances lytic therapy may reveal an underlying stenotic lesion amenable to angioplasty.

Urokinase is the most frequently used agent. The standard dose ranges from 1000 to 2000 units/kg/h and the standard technique is to place a small catheter or open-ended guidewire selectively into the thrombus and to initiate an infusion. Follow-up angiography to assess progress is performed at 4–12 h intervals. Infusion is terminated when the clot dissolves, when there is no further progress at clot dissolution, or when risk of a significant complication outweighs the risk of continuing the therapy.

Coagulation parameters including prothrombin time, partial thromboplastin time, fibrinogen and fibrin degradation products should be followed closely during the infusion period. Serum fibrinogen depletion heralds the development of a systemic lytic state.

Complications include local hemorrhage in the area being treated, distant or diffuse hemorrhage related to development of a systemic lytic state, and pericatheter thrombosis. Risk of the latter can be decreased by systemic heparinization.

Percutaneous transluminal angioplasty

Indications for percutaneous transluminal angioplasty (PTA) in children include main or branch artery stenosis[6], postoperative vascular anastomotic stenosis, and arterial or venous stenosis related to dialysis access, as well as uncommon lesions such as major aortic branch stenosis due to neurofibromatosis or Takayasu's arteritis. Coarctation of the aorta itself is now frequently treated with PTA but this procedure is usually undertaken by interventional cardiologists rather than radiologists.

The standard procedure for an angioplasty begins with a careful initial arteriogram to evaluate the extent of the lesion and to size the vessel precisely. Systemic heparinization is then performed and the lesion is crossed with a guidewire/catheter system. Microdilatation systems such as a balloon mounted on a 0.035-inch diameter guidewire are available, making angioplasty a practical therapeutic option for small children. An appropriately sized balloon is inflated across the lesion. After dilatation an angiogram is performed to assess the adequacy of dilatation and to rule out immediate complications.

Acute technical complications of angioplasty include arterial rupture, dissection with or without thrombosis, and thrombosis with or without distal embolization. Arterial rupture requires urgent surgical intervention. The angioplasty balloon may be inflated across the site of rupture to prevent hemorrhage in the interim. Dissection may require operative intervention if it is flow-limiting. Arterial thrombosis and embolization may be managed percutaneously with lytic therapy. In addition to these technical complications, all of the complications listed above for diagnostic angiography also apply to angioplasty. The most significant delayed complication of angioplasty is re-stenosis[7].

Transjugular intrahepatic portosystemic shunt

Creation of an intrahepatic communication between the portal and hepatic veins is a relatively new interventional radiologic procedure[8]. It provides an alternative to surgical portosystemic shunting and has been used for the following indications: emergency decompression of bleeding esophageal varices, elective or urgent decompression of varices which have failed sclerotherapy, control of ascites due to portal hypertension, and even massive pleural effusion due to portal hypertension. Creation of the transjugular intrahepatic portosystemic shunt (TIPS) can be used to manage the complications of portal hypertension in non-surgical patients and in those awaiting liver transplantation. The need for this intervention in children is uncommon but has been described[8].

Creation of a TIPS is performed from the right jugular approach. A sheath is advanced into the right or middle hepatic vein. Through this sheath, a needle is advanced into the right or left portal vein. The intrahepatic needle tract is dilated over a guidewire with an angioplasty balloon. A vascular stent is then deployed in the tract to hold it open. A satisfactory result is indicated by a post-stent pressure gradient between the portal vein and right atrium of $10-15\,cmH_2O$.

Acute complications of TIPS include pneumothorax, cardiac arrhythmia, intraperitoneal hemorrhage, sepsis, stent thrombosis, portal vein thrombosis and failure. The most common late complication is stenosis at the hepatic vein end of the stent because of intimal hyperplasia. Secondary interventions to maintain stent placement are frequently required. Periodic screening of TIPS function using Doppler ultrasonography is recommended.

Inferior vena cava filter placement

Inferior vena cava (IVC) filter placement is indicated to prevent pulmonary embolus in patients who have had a pulmonary embolus or documented lower extremity or pelvic venous thromboembolic disease and who have the following concomitant problems: failure of anticoagulation to prevent further thromboembolism, a contraindication to anticoagulation, free-floating thrombus above the inguinal ligament, or such pulmonary compromise that the risk associated with further pulmonary embolus is prohibitive.

Fortunately, these problems are unusual in the pediatric population. Placement of an IVC filter in a child has significant implications. Will the filter remain intact for the patient's entire life? Will the filter grow in diameter as the cava grows? Will the ratio of metal to caval lumen cross-sectional area be low enough to avoid caval thrombosis?

A variety of IVC filters are available for use in the USA. These include the Greenfield filter (Meditech, Watertown, Massachusetts), the Bird's Nest filter (Cook, Bloomington, Indianapolis), the Simon–Nitinol filter (Simon Nitinol Co, distributed by B. Braun, Chicago, Illinois), and the Venatech filter (Venatech, Inc, Brookline Massachusetts). Of these, the design which has been in clinical use for the longest time is the Greenfield filter[9]. This is the authors' preferred filter for use in pediatric patients (*Figure 5a, b*).

The procedure begins with an inferior vena cavagram from either the right femoral or right jugular approach to assess caval patency, to identify the level of the renal veins and to exclude caval or renal vein anomaly. A site for filter deployment is chosen and marked. The preferred site for deployment is in the IVC below the level of the renal veins. The filter is deployed at the chosen level after dilatation of the venous access site.

Complications of IVC filter placement include insertion site thrombosis, IVC thrombosis, and failure to prevent pulmonary embolism. In adults, chronic lower extremity swelling occurs in 2–5% and recurrent pulmonary embolism in 2% of cases following Greenfield filter placement. Other rare complications include filter migration and filter leg fracture.

Central venous access

The standard approach to long-term central venous access in children is surgical placement of a Broviac or Hickman catheter (CR Bard Inc., Salt Lake City, Utah) from the subclavian or jugular approach. Whether this procedure is performed by a surgeon or, as is increasingly the case in adults[10], by an interventional radiologist, fluoroscopic guidance and contrast opacification of the subclavian vein during initial access can decrease the risk of pneumothorax and can aid in precise positioning of the catheter tip.

Increasingly, children are outliving the integrity of their central venous system. Maintenance of long-term central venous access in the face of subclavian vein, iliac vein and/or caval thrombosis is a new challenge. Interventional radiologic techniques can be helpful in identifying a venous map for, and in achieving, central venous access in this setting. Translumbar Hickman catheter placement is now well described[11]. In addition, Hickman catheters have been placed from the transhepatic and the intercostal approach (*Figure 6*) in selected cases.

Clinical demand for intermediate-term (2–15 weeks) central venous access is increasing. This demand is driven primarily by the medical system's emphasis on early hospital discharge and is made possible by the proliferation of home health nursing to supervise intravenous therapies in the home setting. The preferred venous catheter for intermediate-term therapy is the peripherally inserted central catheter (PIC catheter). The most common indications are chemotherapy and antibiotic treatment of bacterial endocarditis, osteomyelitis, and chronic pulmonary infections associated with cystic fibrosis.

PIC catheters can be inserted at the bedside via the antecubital vein. Interventional radiologic techniques can be used to place these catheters from a mid-arm brachial vein approach in those who do not have an antecubital vein. This procedure has been performed successfully in children as young as 5 years. The vein is opacified with contrast and punctured under fluoroscopic control. The distance to the junction of the superior vena cava with the right atrium is measured precisely and a 3–5-Fr single- or double-lumen catheter is then passed and fixed to the skin.

The most significant complication of PIC catheter placement is pericatheter thrombosis. If swelling of the arm results, the catheter should be removed. Pneumothorax is not a risk of this procedure.

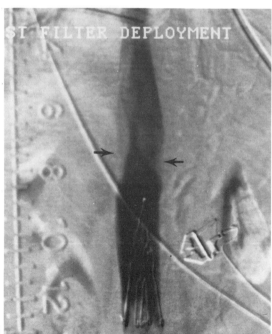

5a

5b

Figure 5   Inferior vena cava filter placement in an 11-year-old girl with systemic lupus erythematosus complicated by both gastrointestinal hemorrhage and lower extremity deep venous thrombosis. (a) Digital subtraction cavagram demonstrating no caval thrombosis. (b) Post-deployment cavagram demonstrating proper positioning of a Greenfield filter below the level of the renal veins (arrows). (Images courtesy of Anna Champlin MD, Albuquerque, New Mexico, USA)

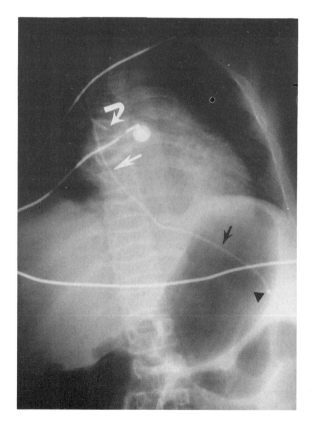

6

Figure 6   Central venous access in a child with IVC and bilateral subclavian vein occlusion. A Hickman catheter has been threaded through the left 11th intercostal vein (black arrow) into the azygos vein (straight white arrow) to lie with its tip in the superior vena cava (curved white arrow). The intercostal vein was chosen because it opacified with contrast medium injected via the left common femoral vein. The arrowhead indicates the venous puncture site

Foreign body retrieval

As the complexity of medical vascular interventions has increased, the frequency of iatrogenically caused intravascular foreign bodies has risen. Typical intravascular foreign bodies include guidewire fragments, catheter fragments, pacemaker fragments and embolization coils. Complications vary with location of the item and include vessel thrombosis, vessel or cardiac chamber perforation and infection. Removal is indicated for both patient care and medicolegal reasons.

Because most intravascular foreign bodies lodge in the central venous or pulmonary vascular tree and are radio-opaque, fluoroscopically-guided percutaneous removal is preferred. A variety of intravascular retrieval devices has been developed. Techniques designed for foreign body retrieval can also be used to reposition the tips of permanent central venous catheters found to be in a suboptimal position on chest radiography performed after placement of the catheter.

The most significant complication of percutaneous foreign body retrieval is cardiac arrhythmia.

NON-VASCULAR INTERVENTION

Non-vascular interventional procedures involve the use of percutaneous catheter and guidewire techniques under imaging guidance in organ systems other than the vascular tree. Procedures include interventions in the urinary tract, the biliary tree and the gastrointestinal tract as well as abscess drainage procedures and fine needle biopsies. In most instances these procedures provide the patient with alternatives to open surgery, which have low associated morbidity rates.

Although non-vascular interventional procedures are similar in many respects to their vascular counterparts, important differences do exist. First, many non-vascular interventional procedures require transgression of the peritoneal space into infected or potentially infected body cavities. Peri-procedural intravenous antibiotics are required to minimize the risk of sepsis during initial access into the stomach, biliary tree, upper urinary tract or into an abnormal fluid collection. Manipulation through an existing tract into these areas (e.g. for a tube change) is less likely to result in bacteremia.

The practice in this unit is to administer broad-spectrum intravenous antibiotics during and for at least 24 h after all initial biliary, gastrointestinal or genitourinary access procedures. For biliary tube changes, the patient is given a single dose of intravenous antibiotic immediately before the procedure. Nephrostomy tube changes are preceded by intravenous antibiotic administration only if the patient's urine appears to be infected, the tube is obstructed and not draining, the patient has a history of post-procedure sepsis, or the patient is immunocompromised. Antimicrobial prophylaxis is not necessary before percutaneous feeding tube change.

The practice of non-vascular interventional radiology demands a high level of commitment to follow-up care on the part of the interventional radiology team and the hospital. A system must be in place to teach patients tube care, to make necessary supplies available, and to allow patients easy access to interventional services on an urgent or emergency basis.

Gastrointestinal intervention

Typical radiologic pediatric gastrointestinal interventions include removal of esophageal foreign bodies, esophageal stricture dilatation, reduction of colonic intussusception, and placement of percutaneous feeding tubes[12]. The first three procedures mentioned have been standard for many years, although new techniques have evolved. The fourth is relatively new and is not as widely accepted.

Esophageal foreign body retrieval is sometimes performed under fluoroscopy using a Foley balloon catheter to drag the object up into the mouth. Foreign bodies can easily be removed by this method provided that the foreign body has not been incorporated into the esophageal wall as evidenced radiographically by airway compression and thickening of the tracheoesophageal stripe. Since the foreign body may be dislodged and introduced into the airway during removal, this method should only be performed when personnel capable of maintaining the airway are immediately available. Some metallic foreign bodies can be removed with a magnetic device. This device can be used to retrieve a ferrous item from the stomach and can decrease the risk of losing the item into the airway as it is withdrawn through the hypopharynx.

Percutaneous placement of gastric and transgastric–jejunal feeding tubes using fluoroscopic guidance was developed in parallel with the more familiar percutaneous endoscopically-guided gastrostomy (PEG) tube placement procedure. Fluoroscopically-guided G-tube placement in a child was first described in 1986 and has been widely used since then in some centers[12].

Percutaneous gastrostomy or gastrojejunostomy tube placement is appropriate if long-term nutritional support is required and if the patient does not need or is not a candidate for an antireflux procedure or pyloroplasty. Placement of a gastrostomy tube (*Figure 7*) is preferred because it is easier to use and maintain than a transgastric–jejunal feeding tube. A gastrostomy tube can also be converted to a 'button' replacement device which many patients and families prefer from a care and cosmetic point of view.

A single-lumen transgastric–jejunal feeding tube is necessary if the patient is at risk of aspiration pneumonia with gastric feeding. A double-lumen gastrojejunostomy tube (*Figure 8a, b*) which provides gastric decompression as well as jejunal feeding should be used only if absolutely necessary because these tubes are particularly prone to malfunction.

The standard procedure is that the stomach is insufflated with air and punctured with a needle. An anchor is placed through the needle to hold traction on the stomach, a guidewire is then placed, the tract dilated, and a self-retaining catheter is inserted.

Percutaneously-placed gastrostomy catheters are typically 8–14 Fr in diameter. If a transgastric–jejunal tube is to be placed, angiographic techniques are used to manipulate a guidewire through the pylorus and around the duodenal sweep into the jejunum. Over this wire, a 6–8-Fr tube is advanced to the desired location. Following the procedure the stomach is decompressed for at least 24 h, hydration and pulmonary toilet are maintained, pain is controlled, and signs of infection must be monitored.

Early complications of percutaneous feeding tube placement include hemorrhage, peritonitis, inadvertent colonic or small bowel perforation, and early dislodgement of the tube before tract formation. As with surgically placed tubes, delayed complications include local wound infection, granulation tissue formation and tube malfunction or dislodgement.

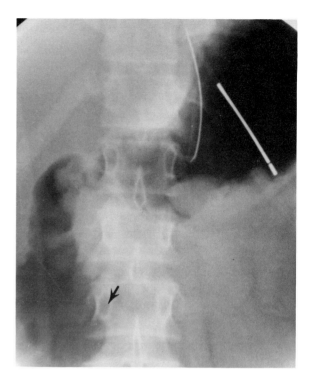

8a

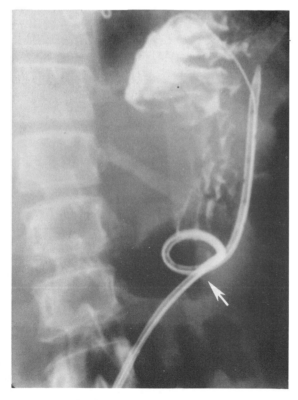

7

Figure 7   Gastrostomy tube placement. A locking pigtail gastrostomy catheter has been placed for supplemental nutrition in a 15-year-old patient with cystic fibrosis. Injection of contrast medium confirms the intraluminal location. The guidewire is still in place. The arrow indicates the gastric puncture site

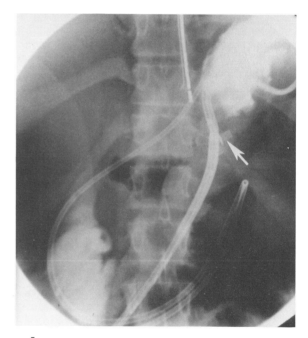

8b

Figure 8   Gastrojejunostomy tube placement to aid in the management of duodenal hematoma causing bowel obstruction. (a) Plain film showing duodenal obstruction (arrow). (b) A double-lumen gastrojejunostomy tube has been placed with a gastric port for drainage and a jejunal limb crossing the point of obstruction for feeding. The arrow indicates a Malecot retention device in the stomach

In addition, gastroesopahgeal reflux can become clinically significant following gastrostomy tube placement. Evidence of this development should be fully evaluated. Transpyloric feeding tube placement or surgical intervention should be pursued if intolerance of gastric feeding develops.

Esophageal stricture dilatation is discussed in the chapter on esophagogastroduodenoscopy on pp. 298–307.

Biliary intervention

Biliary interventional radiologic procedures include diagnostic percutaneous transhepatic cholangiography (PTC), transhepatic biliary drainage, transhepatic biliary stone removal and transhepatic cholangioplasty. The transhepatic approach is most frequently required when the common bile duct is not accessible to the peroral endoscope as is typical following Roux-en-Y choledochojejunostomy. Indications can include biliary anomalies or the presence of intrahepatic biliary stones. In the pediatric population, however, biliary interventions are performed most frequently to treat acute or delayed biliary complications of liver transplantation (*Figure 9a–c*)[13]. Diagnostic PTC is useful for excluding biliary obstruction or leak. Transhepatic drainage is indicated to relieve biliary obstruction or to divert bile drainage from a site of leakage and to stent the leak. Delayed development of biliary strictures may be treated with cholangioplasty. Biliary stones developing after transplantation can be removed through the percutaneous tract.

A recent development in the treatment of biliary strictures is the placement of permanent metallic internal biliary stents. The authors have not used these stents in children because their patency is unlikely to last for the lifetime of the child and they become incorporated into the bile duct wall, adding to the complexity of future biliary surgery.

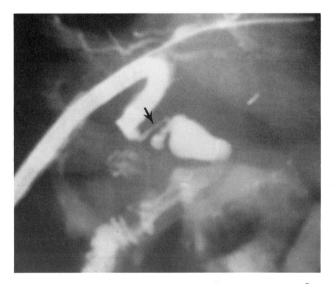

9b

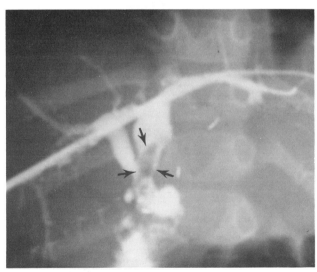

9a

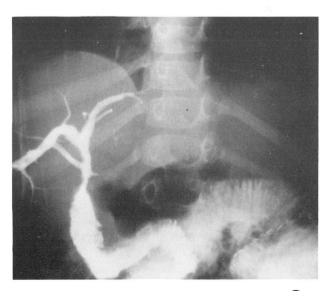

9c

Figure 9   *Elevated bilirubin and fever in a 3-year-old after liver transplantation for treatment of biliary atresia improved following percutaneous transhepatic biliary drainage. (a) Cholangiogram through the transhepatic tract showing a large stone in the hepatic duct (arrows). (b) After stone removal with a percutaneous flexible choledochoscope, repeat cholangiography demonstrated a long hepatic duct stricture (arrow). Balloon dilatation was not curative. (c) Cholangiogram following the surgical revision of the choledochoenteric anastomosis showing a satisfactory result. The percutaneous tube was removed*

Percutaneous access to the biliary tree is performed as in adults with a 22-gauge needle. Self-retaining catheters (6–8 Fr) are preferred for drainage. Complex interventions via the transhepatic approach, such as biliary stone removal, should be delayed until the tract has matured because significant tract dilatation and multiple catheter exchanges through the tract may be necessary.

Acute complications of percutaneous transhepatic biliary access procedures include sepsis, intraperitoneal hemorrhage, hemobilia, bile peritonitis, pneumothorax and colonic perforation. Hemorrhagic complications because of intrahepatic arterial injury may be treated with percutaneous transarterial embolization of the bleeding site. Delayed complications are primarily related to tube malfunction or dislodgement.

Genitourinary intervention

Percutaneous genitourinary interventions in children[14] most frequently involve accessing the kidney and include antegrade pyelography, percutaneous nephros-

tomy, nephroureteral stent placement, stricture dilatation (*Figure 10a–c*), and tract dilatation for nephroscopically-guided stone removal or endopyelotomy. Indications for these procedures include congenital upper urinary tract obstruction, ureteric obstruction after

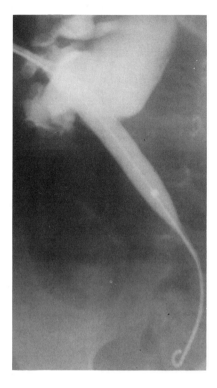

10b

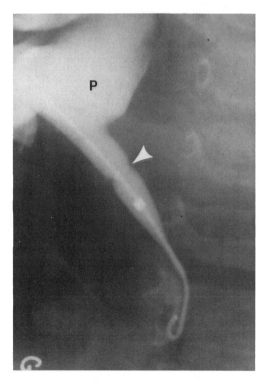

10a

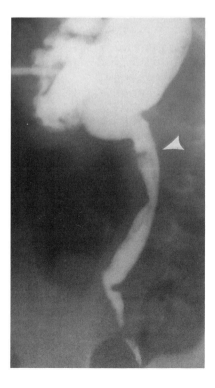

10c

Figure 10   Balloon dilatation of ureteropelvic junction obstruction that recurred after surgery. (a) An angioplasty balloon catheter has been advanced across the junction through a percutaneous nephrostomy tract. The arrowhead indicates a weblike waist on the balloon at the site of the obstruction. P shows the renal pelvis opacified with contrast. (b) Further balloon inflation has resulted in obliteration of the balloon waist. (c) Post-dilatation nephrostogram showing deformity at the site of the dilatation (arrowhead) but patency of the ureter

ureteric reimplantation, upper urinary tract leak, stone, fungal infection requiring irrigation, or any of these entities complicating renal transplantation.

The preferred access to the kidney is through an infracostal posterolateral approach into a lower pole calyx. As for biliary drainage, 6–8-Fr catheters are preferred. Tract dilatation to 18–28 Fr for nephroscopy, endopyelotomy or stone removal is possible even in small children. The infant kidney, however, is frequently too small and too mobile to permit tract dilatation to that degree.

Complications of percutaneous nephrostomy and related procedures include sepsis, hemorrhage (again treatable with percutaneous embolization if a branch renal artery injury is the source of bleeding), urinoma, pneumothorax, hepatic or splenic injury, and colonic perforation.

Percutaneous biopsy and fluid collection drainage

Percutaneous aspiration, drainage and biopsy can be safely performed in most areas of the chest or abdomen.

Percutaneous aspiration is useful to determine whether a collection seen on cross-sectional imaging is sterile or infected. The majority of aspirations in the authors' unit are performed with CT guidance, since this modality offers greater confidence in delineating the bowel and other organs. Fluid collections in children too sick to travel to the CT scanner or large fluid collections are aspirated under ultrasonographic guidance. Aspiration with a thin Chiba needle can be safely performed in any part of the chest or abdomen. Although the thin Chiba needle suffices to aspirate thin fluid collections, aspiration of thicker fluid collections requires a larger caliber needle.

Although aspiration of fluid collections is easily performed, the placement of drainage catheters is more complicated[15]. Several factors must be taken into account when performing this type of procedure, such as access, size and number of fluid collections. Fluid collections which are small and in several locations are not suitable for drainage, while accessible collections of medium to large size are amenable to catheter drainage (*Figure 11*).

Biopsy of intra-abdominal or intrathoracic lesions can easily be done under CT guidance. The initial evaluation is made using a thin Chiba needle for cytology. However, depending upon the location and the tissue, a core biopsy should be obtained.

Potential complications of these procedures include pneumothorax, hematoma, bleeding, fistula formation and infection (accessing fluid collections through the bowel may contaminate a sterile fluid collection). By careful evaluation of the risks involved and the options available in each patient, a decision can be made about the optimal approach.

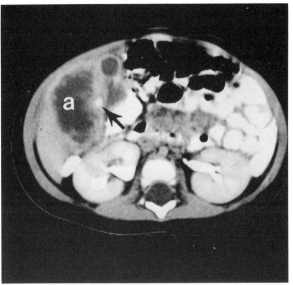

11a

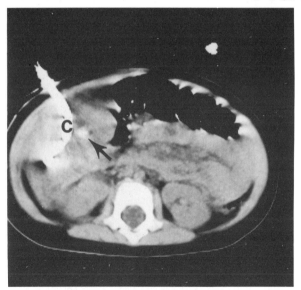

11b

Figure 11   CT-guided abscess drainage. An appendiceal abscess (a) was drained as an emergency. The image after drainage demonstrating the catheter (c) in the collapsed cavity following aspiration of 100 ml of pus. The arrows indicate a calcified appendicolith

Follow-up considerations for non-vascular interventions

Meticulous attention to follow-up care is necessary after any intervention, particularly those resulting in any kind of tube placement such as a biliary drainage tube, percutaneous nephrostomy tube, gastrostomy tube or abscess drainage tube. In children particularly, maintenance of such tubes is fraught with difficulty because the patients as well as their playmates may be active and curious! The patient's primary care-giver must have clear instructions (agreed upon by the interventional radiologist and the primary physician) on how to care for the tube and what to do if the tube should become clogged, broken or inadvertently dislodged.

A routine schedule of prophylactic tube changes can minimize emergency visits related to tube malfunction and minimize the risk of systemic infection because of tube obstruction (*Table 2*).

Table 2   Recommended schedule of prophylactic tube changes for percutaneously placed drainage and feeding tubes. Routine tube changes can be performed on an outpatient basis. The schedule may be modified according to individual patient needs

Tube type	Recommended tube change interval (months)
Gastric	6–9
Transgastric–jejunal	3
Nephrostomy	3
Biliary	1–2
Fluid collection	1–2

Conclusion

Interventional radiology, both vascular and non-vascular, can benefit many pediatric patients. A good working relationship between the interventional radiology service and the pediatric surgery service can ensure that use of these options is efficacious and safe, and that follow-up care is optimal.

References

1. Towbin RB. Pediatric interventional procedures in the 1980s: a period of development, growth, and acceptance. *Radiology* 1989; 170: 1081–90.

2. Cook BA, Bass JW, Nomizu S, Alexander ME. Sedation of children for technical procedures: current standard of practice. *Clin Pediatr* 1992; 137–42.

3. Taylor LM, Troutman R, Feliciano P, Menashe V, Sunderland C, Porter JM. Late complications after femoral artery catheterization in children less than five years of age. *J Vasc Surg* 1990; 11: 297–306.

4. Hemingway AP. Allison DJ. Complications of embolization: analysis of 410 procedures. *Radiology* 1988; 166: 669–72.

5. Repa I, Moradian GP, Dehner LP *et al*. Mortalities associated with use of a commercial suspension of polyvinyl alcohol. *Radiology* 1989; 170: 395–9.

6. Robinson L, Gedroyc W, Reidy J, Saxton HM. Renal artery stenosis in children. *Clin Radiol* 1991; 44: 376–82.

7. Becker GJ, Katzen BT, Dake MD. Noncoronary angioplasty. *Radiology* 1989; 170: 921–40.

8. LaBerge JM, Ring EJ, Gordon RL *et al*. Creation of transjugular intrahepatic portosystemic shunts with the Wallstent endoprosthesis: results in 100 patients. *Radiology* 1993; 187: 413–20.

9. Greenfield LJ, Cho KY, Proctor M *et al*. Results of a multicenter study of the modified hook-titanium Greenfield filter. *J Vasc Surg* 1991; 14: 253–7.

10. Mauro MA, Jaques PF. Radiologic placement of long-term central venous catheters: a review. *J Vasc Intervent Radiol* 1993; 4: 127–37.

11. Lund GB, Lieberman RP, Haire WD, Martin VA, Kessinger A, Armitage JO. Translumbar inferior vena cava catheters for long-term venous access. *Radiology* 1990; 174: 31–5.

12. Malden ES, Hicks ME, Picus D, Darcy MD, Vesely TM, Kleinhoffer MA. Fluoroscopically guided percutaneous gastrostomy in children. *J Vasc Intervent Radiol* 1992; 3: 673–7.

13. Pariente D, Bihet MH, Tammam S *et al*. Biliary complications after transplantation in children: role of imaging modalities. *Pediatr Radiol* 1991; 21: 175–8.

14. Ball WS Jr, Towbin R, Strife JL, Spencer R. Interventional genitourinary radiology in children: a review of 61 procedures. *AJR* 1986; 147: 791–6.

15. Lambaise RE, Deyoe L, Cronan JJ, Dorfman GS. Percutaneous drainage of 335 consecutive abscesses: results of primary drainage with 1-year follow-up. *Radiology* 1992; 184: 167–79.

List of products

Argyle drains, Sherwood Medical Industries Ltd, Crawley, West Sussex, UK

Bear Cub BP 2000 infant ventilator, Bear Intermed Inc, California, USA
Broviac catheter, Bard Access Systems, Salt Lake City, Utah, USA

Conray, Rhône-Poulenc Rorer, Dagenham, Essex, UK
CUSA (Cavitron Ultrasonic Surgical Aspirator), ValleyLab, Boulder, Colorado, USA/ValleyLab UK, London, UK

Dacron, Du Pont, Wilmington, Delaware, USA/Du Pont Pharmaceuticals, Letchworth Garden City, Hertfordshire, UK
Dexon, Davis & Geck, Gosport, UK/Davis & Geck International, c/o Cyanamid International, Wayne, New Jersey, USA
Dinamap, Critikon, USA/Critikon, Bracknell, Berkshire, UK

EEA stapler, Auto Suture, Ascot, Berkshire, UK/US Surgical Corporation, Connecticut, USA
Ethibond, Ethicon, Edinburgh, UK/Ethicon Inc, Somerville, New Jersey, USA

Fletchers' phosphate, Pharmax Ltd, Bexley, Kent, UK

Gastrografin, Schering Health Care, Burgess Hill, West Sussex, UK
Gelfoam, Upjohn, Kalamazoo, Michigan, USA
GIA stapler, Auto Suture, Ascot, Berkshire, UK/US Surgical Corporation, Connecticut, USA

Hitman catheter, Bard Access Systems, Salt Lake City, Utah, USA/Bard Ltd, Crawley, West Sussex, UK
Hypaque, Sanofi Winthrop, Guildford, UK

Intraflo, Abbott Critical Care & Control Systems, California, USA
Ivalon (polyvinyl alcohol particles), Unipoint Industries, North Carolina, USA

Lofric catheter, Astra Tech, Gloucester, UK

Marlex, C P Bard, Massachusetts, USA/Bard Ltd, Crawley, West Sussex, UK
Maxon, Davis & Geck, Gosport, UK/Davis & Geck International, c/o Cyanamid International, Wayne, New Jersey, USA
Mixter forceps, Codman, Bracknell, Berkshire, UK/Codman, Massachusetts, USA

Nurolon (braided polymide), Ethicon, Edinburgh, UK/Ethicon Inc, Somerville, New Jersey, USA

Opsite, Smith & Nephew, Hull, UK

PDS, Ethicon, Edinburgh, UK/Ethicon Inc, Somerville, New Jersey, USA
Penlon Nuffield 200 ventilator, Penlon Intermed, Abingdon, Oxfordshire, UK
Portex tubes, Portex Ltd, Hythe, Kent, UK
Prolene, Ethicon, Edinburgh, UK/Ethicon Inc, Somerville, New Jersey, USA

Redivac drains, Biomet Ltd, Bridgend, South Glamorgan, UK
Replogle tube, Sherwood Medical Ltd, Crawley, West Sussex, UK

Satinsky clamp, Codman, Massachusetts, USA/Codman, Bracknell, Berkshire, UK
Silastic catheters, Vygon (UK) Ltd, Gloucestershire, UK
Steridrapes, 3M, Minneapolis, Minnesota, USA/3M Healthcare Ltd, Loughborough, Leicestershire, UK
Steristrips, 3M, Minneapolis, Minnesota, USA/3M Healthcare Ltd, Loughborough, Leicestershire, UK
Storz cystoscope, Karl Storz Endoscopy America, Culver City, California, USA/Karl Storz Endoscopy, Rimmer Brothers, London, UK
Storz-Hopkins rod-lens telescope, Karl Storz Endoscopy America, Culver City, California, USA/Karl Storz Endoscopy, Rimmer Brothers, London, UK
Storz resectoscope, Karl Storz Endoscopy America, Culver City, California, USA/Karl Storz Endoscopy, Rimmer Brothers, London, UK

TA 55 stapler, Auto Suture, Ascot, Berkshire, UK/US Surgical Corporation, Connecticut, USA
Teflon, Du Pont, Wilmington, Delaware, USA/Du Pont Pharmaceuticals Ltd, Letchworth Garden City, Hertfordshire, UK
Tru-Cut, Travenol Laboratories, Thetford, UK/Deerfield, Illinois, USA

Vicryl, Ethicon, Edinburgh, UK/Ethicon Inc, Somerville, New Jersey, USA

Whitaker hook electrode, Cambac Instruments Ltd, Cambridge, UK

Xeroform, Sherwood Medical, St Louis, Missouri, USA

Index